Spinal Disorders

DIAGNOSIS AND TREATMENT

Edited by

DANIEL RUGE, M.D., Ph.D.

Deputy Director, Spinal Cord Injury Service
Veterans Administration
Washington, D. C.,
Professor of Surgery
Northwestern University Medical School
Chicago, Illinois

AND

LEON L. WILTSE, M.D.

Clinical Professor of Orthopaedic Surgery
University of California School of Medicine
Irvine, California

LEA & FEBIGER / PHILADELPHIA

1977

Library of Congress Cataloging in Publication Data

Spinal disorders.

   Bibliography: p.
   Includes index.
   1. Spine—Surgery.   2. Spinal cord—Surgery. I.   Ruge,
Daniel, 1917-   II.   Wiltse, Leon L. [DNLM: 1. Spine—Surgery.
2. Spinal cord—Diagnosis.   3. Spinal diseases—Diagnosis.
4. Spinal injuries—Diagnosis.   5. Spinal cord diseases—Diagnosis,
6. Spinal cord injuries—Diagnosis.   WE725 S755] RD533.S67   1977
617'.375   77-1875
ISBN 0-8121-0452-8

Published in Great Britain by Henry Kimpton Publishers, London

Printed in the United States of America

Print Number 4 3 2 1

Preface

WHEN the challenge of writing a definitive book on the spine was first posed several years ago, the underlying question was "who is the intended reader of such a book and what should be its special appeal?" The reported literature, both clinical and research in nature, clearly indicated a growing recognition of the fact that this area of human anatomy is quite properly the domain of two surgical disciplines: orthopaedic surgery and neurosurgery. More communication between the two, specifically the sharing of knowledge and experience, was urged. It was along these lines that we proceeded, hopefully acknowledging and presenting the roles of both disciplines.

Often, the areas of responsibility do not divide neatly between disciplines but, rather, call for an integrated approach which benefits from special skills and knowledge which are cooperatively interfaced. Consequently, this book has been prepared under the stewardship of an orthopaedic surgeon and a neurosurgeon, each of whom provided contributions evolving from a singular perspective of his specialty. Overlapping responsibilities and integrated approaches were the focus of considerable collective inquiry.

From this lengthy planning period grew the final model of this book. The transition from idea to reality was a true test, but the support and participation of individuals of great achievement made the task easier. The unselfish sharing of unique experiences and special skills has made the preparation of this manuscript a rewarding and educational experience for the editors. It is hoped that the final product will prove useful to orthopaedists and neurosurgeons alike.

In addition to being greatly indebted to their contributors, the editors wish to thank Mrs. Katherine Trees Livezey for her generous support which permitted the preparation of much of the artwork for this book.

Washington, D.C.　　　　　　　　　　　　　　　　　DANIEL RUGE

Long Beach, California　　　　　　　　　　　　　　LEON L. WILTSE

Contributors

Rush K. Acton, M.D.
   Clinical Associate Professor of Orthopaedic Surgery and of Anatomy,
   University of Miami School of Medicine;
   Active Staff, Jackson Memorial, Variety Children's, Mercy, Baptist, and
   South Miami Hospitals,
   Miami, Florida.

Leslie B. Arey, Ph.D.
   Professor Emeritus,
   Biostructure,
   Northwestern University Medical School,
   Chicago, Illinois.

N. Arumugasamy, M.D.
   Head, Department of Neurosurgery,
   Senior Consultant Neurosurgeon,
   General Hospital,
   Kuala Lumpur;
   Malaysia.

Henry H. Bohlman, M.D.
   Assistant Professor of Orthopedic Surgery,
   Case Western Reserve University School of Medicine;
   Assistant Orthopaedist, Spinal Injury Unit,
   Highland View Hospital;
   Chief of Spinal Injury Unit and of Orthopaedics,
   Veterans Administration Hospital,
   Cleveland, Ohio.

CONTRIBUTORS

D. KAY CLAWSON, M.D.
    Professor and Chairman,
    Department of Orthopaedics,
    University of Washington School of Medicine,
    Seattle, Washington.

THOMAS K. CRAIGMILE, M.D.
    Associate Clinical Professor of Neurologic Surgery,
    University of Colorado Medical School;
    Attending Neurologic Surgeon,
    Colorado General Hospital,
    Veterans Hospital,
    St. Joseph's Hospital, and
    Denver Children's Hospital,
    Denver, Colorado.

RICHARD A. DAVIS, M.D.
    Associate Professor,
    Department of Neurosurgery,
    University of Pennsylvania School of Medicine,
    Philadelphia, Pennsylvania.

HAROLD M. FROST, M.D.
    Department of Orthopaedic Surgery,
    Southern Colorado Clinic;
    Attending Orthopaedic Surgeon,
    St. Mary—Corwin Hospital and
    Parkview Episcopal Hospital,
    Pueblo, Colorado.

GERALD G. GILL, M.D.
    Associate Clinical Professor of
    Orthopaedic Surgery,
    Research Associate,
    University of California Medical School;
    Active Staff, St. Luke's Hospital;
    Attending Staff, University of California
    Medical Center,
    San Francisco, Califoroia.

DONALD R. GUNN, F.R.C.S.
    Clinical Professor of Surgery,
    University of Washington School of Medicine;
    Orthopaedist-in-Chief,
    Harborview Medical Center,
    Seattle, Washington.

ARTHUR K. HODGSON
    Professor of Orthopaedic Surgery,
    University of Hong Kong;
    Queen Mary Hospital,
    Hong Kong.

ROBERT D. KEAGY, M.D.
    Assistant Professor of Orthopaedic Surgery,
    Northwestern University Medical School;
    Attending Staff, Northwestern Memorial Hospital;
    Active Staff, Rehabilitation Institute of Chicago;
    Associate Staff, Weiss Memorial Hospital,
    Chicago, Illinois.

PATRICK J. KELLY, M.D.
    Professor of Orthopaedic Surgery,
    Mayo Medical School,
    University of Minnesota;
    Consultant in Orthopaedic Surgery,
    Mayo Clinic,
    Rochester, Minnesota.

S. HENRY, LaROCCA, M.D.
    Associate Professor,
    Department of Orthopaedic Surgery,
    Tulane Medical Center;
    Visiting Staff, Charity Hospital of Louisiana at
    New Orleans;
    Active Staff, Children's Hospital and Touro Infir-
    mary, New Orleans, Louisiana.

SANFORD J. LARSON, M.D., PH.D.
    Professor and Chairman,
    Department of Neurosurgery,
    Medical College of Wisconsin,
    Milwaukee, Wisconsin.

VALENTINE LOGUE, M.B., B.S., F.R.C.P.,
            F.R.C.S.
    Professor of Neurosurgery,
    London University at the Institute of Neurology,
    The National Hospital,
    Queen Square,
    London, England.

J. VERNON LUCK, M.D.
    Clinical Professor of Orthopaedic Surgery,
    University of Southern California
    School of Medicine;
    Attending Staff,
    Orthopaedic and Good Samaritan Hospitals,
    Los Angeles, California.

JOSEPH T. McFADDEN, M.D.
    Professor and Chairman,
    Department of Neurosurgery,
    Eastern Virginia Medical School;
    Chief, Division of Neurosurgery,
    Medical Center Hospitals,
    Norfolk, Virginia.

PAUL E. McMASTER, M.D.

Clinical Professor of Orthopaedic Surgery,
University of California School of Medicine,
Los Angeles, California;
Senior Consultant in Orthopaedic Surgery,
Veterans Administration Hospital,
West Los Angeles, California.

ROSS H. MILLER, M.D.

Associate Professor of Neurologic Surgery,
Mayo Medical School;
Consultant, Department of Neurologic Surgery,
Mayo Clinic and Mayo Foundation,
Rochester, Minnesota.

DAVID C. G. MONSEN, M.D.

Director of Oncology Services,
Orthopaedic Hospital,
Los Angeles, California.

J. M. MOSIER, M.D.

Associate Clinical Professor of Neurology,
University of California School of Medicine,
Irvine, California.

VERNON L. NICKEL, M.D.

Clinical Professor of Orthopaedic Surgery,
University of Southern California
School of Medicine,
Los Angeles, California;
Professor and Director of Orthopaedics and Rehabilitation,
Loma Linda University;
Chief, Surgical Serivces,
Rancho Los Amigos Hospital,
Downey, California.

HOMER C. PHEASANT, M.D.

Director, Adult Back Clinic,
Orthopaedic Hospital,
Los Angeles, California.

FRANK L. RANEY, JR., M.D.

Associate Clinical Professor
of Orthopaedic Surgery,
University of California Medical Center;
Attending Surgeon, Marshall Hale
Memorial Hospital,
Franklin Hospital, Children's Hospital, and
Mount Zion and Prespyterian Hospital,
San Francisco, California.

LEE H. RILEY, JR., M.D.

Professor of Orthopaedic Surgery,
The Johns Hopkins University School of Medicine;
Orthopaedic Surgeon,
The Johns Hopkins Hospital,
Baltimore, Maryland.

EDWARD J. RISEBOROUGH, M.B., CH. B.
CAPE TOWN

Assistant Professor in Orthopaedic Surgery,
Harvard Medical School;
Senior Associate in Orthopaedic Surgery,
The Children's Hospital Medical Center,
Boston, Massachusetts.

ROBERT A. ROBINSON, M.D.

Professor and Chairman,
Department of Orthopaedic Surgery,
The Johns Hopkins University School of Medicine;
Chief, Division of Orthopaedics,
Johns Hopkins Hospital,
Baltimore, Maryland.

DANIEL RUGE, M.D., PH.D.

Deputy Director,
Spinal Cord Injury Service,
Veterans Administration,
Washington, D.C.;
Professor of Surgery,
Northwestern University Medical School,
Chicago, Illinois.

GEORGE A. SISSON, M.D.

Professor and Chairman,
Department of Otolaryngology and Maxillofacial Surgery,
Northwestern University Medical School;
Chairman, Department of Otolaryngology and Maxillofacial Surgery,
Northwestern Memorial Hospital,
Chicago, Illinois.

EDIR BARROS SIQUEIRA, M.D.

Associate Professor of Surgery,
Northwestern University Medical School;
Attending Surgeon,
Northwestern Memorial Hospital,
Chicago, Illinois.

E. SHANNON STAUFFER, M.D.

Professor and Chairman,
Division of Orthopaedic Surgery and
Rehabilitation,
Southern Illinois University School of Medicine,
Springfield, Illinois.

CONTRIBUTORS

RICHARD N. STAUFFER, M.D.
Instructor, Mayo Medical School;
Consultant in Orthopaedic Surgery,
Mayo Clinic,
Rochester, Minnesota.

JOHN C. STEARS, M.D.
Associate Professor of Radiology,
University of Colorado School of Medicine,
Denver, Colorado.

THEODORE R. WAUGH, M.D.
Professor of Surgery (Orthopaedics),
University of California School of Medicine,
Irvine, California;
Chief of Orthopaedic Surgery,

University of California Medical Center,
Irvine, California.

JACK K. WICKSTROM, M.D.
Professor and Chairman,
Department of Orthopaedic Surgery
Tulane Medical Center;
Attending Surgeon,
Touro Infirmary, Southern Baptist Hospital,
Children's Hospital and Charity Hospital of
Louisiana,
New Orleans, Louisiana.

LEON L. WILTSE, M.D.
Clinical Professor of Orthopaedic Surgery,
University of California School of Medicine,
Irvine, California.

Contents

SECTION I: STRUCTURE

1. Development of the Spine and Spinal Cord   2
   LESLIE B. AREY

2. Anatomy of the Spine   13
   RUSH K. ACTON

3. Neuroanatomy   40
   DANIEL RUGE

SECTION II: DIAGNOSIS

4. Neurologic Evaluation   53
   DANIEL RUGE

5. Radiologic Examination   62
   JOHN C. STEARS

6. Electrodiagnosis of Neuromuscular Disease   76
   J. M. MOSIER

SECTION III: METABOLIC AND INFECTIOUS DISEASES

7. Osteoporoses and Osteomalacias in Spinal Surgery   87
   H. M. FROST

8. Infections of the Spine   96
   PATRICK J. KELLY

9. Tuberculosis of the Spine   102
   A. R. HODGSON

SECTION IV: OPERATIVE APPROACHES

Introduction   115
DANIEL RUGE

10. Laminectomy   117
    DANIEL RUGE

11. Transoral and Transinfrahyoid Cervical Operations   121
    GEORGE A. SISSON

12. Anterolateral Approaches to the Cervical Spine   125
    HENRY H. BOHLMAN
    LEE H. RILEY, JR.
    ROBERT A. ROBINSON

13. Lateral Approach to the Cervical Spine   132
    ERIC K. LOUIE
    DANIEL RUGE

14. The Lateral Extrapleural and Extraperitoneal
    Approaches to the Thoracic and Lumbar Spine   137
    SANFORD J. LARSON

15. Lumbar Spinal Fusion   142
    LEON L. WILTSE

16. Paraspinal Approach to the Lumbar Spine   154
    LEON L. WILTSE

17. Anterior Lumbar Interbody Fusion   162
    FRANK L. RANEY, JR.

18. Osteotomy of the Spine for Fixed Flexion
    Deformity   168
    PAUL E. McMASTER

SECTION V: DEFORMITIES

19. Scoliosis   177
    THEODORE R. WAUGH
    EDWARD RISEBOROUGH

20. Spondylolisthesis and Its Treatment: Conservative
    Treatment; Fusion with and without Reduction   193
    LEON L. WILTSE

21. Spondylolisthesis and Its Treatment: Excision of
    Loose Lamina and Decompression   218
    GERALD G. GILL

22. Congenital Anomalies of the Spine   223
    THOMAS K. CRAIGMILE

SECTION VI: TUMORS

23. Compressive Lesions at the Foramen Magnum   249
    VALENTINE LOGUE

24. Bone Tumors and Tumor-Like Lesions of the
    Vertebrae   274
    J. VERNON LUCK
    DAVID C. G. MONSEN

25. Spinal Cord Tumors   287
    DANIEL RUGE

26. Operating Microscope in Spinal Cord Surgery   295
    ROSS H. MILLER

SECTION VII: SPONDYLOSIS

27. Nonoperative Treatment of the Painful Low Back   301
    LEON L. WILTSE

28. Low Back Pain of Sacroiliac Joint Origin   311
    HOMER C. PHEASANT

29. Spondylosis   315
    DANIEL RUGE

30. Degenerative Diseases of the Thoracic Spine   323
    DONALD R. GUNN

31. An Approach to Failure of Lumbar Spine
Operations   328
     RICHARD N. STAUFFER

SECTION VIII: ROENTGEN SURVEY

32. Roentgen Survey   335

SECTION IX: TRAUMA

33. Head and Neck Injuries from Acceleration-
Deceleration Forces   349
     JACK WICKSTROM
     HENRY LAROCCA

34. Spinal Cord Injuries   357
     DANIEL RUGE

35. The Halo   368
     VERNON L. NICKEL

36. Anterior Open Reduction of the Fractured Cervical
Spine   373
     J. T. McFADDEN

37. Treatment of Fractures of the Thoracolumbar
Spine   380
     E. SHANNON STAUFFER

SECTION X: PAIN

38. Psychologic Aspects of Pain   393
     D. KAY CLAWSON

39. Cordotomy and Rhizotomy for Pain   399
     N. ARUMUGASAMY

40. Percutaneous Cervical Cordotomy for Intractable
Pain   404
     RICHARD A. DAVIS

41. Spinal Implants for Relief of Pain   409
     SANFORD J. LARSON

SECTION XI: SPECIAL CATEGORIES

42. Neurosurgical Management of Spastic Conditions   413
   EDIR B. SIQUEIRA

43. Biomechanics of the Spine and Orthoses   417
   ROBERT D. KEAGY

Index   429

Section I

Structure

1

Development of the Spine and Spinal Cord

LESLIE B. AREY

THE SPINE

IN A HUMAN embryo about three weeks old and 1.5 mm. long, pairs of block-like mesodermal somites begin to appear along each side of the neural groove. At the end of the fifth week, an embryo is 8 mm. long, and possesses the maximum number of 42 somites, nine of which belong to the tail. This appendage is at a relative maximum at the end of the fifth week of development, when it is one-sixth the total length of the embryo. During the succeeding four weeks, it disappears from external view, partly through actual regression. Also, the coccyx, which represents the residual stump of the tail, recedes to a relatively higher position in relation to the bulging buttocks.

From the union of a definite part of each pair of somites will develop a corresponding vertebra. Each somite differentiates into a dorsolateral muscle plate, or myotome, and into a looser ventromedial mass of mesenchyme, which is named the sclerotome (Fig. 1-1 A). It is these latter pairs of masses that give rise to the spine, officially named the vertebral column. The degree of vertebral organization throughout a developing spine progresses in a craniocaudal direction, so that different stages of advance can be found at different levels. Some of the final stages of osteogenesis are not completed until about midway in the third decade of postnatal life. The course of development in the vertebral column occurs in three overlapping periods: (1) blastemal, (2) chondrogenous, and (3) osteogenous.

BLASTEMAL STAGE. Each pair of sclerotomes breaks down into a loose mass of mesenchyme, and both masses migrate toward the notochord and then surround it (Fig. 1-1 B). The now combined mass remains at the same level as the parent somites and corresponding spinal nerves. Each such mass

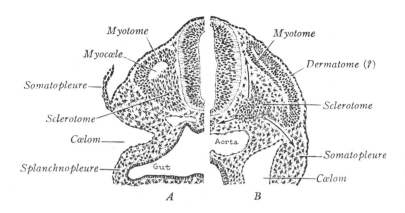

FIG. 1-1. Growth and migration of sclerotomes, shown by transverse sections early in fourth week. A, At 7 somites (×140); B, at 26 somites (×115). (From Arey LB: Developmental Anatomy. 7th Ed. Philadelphia, WB Saunders Co., 1965.)

is bounded cranially and caudally by a pair of intersegmental arteries. The temporary notochord (Fig. 1-3) is a retention of the cellular rod that constitutes the only axial support of Amphioxus, and comprises most of the spine of cyclostomes; but in higher forms it is increasingly replaced by cartilaginous or bony vertebrae. Among mammals the notochord serves as a transient support for the embryo, but it persists permanently only as the so-called pulpy nuclei within the intervertebral discs.

In embryos 5 mm. long and four weeks old, the more cranial of the serially arranged segmental masses of mesenchyme are already proliferating in their caudal portions, so that a cranial less dense half and a caudal denser half are seen strikingly (Fig. 1-2 A). A fissure then appears that separates these parts, and the caudal, denser half of each total sclerotomic mass recombines with the now separate cranial half of the mass just behind it (Fig. 1-2 B). These new combinations, and not the original total sclerotomes, become the primordia of the definitive vertebrae. The denser portion is the dominant part of the vertebral primordium. It shares in the formation of the body of a vertebra, and, almost unaided, gives rise to the outgrowths that become the vertebral arch, transverse processes, and ribs.

Growth of the paired sclerotomic masses in a medial direction, so as to surround the notochord and establish the basis of a vertebral centrum, is an important first step in the development of vertebrae. But two additional directions of growth occur from each side of each conjoined sclerotomic mass (Figs. 1-1 B and 1-3). One is dorsally flanking and ultimately enclosing the neural

tube, thereby producing the basis of the vertebral arch and spinous process. The other growth direction is laterally, thereby producing a pair of primitive transverse processes (and their extensions, the rib primordia).

The recombinations of sclerotomic masses, as already described, create new, definitive intervertebral spaces between the organizing vertebrae. Mesenchyme derived from the denser (now cranial) portion of each body condenses, and becomes an intervertebral disc located within each such interspace. It is at these intervals, now aligned with the middle of the respective pair of myotomes, that surviving remnants of the notochord become incorporated into the disc by the beginning of the third month. They contribute to the formation of the persistent pulpy nuclei. Addition to this pulpy substance comes from a mucogelatinous degeneration centrally within the disc itself.

One general result of the sclerotomic recombinations is that the accompanying pairs of arteries, originally intersegmental in position, now assume a new relationship by coursing midway across the vertebral bodies. Moreover, each myotome now agrees with halves of successive vertebrae, and the segmental nerve to that myotome comes to lie at the level of an intervertebral disc. Such a myotomic and vertebral alternation is a necessary arrangement that permits the presently differentiating intervertebral muscles to bend the spine.

CHONDROGENOUS STAGE. There are four centers of chondrification in each blastemal prevertebra (Fig. 1-3): One appears in each growing arch rudiment, even

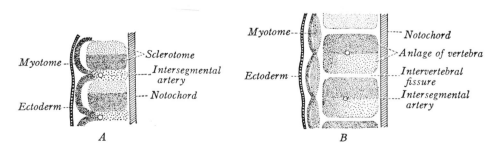

FIG. 1-2. Early stages in organization of vertebrae, shown by frontal sections through left somites (×75). A, At 4 mm.; B, at 5 mm. (From Arey LB: Developmental Anatomy. 7th Ed. Philadelphia, WB Saunders Co., 1965.)

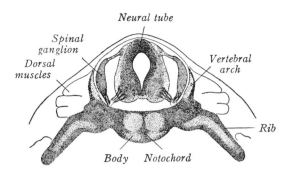

FIG. 1-3. Vertebra and ribs, in transverse section at 13 mm., showing centers of chondrification (×18). (From Arey LB: Developmental Anatomy. 7th Ed. Philadelphia, WB Saunders Co., 1965.)

though these as yet flank only the ventral half of the spinal cord. Another pair of centers arises in the primitive body. All centers are demonstrable in the higher levels of the trunk in embryos 13 mm. long and about six weeks old; the process of chondrification progresses along the primitive spine in a craniocaudal direction. Growth enlarges all of these centers, but the spread is particularly impressive in the laggardly elongating halves of a total arch; these cartilaginous plates do not meet dorsally until well into the third fetal month. The several processes of a cartilaginous vertebra are secondary outgrowths.

Joints begin to appear in the second month. They arise as cavities surrounded by blastemal tissue that converts into joint capsules. Also from the tissue surrounding the cartilaginous vertebrae are developed the various ligaments of the spine.

Specializations occur in the several regional groups of vertebrae, but these are mostly quantitative differences. Quite otherwise are specializations in the first and second cervical vertebrae. When the atlas is developing, its centrum differentiates typically, but is soon taken over by the centrum of the axis; thereafter, it serves as its peg-like extension, the dens. The missing region of the atlas, originally occupied by its body, is filled in by a condensed tissue that also becomes chondrified. In the coccygeal region, only the arch processes of the first pre-vertebra give rise to cartilaginous, wing-like plates; these are known as the cornua.

Costal processes are originally continuous with the blastemal tissue of a vertebra, and a center of chondrification appears in each at about the time when the main vertebral centers are arising (Fig. 1-3). Such processes typically extend into the interspaces between successive myotomes. In the neck, the ribs are tiny, forming ventral borders to the transverse foramina; in the thorax, they become long bars; in the lumbar region, they are relatively short, robust stubs; in the sacral region, they become modified into flat plates. Only in the first of the coccygeal vertebrae are there any representatives of ribs.

OSTEOGENOUS STAGE. Vertebrae in general produce three primary centers of ossification, and these correspond to the general locations of the earlier chondrogenous centers. There is a center for each hemi-arch and one for the centrum, although the latter sometimes is double or becomes so (Fig. 1-4). The first centers appear during the third fetal month in cervical, thoracic, and lumbar vertebrae, but sacral centers do not arise until near mid-term and coccygeal centers only postnatally. The onset of ossification in vertebral arches progresses consistently from cervical levels caudalward; on the contrary, the sequence of centers for the

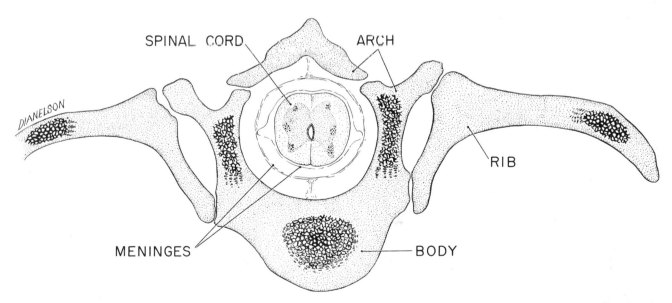

FIG. 1-4. Thoracic vertebra and ribs, in transverse section in fourth month, showing centers of ossification in cartilage (×33).

bodies advances slowly in a cranial direction but quickly caudal-ward.

At birth, the spreading osteogenesis from primary centers is still incomplete, and each hemi-arch, with its corresponding vertebral body, is separated by a plate of cartilage. During the first postnatal year, most of the ossifying hemi-arches become united dorsally, whereas the completed arches do not join the vertebral bodies until the third to sixth year. Hemi-arch union occurs earliest in the lumber region; arch-body union takes place earliest in the thoracic region. The center of ossification in the body of the cartilaginous vertebra gives rise to most of the definitive body; the two centers in the total arch produce the dorsolateral parts of the body, the greater part of the primary bony arch, and all of its various processes.

The atlas develops a center in each hemi-arch, but the bones do not meet dorsally until the third postnatal year. The ventral, secondarily restored portion of the atlas acquires a center (and sometimes apparently two centers) during the first post-natal year. The union of the arch and this substitute ventral component occurs between the fifth and ninth year.

The vertebral arch and body of the axis develop essentially as in other cervical vertebrae. The captured dens becomes ossified from paired centers which appear in the fifth fetal month and soon merge. Between the third and sixth years, all of the separate components of the axis meet and fuse.

The various sacral centers arise between the third and eighth fetal month, while all but one of the fusions occur in the second to sixth year. Especially tardy is the dorsal union of the two hemi-arches of each vertebra; this is delayed until the seventh to tenth year. Between puberty and about the twenty-fifth year, the sacral vertebrae unite progressively into a composite bony unit.

The coccygeal vertebrae are unique in that ossification delays an appearance until after birth, and then the spread in each vertebra advances from the single center. The first vertebra usually develops its center during the first postnatal year. The center of the second vertebra arises between the fifth and tenth years, and those of the third and fourth vertebrae appear, respectively, just before and just after puberty.

Long after birth secondary epiphysial centers organize, and the times of appearance agree well in cervical, thoracic, and lumbar vertebrae. One of these centers develops at the time of puberty in each still-persisting layer of cartilage covering the cranial and caudal ends of a body. Each ossifying region produces an epiphysial disc, and these plates (peculiar to mammals) fuse with the centra in the eighteenth to twenty-third year. In young fetuses, the cervical centra are much longer than those of the lumbosacral region, but at the cessation of epiphysial growth, vertebrae are longer in the lumbar region than elsewhere. Similarly, the tips of the bony spinous transverse and articular processes of each vertebra are still covered by cartilage postnatally. A secondary center arises in each of these, and their times of origin and fusion correspond with those of the developing discs of the bodies.

The body of the axis produces a single epiphysis at puberty, and it joins the body at 20 to 25 years. The apex of the dens also develops a center; it appears at two to six years, and its bony mass joins the main part of the dens before the twelfth year.

The bodies of sacral vertebrae develop epiphysial centers at puberty, and fusions between them occur at 18 to 25 years. The spinous processes acquire centers at 18 years, and fusions occur at 20 to 25 years. Each pars lateralis of the sacrum, which is a flat, plate-like rib, gains a center along its lateral extremity at 13 to 19 years, and fusions occur at 15 to 21 years. The fibrocartilaginous intervertebral discs of the sacrum also ossify. Ultimately the consolidating components produce a unified mass by the twenty-fifth year.

Some reports have recorded the occurrence of epiphysial plates for the coccygeal vertebrae, and also a pair of such centers for the horns of the first vertebra in the series. The three more caudal vertebrae join into a composite unit before middle life, and fusion with the first vertebra follows somewhat later. In old individuals, the entire coccyx not infrequently unites with the sacrum, and this happens more often in Caucasians than in Negroes; such fusion predominates in female Caucasians and male Negroes.

Terrestrial life for animals introduced many functional changes, and man has altered conditions still further by adopting an erect posture. This position and the modified locomotion that accompanies it have made necessary certain correlated adaptations. A narrowing of the spine occurs both in the upper thoracic region and toward its lower end. The former is correlated with the presence of ribs and a sternum, which help in relieving the spine in its function as a support; similarly, the transference of weight to the pelvis relieves the lower spine. The C-shaped curvature of the spine in the cramped fetus straightens in the newborn. The permanent curves of the spinal column appear partly through the pull of muscles, and these are not prominent until posture becomes erect.

CAUSAL FACTORS. The course of bone development and the assumption of characteristic form by different bones are inherent and determined through gene action. Bones are self-differentiating organs in which the histogenesis and morphogenesis of the cartilaginous model and its early replacing bone are not dependent on mechanical or environmental influences. Yet extrinsic influences are of real importance in furnishing the conditions necessary to normal development, and, as mechanical forces, in producing the final perfections of form that are required of a functioning skeleton.

The proper development of a cartilaginous axis in an embryo depends on the presence of the spinal cord. It exerts an influence over the modeling and proportions

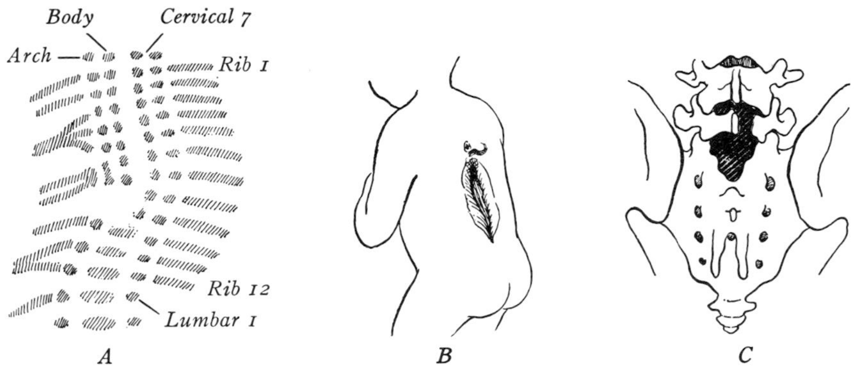

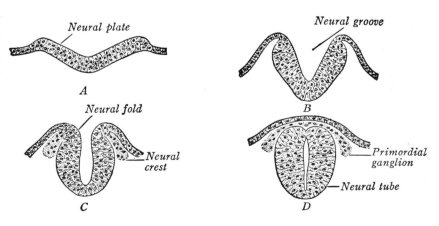

FIG. 1-5. Anomalies of spine. *A*, Irregular segmentation, shown by x-ray examination at five months; *B*, cleft spine, exposing flat spinal cord; *C*, cleft spine at lumbosacral junction. (From Arey LB: Developmental Anatomy. 7th Ed. Philadelphia, WB Saunders Co., 1965.)

of the vertebral arches and over the jointing of its vertebral segments. The notochord is not a positive factor in these governing activities.

ANOMALIES. Remnants of the notochord may persist within the spine and give rise to chordomas. With the exception of the cervical region, numeric variations above or below the normal number of vertebrae are not infrequent. Such variations occur in embryos as well as in adults, and the frequency in both is probably the same. The change to a secondary type of segmentation that results in a definitive spine may be carried out irregularly, so that a half-vertebra is missing or is not joined to its mate (Fig. 1-5 *A*); successive vertebrae may fuse unsymmetrically, and their relations to ribs are then similarly irregular.

Most vertebral defects are due either to the absence of certain cartilages or bony centers or to the imperfect fusion of otherwise well-formed components. The nonunion of the dorsal ends of the paired vertebral arches is rachischisis, or cleft spine, also known as spina bifida (Fig. 1-5 *B*, *C*). An extensive involvement of the spine is much less common than are relatively localized defects, which tend to favor lumbar or sacral locations. Rarely, such an abnormality may be so severe as to be directly observable (Fig. 1-5 *B*). More frequently, it may be complicated by a concomitant herniation of the meninges and elevation of the integument (Fig. 1-13 *B*). A simple concealed cleft is designated as spina bifida occulta (Fig. 1-5 *C*).

THE SPINAL CORD

At the end of the third week of human development, the ectoderm of the three-layered embryonic disc thickens along the midline into a neural plate (Fig. 1-6 *A*). Through localized growth, this plate straightway produces a pair of neural folds that flank a medially-coursing neural groove (*B*, *C*). The two folds meet and fuse (*D*), at first about midway of the length of the early embryo, then simultaneously in cranial and caudal directions until a complete closed neural tube is attained. Even before this folding and closure are completed at the end of the fourth week, a larger brain region is easily distinguishable from a more slender precursor of the spinal cord. At the time of complete closure, the spinal cord extends caudad only through the future thoracic level. Elongation into lumbar and sacro-coccygeal levels reaches terminal growth concomitant with the addition of the lower regions of the body.

The junctional tissue, where the neural plate and ordinary ectoderm abut, is not taken up into the wall of the neural tube; instead, when the neural tube detaches from the ordinary ectoderm, the flanking strips of junctional tissue also detach and separate into two longitudinal bands known as the neural crests (Fig. 1-6 *C*, *D*). They lie alongside each dorsolateral wall of the neural tube and promptly consolidate segmentally into a series of paired masses that represent the primordia of future craniospinal ganglia (Fig. 1-7).

FIG. 1-6. Origin of the neural tube and neural crests, shown by transverse sections from early embryos (×125). (From Arey LB: Developmental Anatomy. 7th Ed. Philadelphia, WB Saunders Co., 1965.)

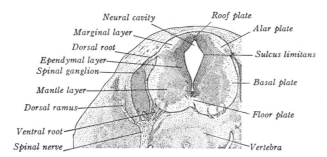

FIG. 1-7. Organization of spinal cord and spinal nerve, shown by transverse section at 10 mm. (×30). (From Arey LB: Developmental Anatomy. 7th Ed. Philadelphia, W. B. Saunders Co., 1965.)

These agree in position with the emerging myotomic (muscle) plates of the mesodermal somites.

EARLY INTERNAL ORGANIZATION. The wall of the neural tube thickens rapidly and exhibits a progressive differentiation into three concentric zones. These zones are clearly established in an embryo 8 mm. long and five weeks old (Fig. 1-7). An internal zone bordering the central canal of the tube constitutes the ependymal layer; its cells become the supporting elements that bear this distinctive name. A middle, thicker zone is named the mantle layer; in it will differentiate the multipolar nerve cells that characterize the gray substance of the brain and spinal cord. A peripheral zone, relatively noncellular and presently composed largely of nerve fibers, is the marginal layer; when many of its fibers gain a myelin sheath, it is called appropriately the white substance. In this way, the early neural tube becomes a three-layered tube both structurally and functionally.

Also, in an embryo of five weeks the neural tube specializes both structurally and functionally into six longitudinal strips or bands (Fig. 1-7). The primitive dorsal and ventral walls are primarily ependymal and neuroglial in structure and do not participate in the marked thickenings that characterize the lateral walls. These dorsal and ventral strips are named, respectively, the roof plate and the floor plate. They are essentially non-nervous, although their thin marginal zones become the pathways for commissural nerve fibers. Midway on the inner surface of each lateral wall is a groove, the sulcus limitans, which is an important landmark (Fig. 1-7). It indicates the subdivision of the wall into a dorsolateral pair of so-named alar plates (essentially sensory and coordinating in function) and into a thicker ventrolateral pair of basal plates (primarily motor in function). An understanding of the concentric and longitudinal organizations of the early neural tube is fundamental to a proper appreciation of its later specializations.

CELL SPECIALIZATION. Originally the neural plate is composed of undifferentiated, proliferative epithelium.

Its daughter cells enter into two lines of specialization (Fig. 1-8). One path leads toward the production of neuroblasts that differentiate further into multipolar nerve cells. The other course is toward ependymal cells and neuroglial cells; these constitute the distinctive supporting tissue of the central nervous system. Only astrocytes and oligodendrocytes are glial end-products. Microglia are secondary invaders of the neural tube, tracing origin to the surrounding mesenchyme.

The neural crest is a versatile tissue, giving rise to various elements besides the distinctive unipolar sensory cells of spinal ganglia. Among the other products are satellite elements (encapsulating all ganglion cells), autonomic ganglion cells, Schwann cells of neurilemma sheaths, melanocytes of the skin, and the medullary cells of the suprarenal glands.

Ventral root axons of motor neuroblasts in the mantle layer are emerging from the ventrolateral walls of the spinal cord as early as the fourth week (4 mm. embryo) of development (Fig. 1-9 A). They occur in segmental groups that become the ventral roots of spinal nerves. Slightly later, sensory neuroblasts of the spinal ganglia send processes both inward into the spinal cord (dorsal root fibers) and outward to join the corresponding ventral root fibers and produce a composite bundle, the trunk of a spinal nerve (B). By the fifth week of development, the spinal nerves of each side form a nearly complete series in alignment with the myotomic plates of correspondingly located mesodermal somites. Also at this time, the beginnings of the brachial and lumbosacral nerve plexuses are indicated.

Between the fourth month of fetal life and the third month following birth, a fatty myelin sheath begins to appear about many peripheral nerve fibers. It is a product of the cellular units, or Schwann cells, of the neurilemma sheath, and is deposited in layers corresponding to the individual extents of such spirally-wrapped elements. In the central nervous system, there is no typical neurolemma sheath investing the nerve fibers; yet many of these fibers do acquire a similar

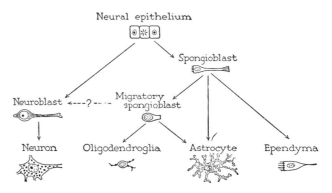

FIG. 1-8. Diagram showing lineage of cells differentiating in neural tube. (From Arey LB: Developmental Anatomy. 7th Ed. Philadelphia, WB Saunders Co., 1965.)

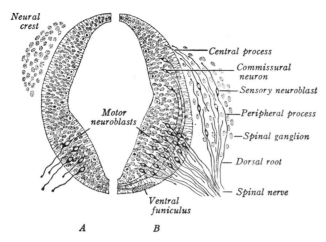

FIG. 1-9. Growth of neuroblasts and spinal nerve shown by transverse hemi-sections of spinal cord. *A,* At 4 mm. (×225); *B,* at 5 mm. (×140). (From Arey LB: Developmental Anatomy. 7th Ed. Philadelphia, W. B. Saunders Co., 1965.)

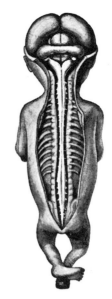

FIG. 1-10. Dorsal dissection, exposing spinal cord at three months (×1). (From Arey LB: Developmental Anatomy. 7th Ed. Philadelphia, W. B. Saunders Co., 1965.)

spiral myelin sheath. Here rows of glial cells, identified as oligodendrocytes, are believed to substitute for the Schwann cells of peripheral nerves.

EXTERNAL FORM. In the absence of a special boundary between the brain and spinal cord, the latter can be considered to begin at the level of the first pair of spinal nerves. For a time, the spinal cord is a tube that tapers gradually to a caudal ending at the tip of the spine. In the fourth month, it enlarges at the levels of the pairs of nerve plexuses that supply the upper and lower limbs (Fig. 1-10). These swellings (the cervical and lumbosacral enlargements) result from the presence of additional sensory and motor neurons at these levels, and from the occurrence there of shorter segments between successive pairs of spinal nerves.

After the third month, the spine grows faster than the spinal cord. Since the cord is anchored by the brain within the skull, this disproportion in the rate of growth has an important result. During subsequent growth, the vertebrae of necessity shift caudad along the spinal cord. This movement drags down inside the vertebral canal the nerve roots that have to retain the same exits between vertebrae that were originally directly opposite their sites of origin (Fig. 1-11). For this reason, the spinal cord proper appears to recede progressively up the vertebral canal until at birth it ends at the level of the third lumbar vertebra, and in the adult opposite the first lumbar vertebra. Thus, the roots of the lumbar, sacral, and coccygeal nerves leave the cord at fairly high levels; continuing downward within the vertebral canal, the nerves emerge between vertebrae at increasingly lower levels. As might be expected, the thoracic nerves are displaced to a less degree, while the cervical nerves incline but little in a caudal direction.

The tip of the neural tube retains its terminal connections with the connective tissue of the skin during this period of unequal growth; hence, it becomes stretched and de-differentiated into a slender, fibrous strand known as the filum terminale (Fig. 1-11). The obliquely coursing spinal nerves, surrounding the filum terminale, constitute the cauda equina, which was so named because of its fancied resemblance to a horse's tail. A trace of the original saccular termination of the neural tube in the integument is recognizable at birth. It constitutes the coccygeal vestige, located near the tip of the coccyx; its site is frequently marked superficially by a dimple or pit in the skin where attachment occurs.

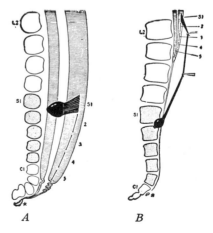

FIG. 1-11. Diagrams illustrating dislocations through unequal growth of spine and spinal cord (after Streeter). *A,* At nine weeks (×6); *B,* at six months (×1). (From Arey LB: Developmental Anatomy. 7th Ed. Philadelphia, W. B. Saunders Co., 1965.)

The central nervous system is relatively large throughout the fetal period, and at birth it still represents 10 per cent of the body weight as against 2 per cent in the adult. The spinal cord relatively outgrows the brain during the postnatal years, increasing from 0.9 per cent of the brain weight to an ultimate 2 per cent. After the cessation of neuron production, shortly after birth, an important factor in the further increase in bulk of the spinal cord and brain is the thickening of myelin sheaths. Some of these investing sheaths are already present at birth, but at best they are still thin.

INTERNAL ORGANIZATION. The wall of the spinal portion of the early neural tube thickens so rapidly that in the fourth week of development the typical three concentric layers have already made their appearance. Coincidental with continued growth comes a relative narrowing of the internal canal. For a short time, this cavity is somewhat diamond-shaped in section, its lateral angle (sulcus limitans) on each side subdividing the lateral walls into plainly seen alar and basal plates (Fig. 1-7). The roof and floor plates are relatively thin and poor in cells.

EPENDYMAL LAYER. This innermost stratum is a prominent component of the early neural wall, and comprises much of the roof plate and floor plate (Fig. 1-7). As the alar plates continue to thicken, the roof plate is obliterated, as such, and the facing ependymal layers of this region unite progressively into a median seam, the posterior median septum (Fig. 1-12). This fusion steadily reduces the dorsal extent of the central canal; in the fourth month, the cavity has become limited to a relatively small definitive lumen at the most ventral extent of the original canal.

As the proliferative activity within the neural tube advances, the rapidly bulging walls of the basal plates overlap the laggard floor plate, and produce the progressively deepening furrow known as the anterior median fissure of the spinal cord (Fig. 1-12). Here the ependymal cells of the thin floor plate retain their original radial orientation and extend to the surface of the cord.

MANTLE LAYER. Neuroblasts are the important and conspicuous constituents of this zone, which lacks myelinated nerve fibers, and hence receives the name *gray substance*. Increase in mass of this tissue depends upon cell division and subsequent growth; when the proliferation ceases shortly after birth, the gray substance nears its definitive size. In embryos of 10 mm., a thickening in each basal plate becomes prominent ventrolaterally. Its cells constitute the ventral gray columns which, in considerably later stages, supply migrant cells that organize also lateral gray columns (Fig. 1-12). The grouping of cells in the ventral column is such that the cells of origin of somatic motor fibers (which are distributed to muscles of somite origin) lie ventral and median to cells whose axons (general visceral motor) become preganglionic autonomic fibers. In embryos of 20 mm., a dorsolateral thickening in each alar plate contains neuroblasts aggregating as the dorsal gray columns.

These proliferations in the alar and basal plates produce, respectively, the receptive and motor cells characteristic of these columns. Fetuses in the mid-fourth month of development have their gray substance arranged in what is essentially the permanent form of cell groups.

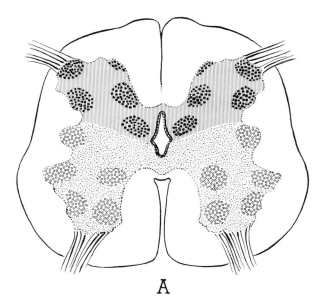
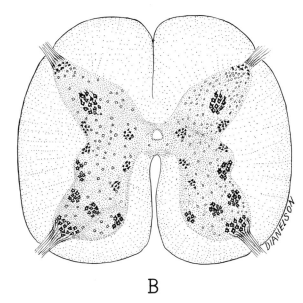

A   B

FIG. 1-12. Advancing organization of spinal cord following early stage shown in Fig. 1-7. *A,* At three months ($\times 70$); *B,* at term ($\times 20$). Paired columns of white substance are demarcated by nerve roots. Sensory and motor regions of gray substance (and their differentiating nuclei) are shown in *A* by hatched and stippled fields. Later distribution of gray nuclei is illustrated in *B*.

MARGINAL LAYER. This zone is primitively a meshwork made up of the processes of ependymal and neuroglial cells. Into it grow the axons of nerve cells differentiating progressively in the mantle layer. These axons are ascending and descending fibers, and their presence causes the marginal layer to thicken markedly. The acquisition of a myelin sheath by many of the fibers of this zone is responsible for the appearance of a conspicuous layer of white substance at the periphery of the spinal cord.

Myelin deposition begins at four months of fetal life, and is not completed in some tracts until the second postnatal year. It occurs first in the cervical cord, and then extends progressively to lower levels. Deposition of myelin begins close to the nerve cell, and spreads along the fiber until near its termination. The continued deposit of myelin produces progressively thicker sheaths, and this accounts for the steadily increasing size of the marginal layer even into adolescence. Myelinization commences at widely varying times in different fiber systems. In general, it appears first in those nerve tracts that function earliest or are the oldest ones phylogenetically. There is good evidence that tracts become completely myelinated at about the time they become fully functional.

The white substance is subdivided by the dorsal and ventral roots into dorsal, lateral, and ventral funiculi (Fig. 1-12). These, in turn, are arranged in functional tracts whose general relations and proportions are attained at the middle of the fetal period. The earliest tracts of fibers differentiate early in the second month for the purpose of distributing dorsal root fibers within the cord and linking together the nerve centers of the cord itself. In the third month, long association tracts of two kinds come into existence. Some begin with cell bodies in the cord, and ascend to the brain; these serve to relay to the fore-, mid- and hind-brain the sensory impulses arriving in the cord from without. Others originate in the mid- and hind-brain, and descend, thereby making possible an influence of higher centers over lower ones. Finally, in the fifth month, the corticospinal tracts begin growing downward from the motor cortex. It is through these neurons that the brain controls the motor cells of the spinal cord.

THE MENINGES. These closed coverings of the brain and spinal cord arise largely, at least, as condensations of the neighboring mesenchyme (Fig. 1-4). The tough dura mater has become a distinct fibrous membrane at eight weeks. The delicate pia-arachnoid, also apparently of mesenchymal origin, may receive some migrant cells from the neural crest; yet the existence and extent of this contribution remain unsettled.

CAUSAL FACTORS. The tissue of the early notochord acts as an inductor in influencing the overlying ectoderm to become a neural plate and the neural crests. It does this by secreting an evocating fluid that imposes an appropriate pattern-forming response, irreversible in nature. Moreover, it is held that gradients exist along the length of the notochord, and that these correspond to varying concentrations of a head-organizing substance and a trunk-organizing substance. Such graded differences in the composition of the secreted fluid at local levels establish a craniocaudal quantitative polarity responsible for calling forth regional specializations. The result is the production of the serial divisions of the brain and spinal cord.

A thick neural plate arises when cells are pushed, at least in part passively, toward the midline by an expanding movement taking place in the adjacent ectoderm. By contrast, the folding of the neural plate into a tube is essentially an active process, but the exact mechanics of the act is not wholly understood. The normal presence and positions of the notochord and somites with respect to the early spinal cord are actively responsible for its characteristic shape, proportions and bilateral symmetry. The formative effects of the notochord and somites are antagonistic, but their locations are such that somites induce the thick lateral walls of the spinal cord while the notochord is responsible for the thin floor plate.

The neural tube and neural crest are not inherently metameric. The segmental arrangement of the spinal nerves is a secondary acquisition that is dependent on the presence of the primary metamerism established by the presence and arrangement of myotomes. The size of ganglia and the number of ganglion cells differentiated in them depend on the size of the skin area supplied. Similarly, but less precisely, the number of motor neurons at a particular level of the cord develop in relation to the number of units to be innervated. All of these dependent relations are subject to experimental proofs.

After the closure of the neural tube, distinctive histogenetic fates become assigned to its unspecialized cells. Yet the specific factors that determine and direct the divergent courses of differentiation into forming neuroblasts, glioblasts, and ependymal cells are not known. Also undetermined is why certain neuroblastic groups arise only in particular locations. Nerve fibers can reach their appropriate destinations even when their normal pathways are blocked, or when the target-organ has been displaced to a strange location. The nerve fibers act as if attracted; yet this guidance is nonspecific, since a nasal placode, for instance, can substitute for a myotome. The guiding force is neither chemical nor electrical, as once believed. The directed axonal growth, both sensory and motor, is apparently a response to the presence of a local region undergoing intensive mitotic activity. At an early stage of embryonic development, the path of neuron growth to terminal sites is short and direct; this circumstance simplifies the problem of appropriate directional growth.

ANOMALIES. Striking malformations of the spinal cord and its investing membranes often accompany a cleft spine. The cord may be widely exposed, like an

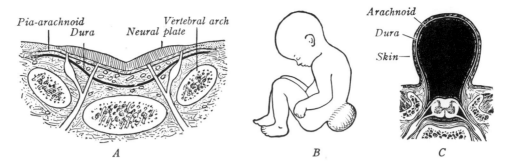

FIG. 1-13. Anomalies of spinal cord. *A,* Unclosed and retarded spine and spinal cord, shown in transverse section; *B, C,* meningocele, shown in side view and in vertical section. (From Arey LB: Developmental Anatomy. 7th Ed. Philadelphia, W. B. Saunders Co., 1965.)

unclosed neural plate (myeloschisis, Fig. 1-13 *A*), or it may be practically absent (amyelus). Herniation of the membranes, with or without participation of the cord, is made possible by an unclosed spine. The most common location is in the lumbosacral region (*B*), and the skin-covered sac may vary from the size of an orange to one too small to be visible externally. A meningocele denotes a simple fluid-filled sac, bounded by the protruded membranes (*C*). A meningomyelocele includes the local cord in the herniated cavity. Duplication of the central canal, especially toward its caudal end, sometimes occurs. It results from dual tunneling of the solid, growing end of the cord, since a lumen through folding does not extend below thoracic levels. A pilonidal sinus begins as a dimple where the original tip of the neural tube inserted into the integument.

2

Anatomy of the Spine

RUSH K. ACTON

OUR PRESENTATION of the anatomy of the spine encompasses that of the skin and related structures, the bony supporting structures with their cartilaginous components, and the muscles and muscle groups that fix and move the parts of the spine. Vascular structures and elements of the peripheral nervous system, as they relate to the aforementioned structures, also are discussed.

SKIN

The human skin provides cover, containment, and protection for the musculoskeletal structures and organs of the body, serving to prevent dehydration within the limits of the environmental conditions surrounding the body. It further provides the organ most directly related to man's environs, and contains specialized organs of perception of the physical conditions around him. It plays a role in the regulation of body temperature. The skin overlying the spine serves to cushion the weight of the body as it rests supine, often for as long as one-third of each day. It consists of a deep layer of dermis, dense connective tissue derived from the embryonal mesoderm, and a superficial layer or epidermis derived from the primitive ectoderm. Even at birth, the dermis is thicker over the major portion of the spine in keeping with its hard use. Sebaceous glands opening into hair follicles and sudoriferous or sweat glands are present throughout the skin of the body, including the back, but are most numerous in specialized areas.

The sensation of the back is derived mainly from the posterior primary rami of the spinal nerves with branches coming around the trunk from the ventral rami bilaterally. Each spinal nerve is formed by the ventral or motor root and the dorsal or sensory root, and immediately divides into ventral and dorsal rami. The latter split into medial and lateral branches, pierce and supply the overlying muscles, and terminate in sensory organs of the skin. The first and last two cervical and last two lumbar posterior rami ordinarily do not have cutaneous branches, but the rest supply sensation over the entire spine from head to tailbone (Fig. 2-1).

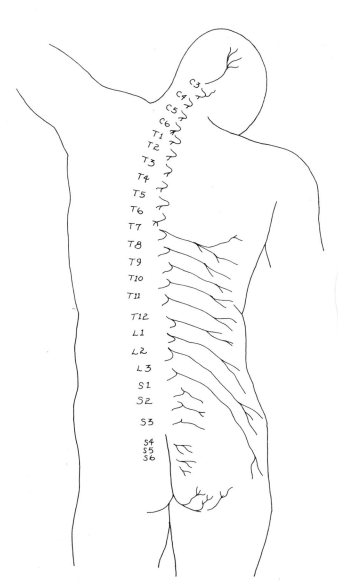

FIG. 2-1. General pattern of cutaneous branches of dorsal divisions of spinal nerves. Note that dorsal primary rami form medial and lateral branches, and that generally speaking medial branches pierce muscles to supply skin of back above mid-dorsal region. Lateral branches tend to supply skin of back below this level.

VERTEBRAE AND INTERVERTEBRAL DISCS

The support structures of the spine are composed of some 33 individual units which share certain common characteristics as vertebrae, and yet are grouped in five general classifications according to site and special characteristics (Fig. 2-2). Although there are generally seven cervical vertebrae, 12 thoracic vertebrae, five lumbar vertebrae, five sacral vertebrae, and three to five coccygeal vertebrae, the total number can vary as well as the proportionate numbers in each division. The concept of the unit, which consists of any two adjacent vertebrae with the intervening disc, takes into account the adjoining facet joints as well as the intervertebral disc joint in the relationship of the two vertebrae as a single unit. This concept has some merit, particularly in view of the fact that the embryonic origin of the vertebrae consists in the splitting of the original segments of mesenchyme or sclerotomes into two halves and union of the upper half of one with the lower half of the other. It is more logical, however, to consider each vertebra as a unit in itself.

A single vertebra, with the exception of the first cervical vertebra, always has a body and a bony or neural arch. The body is generally somewhat cylindrical or spool-shaped in contour. The bony arch consists of two paired pedicles, two paired laminae to roof over the canal, and seven bony projections or processes on each arch (a pair of transverse processes, a spinous process, and four articular processes, two superior and two inferior). Rowe and Roche noted in studying x-ray evidence of ossification of the neural arch that the pedicles and body do not fuse until the age of three to six years. The importance of this fact is that oblique views could superimpose the neurocentral synchondrosis in such a way as to suggest fracture or defect in the arch.

Each vertebra is joined to its fellow anteriorly by a rubbery intervertebral disc, forming a slightly movable articulation or amphiarthrosis (Fig. 2-3). Posteriorly there are paired facet joints between adjacent vertebrae, which are true diarthroses or freely movable articulations. These latter joints are the arthrodial or gliding type. Like all freely movable articulations, they have a joint capsule lined with synovium enclosing the two articular apposing surfaces. A typical pair of adjacent vertebrae then, except for the first two cervical, has a controlled type of motion. This is a modified flexion and extension permitted by the capability of the intervertebral disc to deform and alter its shape, guided by the limited motion of the facet joints, and controlled by adjacent ligamentous and muscular structures. The vertebral body itself consists of cancellous or spongy bone surrounded by a cylinder of cortical bone and capped at both ends by hyaline cartilage, which adjoins the intervertebral disc. It should be noted that the

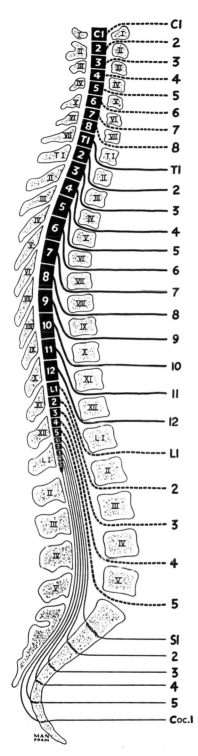

FIG. 2-2. Sagittal view of spine. In this drawing of hemisected spine, note that cord terminates at upper end of L2, continuing into narrow filament of filum terminale. Primary dorsal and sacral curves are convex anteriorly, whereas secondary cervical and lumbar curves are convex posteriorly. (From Haymaker, W., and Woodhall, B.: Peripheral Nerve Injuries. 2nd Ed., Philadelphia, W. B. Saunders, 1953.)

growth of a vertebral body takes place through the usual epiphyses capping the ends of the body just as epiphyses cap the ends of any long bone. Not to be confused with the true epiphyses, however, are the traction apophyses called vertebral ring apophyses by Bick and Copel, and, earlier, randleiste by Schmorl. These discrete structures have been shown to calcify at age six, ossify at 13, and fuse to the vertebral body at approximately age 17.

While there are more or less 33 vertebrae in the human spine, there are 24 presacral vertebrae and 23 intervertebral discs. There may be rudimentary disc formations related to the sacrococcygeal vertebrae, but the presacral intervertebral discs are fully developed and more or less alike anatomically except for differences in thickness.

The fusion of the first two cervical vertebrae into a single dens eliminates a disc for this interspace. The remainder of the presacral discs are named for the vertebrae above. The lowest fully developed disc is commonly called the lumbosacral disc. The intervertebral disc serves as an amphiarthrosis or slightly movable joint between the vertebrae as well as a shock absorber. Its capacity to transmit and modify stresses hydrodynamically serves this purpose well while it is intact. The healthy disc has the capacity to imbibe and to release water, and thus to be deformed and reformed upon release of stress. It consists of the nucleus pulposus and its limiting membrane, the anulus fibrosus. The nucleus is a mucoid, gelatinous remnant of the notochord, containing as much as 77 per cent water in the fully developed fetus and diminishing by at least one-fourth its water content in the elderly. In addition, the water content may diminish drastically in the relatively young individual as a result of pathologic drying-out processes and degeneration, predisposing to the disruption and displacement of fragments of the disc as in the "herniated disc syndrome."

Lysell studied specimens from cadavers of all ages by means of three-dimensional x-ray to show cervical intersegmental motion. He noted considerable differences in range of motion attributable to early degeneration of intervertebral discs. As early as the fourth or fifth year of age, fissure formation was noted, with vascularized tongues of connective tissue and subsequent spur formation. As the disc progressively loses moisture, bulk, and height, it is replaced by scar and eventually by bone, particularly in the C4, C5 and C6 interspaces at the site of greatest sagittal motion.

The anulus fibrosus consists of fibrocartilaginous circular plates, fibers of which stream obliquely to attach in concentric rings to the adjacent cartilaginous end plates of the vertebral bodies. These fibers crisscross as if to give greater strength to the union. Coventry et al. have shown that some fibers blend into the anterior and posterior longitudinal ligaments, and others pass over the rim of the body to insert into the adjacent bone.

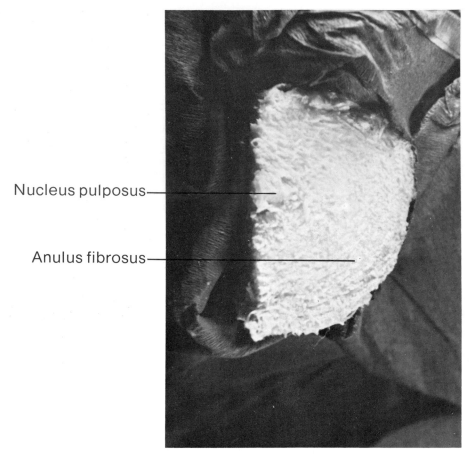

Nucleus pulposus

Anulus fibrosus

FIG. 2-3. This transverse section of a hemisected mid-lumbar disc specimen shows concentric lamellae arranged around eccentric nucleus pulposus.

Overhassler performed microangiographic studies of the arteries at the intervertebral disc margins, and found that this blood supply diminished progressively with age. Vessels regularly penetrated from the vertebral body into the disc at birth, but were sparse in children and absent in adults.

At the upper end of the spinal column, the seven cervical vertebrae have the specialized function of supporting and placing the head in position relative to man's environment for best perception of sight and sound (Fig. 2-4). The control center of the body in the cranium and the upper end of the digestive tube must have support and protection. These vertebrae are the smallest in volume of any of the vertebrae, and, as expected, the greatest range of motion is possible in this segment of the column. All seven cervical vertebrae have a foramen in the transverse process, distinguishing them from all other vertebrae. The vertebral artery and vein and sympathetic nerves take passage through these openings in the upper six cervical vertebrae, and the vertebral artery occasionally pierces the foramen in the seventh on the left side. The vein may pass through this foramen on both sides of the seventh cervical vertebra. The third, fourth, fifth, and sixth cervical vertebrae are fairly similar (Fig. 2-5). All have relatively short, usually split spinous processes with two bony knobs extending posteriorly instead of one. The cervical spinous processes are the shortest of any of the vertebrae, becoming longer, however, in the fifth and especially the sixth (Fig. 2-6).

The first, second, and seventh cervical vertebrae are unique and deserve special descriptions. The first cervical vertebra supports the head on its superior articular processes as the mythical Atlas supports the world on his shoulders, and is thereby named the atlas. It lacks a body and instead pivots about a bony process called the dens (odontoid process) which is essentially the bodies of C1 and C2 vertebrae fused into one bony mass. It has a very small tubercle posteriorly in lieu of a spinous process, but it serves as one. All spinous processes in the cervical spine receive a sagittal sheet of fibrous tissue called ligamentum nuchae, which continues its attachment to the supraspinal ligament, spanning the base of the skull and the spinous process of the seventh cervical vertebra. A typical spinous process on the atlas would block motion between the skull and the atlas. Thus the

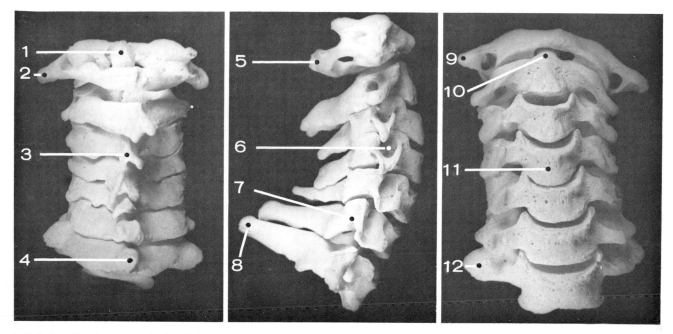

FIG. 2-4. Articulated cervical spine: *1*, dens; *2*, transverse process C1; *3*, bifid spinous process C3; *4*, spinous process C7 (vertebra prominens); *5*, posterior tubercle C1; *6*, intervertebral foramen; *7*, lateral mass C6; *8*, spinous process C7; *9*, transverse process C1; *10*, base of odontoid process; *11*, body of C4; *12*, transverse process C7.

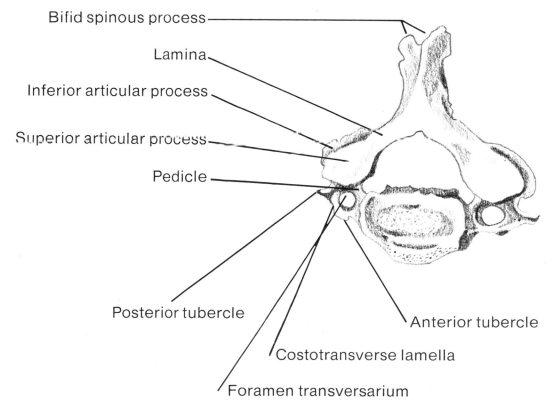

Bifid spinous process

Lamina

Inferior articular process

Superior articular process

Pedicle

Posterior tubercle

Anterior tubercle

Costotransverse lamella

Foramen transversarium

FIG. 2-5. Fourth cervical vertebra from above.

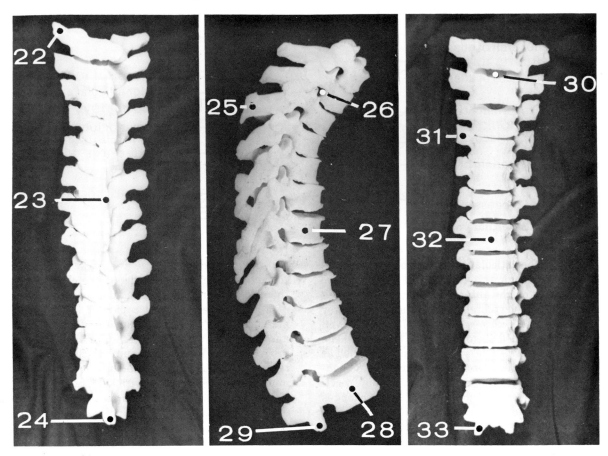

FIG. 2-9. Articulated thoracic spine: *22*, transverse process T1; *23*, spinous process T6; *24*, spinous process T12; *25*, spinous process T3; *26*, intervertebral foramen; *27*, body of T7; *28*, body of T12; *29*, inferior facet T12; *30*, intervertebral disc space T1-T2; *31*, transverse process T4; *32*, body of T7; *33*, inferior facet T12.

Since there are no ribs to articulate with the lumbar vertebrae, there are no facets on the vertebral body. Whereas the pedicles arise from the upper posterior bodies of the thoracic vertebrae, they tend to move down in the lumbar region slightly, remaining in the upper half of the posterior surface of the lumbar vertebrae. The intervertebral foramina are openings through which the paired spinal nerves pass out from the vertebral canal. In the lumbar region, they are largely made up of the so-called inferior vertebral notch, which is merely the grooved undersurface of the pedicle plus adjacent posterior body of the vertebra. In addition, the intervertebral foramen comprises the opening posterior to the lumbar disc and a small superior vertebral notch on the upper surface of each lumbar pedicle. The relative high placement of the pedicle on the body of each lumbar vertebra allows the nerve root of that level to escape through the foramen adjacent to the bony body. Thus, the posterior displacement of a given lumbar disc generally does not involve the nerve root escaping from that numbered level, but rather the one numbered below. The lumbar spinous processes are much thicker,

shorter, and more horizontally directed than those above and have greater stress on them in their function as bases of attachment for ligaments and muscles supporting the entire mobile spine and its appendages. The span of the transverse processes of the lumbar vertebrae increases from approximately 6 cm. in the upper lumbar spine to as much as 8 or 9 cm. in the lowest lumbar vertebra (Figs. 2-13 and 2-14). Two of the posterior muscles of the abdomen arise from these important lumbar transverse processes. The psoas major arises from the anterior surface of all of the lumbar transverse processes. The quadratus lumborum attaches to the apices of the transverse processes of the first four lumbar vertebrae and sometimes from the upper border of the transverse processes of the lower four. The plane of the facet joints of the lumbar vertebrae beginning with the T12-L1 facet articulation is generally sagittal, but it tends to turn gradually in the coronal direction, not quite succeeding at the lumbosacral facet joints. This is in keeping with the flexion-extension action that takes place in the relatively mobile lumbar spine, allowing a little lateral

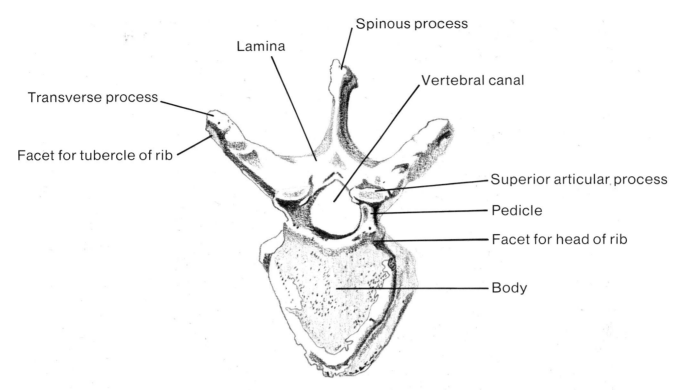

FIG. 2-10. Seventh thoracic vertebra from above.

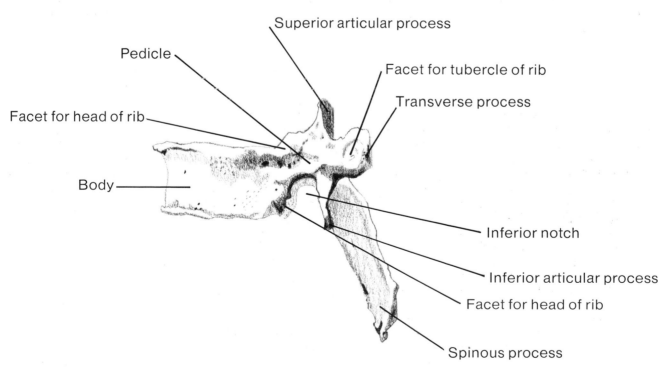

FIG. 2-11. Seventh thoracic vertebra, lateral view.

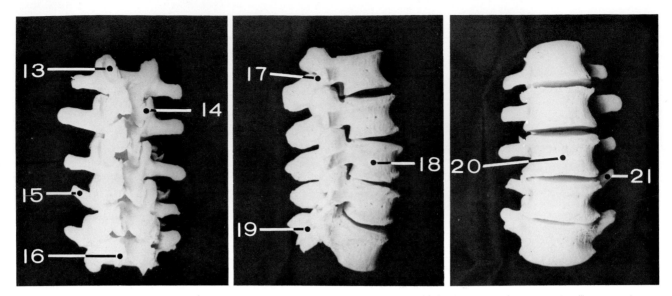

FIG. 2-12. Articulated lumbar spine: *13,* superior facet L1; *14,* facet joint L1-L2; *15,* transverse process L4; *16,* spinous process L5; *17,* transverse process L1; *18,* body of L3; *19,* transverse process L5; *20,* body of L3; *21,* transverse process L4.

bend at the lumbosacral articulation. The transverse processes of the thoracic spine lie posterior to the facet joints, whereas those of the lumbar spine lie anterior, and the latter are homologous with the dorsal ribs. A tubercle named the mamillary process lies on the posterior surface of the superior articular process of each lumbar vertebra. Another tubercle called the accessory process lies at the posterior base of the transverse process of the lumbar vertebra.

The five sacral elements of embryonic life are generally united into a single large triangular sacrum in the adult (Fig. 2-15). This bone lies wedge-like between the two innominate bones completing the ring of the bony pelvis and serving as a suitable base for the entire movable spinal column. The sacrum is slung into its pelvic base by powerful ligaments and acts as a slightly movable base relative to the pelvis for all the superimposed structures. The upper three elements of the

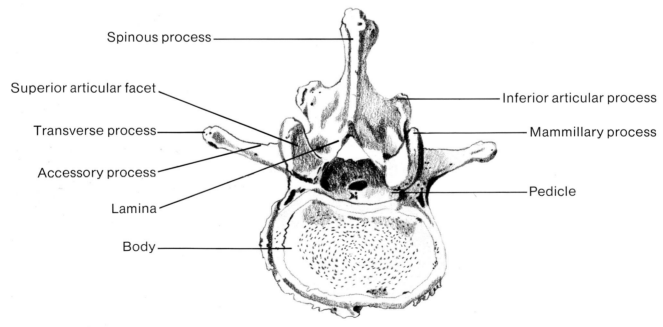

Spinous process

Superior articular facet

Transverse process

Accessory process

Lamina

Body

Inferior articular process

Mammillary process

Pedicle

FIG. 2-13. Third lumbar vertebra from above.

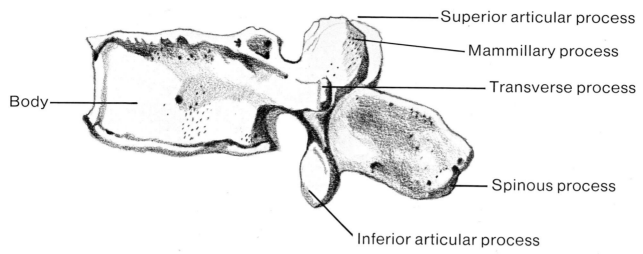

FIG. 2-14. Third lumbar vertebra, lateral view.

sacrum may be considered the keystone in an arch radiating upward from the acetabular components of the pelvis. The presacral spine, therefore, sits upon the summit of this arch. The spinous processes are represented in the sacrum by several rudimentary tubercles lying on the middle sacral crest and bordered on each side by a sacral groove formed by the fused laminae (Fig. 2-16). The articular processes of the mobile vertebra are represented in the sacrum by fused masses making up the sacral articular crest just lateral to the groove. In lieu of a single intervertebral foramen, as is present in the movable spine, there are anterior and posterior sacral foramina through which pass respectively anterior and posterior divisions of the sacral nerves. Lateral to the posterior sacral foramina the representatives of the transverse process consist of a series of tubercles making up the lateral crests of the sacrum. On the anterior surface of the sacrum, facing the pelvis, are the fused bodies of the sacral elements, each fusion represented by a ridge, the anterior sacral foramina, and the lateral parts of the sacrum. The coccyx, or tailbone, is formed of three to five rudimentary vertebrae, often the lowest portion being the size and shape of a pea. The coccygeal elements are representative of only the bodies without the processes and often are fused in part or whole (Fig. 2-17).

Hallock noted that the lumbosacral angle, as measured from the superior surface of the sacrum, is on the average about 42 degrees with the horizontal. As this angle increases by a more horizontal position of the sacrum along with increased lordosis, great shearing forces develop on the lumbosacral disc and ligaments aggravated by anterior displacement of the center of gravity. Some flexibility of this angle is possible, especially in the young, and the abdominal muscles and gluteus maximus can actively decrease the angle and the subsequent strain.

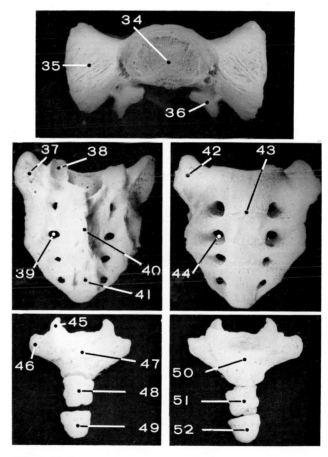

FIG. 2-15. Sacrum and coccyx: 34, body of sacrum; 35, ala; 36, articular process; 37, ala; 38, articular process; 39, posterior sacral foramen; 40, medial sacral crest; 41, sacral hiatus; 42, ala; 43, body of sacrum, junction S1–S2; 44, ventral sacral foramen; 45, cornu; 46, transverse process; 47, first coccygeal segment; 48, second segment; 49, third segment; 50, first segment; 51, second segment; 52, third segment.

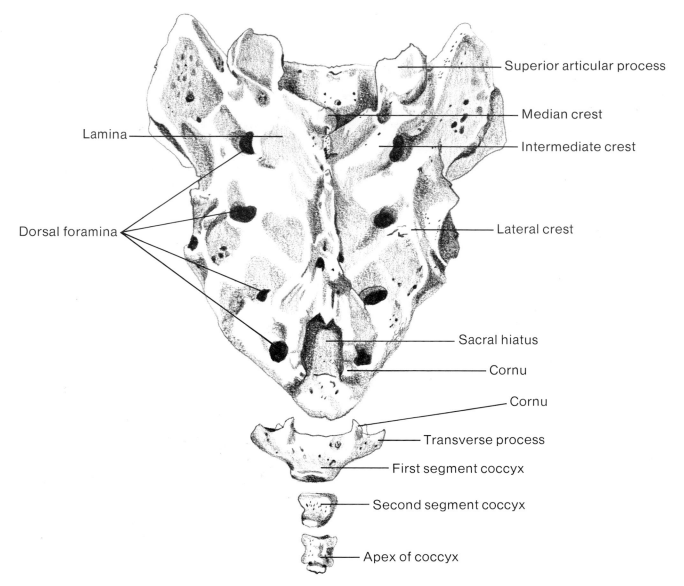

FIG. 2-16. Sacrum and coccyx; dorsal surface.

LIGAMENTS

The so-called inter-central ligaments connecting the vertebral bodies across the slightly movable intervertebral discs are the anterior and posterior longitudinal ligaments. The joints of the bony or neural arches are freely movable and are joined by the supraspinal ligaments (ligamentum nuchae in the cervical region), ligamentum flava, interspinal ligaments, and intertransverse ligaments. In addition, there are some specialized ligaments that bind together the skull and the first two cervical vertebrae.

The anterior and posterior longitudinal ligaments extend from the second cervical vertebra to the sacrum, providing strong support against flexion and extension

stresses, and leaving the lateral aspects of the vertebral bodies relatively free and unprotected. Coventry et al. note that the anterior ligament is by far the stronger of the two and probably accounts for the frequency of posterolateral protrusion of herniated intervertebral discs. In addition, the attachments of the anulus are more firmly fixed to the anterior ligament than to the posterior. The anterior ligament consists of longitudinal fibers spanning one to five vertebrae, and actually receives strong fibers from the anulus fibrosus. Its thickness increases over the concavities of the anterior surface of each vertebra as the fibers interlace and tend to layer and to fill up the shallow space more nearly flush with the surface over the discs. The posterior longitudinal ligament consists of fibers spanning one to four vertebrae and again tightly interlaced. The posterior ligament lies anteriorly within the bony neural arch. It narrows between the pedicles over the posterior body of the vertebra, and the concavity here is partially filled with the confluence of veins that drain the vertebral bodies, the basivertebral veins. These large venous channels collect blood from the spongy bone of the bodies and communicate with the anterior internal vertebral venous plexus in relation to the anterior longitudinal ligament.

The ligaments related to the bony neural arches are more or less continuous bands of dense fibrous tissue which seek attachment at all bony prominences as is characteristic of connective tissue. At these points of attachment to bone, the sheets tend to specialize as ligaments and are named according to the bony attachments. That portion which spans the tips of all the spinous processes is called the supraspinal ligament, and it is made up of fibers spanning one to four vertebrae, and these fibers are densely interwoven and interlaced. Fibrocartilaginous caps receive these fibers at the tip of each spinous process, and as is true with the small segmental muscles spanning the bony arches, these ligaments have relatively less function in the stable thoracic region. In the lumbar region, the supraspinal ligament is strong, dense, and heavily woven with fibers. In the cervical region, it becomes the ligamentum nuchae, a powerful sagittal sheet spanning the external occipital protuberances to the tip of the spinous process of the vertebra prominens. It thus provides a septum filling the lordotic curve posterior to the spinous processes of the cervical vertebrae.

The interspinal ligaments fill the space between the spinous processes and bridge and continue into the

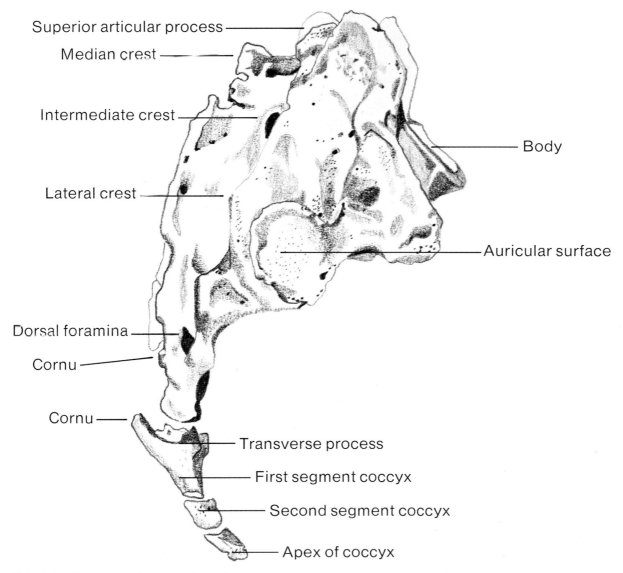

FIG. 2-17. Sacrum and coccyx, lateral view.

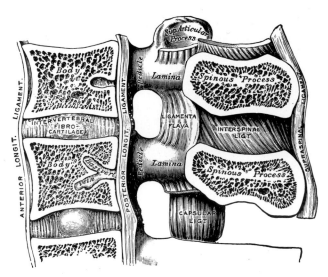

FIG. 2-18. Median sagittal section of two lumbar vertebrae and their ligaments. (From Gray's Anatomy, Lea & Febiger.)

supraspinal ligaments posteriorly and the ligamenta flava anteriorly. Again, they are best developed in the lumbar region. In the cervical region, the interspinous spaces are less significant, and the powerful ligamentum nuchae takes over the elastic resistance to vertebral flexion from the interspinales. The inter-

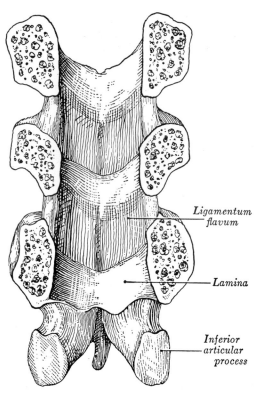

FIG. 2-20. Ligamenta flava of lumbar region. Anterior aspect. (From Gray's Anatomy, Lea & Febiger.)

transverse ligaments connect the transverse processes of the entire spine, but serve little function and are, accordingly, small. There is little need for passive elastic resistance to lateral bend movement of any part of the spine.

The ring-like opening of the atlas vertebra surrounded by the anterior and posterior arches and lateral masses is narrowed to a smaller nearly circular opening anteriorly by the powerful fibers of the transverse ligament of the atlas (Fig. 2-21). This ligament attaches to the small bony tubercle which lies just medial to the anteromedial portion of the lateral mass. Vertical fibers

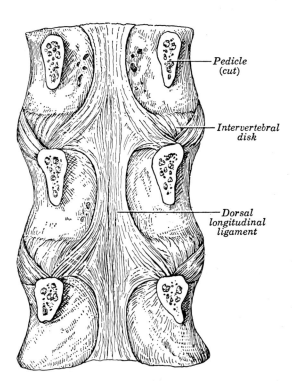

FIG. 2-19. Posterior longitudinal ligament of vertebrae in lumbar region. (From Gray's Anatomy, Lea & Febiger.)

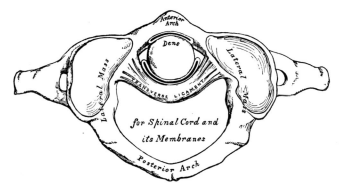

FIG. 2-21. Articulation between dens and atlas. (From Gray's Anatomy, Lea & Febiger.)

bisect the transverse ligament and pass superiorly to the basilar portion of occipital bone and inferiorly to the posterior surface of the body of the second cervical vertebrae, forming the cruciate ligament of the atlas. Because of the unique requirements of pivotal motion between the first two vertebrae, the ligamentum flava is not present here, but is replaced by the posterior atlantoaxial ligament, which spans the lamina of C2 vertebra with the corresponding posterior arch of C1 vertebra. The corresponding structure between the atlas and the skull is the posterior atlantooccipital membrane, which attaches the posterior arch of C1 to the posterior border of the foramen magnum (Fig. 2-22).

The anterior longitudinal ligament continues superiorly between the anterior surface of the body of C2 and the anterior arch of C1 as the anterior atlantoaxial ligament. Fibers then continue the line of attachment of the anterior longitudinal ligament as the anterior atlantooccipital membrane to the anterior border of the foramen magnum. A strong cord-like bundle of fibers strengthens the two ligaments spanning the skull and the first two cervical vertebrae anteriorly and lies in the midline of the two ligaments. The posterior longitudinal ligament continues superiorly from the body of C2, covering the posterior surface of the cruciate ligament on its way to the anterior border of the foramen magnum. This portion of posterior ligament is called the tectorial membrane. Anterior to the cruciate ligament lie three cords which further stabilize the relationship of skull and C2 and serve as checkreins. Two alar ligaments pass laterally as heavy cord-like ligaments from the superior portion of odontoid to the

medial sides of the occipital condyles, while an apical odontoid ligament extends from the superior extreme of the odontoid process to the anterior border of foramen magnum.

Moreover, all of the articular capsular ligaments enclosing the facet joints of the entire spine must be considered as ligaments. The articular capsular ligaments of the atlantooccipital facet joints are reinforced by strong fibers which span the jugular process of occipital bone to the atlas adjacent to its lateral masses.

JOINTS

The joints of the human body are either movable to some degree or not at all, and are variously classified as immovable, slightly movable, or freely movable. Both slightly movable and freely movable joints are represented in the spine. Although motion in the various freely movable joints is classified as flexion, rotation, gliding, and so on, it is safe to say that no joint in the human body is limited to a single pure type of motion, but rather a combination of many types. The intervertebral discs of fibrocartilage represent the so-called slightly movable joints, sometimes called amphiarthroses. At the superior end of the spine, the relationship of the condyles of the atlas to the skull represents a condyloid articulation. The rotation of the ring-like atlas about the dens of the axis represents the trochoid or pivot motion, and the facet joints generally represent a modified type of gliding or arthrodial motion.

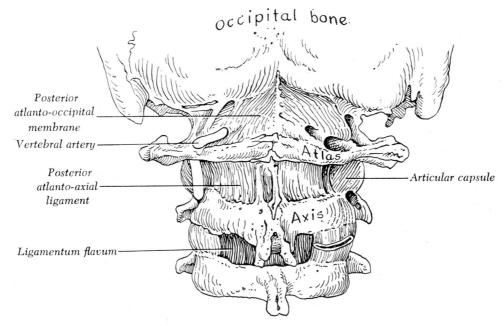

FIG. 2-22. Posterior atlantoöccipital membrane and atlantoaxial ligament. (From Gray's Anatomy, Lea & Febiger.)

MUSCLES

Superficial Muscles

The muscles that act upon the spine may be classified in many ways, such as superficial and deep, extrinsic and intrinsic, groups of muscles with generally the same fiber direction, or groups of muscles according to innervation. In any event, the most superficial muscles encountered in the spine are the two muscles that virtually clothe the intrinsic or deep muscles posteriorly, and indeed must be divided in order to expose these latter muscles (Fig. 2-23). These are the paired trapezius and the latissimus dorsi.

TRAPEZIUS. One of the functions of the trapezius muscle is to control the placement and fixation of the shoulder girdle when the spine is fixed, and thus control the placement of the base of action of the upper ex-

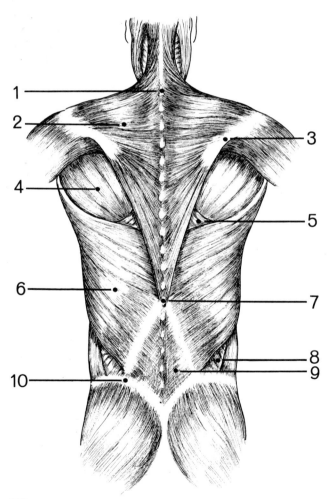

FIG. 2-23. Extrinsic muscles of spine: *1*, spinous process C7; *2*, trapezius; *3*, spine of scapula; *4*, infraspinatus; *5*, triangle of auscultation; *6*, latissimus dorsi; *7*, spinous process T12; *8*, lumbar triangle; *9*, lumbodorsal fascia; *10*, crest of ilium.

tremity. From this somewhat mobile base, the hand exhibits a wide range of motion. The trapezius spans the entire cervicodorsal spine longitudinally from the external occipital protuberance on the posterior skull all the way to the twelfth thoracic vertebra. It attaches to the spinous processes of all the cervical and thoracic vertebrae, but the cervical attachments from the base of the occiput to the C7 spinous process are by way of the powerful ligamentum nuchae. The fibers of each side of the trapezius converge to a broad attachment in a U-shaped manner from the posterior border of the lateral one-third of the clavicle along the medial margin of the acromion and the posterior border of the spine of the scapula, the final attachment being at a tubercle at the apex of the smooth triangular surface on the medial border of the spine. The two halves of the trapezius muscle form a figure called in Greek, a trapezion, translated as a little table or an irregular four-sided figure. Thus, its name applies to the figure formed by the two muscles considered together. The insertion of the trapezius is coextensive with the origin of the powerful deltoid muscle and continues the line of pull from the occiput and cervicodorsal spine to the deltoid tuberosity on the lateral aspect of the humerus.

The scapula, however, is more than an intermediary sesamoid en route from spine to humerus. The scapula is actually supported and controlled by 15 muscles with at least 11 different innervations. Its muscles assist the powerful trapezius in rotation, depression, elevation, adduction, or fixation of this portion of the shoulder girdle, which pivots on the lateral end of the clavicle anteriorly and glides along the chest wall to achieve its range of motion. A principal innervation of the trapezius is the eleventh cranial nerve, assisted by anterior primary divisions of the third and fourth cervical nerves. The trapezius may attain a high degree of bulk and tone from a specific training effect and give a bull-necked appearance if well developed. The span of the trapezius commonly measures 15 inches or more in the transverse and longitudinal axes, even in a small adult.

LATISSIMUS DORSI. The lower corner of the origin of the trapezius overlaps, the origin of the latissimus dorsi for the length of six vertebrae. The latissimus attaches to the spinous processes of the lower six thoracic vertebrae and to all the lumbosacral vertebrae and supraspinal ligaments thereon, as well as the posterior crest of the ilium and the lower three or four ribs. Its origin is a posterior layer of lumbodorsal fascia, which invests the sacrospinalis muscle posteriorly. These fibers converge as they pass laterally, picking up muscle fibers from the lower angle of the scapula as they pass around this bone, and twisting and rotating to insert at the inferior portion of the intertubercular groove of the humerus in a conjoined tendon with the teres major. Its innervation is the thoracodorsal or long subscapular nerve.

Whereas the function of the trapezius is complex and variable, depending on which portions are acting and which antagonists are apposing, its main purpose, assisted by the other 14 muscles, seems to be to place the scapula at any desired point in its range of excursion over the posterior chest wall, and to fix it for a base from which the upper extremity can operate. The latissimus dorsi, however, internally rotates the humerus and extends and adducts it, pulling the shoulder down and back if the spinal origin is fixed and the arm is free. Conversely, if the individual is supporting himself on both hands, the latissimus dorsi helps to support the trunk hanging from the tendinous insertion in the bicipital groove.

SERRATUS MUSCLES. Next, we encounter the two accessory muscles of respiration, the serratus posterior superior and inferior, whose total function appears to be to enlarge the rib cage by pulling its proximal and distal portions in opposite directions when the spine is fixed. Essentially, the serratus posterior superior has an aponeurotic origin from the spinous processes of C7 and T1 through T3, dropping down two levels on passing obliquely inferolaterally to attach to the second through fifth ribs lateral to their angles. The serratus posterior inferior arises from the aponeurotic origin of the T11, T12, L1, and L2 vertebrae and rises up two levels, passing obliquely superolaterally to attach to the lower four ribs lateral to their angles. These inspiratory muscles are among the few exceptions to posterior primary ramus innervation of the back muscle, being innervated by the upper three or four and lower three or four anterior primary rami, respectively, in the thoracic region.

Scapula

The scapula is slung superomedially and medially by the levator scapulae, the rhomboid minor, and the rhomboid major. The levator scapulae, as the name implies, is a scapular elevator and arises from the transverse processes of the upper four cervical vertebrae, passing almost vertically to the vertebral border of the scapula from the medial angle to the triangular smooth surfaces at the base of the spine. The third and fourth cervical nerves and often the dorsal scapular nerve innervate this muscle. The dorsal scapular nerve innervates consistently the two rhomboid muscles. The rhomboid minor arises from the spinous processes of C7 and T1, passing obliquely downward to the base of the triangular smooth surface. The rhomboid major spans the gap from the spinous processes of the next four thoracic vertebrae to the remainder of the vertebral border of the scapula to its inferior angle. A glance at the skeleton will clearly establish the suspensory and adductor action of the rhomboid muscles in placing or fixing the scapula.

Deep Muscles

Because of the complex, compound, or multiple attachments, as well as a great degree of blending and dividing of fiber bundles through the course of these muscles, it becomes academic to separate the intrinsic or deep muscles of the back in the same manner in which one would separate the muscles of the extremity. Nonetheless, these powerful back muscles all span the posterior aspect of the axis of flexion of the small joints of the spine, and are therefore, among other things, extensors of the spine to a greater or lesser degree. In addition, they fix or move the head as well as segments of the spine. Since all are lateral to the midline, they are also able to bend laterally, rotate, or combine complex motions of the spine.

SPLENIUS MUSCLES. Splenius capitis (Gk. *splenion*, bandage) attaches superiorly to the occiput below the lateral third of the superior nuchal line under the sternomastoid attachment and also into the mastoid process of the temporal bone. The lower attachment is to the lowest cervical and upper four thoracic spinous processes. The origin of the splenius cervicis spans the spinous processes of T3 through T6 vertebrae, diverging to attach to the posterior tubercles of the upper few cervical vertebrae, usually at least two or three.

ERECTOR SPINAE. The powerful sacrospinalis or erector spinae fills the shallow trough along each side of the spinous processes overlying the laminae and transverse processes of the entire spine. This muscle is divided into three longitudinal divisions on each side, and each of these has three subgroups named after the major group of vertebrae. The three longitudinal columns diverge from a single common tendinous origin from the midline of the sacrum, lumbar, and lower two thoracic vertebrae by spinous processes as well as the inner lip of the iliac crests and sacral crests. The lateral column of fibers approximately at the level of the angles of the ribs is called the *iliocostalis*. The intermediate column at the level of the junction of the transverse processes and rib tubercles is called the *longissimus*. The medial *spinalis* group lies alongside the spinous processes. All three groups have thoracic and cervical divisions, but the iliocostalis also has a lumbar division, and the other two have a capital division. In other words, the more medial two groups are represented at the highest level up to the skull, and the more lateral group only as far as the cervical region. All of the sacrospinalis muscle fibers are innervated by posterior primary rami. All of them act either to extend actively the various segments of spine or to fix one or both sides of the spine for other muscles to act from the fixed region or to provide a controlled flexion by acting as an antagonist to gravity. Davis, Troup, and Bernard found that when a man bends to pick up a load, the erector spinae fibers are relatively silent by electromyographic testing until the weight is raised about

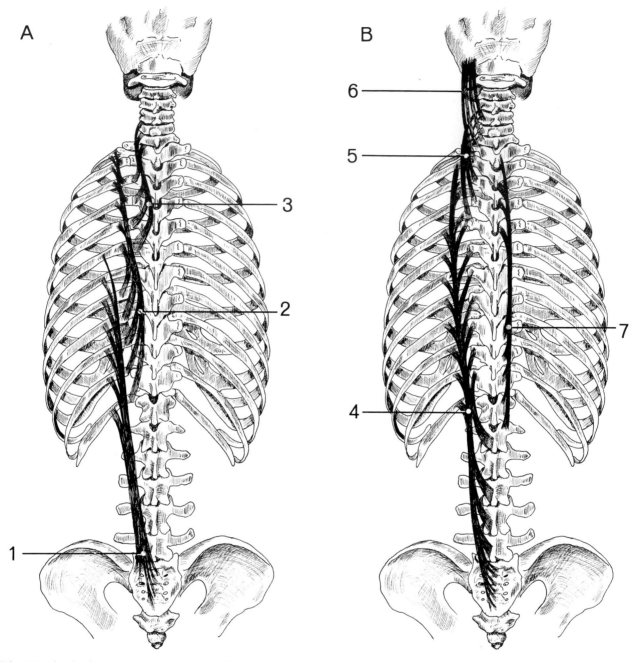

FIG. 2-24. Intrinsic muscles of spine: *1, iliocostalis lumborum; 2, iliocostalis thoracis; 3, iliocostalis cervicis; 4, longissimus thoracis; 5, longissimus cervicis; 6, longissimus capitis; 7, spinalis thoracis; 8, semispinalis thoracis; 9, semispinalis cervicis; 10, semispinalis capitis; 11, multifidus; 12, rotators; 13, interspinales.*

one-third of the way. Until this point, the intervertebral compressive forces are maximal, and the intra-abdominal pressure increases to provide a stabilizing force for the spine and to resist trunk flexion and to mitigate the intervertebral compressive forces. However, from this point, as the body straightens with the load, there is a continuous active extension of the muscles of the lumbar spine.

Morris et al., in studying the electromyographic activity of the intrinsic muscles of the back, found the longissimus dorsi to be in continuous activity in the erect posture, whereas other tested intrinsic muscles of the spine showed intermittent activity with shifts of the center of gravity. In flexion and extension of the spine, the erector spinae, rotatores, and multifidus actively resisted gravity but rested in complete extension. In lateral bend, the erector spinae was active bilaterally. Generally the balance of muscle contraction

C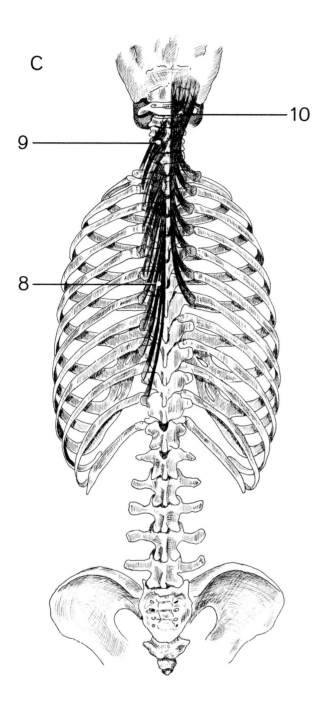

D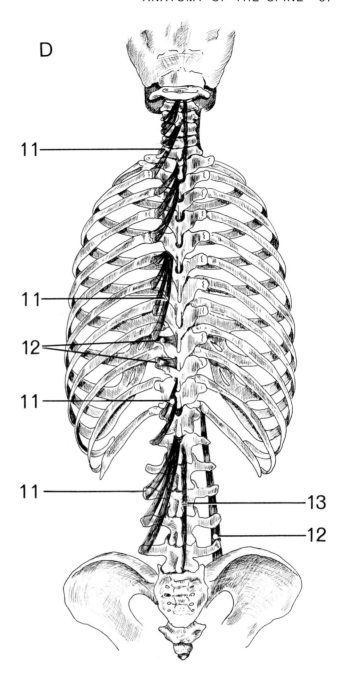

assisted gravity actively, pulling the spine to one side, but occasionally the major contraction worked opposite to gravity, lowering the trunk in a controlled lateral bend. The subjects tested were able to stand flexed at the waist with the intrinsic back muscles silent electromyographically, thus maintaining support of the back by ligaments only.

Asmussen and Klausen tested the abdominal muscles and erector spinae in the lumbar region by electromyographic electrodes and found that the two groups of muscles worked alternately as antagonists in the erect posture while rocking in flexion and extension, and that only one set of the two possible groups was active when the body was in quiet stance.

Lucas and co-workers studied the relation of the trunk to the stability of the spine. When a weight of 200 pounds is lifted with the body in the flexed position, a force greater than 2000 pounds would be placed on the lower lumbar spine if the thorax and abdomen played no part. When weights as high as 100 or 200 pounds are lifted, the muscles of the abdominal wall, diaphragm, and chest wall contract simultaneously, providing a relatively sturdy cylindrical unit to assist the spine in resisting deformity.

TRANSVERSOSPINAL MUSCLES. The muscles proximal and deep to the erector spinae may be grouped as transversospinalis muscles and, as the name implies, pass from the transverse processes of any given vertebra or vertebrae superomedially to the spinous process of one or more above. They may be divided into three groups of transversospinal muscles which span progressively fewer vertebrae and are, therefore, changing from a nearly longitudinal direction in the first group to a nearly horizontal direction in the third group. The *semispinalis* muscle bundles span from four to six vertebrae, the *multifidus* from two to four, and the *rotatores* from one to two. If we consider four regions of these muscles in longitudinal succession—capital, cervical, thoracic, and lumbar—the semispinalis group is represented in the upper three divisions and the multifidus and rotatores in the lower three divisions. In other words, the semispinalis group is not present below the thoracic region and the multifidus and rotator groups are not present above the cervical region. Actually, the latter two span the spine from sacrum to second cervical vertebra (Fig. 2-24).

Since the iliocostalis, or lateral third of each erector spinae group, lies at the level of the angle of the ribs, only the two medial portions of erector spinae, i.e., spinalis and longissimus, cover the semispinalis muscles in the dorsal region. The regional divisions of semispinalis are generalizations, as is true for all these groupings. Nonetheless, the thoracic portion spans the transverse processes of the lower six thoracic vertebrae, perhaps excluding the lowest one or two, through the spinous processes of C6 to T4. The cervical portion of semispinalis spans from the transverse processes of the upper six thoracic vertebrae through the spinous processes of the cervical, excluding the first and the last two. The capital portion has a broad origin from the transverse or articular processes of C4 to T6 and attaches into the occiput between the superior and inferior nuchal lines, producing the most extensive insertion of any of this muscle group.

The multifidus spinae group originates on transverse processes and each fasciculus spans two to four vertebrae on the way to its insertion on the spinous process above. Multifidus and rotatores actually fill the trough on either side of the midline of the vertebrae from sacrum to axis. Deepest in this general classification are the rotator spinae whose fasciculi arise from the transverse process passing to the spinous process one or two levels above.

If one traces the attachments on the skeleton of any portion of these muscles, it becomes apparent that there is a regular progression of fiber direction from horizontal to vertical between these three groups of transversospinal muscles as well as within the groups. Some fibers in the semispinalis group which span six vertebrae are within less than ten degrees of longitudinal in direction. Successive fibers pass progressively more obliquely until the short rotator muscles in the thoracic region are virtually horizontal, spanning the tip of the transverse process of one vertebra to the spinous processes of the one above. In the dorsal spine, the tip of each spinous process lies between or slightly below the transverse processes of the vertebra below. All of these muscles span the axis of flexion of any paired intervertebral unit posteriorly; therefore they extend the vertebral column. Because of their obliquity to the long axis of the spine, they are also rotatores, turning the point of insertion to the opposite side. The final group of fibers running essentially longitudinally comprise the *interspinales*, attaching, as the name implies, to the spinous processes of adjoining vertebrae, and *intertransversarii*, which attach to the transverse processes in a similar manner.

As one would expect, such muscles have little function in the relatively rigid portions of the spine, such as the dorsal, and none in the fused sacral units. Their greatest function is in the most mobile segments of the cervical region, where their development is extensive. They are also present in the second most mobile portion of the spine, the lumbar region, and both cervical and lumbar segmental muscles extend into the adjoining bordering thoracic vertebrae. Because of their relations to and distance from the axes of flexion and lateral deviation, respectively, the interspinales are extensors of the vertebral column, efficiently performing this function from a rather long lever arm, and the intertransversarii are lateral benders of the column.

According to Arkin, unilateral spasm of the intertransverse muscles can produce a scoliotic type curve concave to the affected side, though he feels this plays no part in structural scoliosis. Despite our limited knowledge of the individual actions of any of these complex, interwoven intrinsic muscles, it is certain that lateral bend is seldom pure and often comprises a combination of bending, torsion, and side-slipping, depending on which antagonists are relaxed or working synergistically with the agonist muscles. The direction, type, and extent of motion also depend on the shapes of adjoining articular surfaces and range of movement permitted by capsule and ligament.

SUBOCCIPITAL MUSCLES. Finally, a special group of muscles is located in the suboccipital region, for which they are named (Fig. 2-25). There are two *posterior capital erectors*, major and minor, and two *oblique capital muscles*, superior and inferior. These muscles define and bound the suboccipital triangle and are innervated by a portion of the posterior ramus of the suboccipital nerve. The latter, which is the dorsal primary division of the first cervical nerve, leaves the spinal canal above the posterior arch of C1, passing between it and the vertebral artery to enter this triangle. It also innervates the semispinalis capitis. All of the suboccipital muscles, except the obliquus capitis inferior, attach to the occiput on or between the nuchal lines and are thus head extensors. The rectus capitis posterior major rotates the head in addition, and the

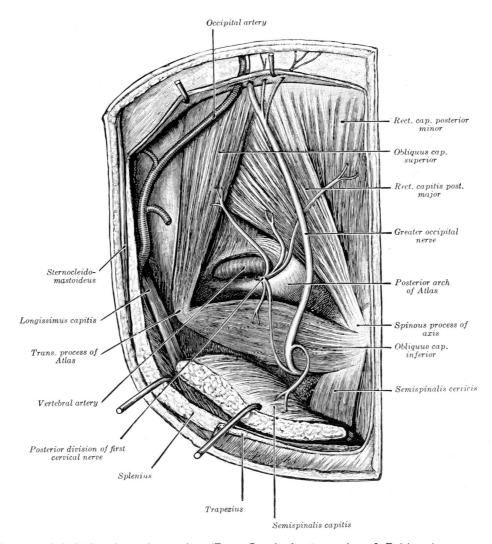

Occipital artery

Rect. cap. posterior minor

Obliquus cap. superior

Rect. capitis post. major

Greater occipital nerve

Posterior arch of Atlas

Spinous process of axis

Obliquus cap. inferior

Semispinalis cervicis

Sternocleido-mastoideus

Longissimus capitis

Trans. process of Atlas

Vertebral artery

Posterior division of first cervical nerve

Splenius

Trapezius

Semispinalis capitis

FIG. 2-25. Left suboccipital triangle and muscles. (From Gray's Anatomy, Lea & Febiger.)

obliquus capitis superior bends it laterally. The obliquus capitis inferior also rotates the atlas and thus the head secondarily.

All of these intrinsic spinal muscles are innervated by dorsal primary divisions of the spinal nerves. The anterior primary divisions of the spinal nerves pass around the trunk to provide motor and sensory innervation to the body wall.

EXTRINSIC MUSCLES ACTING ON THE SPINE. Since every muscle that spans a freely movable joint exerts some action on that joint, we must include among those muscles acting on the spine the following:

1. The *sternocleidomastoid* muscle has two fleshy heads of origin from the medial clavicle and sternum and passes obliquely across the anterolateral side of the neck to insert into the mastoid process of the temporal bone just posterior to the external ear and into the occipital bone and superior nuchal line. The sternomastoid muscle, which is innervated by the spinal accessory nerve and by anterior rami of C2 and C3 nerves, can rotate the head, point the chin, bend the neck and head laterally, or flex the cervical capital region, depending on synergistic or antagonistic action of certain other muscles.

2. The *infrahyoid* or "strap" muscles are the sternohyoid, the sternothyroid, the thyrohyoid, and the omohyoid muscles, because in their upward continuations past the hyoid bone via the four suprahyoid muscles all have an action on the cervical capital region depending on fixation. This action is essentially negligible in view of the fact that, despite their anterior spanning of the cervical vertebrae, a much more powerful sternomastoid muscle spans these joints from a further distance, thus having a greater lever arm and a more direct attachment.

3. The *anterior vertebral muscles* are innervated by cervical nerves according to the levels they span. The ventral primary divisions of the upper four cervical

nerves form a cervical plexus, whose deep muscular branches supply the muscles in question. Longus colli lies on the anterior surface of the vertebral bodies from C2 to T3 and can arbitrarily be considered as having three sections, superior oblique, inferior oblique, and vertical. The anterior vertebral muscles are neck flexors and rotatores, depending on adjoining muscle action at the time. Longus capitis continues the direct line of pull from anterior scalene to the undersurface of the skull and the inferior surface of the basilar portion of occipital bone, and thus flexes and slightly rotates the head (Fig. 2-26). Rectus capitis anterior runs parallel and deep to longus capitis, spanning C2 and the base of the occiput just anterior to the foramen magnum. Rectus capitis lateralis continues the line of pull of the intertransversarii. It can stabilize the skull or bend it laterally.

4. The *lateral vertebral muscles.* The anterior, middle, and posterior scalenes have functions of placing and fixing the head and neck. The roots of the brachial plexus emerge laterally from between the anterior and middle scalenes. The anterior scalene attaches to the anterior tubercles of transverse processes C3 through C6 and to the scalene tubercle on the inner border of the first rib and the adjacent ridge. A middle scalene

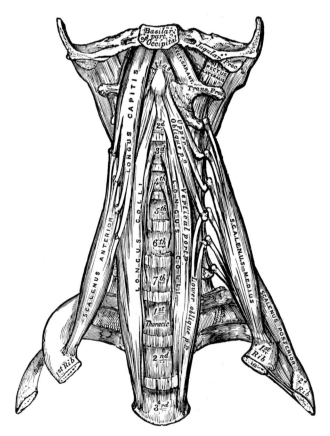

FIG. 2-26. Ventral vertebral muscles. (From Gray's Anatomy, Lea & Febiger.)

attaches to the posterior tubercles of the transverse processes of the lower six cervical vertebrae inserting into the upper first rib between the tubercle and the subclavian groove. A posterior scalene arises from the posterior tubercles and transverse processes of the lower three cervical vertebrae attaching into the second rib. These muscles can be accessory respiratory muscles elevating the apex of the chest cavity by their rib attachments. They can also produce lateral bend of the vertebral column or a complex rotation-flexion action. The abdominal muscles, obliquus externus and internus as well as the transverse abdominis and the rectus abdominis, act as flexors or rotatores of the spine by the axes they span. Quadratus lumborum, the very efficient fixer of the chest via the twelfth rib, which spans to the posterior crest of the ilium, can also bend the thorax laterally on the pelvis by unilateral action. Psoas minor, sometimes known as psoas parvus, when present, attaches to the sides of the body of T12 and L1 and spans to the iliopectineal eminence. It thus flexes and possibly rotates the lumbar spine and bends it laterally.

The iliopsoas is made up of two muscles. The iliacus arises from the superolateral two-thirds of the iliac fossa. The psoas major originates from all of the lumbar transverse processes and by means of fibrous slips and tendinous arches from the lumbar and lowest thoracic vertebrae. Its conjoined tendon spans the hip joint to insert on the lesser trochanter of the femur, thus attaching spine, pelvis, and femur together by powerful muscle fibers.

MUSCLE ACTION

Some generalizations about muscle action are in order. A muscle cannot act by pushing. It can only act by contracting its fibers and shortening the distance between any two points of its attachment. Movements of any of the diarthrodial, or freely movable, joints in the body are complex, but for simplification we tend to classify muscles as flexors, extensors, etc. This classification, in effect, places an imaginary axis through the joint. If it is a simple hinge joint, muscles that lie anterior to the axis would flex the joint, and those that lie posterior to the axis would extend the joint with varying degrees of efficiency, depending on the line of pull and the perpendicular distance to the axis. A rotator would lie on the medial or lateral side of a vertical axis through the joint, and would thus achieve medial or lateral rotation accordingly. An adductor or an abductor would similarly lie medial or lateral to the axis of adduction and abduction. There are few pure flexors, extensors, or rotatores, that is, muscles that do not have more than one action on a joint. A muscle has to have some dimension and bulk, and would have to exert a pure line of pull precisely related to the imaginary axis in order to achieve a singular effect upon a joint. Also, the action of muscles across the joint depends on the position of the bones of the joint at the time of the action. If we consider the anatomic position or the so-called neutral position of the joint in which it lies at mid-range with ligaments relaxed under the least tension, this is the logical position for describing the supposed action of the muscle. Portions of a muscle such as the deltoid may lie on opposite sides of the joint, and if capable of acting separately, could theoretically provide both agonist and antagonist. Except under experimental conditions of electrical muscle stimulation, as with implanted electrodes, a single muscle seldom, if ever, operates in an isolated manner. Muscles tend to act synergistically. As the agonist contracts, the antagonist relaxes in a controlled manner to permit the motion to occur. In addition, groups of muscles tend to act together to achieve the same or a combined type of motion.

In studying the action of the muscles of the spine, we speak of a group of muscle fibers that attach to two points as if it were acting in an isolated manner, but we can never forget the above maxims regarding this action. Some of the most graphic demonstrations of intrinsic muscle action of the spine are seen in the severe paralytic spine. Garrett, Perry, and Nichol, in their work on stabilization of the collapsing spine, have

presented many cases of partial and complete paralysis of the intrinsic muscles of the neck and back. If the paralysis is asymmetric, paralytic scoliosis results. If the paralysis is total, the spine collapses in the erect posture within the limits of stretch of the supporting ligaments. All of the intrinsic muscles of the spine lie posterior to the axis of flexion of any two adjacent vertebrae. Since none of them lies purely in the midline over the dorsum of this joint, they are also individually lateral flexors or rotatores. A straight spine in the anterior posterior view is dependent upon a balanced pull of these muscles throughout the growth period. Whatever the cause of asymmetry of pull in idiopathic scoliosis, for example, the curve may progress at least until such time as growth is complete with an ever-increasing mechanical advantage of the muscles on the concave side of any given curve. The initial function of any given bundle of muscle fibers changes with the changing position of the adjacent vertebrae. Extensors thus become progressive deforming forces, vertebrae rotate and bend laterally into increasing curves, and growing bone responds in accordance with Wolf's Law, producing wedging deformities of the body of the vertebrae.

Klausen studied the form and function of the loaded

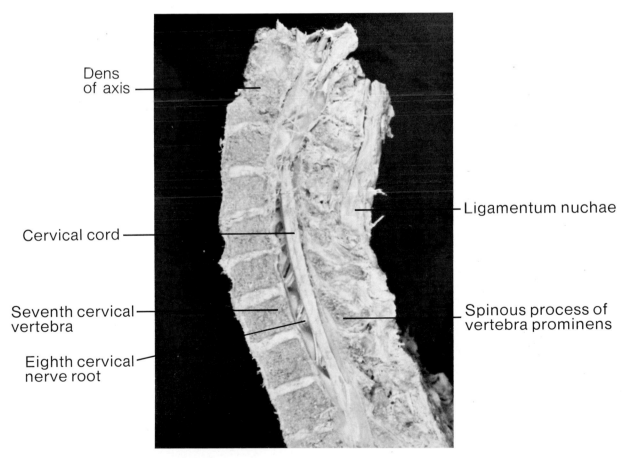

Dens of axis —

Cervical cord —

Seventh cervical vertebra —

Eighth cervical nerve root —

— Ligamentum nuchae

— Spinous process of vertebra prominens

FIG. 2-27. Hemisected cervical spine and cord.

human spine in which he not only took measurements of motion, but studied the trunk muscles with electromyography. The position of any segment of the spine is dependent upon the weight of that portion of the body above that level and its line of gravity in relation to the axis of movement of the adjacent joints. The resistance to compression of the intervertebral disc, plus muscle and ligamentous pull on adjacent joints, counterbalances the tendency of any particular segment to become displaced. Thus—depending on the posture and erect position of the spine—the abdominal wall muscles, the deep one-joint muscles of the back, or the more oblique multi-joint muscles contract to balance the pull of gravity. A resistance to compression of the intervertebral disc provides a counteracting force in addition.

Morris, Benner, and Lucas reported an electromyographic study of the intrinsic muscles of the back. Studies were done of the deep back muscles in the lower thoracic and lumbar region, specifically the erector spinae, the multifidus, and the rotatores. When the body was in the standing position the longissimus dorsi showed constant activity, whereas changes in the center of gravity, produced by a slight shift in body weight or position, caused other muscles in the area to become active. The erector spinae muscles, the rotatores, and the multifidus showed electrical activity in opposing the force of gravity while the body was bending at the waist, but they were totally at rest with the body in a relaxed, completely extended position. A synergistic relaxation and contraction of opposing muscles occurred to permit and sustain changes of position in flexion, extension, lateral bend, and rotation. Thus the components of the paraspinal muscles, as previously believed, generally act as a group in maintaining or controlling flexion, extension, lateral bend, and rotation of the body, but they also perform discrete acts as separate muscles when required.

BLOOD SUPPLY

Blood is supplied to the spinal column by way of a series of ring-like anastomoses that occur at the midportion of each vertebra. The principal divisions of this system are the segmental vessels, which arise from the vertebral artery in the cervical region, from the aorta in the thoracic and lumbar regions, and from the lateral sacral arteries in the sacral region. Each segmental vessel divides into ventral and dorsal branches at the

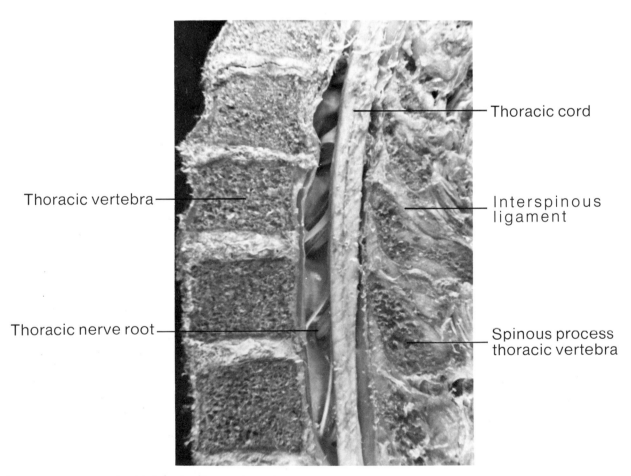

Thoracic cord

Thoracic vertebra

Interspinous ligament

Thoracic nerve root

Spinous process thoracic vertebra

FIG. 2-28. Hemisected mid-dorsal spine and cord.

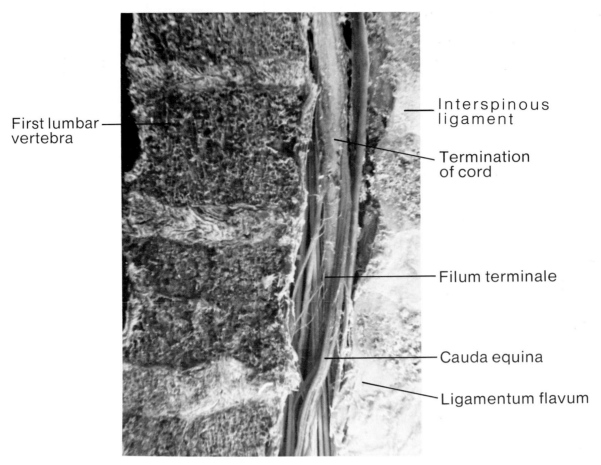

First lumbar vertebra

Interspinous ligament

Termination of cord

Filum terminale

Cauda equina

Ligamentum flavum

FIG. 2-29. Hemisected lumbar spine and cauda equina.

ventrolateral aspect of the body of each vertebra. The ventral branch courses laterally to supply the walls of the trunk, chest, and neck, whereas the dorsal branch gives off a spinal artery and continues dorsally to supply the muscles and soft tissues adjacent to the spinal column. The spinal artery enters the intervertebral foramen and gives off a rich anastomosis to the bony neural arch as well as to the cord, its coverings, and the vertebrae.

Willis reported in 1948 on the nutrient arteries of the vertebral bodies, which were previously thought to enter the anterior surface of the body of the vertebra. The principal nutrition of the vertebral body was shown to be supplied by the most anterior of these three branches. Four of these vessels converge on the center of the posterior surface of any given vertebra from the four adjacent intervertebral foramina. The vessels entering this nutrient foramen from this layer of loose connective tissue deep to the posterior spinal ligament then diverge into the substance of the cancellous bone of the body of the vertebra. Ferguson studied the circulation in fetal and infant spines and reported on his findings in 1949. He injected the arteries, sectioned the spines in three different planes, and also dissected them. His work confirmed the principal supply from the

dorsal aspect of the vertebral body and, in addition, described small arteries entering the anterior aspect of the individual vertebral body from the respective segmental vessel.

Small vessels also were described which apparently perforated the cartilaginous plate, permitting capillary vessels to enter the anulus fibrosus, but these branches are not present in the *adult* intervertebral disc.

NERVES

On each side of the spine 31 spinal nerves arise from the cord by the ventral motor and dorsal sensory roots, and emerge from the intervertebral foramen at every level. Eight pairs are cervical, twelve thoracic, five lumbar, five sacral, and one coccygeal. Each spinal nerve has a dorsal and ventral primary division. The dorsal primary branches pass directly posteriorly and therefore innervate the intrinsic muscles of the spine and supply sensation to the skin overlying these muscles (Figs. 2-27, 2-28, 2-29, and 2-30).

The skin that covers the remainder of the body, that is, the limbs and ventrolateral trunk, is supplied by the sensory branches of the ventral primary division of the

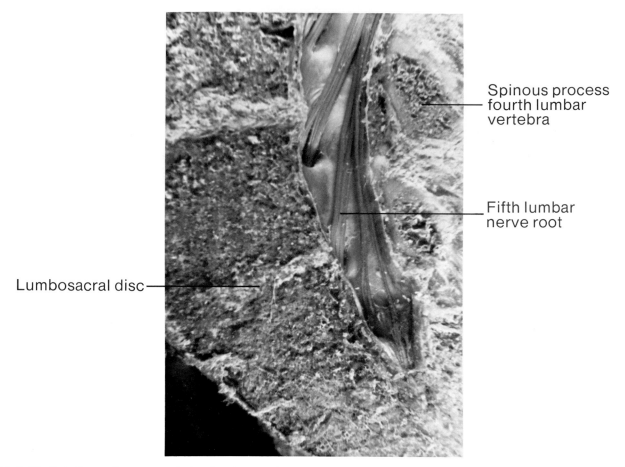

Spinous process
fourth lumbar
vertebra

Fifth lumbar
nerve root

Lumbosacral disc

FIG. 2-30. Relations of nerve roots to disc in canal.

spinal nerves. Thoracic ventral primary divisions are called intercostal nerves, except for the last, which is the subcostal. The intercostal nerves supply the ventro-lateral trunk. The upper two or three intercostal nerves supply innervation to the medial arm via the inter-costobrachial branches. The remainder of the ventral primary divisions contribute to complex plexus arrangements. The superior four cervical nerves make up the cervical plexus. Its branches emerge from an area the size of a dime posterior to the midpoint of the sterno-cleidomastoid muscle to go in all directions posteriorly. The branches provide sensory innervation for the face and the neck down over the clavicle. The last four cervical and first thoracic contribute branches to form the brachial plexus which provides motor and sensory innervation of the upper extremity.

The lumbar plexus is made up of ventral primary divisions of T12 through L4. The sacral coccygeal plexus consists of a portion of the ventral primary division of L4 through the sacral and coccygeal branches. These combine to form motor and sensory innervation for the lower extremity.

Pedersen and associates dissected and described in detail the sinuvertebral nerves, which were previously described by others and first reported in detail by von Luschka. These branches arise from the spinal nerve distal to the ganglion or, with the rami communicantes, enter the spinal canal to supply the posterior longitudinal ligament, dura, periosteum, and blood vessels. They contain sensory fibers.

References

1. Arkin AM: The mechanism of rotation in combination with lateral deviation in the spine. J Bone Jt Surg *32A*:180–188, 1950.
2. Asmussen E, Klausen K: Form and function of the erect human spine. Clin Orthop, *25*:55–63, 1962.
3. Bick EM, Copel JW: Longitudinal growth of the human vertebra. J Bone Jt Surg *32A*:803–814, 1950.
4. Coventry MB, Ghormley RK, Kernohan JW: The intervertebral disc: Its microscopic anatomy and pathology. J Bone Jt Surg *27*:105–112, 1945.
5. Davis PR, Troup JD, Bernard JH: Movements of the thoracic and lumbar spine when lifting. J Anat *99*:13–26, 1965.
6. Ferguson WR: Some observations on the circulation in foetal and infant spines. J Bone Jt Surg *32A*:640–648, 1950.

7. Gray H: Anatomy of the Human Body. Ed 27, Philadelphia, Lea & Febiger, 1959.

8. Hallock H.: Low Back Lesions—Anatomical Considerations. American Academy of Orthopaedic Surgeons Instructional Course Lectures, Vol. IV 87-89, Ann Arbor, JW Edwards, 1948.

9. Hassler O: The human intervertebral disc. Acta Orthop Scandinav *40*:765-772, 1970.

10. Hollinshead WH: Anatomy of the spine: points of interest to orthopaedic surgeons. J Bone Jt Surg *47A*:209-215, 1965.

11. Klausen K: The form and function of the loaded human spine. Acta Physiol Scand *65*:176-190, 1965.

12. Lucas DB: Mechanics of the spine. Bull of the Hosp for Jt Dis *31-2*:115-131, 1970.

13. Lysell E: Motion in the cervical spine. Acta Orthop Scand *123*:7-61, 1969.

14. Morris JM, Lucas DB, Bresler B: Role of the trunk in stability of the spine. J Bone Jt Surg *43A*:327-351, 1961.

15. Morris JM, Benner G, Lucas DB: An electromyographic study of the intrinsic muscles of the back in man. J Anat *96*:509-520, 1962.

16. Orofino C, Sherman MS, Schechter D: Luschka's joint—a degenerative phenomenon. J Bone Jt Surg *42A*:853-858, 1960.

17. Overton LM, Grossman JW: Anatomical variations in the articulation between the second and third cervical vertebrae. J Bone Jt Surg *34A*:155-161, 1952.

18. Pedersen HE, Blunck CFJ, Gardner E: The anatomy of lumbosacral posterior rami and menigeal branches of spinal nerves (sinu-vertebral nerves). J Bone Jt Surg *38A*:377-391, 1956.

19. Rowe GG, Roche MB: The lumbar neural arch. J Bone Jt Surg *32A*:554-557, 1950.

20. White AA III: Analysis of the mechanics of the thoracic spine in man. Acta Orthop Scand *127*:8-88, 1969.

21. Willis TA: Nutrient arteries of the vertebral bodies. J Bone Jt Surg *31A*:538-540, 1949.

3

Neuroanatomy

DANIEL RUGE

THOUGH the neural tube is modified greatly to form the brain and brain stem, it is changed little to form the spinal cord. The structure of the latter is quite constant throughout its length, but is altered to accommodate the varying numbers and types of neurons introduced. Continuous with the medulla oblongata, the spinal cord takes the form of a slightly flattened cylinder ensheathed by the three meninges: the pia mater which clings to the cord, the arachnoid which contains the cerebrospinal fluid, and the outermost layer, the dura mater.

In the embryo, the spinal cord fills the total length of the vertebral canal, but at birth the tip of the cord has ascended to the level of the third lumbar vertebra. After birth, the spinal cord continues to grow more slowly than the vertebral column so that by adult life it lies within the upper two-thirds of the vertebral canal and terminates caudally as the conus medullaris between the first and second lumbar vertebrae (Fig. 3-1). Only rarely does the conus extend farther down the canal. The pia mater continues caudally from the tip of the conus as a non-neural thread—the filum terminale—to the terminal end of the vertebral column where it is anchored. The arachnoid and dura mater continue as tubular sheaths to the level of the second sacral vertebra where they join the filum terminale.

Six longitudinal furrows are found on the surface of the cord. The deep anterior median fissure is the most definite and extends into the ventral surface approximately one-third of its anteroposterior diameter. This fissure and the shallow posterior median sulcus divide the cord into symmetric lateral halves. On both sides the broad, shallow anterolateral sulcus is the site of emergence of the ventral nerve rootlets. Similarly corresponding to the line of origin of the dorsal nerve rootlets is the narrower but rather deep posterolateral sulcus.

40

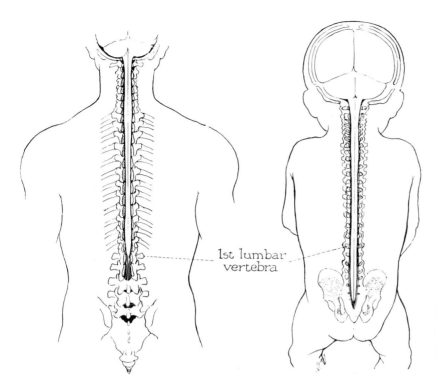

1st lumbar
vertebra

FIG. 3-1. Diagram shows extent of spinal cord in relation to spinal canal in a man and in an infant. (From Davis L, and Davis RA: Principles of Neurological Surgery. Philadelphia, WB Saunders Co., 1963.)

Ribbon-like bands of pia mater are attached to the spinal cord bilaterally and incompletely divide the subarachnoid space into anterior and posterior compartments, hence separating the ventral and dorsal roots. Their attachment to the cord is continuous, but laterally each gives off a series of fine, tooth-like projections called dentate ligaments, which midway between the exits of adjacent nerves pierce the arachnoid and attach to the dura mater holding the cord in position. There are approximately 21 pairs of these ligaments extending from the foramen magnum to the level of the first lumbar vertebra. The last dentate ligament at the level of the L1 vertebra assumes a fork-like shape with an outer prong about one centimeter long (it may be three to four centimeters long) which is attached at its end to the dura.[9] Its inner prong attaches to the pia on the lateral aspect of the cord and runs downward to the tip of the conus medullaris. Elsberg notes that the first lumbar dorsal root may be identified because it rests upon this fork-shaped dentate ligament.

At the intervertebral foramina, dorsal and ventral roots merge to form the spinal nerves, and it is at this point that the ganglia of the dorsal roots are situated. The arachnoid and dural layers form a sleeve to cover each combined dorsal and ventral root, and the dura mater becomes continuous distally with the epineurium of the peripheral nerve.

There are eight segments in the cervical portion of the spinal cord and one would anticipate that there would be eight bilateral pairs of dorsal and ventral roots emerging to form eight spinal nerves on each side. Actually the first pair may be absent or attenuated, but what there is

emerges between the occiput and the atlas. The second cervical nerve emerges between the atlas and axis, and all succeeding nerves pass through intervertebral foramina which are situated just anterior to the posterior articular facets uniting the vertebrae. In the cervical region, the nerve is named after the vertebra below its emergence, except for the eighth cervical nerve, which leaves between the C7 and T1 vertebrae. Beginning with the first thoracic nerve, the emerging nerves are identified with the vertebra above their exits.

In the cervical and upper thoracic spine, the spinal roots and nerves emerge at right angles to the cord. However, due to the ascent of the cord within the vertebral canal, all the others take a downward course which becomes more pronounced at lower levels. In the adult, the twelve segments of the thoracic cord are contained in the upper nine thoracic vertebrae, the five lumbar segments are contained within the tenth and eleventh thoracic vertebrae, and the five sacral segments and one coccygeal segment of the spinal cord are within the twelfth thoracic and first lumbar vertebrae. It follows then, that the lower the level of the origin of the nerve, the greater the distance between its origin and point of exit. The spinal nerves constituting the cauda equina are within the lumbar vertebral canal and emerge from the foramina of the lumbar spine or pass under the sacral apertures. These roots are so arranged that those arising at the higher levels lie lateral to those arising at lower levels. In spite of this organized pattern, it is difficult to identify the nerve roots unless one can see the points of emergence from the vertebral canal (Fig. 3-2).

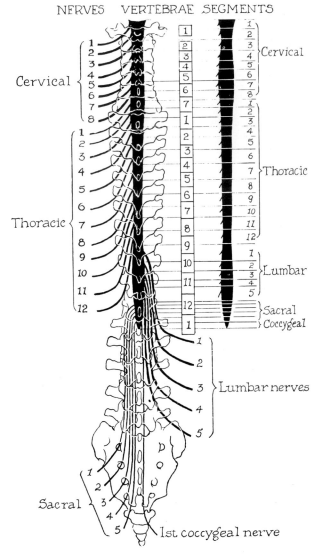

FIG. 3-2. Diagram shows relation of spinal nerves and segments of spinal cord to vertebral spinous processes. (From Davis L, and Davis RA: Principles of Neurological Surgery. Philadelphia, WB Saunders Co., 1963.)

In cross section the spinal cord can be separated into two major zones, the gray matter and the white matter (Fig. 3-3). The former contains much of the intrinsic vascular supply of the spinal cord in addition to the neuron cell bodies and hence is darker than the white matter which contains the long fiber tracts insulated with glistening white myelin sheaths.

GRAY MATTER

The gray matter is composed of groups of nerve cell bodies which form longitudinal columns in the center of the spinal cord. Cross sections of the spinal cord at different levels show varying H-shaped patterns of gray matter, which can be separated into dorsal, intermediate, and ventral columns. Many cells of the spinal cord are required to supply the upper and lower extremities, accounting for the enlargement of the gray matter in the cervical and lumbar regions. The thoracic and upper lumbar segments that supply only the trunk have a lateral projection in the intermediate portion containing autonomic neurons, the axons of which enter the sympathetic ganglia.

Dorsal Column (Horn) Gray

The dorsal column gray contains cells which receive impulses from the dorsal roots. The fibers carrying the impulses to the dorsal horn have their cell bodies in the dorsal root ganglia and may be subdivided conveniently into short, intermediate, and long fiber systems according to the distance they travel prior to synapse.

The short dorsal root fibers enter the substantia gelatinosa either by traversing the tract of Lissauer (dorsolateral fasciculus) or by first ascending or descending in the tract of Lissauer for a segment or two. Intermediate posterior root fibers pass into the dorsal horn and proceed up the dorsal column for varying distances, after which they turn ventrally to terminate in the nucleus proprius. Long dorsal root fibers do not enter the dorsal column gray, but enter the lateral aspect of the posterior funiculus and pass upward via the fasciculus gracilis and the fasciculus cuneatus. Incoming dorsal root fibers also may take a course along the ventral edge of the posterior column to reach the nucleus dorsalis (Clarke's column) situated at the base of the dorsal column gray. Other dorsal root fibers terminate rather diffusely in the posterior funicular gray, chiefly in Stilling's nucleus and the posterior commissural nucleus.

Intermediate Column Gray

The intermediate column gray lies lateral to the central canal of the spinal cord and is present only in the lower cervical, thoracic, lumbar, and sacral portions of the cord. The cell bodies of the sympathetic neurons lie in the intermediolateral nucleus of the lateral horn of the intermediate column gray in spinal cord segments T1 to L3. Their axons exit via the ventral roots as sympathetic preganglionic fibers which course through the white rami communicans to synapse in the prevertebral and paravertebral ganglia with postganglionic fibers, which subsequently pass via the gray rami communicans to their sites of innervation. The sacral parasympathetic cell column is similarly situated in cord segments S2 to S4. Fibers from this column pass out of the spinal cord in the corresponding ventral roots to end on postganglionic neurons near, on, or in the organs which developmentally reside in the pelvis.

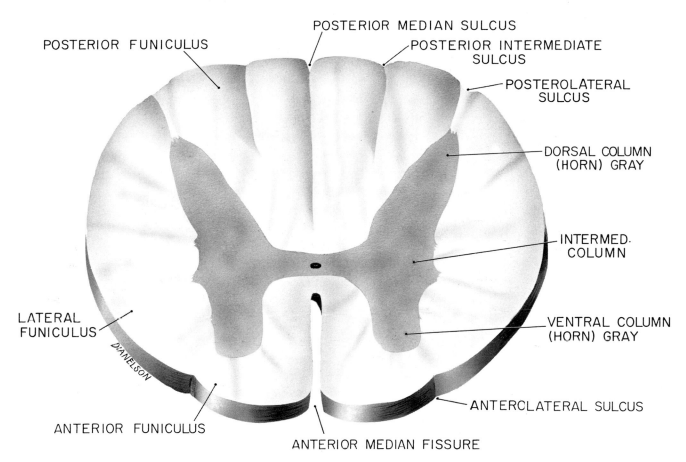

POSTERIOR MEDIAN SULCUS

POSTERIOR INTERMEDIATE SULCUS

POSTERIOR FUNICULUS

POSTEROLATERAL SULCUS

DORSAL COLUMN (HORN) GRAY

INTERMED. COLUMN

VENTRAL COLUMN (HORN) GRAY

ANTEROLATERAL SULCUS

LATERAL FUNICULUS

ANTERIOR FUNICULUS

ANTERIOR MEDIAN FISSURE

FIG. 3-3. Sulci, and gray and white matter of spinal cord.

Ventral Column (Horn) Gray

The ventral column gray contains relatively large multipolar motor neurons with coarse Nissl granules characteristic of efferent cells. While their dendrites spread out rather widely in all directions, some actually passing through the anterior commissure into the contralateral side of the cord, the majority of their axons leave the spinal cord by the ipsilateral ventral roots. While small deep muscles of the spine are innervated by axons from the dorsomedial cells, the superficial muscles of both spine and abdomen are innervated by the ventromedial cells. The axons of the retrodorsal cells send impulses to the small muscles of the hands, fingers, feet, and toes, while the adjacent dorsolateral cells innervate the larger muscles of the forearm, hand, leg, and foot. The ventrolateral cells send axons to the shoulder, upper arm, hip, and thigh.

WHITE MATTER

The white matter differs slightly in its course through the length of the spinal cord. Since the number of sensory fibers increases at higher levels as new fibers are added, and the number of motor fibers decreases at lower levels as fibers terminate in the gray matter, the quantity of white matter is greater at higher levels.

The white matter is contained within the posterior, lateral, and anterior funiculi, and their slight variation accommodates the size and shape of the gray matter as well as the additions of ascending fibers and terminations of descending fibers. The long tracts travel in the funiculi, but one cannot distinguish one tract or set of tracts from the other. The posterior funiculus contains only ascending sensory fibers, while the anterior and lateral funiculi contain ascending sensory pathways and descending motor or motor facilitory pathways.

Ascending Sensory Pathways (FIG. 3-4)

Pain and Temperature Pathways

LATERAL SPINOTHALAMIC TRACT. Fibers entering from the ganglion of the dorsal root proceed to the tip of the dorsal column gray and bifurcate to ascend (and descend) for one or two segments in Lissauer's tract (dorsolateral fasciculus). Throughout their course of

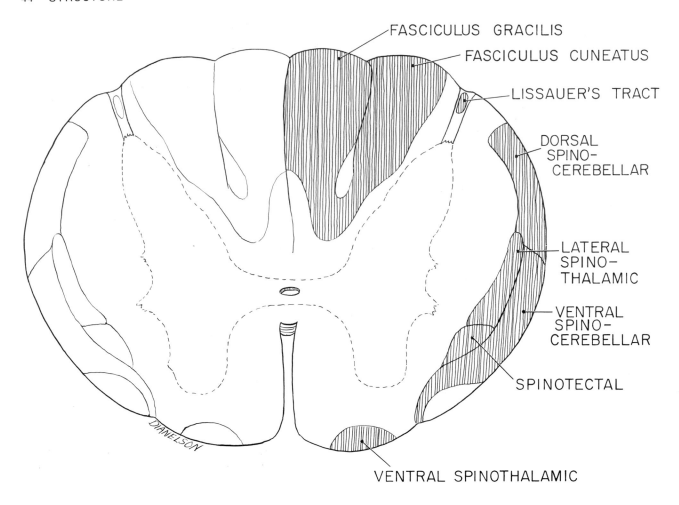

FASCICULUS GRACILIS

FASCICULUS CUNEATUS

LISSAUER'S TRACT

DORSAL SPINO-CEREBELLAR

LATERAL SPINO-THALAMIC

VENTRAL SPINO-CEREBELLAR

SPINOTECTAL

VENTRAL SPINOTHALAMIC

AFFERENT PATHWAYS (sensory)

FIG. 3-4. Important sensory afferent pathways.

ascent (and descent), these fibers terminate in the nucleus posteromarginalis, substantia gelatinosa, and nucleus proprius of the dorsal column gray. Though the individual fibers distribute to no more than three segments, when added one on top of the other, they may be considered as a tract that extends the entire length of the cord. Though the exact origin of the lateral spinothalamic tract is in question, it may arise from neurons that synapse with cells of Lissauer's tract and subsequently decussate through the anterior white commissure before ascending the spinal cord. Lamination of the lateral spinothalamic tract occurs with the cervical fibers situated most anteriorly and medially, and the thoracic, lumbar, and sacral segments more posteriorly and laterally, in that order. In addition the fibers carrying pain are located slightly anterior to those conveying temperature. At the level of the medulla oblongata (or even as low as C1 or C2) the tract is joined by fiber coming from the spinal nucleus of the trigeminal nerve. The fibers of the lateral spinothalamic tract end in the ventral posterolateral nucleus

of the thalamus, while those from the spinal nucleus of the trigeminal nerve enter the ventral posteromedial nucleus.

SPINOTECTAL TRACT. The site of origin in the posterior horn is unknown, but from lower thoracic levels and upward, fibers decussate at the anterior white commissure and ascend in the anterior and lateral columns adjacent to the lateral spinothalamic tract, eventually projecting to the superior colliculus and the lateral regions of the central gray of the midbrain. Their close association with the lateral spinothalamic tract suggests that they function in transmitting pain.

VISCERAL PAIN PATHWAYS. Axons carrying visceral pain impulses enter the spinal cord through the lateral portion of the dorsal root and terminate in the visceral gray of the dorsal column gray. Secondary visceral neurons ascend, crossed and uncrossed. It is believed that there are many synapses in this ascent and that the fibers travel within the visceral gray matter of the dorsal column gray as well as the adjacent white matter.

Touch, Pressure, and Position Sense Pathways

VENTRAL SPINOTHALAMIC TRACT. The cell bodies of the neurons concerned with light touch and pressure sensation lie in the dorsal root ganglion, and their axons enter the spinal cord in the middle of the dorsal roots to synapse with the small cells of the nucleus proprius. Most of the fibers of this nucleus cross to the opposite side in the ventral white commissure to form the contralateral ventral spinothalamic tract in the ventral aspect of the cord, though some contribute to the ipsilateral ventral spinothalamic tract. These fibers are also laminated, so that those originating from the most caudal segments of the spinal cord are situated laterally with respect to those from more rostral segments. At the level of the lower pons, these fibers join the medial lemniscus and terminate in the ventral posterolateral nucleus of the thalamus.

DORSAL WHITE COLUMN: FASCICULUS GRACILIS AND FASCICULUS CUNEATUS. The cell bodies of the neurons concerned with discriminative tactile sensation (two-point tactile discrimination) and kinesthetic sense (position and movement) are also found in the dorsal root ganglia and they send their long axons into the cord within thick medullary sheaths directly to the ipsilateral dorsal white funiculus (fasciculus gracilis for sacral, lumbar, and lower thoracic contributions and fasciculus cuneatus for upper thoracic and cervical contributions).

The fibers from the lowermost (sacral) dorsal root ganglia assume a dorsomedial position for the ascent, whereas fibers from the uppermost (cervical) dorsal root ganglia lie ventrolaterally in the posterior columns. The fibers of the fasciculi gracilis and cuneatus terminate in the nuclei gracilis and cuneatus, where they synapse with internal arcuate fibers, which decussate with the medial lemniscus and end in the ventral posterolateral nucleus of the thalamus.

Whereas the epicritic modalities of tactile discrimination and kinesthetic sense are transmitted by the fasciculi gracilis and cuneatus, which are uncrossed throughout the extent of the spinal cord, the affective modalities of temperature and pain are transmitted by the lateral spinothalamic tract, which decussates near the level of entry of the dorsal root in the cord. Both tracts send fibers to the ventral posterolateral nucleus of the thalamus. From there, fibers of the posterior limb of the internal capsule travel to the postcentral (sensory) gyrus of the cortex.

Pathways for the Sensation of Muscle Tone: the Spinocerebellar Systems

DORSAL SPINOCEREBELLAR TRACT. Cell bodies within the dorsal root ganglion send axons via the medial fibers of the dorsal root to the ipsilateral dorsal column of Clarke in the dorsal column gray. Because Clarke's column exists only in segments L3 to C8 of the spinal cord, sacral contributions ascend in the dorsal white column before entering Clarke's column. After the fibers have reached Clarke's column, they bifurcate and extend rostrally and caudally within it. Secondary neurons within this column send axons to the ipsilateral spinocerebellar tract, which occupies a peripheral location on the dorsolateral surface of the cord. Within this tract, the fibers ascend uncrossed to the medulla and to the cerebellum via the inferior cerebellar peduncle. Implicated in the maintenance of coordinated posture and movement, the dorsal spinocerebellar tract receives sensory input primarily from the muscle spindles and Golgi tendon organs of the lower extremities.

CUNEOCEREBELLAR TRACT. Serving the same purpose as the dorsal spinocerebellar tract for the upper extremities and the neck, the cuneocerebellar tract is comprised of fibers of the fasciculus cuneatus which synapse in the ipsilateral accessory cuneate nucleus with posterior external arcuate fibers, which enter the cerebellum by the inferior cerebellar peduncle.

VENTRAL SPINOCEREBELLAR TRACT. Other cell bodies within the dorsal root ganglion send axons to the ipsilateral dorsal column gray. Secondary neurons in this dorsal column send some axons to the ipsilateral ventral spinocerebellar tract, but most go to the contralateral spinocerebellar tract. The ventral spinocerebellar tracts occupy a peripheral position in the ventrolateral surface of the cord just anterior to the dentate ligament. It is believed that many of the fibers that cross over within the spinal cord cross back within the cerebellum; consequently, the projection from cord levels to the cerebellum via the superior cerebellar peduncle is essentially ipsilateral. This tract may relay information concerning the movement of groups of muscles and the posture of entire limbs.

Descending Motor and Motor Facilitory Tracts (FIG. 3-5)

Lateral Corticospinal Tract (Pyramidal Tract)

The vast majority of motor fibers descending from the precentral gyrus of the cerebral cortex make their decussation at the junction of the inferior medulla and superior portion of the cervical spinal cord. It is believed that nearly all of these fibers make up the lateral corticospinal tract which lies in the dorsolateral portion of the cord. At the pyramidal decussation the fibers destined for control of arm movement cross over at a higher level than those destined for control of leg movement, and within the lateral corticospinal tract,

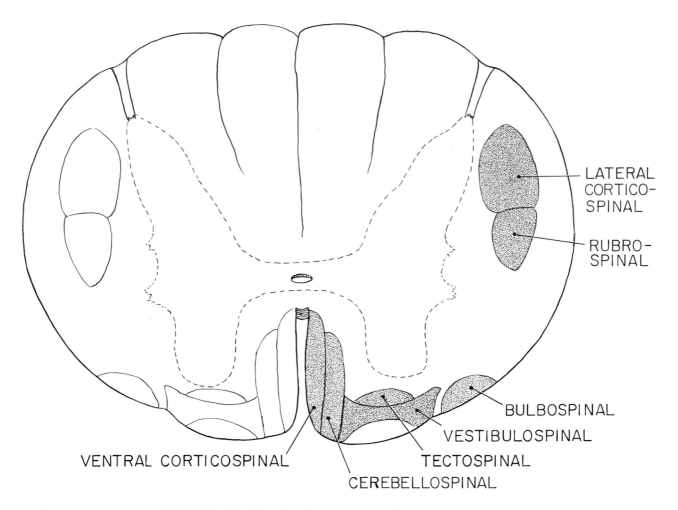

LATERAL CORTICO-SPINAL

RUBRO-SPINAL

BULBOSPINAL

VESTIBULOSPINAL

TECTOSPINAL

CEREBELLOSPINAL

VENTRAL CORTICOSPINAL

EFFERENT PATHWAYS (motor)

FIG. 3-5. Important motor efferent pathways.

fibers serving the upper extremities are deep to those serving the lower extremities. This tract is concerned primarily with initiating voluntary movements of the extremities.

As the corticospinal fibers enter the ventral column gray, over half of them terminate in the cervical cord and the remaining fibers divide approximately equally between the thoracic and lumbar areas.

Ventral Corticospinal Tract

Corticospinal fibers that do not decussate at the pyramids retain their anteromedial location as they descend to lower cervical and upper thoracic levels of the cord, forming the ventral corticospinal tract which lies adjacent to the ventral median fissure. Subsequently these fibers cross over to the contralateral ventral gray column by the anterior white commissure to provide the motor fibers responsible for controlling the neck and trunk.

Rubrospinal Tract

This poorly developed tract has fibers arising in the red nucleus which decussate immediately at the ventral tegmental decussation. Those fibers that enter the spinal cord have already assumed a position ventral to the lateral corticospinal tract and, like the latter, discharge into the ventral column gray. This tract probably does not extend over a large length of the spinal cord (not demonstrated below thoracic levels in man), but it is accompanied by bundles from the midbrain, which do have a distal descent in the same position within the cord. It is suspected that the rubrospinal tract controls the muscle tone of flexor muscle groups.

Tectospinal Systems

MEDIAL TECTOSPINAL TRACT. Fibers originating in the superior colliculus and decussating at the dorsal tegmental decussation descend within the cervical portion of the spinal cord as the medial tectospinal tract, which lies in the white matter just deep to the ventral column gray. This tract's function is concerned with turning the head and moving the upper extremity in response to visual and perhaps auditory stimuli which reach the superior colliculus.

LATERAL TECTOTEGMENTOSPINAL TRACT. Also originating in the superior colliculus, the lateral tecto-tegmentospinal tract lies just lateral to the intermediate column gray. It is believed that its fibers serve movements of the head, but there are other fibers which end in relationship to preganglionic neurons with cell bodies in the first and second thoracic levels of the intermediolateral cell column. Such preganglionic fibers leave the cord with the ventral roots and turn into the chain ganglia through the white rami to ascend to the superior cervical ganglion.

Cerebellospinal Tract

This tract, which is limited to the cervical spinal cord, lies close to the anterior median fissure in a bundle named the sulcomarginal fasciculis and is concerned with change in the position of the head.

Vestibulospinal Systems

MEDIAL VESTIBULOSPINAL TRACT (MEDIAL LONGITUDINAL FASCICULUS). Arising from the vestibular area, the medial vestibulospinal tract descends just dorsal to the medial tectospinal tract in the spinal cord and is limited to cervical levels. The fibers end around motor neurons that supply neck and upper extremity muscles. This tract, known as the medial longitudinal fasciculus at higher levels, aids in maintaining equilibrium.

VENTROLATERAL VESTIBULOSPINAL TRACT. The ventrolateral vestibulospinal tract, which also originates in the vestibular area, descends in the ventral white funiculus of the spinal cord. It descends the entire length of the spinal cord and aids in maintaining equilibrium.

Reticulospinal Systems

The reticular system is complex and at present its precise anatomy is unknown. Some of the fibers have definite autonomic functions, and it has been shown that important efferent respiratory impulses travel in fibers that are located in the ventral quadrants of the cord near the spinothalamic tracts. Belmusto et al. concluded that the fibers concerned with respiration in man occupied an area from C1 to C3 between 3 and 5.5 mm. from the lateral margin of the cord.[2] Nathan located the efferent respiratory pathway 2 to 4 mm. from the surface of the cord in the region of the ventral horn and roots.[17] The reticulospinal tracts have also been implicated in the control of muscle tone, voluntary movement, cortically induced movement, and reflex activity.

LATERAL RETICULOSPINAL TRACT. Derived from primarily uncrossed fibers originating in the reticular formation of the medulla, the lateral reticulospinal tract lies in the lateral funiculus close to the intermediolateral cell column and, as one might expect, some of the components end in relation to the cells of this column. Preganglionic neurons of this column send out fibers through the upper thoracic ventral roots into the sympathetic ganglia and ascend to the upper cervical ganglion. Postganglionic fibers supply sweat glands of the face.

VENTRAL RETICULOSPINAL TRACT. The reticular formation of the pons serves as the origin for the uncrossed fibers comprising the ventral reticulospinal tract, which descends in the ventrolateral funiculus of the spinal cord. Impulses over this tract produce sweating on the extremities and trunk. The connection to lower sympathetic ganglia follows a pattern similar to that of the lateral tract to the upper thoracic ganglia.

VENTROLATERAL RETICULOSPINAL TRACT. The ventrolateral reticulospinal tract, having its origin in the respiratory centers of the brain stem, descends in the ventrolateral white column of the spinal cord.

Intersegmental Pathways

Fasciculi Proprii

There is a great deal of independent activity within the spinal cord. Intersegmental activity, as well as reflex activity, is modulated by higher centers, but also occurs independently. Cell bodies situated along the border of the gray matter give off axons, which collected in bundles pass upward and downward in the adjoining white matter bringing the various segments of gray matter into communication with each other. These spinospinal fibers found in all the funiculi adjacent to the gray matter comprise the fasciculi proprii.

ARTERIAL SYSTEM

The vascular supply of the spinal cord is quite complex (Fig. 3-6), in both its origin and its final pattern on and in the cord. The extraspinal arterial vasculature arises symmetrically and bilaterally as segmental vessels from the aorta and branches of the subclavian and internal iliac arteries. The subclavian arteries contribute to vertebral arteries and thyrocervical and costocervical trunks.

Branches from the vertebral arteries form the rostral origins of the anterior spinal artery and posterior spinal arteries, and are major suppliers of blood to the spinal cord. In addition, each vertebral artery may give off segmental arteries to the upper five cord segments, but as a rule there are very few anterior and posterior radicular vessels at the upper three cervical levels.

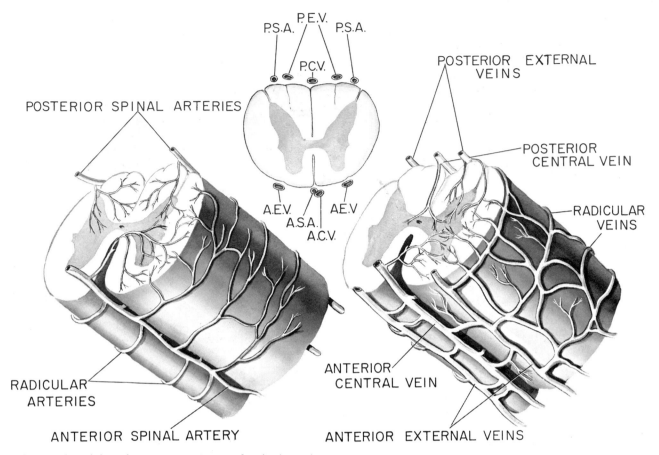

FIG. 3-6. Arterial and venous systems of spinal cord.

The segmental arteries to the inferior cervical cord originate from the ascending cervical arteries, which are branches of the thyrocervical trunks. The costocervical trunks give off several pairs of intercostal arteries which nourish the upper thoracic region. The aorta gives off intercostal and lumbar arteries, some of the terminations of which enter the cord. The internal iliac arteries supply blood via the iliolumbar and lateral sacral arteries to the lower cord.

The origins of the anterior spinal artery actually begin within the calvarium. Just caudad to the point at which the vertebral arteries merge to form the basilar artery, each vertebral artery gives off a branch that runs downward in front of the medulla oblongata. At the level of the foramen magnum, these two branches merge to form a single anterior spinal artery which extends along the anterior surface of the cord. It lies over the anterior median fissure, not within it, and is covered by pia mater. While this artery extends the length of the cord, it is not always continuous. It becomes quite narrow in the upper thoracic cord, and often deviates to either side to receive branches.

Each vertebral artery also yields a branch near the lateral margin of the medulla oblongata to become a posterior spinal artery. These arteries are distinct at their origins but, as they proceed downward, they form plexiform channels running longitudinally on the dorsal surface of the cord, being bounded laterally by the posterior roots.

Reinforcements to the anterior and posterior spinal arteries accompany the nerve roots and are known as radicular arteries. Since most of them end in a nerve root or dorsal root ganglion and only some of them go to the spinal cord, Gillilan has suggested that the latter be called segmental medullary arteries.[10] There are generally considered to be only six to eight important anterior medullary arteries and a slightly larger number of important posterior medullary arteries. The levels at which the important segmental arteries leave the aorta, as determined by segmental vessels, and give off important medullary arteries are subject to much individual variation. The most consistent and important of the anterior medullary arteries is the great anterior medullary artery of Adamkiewicz, which usually approaches the cord on the left side with an anterior root between T8 and L3. The descending branch of the artery of Adamkiewicz is larger than the ascending branch, and the entire artery is obviously important. According to Austin, it is the most caudad ventral artery in any spinal cord, and may be responsible for one-quarter to one-half of the blood supply.

In the upper and mid-cervical portions of the cord,

the flow in the anterior spinal arteries is caudad, but because of the great variations in the arterial anatomy, one cannot be certain of the direction in other areas. Some of the anterior medullary arteries divide into ascending and descending branches, and constitute a part of the anterior spinal artery. According to Suh, the lumbar radicular vessels are an important source of blood for a major part of the thoracic cord, so presumably there the flow is cephalad.[22]

The intrinsic spinal cord vasculature consists of the anterior spinal artery and the paired posterior spinal arteries and their branches. At intervals of about 2 mm., the anterior spinal artery gives off central branches (central arteries or sulcocommissural arteries), which in turn branch both peripherally and centrally. According to Herren and Alexander, each of these central arteries supplies only one side of the cord, either the right or the left.[14] Bolton states that the posterior spinal arteries nourish only the posterior portion of the posterior columns and the posterior horns, while the anterior spinal arteries supply the rest of the cord, both gray and white matter.[5] He also credits the anterior spinal artery as being the main source of blood to the posterior spinal arteries below the upper thoracic level. There are centrifugal and centripetal arteries in the substance of the spinal cord. The central arteries and their branches comprise the centrifugal group, in that their main stems penetrate into the deeper areas and branch out in a peripheral direction, whereas the centripetal arteries are formed from the peripheral arteries, which lie in the pial network on the surface of the cord. The centrifugal system, which receives blood from the central or sulcocommissural arteries, is particularly important in nourishing the gray matter, and is partially responsible for its color. The quantity of gray matter in the upper thoracic cord is scant, and so the needs for blood at this level are less. According to Herren and Alexander, the lumbar cord receives the richest supply, but the cervical region fares considerably better than does the thoracic.

The arterial system of the spinal cord does not have an extensive collateral circulation and, therefore, places much of the load on the extraspinal arterial sources. Any condition that interferes with the flow of blood over one or more of the important radicular arteries may produce serious neurologic consequences, but unfortunately it is impossible to know which roots carry the essential vessels.

VENOUS SYSTEM

Six main longitudinal channels receive venous blood from the interior of the spinal cord. A rather extensive venous plexus is formed so that there are numerous interconnections.

The greatest source of venous blood is from and around the gray matter. Much of the blood from the gray matter is emptied into the central vein, and from there enters the anterior central vein, which lies adjacent to the anterior spinal artery. There are also radial veins which arise at the periphery of the gray matter and pass through the white matter to join the coronal venous plexus in the pia mater. While some of this empties into the anterior central vein, some goes to the other five longitudinal channels. The two anterior external veins lying on the anterolateral sulci aid in collecting blood from the anterior portion of the cord and possibly additional portions of the lateral columns. Three veins lie on the posterior surface of the cord and, with their anastomoses, make up the posterior venous trunk: the posterior central vein and the two posterior external spinal veins. They drain the greater portion of the dorsal aspect of the cord, but it is believed that many veins drain directly into the posterior radicular veins.

There are approximately 40 anterior and posterior radicular veins in the human spinal cord. The portions of the nerve roots adjacent to the spinal cord have several small venous channels which are on and within the nerve root bundles. They merge to form a single vein which then enters the longitudinal venous sinuses, and drains into vertebral, intercostal, lumbar, and sacral veins. Ultimately, of course, the venous blood flows to the vena cava.

References

1. Austin, G: The Spinal Cord. Springfield, Charles C Thomas, 1972, ed 2.
2. Belmusto L, Brown E, Owens G: Clinical observations on respiratory and vasomotor disturbances as related to cervical cordotomies. J Neurosurg *20*:225-232, 1963.
3. Belmusto L, Woldring S, Owens G: Localization and patterns of potentials of the respiratory pathway in the cervical spinal cord in the dog. J Neurosurg *22*:277-283, 1965.
4. Bing R: Compendium of Regional Diagnosis in Lesions of the Brain and Spinal Cord. Translated and edited by W Haymaker. Saint Louis, CV Mosby Co., 1940.
5. Bolton B: The blood supply of the human spinal cord. J Neurol Psychiat *2*:137-141, 1939.
6. Bowden REM, Abdullah S, Goodring MR: Anatomy of the cervical spine, membranes, spinal cord, nerve roots and brachial plexus. *In* Cervical Spondylosis. Edited by WR Brain and M Wilkinson. Philadelphia, WB Saunders, 1967.
7. Crosby EC, Humphrey T, Lauer EW: Correlative Anatomy of the Nervous System. New York, Macmillan, 1962.
8. Davis L, Davis RA: Principles of Neurosurgical Surgery. Philadelphia, WB Saunders, 1963.
9. Elsberg CA: Diagnosis and Treatment of Surgical Diseases of the Spinal Cord and Its Membranes. Philadelphia, WB Saunders, 1916.
10. Gillilan LA: The arterial blood supply of the human spinal cord. J Comp Neurol *110*:75-103, 1958.
11. Grant JCB: A Method of Anatomy. Baltimore, Williams and Wilkins, 1944, ed 3.
12. Gray H: Anatomy of the Human Body. Edited by CM Goss. Philadelphia, Lea and Febiger, 1973, ed 29.

4

Neurologic Evaluation

DANIEL RUGE

EVERY patient with symptoms suggesting disease of the spine or spinal cord is deserving of a complete examination, not limited to the function of the cord and cauda equina. The state of the brain and peripheral nervous system modulates signs ordinarily ascribed to the cord and cauda equina. It is, however, our purpose to concentrate on the important findings that will aid in evaluation of the patient with neural disease within the vertebral column.

Haymaker states that when one is confronted with evidence of injury to the spinal cord, two aspects of localization should be considered: (1) the site of the lesion in the transverse plane and (2) the site of the lesion in the longitudinal plane.[8] After one has decided whether it is central or peripheral, dorsal or ventral, right or left, one should determine the segment or segments involved. Occasionally, one will be aided by symptoms, particularly those of a sensory nature.

A working knowledge of the major sensory and motor pathways outlined in Chapter 3 will aid the examiner in assessing the site of the lesion, particularly in the transverse plane. The standard sensory charts (Figs. 4-1 and 4-2) and the charts of Haymaker and Woodhall, which delineate the segmental innervation of muscles (Tables 4-1 to 4-4), are useful in localizing the level of a lesion.

Trauma and the rare vascular lesions produce signs abruptly and are more inclined toward creating complete lesions. It is always wise, when one suspects a complete transverse lesion, to test sensation of the sacral dermatomes, because "sacral sparing" indicates that the lesion is incomplete. Pinprick is the most reliable sensory modality, and one may begin stimulation at the toes and work upward, asking the patient to report when he perceives pain, thus establishing a general idea of the level of the lesion. A

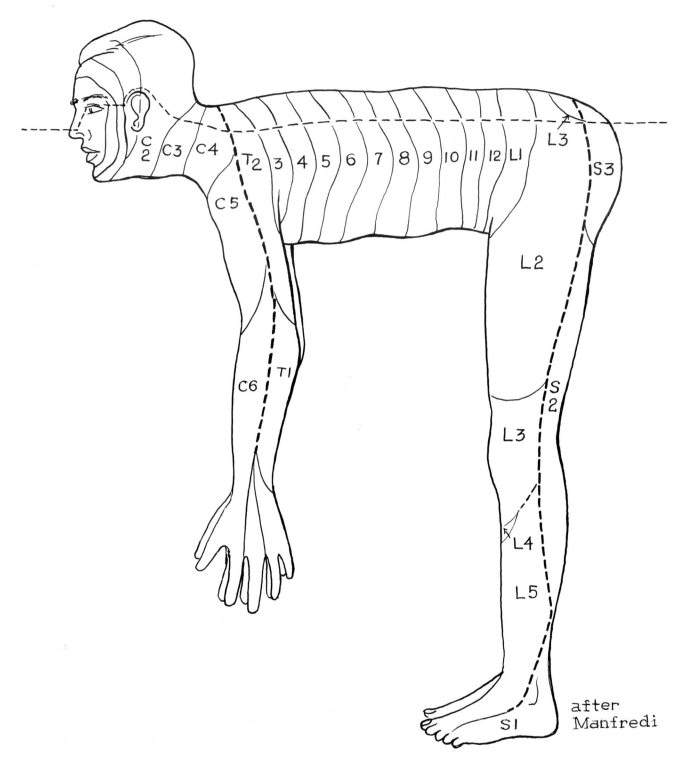

FIG. 4-1. Sensory dermatomes in lateral aspect of body. (From Haymaker W, and Woodhall B: Peripheral Nerve Injuries. Philadelphia, WB Saunders Co., 1953, ed 2.)

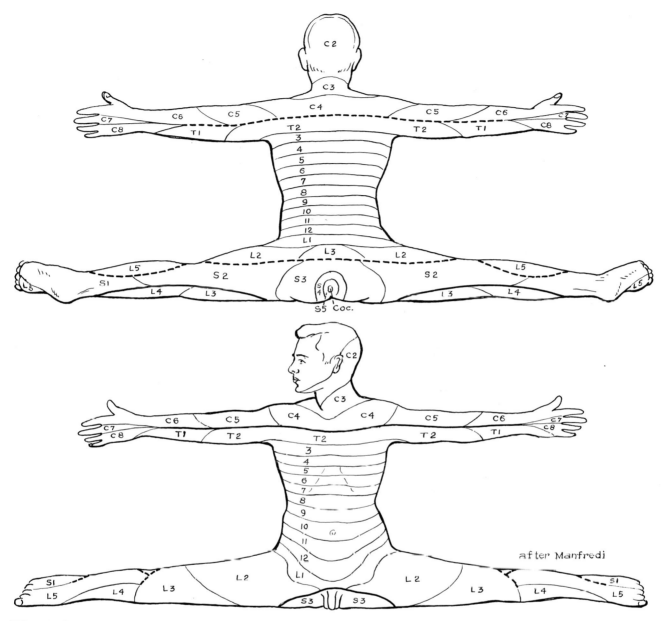

FIG. 4-2. Sensory dermatomes in posterior and anterior aspects of body. (From Haymaker W, and Woodhall, B: Peripheral Nerve Injuries. Philadelphia, WB Saunders Co., 1953, ed 2.)

simple rule is to consider the inguinal line as the L1 spinal cord level; the umbilicus as T10; the nipple line as T5; the little finger as C7, and the thumb as C5.

Light touch may be evaluated by the use of cotton, and localized vibratory function by the tuning fork, the latter being particularly valuable for determining lesions affecting the dorsal white columns.

To corroborate information obtained through the various sensory tests, specific muscles may be examined. Immediately following the onset of compression of the spinal cord, as in trauma to the spine, the muscles of the limbs may exhibit a flaccid paralysis owing to spinal shock. In patients with upper motor neuron lesions (e.g.,

lesions of the long motor tracts), the muscles innervated by segments below the level of the lesion eventually become spastic with increased muscle tone and hyperreflexia. By contrast, patients with lower motor neuron lesions (e.g., lesions of the ventral roots or the ventral gray horn cells) will continue to have flaccid paralysis and eventually atrophy of the affected muscles. Examination of the superficial and deep reflexes as well as pathologic reflexes, such as the Babinski sign, is helpful in determining the extent of lateral corticospinal tract involvement.

In a complete transverse cord lesion, the area controlled by the cord distal to the site of the injury remains

TABLE 4-1.

SPINAL SEGMENTS								
C1	C2	C3	C4	C5	C6	C7	C8	T1
Sternomastoid†								
	Trapezius†							
		Levator scapulae						
				Teres minor				
				Supra-spinatus				
				Rhomboids				
				Infraspinatus				
				Deltoid				
				Teres major				
				Biceps				
				Brachialis				
				Serratus anterior				
				Subscapilaris				
				Pectoralis major				
					Pectoralis minor			
					Coraco-brachialis			
					Latissimus dorsi			
						Anconeus		
						Triceps		

Tables 4-1 to 4-4 from Haymaker, W., and Woodhall, B.: Peripheral Nerve Injuries. Philadelphia, WB Saunders Co., 1953, ed. 2.

TABLE 4-2.

SPINAL SEGMENTS

Muscle	C5	C6	C7	C8	T1
Brachioradialis	X	X			
Supinator	X	X			
Pronator teres		X	X		
Ext. carpi radial. longus & brevis		X	X		
Flexor carpi ulnaris		X	X		
Flexor carpi radialis		X	X		
Ext. digitorum			X	X	
Ext. carpi ulnaris			X	X	
Ext. indicis			X	X	
Ext. digiti 5			X	X	
Ext. pollic. longus			X	X	
Ext. pollic. brevis			X	X	
Abductor pollicis longus			X	X	
Palmaris longus			X	X	X
Pronator quadratus			X	X	X
Flexor digitorum sublimis			X	X	X
Flexor digitorum profundus			X	X	X
Flexor pollicis longus			X	X	X
Opponens pollicis				X	X
Abduct. pollic. brevis				X	X
Flexor pollicis brevis				X	X
Palmaris brevis				X	X
Adductor pollicis				X	X
Flexor digiti 5				X	X
Abductor digiti 5				X	X
Opponens digiti 5				X	X
Interossei				X	X
Lumbricals			X	X	X

TABLE 4-3.

SPINAL SEGMENTS						
L1	L2	L3	L4	L5	S1	S2
Iliopsoas	Iliopsoas	Iliopsoas	Iliopsoas			
	Gracilis	Gracilis	Gracilis			
	Sartorius	Sartorius	Sartorius			
	Pectineus	Pectineus	Pectineus			
	Adductor longus	Adductor longus	Adductor longus			
	Adductor brevis	Adductor brevis	Adductor brevis			
		Adductor minimus	Adductor minimus			
		Quadriceps femoris	Quadriceps femoris			
		Adductor magnus	Adductor magnus	Adductor magnus	Adductor magnus	
		Obturator externus	Obturator externus	Obturator externus		
			Tensor fasciae latae	Tensor fasciae latae	Tensor fasciae latae	
			Gluteus medius	Gluteus medius	Gluteus medius	
			Gluteus minimus	Gluteus minimus	Gluteus minimus	
			Quadratus femoris	Quadratus femoris	Quadratus femoris	Quadratus femoris
			Gemelli	Gemelli	Gemelli	Gemelli
			Semitendinosus	Semitendinosus	Semitendinosus	Semitendinosus
			Semimembranosus	Semimembranosus	Semimembranosus	Semimembranosus
				Piriformis	Piriformis	Piriformis
				Obturator internus	Obturator internus	Obturator internus
				Biceps femoris	Biceps femoris	Biceps femoris
				Gluteus maximus	Gluteus maximus	Gluteus maximus

TABLE 4-4.

SPINAL SEGMENTS			
L4	**L5**	**S1**	**S2**
Tibialis anterior →	→		
Popliteus →	→	→	
Plantaris →	→	→	
	Peroneus tertius →	→	
	Extensor digitorum longus →	→	
	Abductor hallucis →	→	
	Flexor digitorum brevis →	→	
	Flexor hallucis brevis →	→	
	Extensor hallucis brevis →	→	
	Flexor digitorum longus →	→	→
	Peroneus longus →	→	→
	Peroneus brevis →	→	→
	Tibialis posterior →	→	→
	Flexor hallucis longus →	→	→
		Extensor hallucis longus →	→
		Soleus →	→
		Gastrocnemius →	→
		Extensor digitorum brevis →	→
		Flexor digitorum accessorius →	→
		Adductor hallucis →	→
		Abductor digiti quinti →	→
		Flexor digiti quinti brevis →	→
		Interossei →	→
	Lumbricals →	→	→

paralyzed insofar as volitional control is concerned. Although reflexes of the spinal cord remain absent at the level of the injury, there is usually return of increased reflex activity in the segments below the injury. In rare instances, however, when a descending vascular lesion affects the cord distal to the site of injury, flaccidity may be permanent.

The patient with a complete transection of the spinal cord at the level of C3 or above will not survive. Lesions in the area of the foramen magnum cause mixed signs and symptoms owing to paralysis of one or more of the cranial nerves on one side as well as compression of the spinal cord.

Lesions in the upper segments of the cervical cord may produce pain and paresthesias in the occipital or cervical region along with nuchal rigidity. There is weakness and wasting of the neck muscles accompanied ultimately by spastic tetraplegia, but occasionally the contralateral upper extremity may be spared. There may also be some trigeminal symptoms. It has frequently been observed that patients with partial lesions at C1, C2, or C3 have a greater weakness in the upper than in the lower extremities.

Involvement at C4-C5 is characterized by the arms lying motionless at the patient's sides, and sensory examination discloses no sensibility in the upper extremities.

If the lesion is at C5-C6, the arms are held at right angles to the long axis of the body with the elbows moderately flexed and the forearms rotated externally, placing the hands at the level of the head. Atrophy ultimately involves the deltoid, biceps, supinators, and rhomboids.

A lesion at C6-C7 spares the innervation of the biceps muscle, and the arms are in flexed position across the chest with the motionless hands partially closed, whereas a lesion at C7-T1 may permit considerable movement of the upper extremities.

Bowden et al. have prepared a chart which ascribes function at the joints of the upper extremities to the spinal nerve in a helpful manner[4]:

Shoulder
Abduction and lateral rotation	C5
Abduction and medial rotation	C6, 7, 8

Elbow
Flexion	C5
Extension	C7, 8

Forearm
Supination	C6
Pronation	C7, 8

Wrist
Flexion and extension	C6, 7

Digits
Flexion and extension by long muscles	C7, 8
Intrinsic muscles	C8, T1

In the thoracic cord, the diagnosis is aided greatly by the determination of the sensory level. The abdominal skin reflexes are absent below the level of the lesion, and the Beevor sign may be helpful in pointing to paresis of lower abdominal muscles.

Lesions in the lumbar region may be localized by the level of the sensory loss and motor weakness. Injuries involving the first and second lumbar segments cause a loss of the cremasteric reflexes, but the abdominal skin reflexes are present, and the deep tendon reflexes of the lower limb are increased.

If the lesion affects the third and fourth segments of the lumbar cord, and does not involve the roots of the cauda equina, there is weakness in the quadriceps muscles, loss of the patellar reflex, and possibly increase of the Achilles reflex. But, more commonly, lesions at this level also involve the cauda equina, and there is a flaccid paralysis of the lower extremities with loss of both knee and ankle reflexes.

The initial symptoms of lesions of the conus and cauda equina are pain in the lower back, possibly sciatica, and probably incontinence and impotence. Fasciculations are observed in the musculature of the lower extremities, and they indicate that atrophy will soon appear.

Incomplete lesions may present themselves in a variety of ways, but certain syndromes are of special interest and frequently are helpful in diagnosis.

BROWN-SEQUARD SYNDROME. True hemisection of the spinal cord and signs suggesting a true hemisection are rare. It has, however, become quite common to use the term "modified Brown-Sequard" to describe the patient who has an ipsilateral paralysis and contralateral sensory loss. Were one to examine for fine tactile discrimination, position, and vibratory sensibility, these would be lost ipsilaterally owing to involvement of the dorsal white columns. Destruction of the lateral spinothalamic tract produces contralateral loss of the important modalities of pain and temperature, and destruction of the ventral spinothalamic tract at least reduces the appreciation of general tactile sensibility contralaterally.

Destruction of the pyramidal (lateral corticospinal) and extrapyramidal systems results in an initial flaccid paralysis on the side of the lesion, which later becomes spastic.

Destruction of the reticulospinal tract and tegmentospinal systems will produce miosis, ptosis, enophthalmos, and dryness of facial skin ipsilaterally (Horner's syndrome), owing to interruption of fibers destined to leave the upper thoracic levels.

CENTRAL CORD LESIONS. Syringomyelia, intramedullary cord tumors, and the acute central cervical cord syndrome described by Schneider et al. are examples of this type of lesion.[15] If the lesion affects the inferior portion of the cervical spinal cord, examination of the patient discloses proportionately more motor impairment in the upper extremities than in the lower, because the more rostral parts of the body are supplied by tracts situated near the center of the cord. Should the lesion affect the anterior horn cells, flaccidity and atrophy are present in the upper extremities. Injury to the corticospinal tracts may cause spasticity in the lower extremities if the peripheral lamellations of the corticospinal tract are involved. Also noted with central cord lesions are hypesthesia and hypalgesia to a level consistent with the lesion, and partial loss of touch and vibration, but preservation of the sensations of motion and position.

Bell has ascribed the term "cruciate paralysis" to conditions resembling the effects of central cord lesions.[1] His patients had midline lesions on the anterior aspect at the junction of the medulla and cervical cord, where the superficially located fibers of the pyramidal tract decussate. Since fibers supplying the arms decussate at a point superior to the point of decussation of those supplying the legs, selective compression (e.g., by the nearby dens) of the arm fibers may cause a disproportionate weakness in the arms with relative sparing of the legs.

Alternatively, a laterally placed lesion involving the crossed arm and uncrossed leg fibers at the pyramidal decussation might result in ipsilateral arm and contralateral leg paralysis, and Wallenberg has named this condition "hemiplegia cruciata."[18]

ANTERIOR CORD LESIONS. Compression of the anterior aspect of the cord by dislocated bone fragments resulting from trauma, herniation of the nucleus pulposus and anteriorly situated tumors are some of the causes of the acute anterior spinal cord syndrome described by Schneider.[13] The syndrome is characterized by complete paralysis below the level of injury with corresponding hypesthesia and hypalgesia, but with preservation of touch, position, and some vibration sensation. Presumably, this dissociation of sensations is due to involvement of the ventral and lateral spinothalamic tracts with concurrent sparing of the dorsal white columns.

AMYOTROPHIC LATERAL SCLEROSIS. This progressive degenerative disease typically destroys the corticospinal tracts and the anterior horn cells at cervical levels resulting in flaccid paralysis of the arms and spastic paralysis of the legs. Later, functional disturbances of the bowels and bladder result from involvement of descending autonomic pathways.

SUBACUTE COMBINED DEGENERATION. Demyelination of the fibers of the posterior and lateral funiculi, as in Friedreich's disease, multiple sclerosis, and subacute combined degeneration, results in loss of tactile discrimination and ataxia characteristic of dorsal white column lesions and spastic paralysis characteristic of injury to the lateral corticospinal tract. The extent of involvement of the dorsal spinocerebellar tract varies, and visceral disturbances may result from interruption of the descending autonomic fibers.

References

1. Bell HS: Paralysis of both arms from injury of the upper portion of the pyramidal decussation: "cruciate paralysis." J Neurosurg 33:376–380, 1970.
2. Bing R: Compendium of Regional Diagnosis in Lesions of the Brain and Spinal Cord. Translated and edited by W Haymaker. Saint Louis, Mosby, 1940, ed 11.
3. Bors E, Comarr AE: Neurological Urology. University Park Press, Baltimore, 1971.
4. Bowden REM, Abdullah S, Gooding MR: Anatomy of the cervical spine, membranes, spinal cord, nerve roots and brachial plexus. In Cervical Spondylosis. Edited by WR Brain, M Wilkinson. Philadelphia, WB Saunders, 1967.
5. Brown-Sequard E: Experimental Researches Applied to Physiology and Pathology. New York, H Bailliere, 1853.
6. Foerster O: The dermatomes in man. Brain 56:1–39, 1933.
7. Haymaker W: Bing's Local Diagnosis in Neurological Diseases. St. Louis, CV Mosby, 1969, ed 15.
8. Haymaker W, Woodhall B: Peripheral Nerve Injuries. Philadelphia, WB Saunders, 1953, ed 2.
9. Kahn EA: Spinal cord injuries. J Bone Joint Surg 41A:6–11, 1959.
10. Merritt HH: A Textbook of Neurology. Philadelphia, Lea & Febiger, 1967, ed 4.
11. Rand RW, Crandall PH: Central spinal cord syndrome in hyperextension injuries of the cervical spine. J Bone Joint Surg 44A:1415–1422, 1962.
12. Ruge D: Spinal Cord Injuries. Springfield, Charles C Thomas, 1969.
13. Schneider RC: The syndrome of acute anterior spinal cord injury. J Neurosurg 12:95–122, 1955.
14. Schneider RC, Cherry G, Pantek H: The syndrome of acute central cervical spinal cord injury with special reference to the mechanisms involved in hyperextension injuries of the cervical cord. J Neurosurg 11:546–577, 1944.
15. Schneider RG, Thompson JM, Bevin J: The syndrome of acute central cervical spinal cord injury. J Neurol Neurosurg Psychiat 21:216–227, 1958.
16. Taylor RG, Gleave JRW: Incomplete spinal cord injuries with Brown-Sequard phenomena. J Bone Joint Surg 39B:438–450, 1957.
17. Truex RC, Carpenter MB: Human Neuroanatomy. Baltimore, Williams and Wilkins, 1969, ed 6.
18. Wallenberg A: Anatomischer befund in einemals "acute bulbaraffection (embolic der art. cerebellar post. inf. sinister?)" beschriebenen falle. Arch Psychiat 34:923–959, 1901.

5

Radiologic Examination

JOHN C. STEARS

A REVIEW of the fundamental anatomic features of the spinal skeleton will precede a discussion of its radiographic evaluation. Both are necessary to provide a complete concept of the potential and detail of radiographic analysis.

REVIEW OF ANATOMIC FEATURES

The spine, from the craniovertebral junction to the coccyx, consists of 24 mobile vertebrae, 25 intersegmental articulations from occiput to sacrum, 25 pairs of segmental spinal nerves related to the mobile vertebrae, and 2 composite vertebrae (the sacrum and coccyx) with their own segmental nerves.

The 1st to the 7th cervical roots each exit rostral to the vertebral arch of the identically numbered vertebra. C8 roots exit at the C7-T1 intervertebral foramen. The roots T1 through L5 depart caudal to each respective identically numbered vertebral arch.

The vertebral bodies progressively enlarge caudal to C3. The intervertebral spaces slowly increase in rostrocaudal height from C2 to C7 (or T1), decrease to T2, remain uniform to T10, and then progressively widen to L5. L5-S1 interspace is usually narrower, but variable. The vertebral (or neural) arch varies in its intrinsic anatomy and in its relation to the vertebral body at different levels. The pedicles C3 to C7 emerge from the body at a 45- to 50-degree posterolateral angle from the sagittal plane, resulting in a relatively lateral position of the pars interarticularis, a wide canal side-to-side, long laminae, and intervertebral foramina directed anterolaterally at 55 to

60 degrees from the sagittal plane. By comparison the thoracic and lumbar pedicles are directed only 5 to 10 degrees lateral from straight backward, the major arch elements lie behind the body, the laminae are relatively shorter though vertically elongated, and the intervertebral foramina are directed approximately laterally. The plane of the neural arch, relative to the mid-body axial plane, lies between 0 and 10 degrees caudally, depressed dorsally throughout, that is, the closest aspect of the midline ventral laminar fusion lies at, or only slightly caudal to, the mid height of the canal aspect of the body. This means that the vertebral canal, sheathed ventrally by the posterior longitudinal ligament across bone and anulus fibrosis, and sheathed dorsally by ligamentum flavum, has ligamentum flavum (not bone) directly opposite the interspace. The apophysial joints and other differential features will be described subsequently, area by area and projection by projection (Fig. 5-1).

RADIOGRAPHIC PRINCIPLES AND METHODS

In the interest of thoroughness, the radiographic examination of the spine should include:

1. Frontal, lateral, and oblique (in cervical and lumbar regions) views of the vertebrae.

2. An optimal anatomic view of each vertebra, that is, without circumaxial rotation and side-to-side (coronal plane) tilting.

3. A view of the vertebrae as a group in neutral alignment.

4. On occasion, a view of vertebral functional relationships. This requires flexion-extension bending in the sagittal plane, side-to-side tilting in the coronal plane, circumaxial rotation about the longitudinal axis, and changes with weight-bearing.

The utilization of the obligatory divergent quality of the x-ray beam (from an anode source 0.5 to 2.0 mm. in diameter to one several inches wide at a distance of 40 inches) helps to compensate for normal or abnormal spinal curvatures. Thus the beam is ideally projected into the concavities of the curvatures. In frontal views, therefore, the thoracic and sacral spine projection is anteroposterior (AP), but the cervical and lumbar projection is postero-anterior (PA). Oblique views follow the same rationalization.

Total spinal segments should be included in first projections, the "coned-down," detailed, or special projections being reserved for certain designated areas.

Stereoscopy is used to separate images spatially, especially in cervical lateral projections and lumbosacral frontal projections. Its value is considerable in the study of traumatic injuries.

Tomography, an adjunct to routine radiographic study, is usually available in only the standard projections. Rarely are the special machines available for

Pedicle

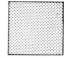
Pillar (Lateral Mass)

Laminar Arch — Spinous Process
A

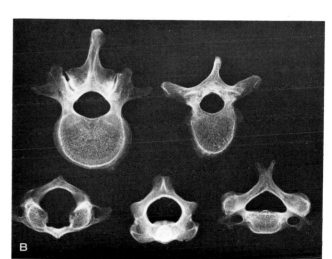

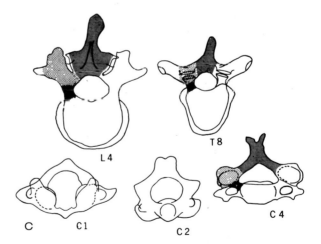

FIG. 5-1. A, Shading code used on all line drawings in this chapter; B, transaxial radiographs of dried separated vertebrae at typical levels; C, shaded line drawings of vertebrae shown in B.

transaxial plane tomography. Results of the latter are informative, although film quality is seriously lacking. The future application of Computerized Axial Tomography (CAT) to the spine is an exciting prospect.

Fluoroscopic observation of cervical spine function is preferable to standard stress films; the graded function evaluation is safer. In the study of the thoracic and lumbar area, however, nonfluoroscopic stress films may be more practical.

CERVICAL SPINE

The radiographic anatomy of the spine will now be considered in segments, and in context of the specific usual projections. Brief notes regarding patient and beam positioning are included.

LATERAL PROJECTION (Fig. 5-2). This projection permits clear evaluation of the vertebral body, the lateral mass or pillar, the apophysial joints, the vertebral canal, and the spinous process. C1 and C2 are special (rotary) function atypical vertebrae, C3 through C6 are typical, and C7 shows some transitional features. The anatomy of the typical vertebra is shown as two quadrangles or parallelograms and an adjacent elongated ovoid spinous process. These parallelograms need to be defined according to the alignment of their long

(AP) axis with the transaxial plane of each vertebra. (The latter is defined as a plane perpendicular to the mid aspect of the dorsal vertebral body surface.) Thus the ventral quadrangle represents the body, slopes ventrocaudally approximately 5 to 7 degrees, and has a concave caudal surface and a slightly convex rostral surface. The caudal vertebral plate is longer than the rostral (AP), and the antero-inferior beak is prominent. The second quadrangle is the lateral mass or pillar; it includes the pars interarticularis and the superior and inferior articular processes and facets. This angles dorsocaudally at 37 degrees at C3, increasing to about 45 degrees at C6. Thus the two quadrangles are at 42- to 52-degree angles, and the dorsal quadrangle is more rostral than the ventral. The apophysial facets below C3 lie in this same 37- to 45-degree transverse oblique-coronal plane and so are optimally identified in lateral projection. The C2-3 apophysial joints (as defined by direction of the facet of the inferior or donor articular process) are directed slightly medial to forward, and are often not clearly opened in lateral projection. From C3 to C6 the lateral mass quadrangle is circular in cross-section and resembles a cylinder with oblique flat-cut rostral and caudal ends. The name pillar seems appropriate. The pedicle is poorly defined (or undefined).

The transverse process, with its anterior and posterior tubercles and spout (costotransverse plate), is

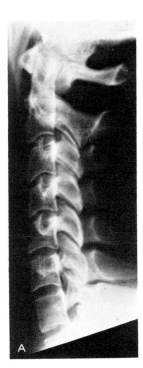 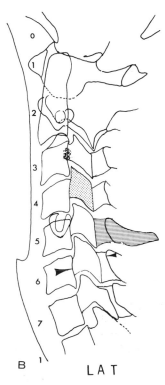 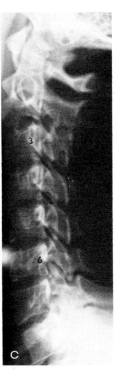

LAT

FIG. 5-2. *A*, Lateral cervical spine; *B*, shaded line drawing of *A*; *C*, lateral cervical spine with diffuse axial rotation of 5 to 10 degrees.

projected entirely anterior to the vertebral canal, over the dorsorostral two-thirds of the body. Uncommonly elongated anterior tubercles may project anterior to the ventral body surface, a feature increased with circumaxial rotation.

The uncinate process from the lateral rostral body is seen as a setting sun peering over the body plate, superimposed on the transverse processes.

The laminae are seen obliquely dorsal to the pillar over a distance of several millimeters. The only laminar tangent is the arcuate, caudodorsally directed, angled base of the spinous process; this is the ventral laminar fusion (VLF). The bony vertebral canal in sagittal dimension is, therefore, the minimum distance from the dorsal surface of the body to the VLF. This occurs at mid-body level, measures in low 20s at C1, and converges to 14 to 18 mm. at C3 and below (uncorrected for magnification, 72-inch tube-film distance). The ligamentum flavum smooths out the interlaminar aspect of the dorsal vertebral canal, and lies in the transaxial plane behind the intervertebral space.

At C7 the transverse process is less visible, although it is actually longer. The pillar of C7 is ventrodorsally elongated, and the apophysial joint consumes only the ventral two-thirds of the apparent rostral surface of the C7 pillar. An indentation may mark the dorsal end of the facet. These features may lead to the erroneous diagnosis of a C7 pillar vertebral fracture, or of subluxation of C6 ventrally on the C7 pillar.

The spinous processes are massive at C2, small at C3 and C4, and enlarge and elongate through C7 and into even longer thoracic spines.

C1, which has no apophysial joints, has two lateral masses saddle-bagging the dens. These lateral masses bear rostral biconcave occiput-C1 joints, and caudal flat C1-C2 joints. Neither pair of joints is seen to be open in lateral projection, except by tomography. The lateral mass is poorly seen ventrally, but dorsally it projects over and dorsal to the dens, more dorsal rostrally. The C1 anterior arch is an ovoid-triangle tangent on lateral view, with a flat base separated 1 to 2 mm. from the dens (odontoid), opened by stress to a maximum of 2 to 3 mm. in the adult and 5 mm. in young children. The anterior arch-dens space may be parallel, but often is wider rostrally by a factor of 2 or 3.

C2 has a central body, a dens, and a compound lateral mass of confluent body, pedicle, and semi-pillar. Superiorly it bears facets for the C1-2 joints, on the shoulders of its "lateral masses." It has true inferior articular processes and apophysial facets, though as noted, the C2-3 apophysial joint may be unclear on lateral view. The dorsal surfaces of C2 body and dens are continuous in a linear or rostrodorsally angled course. The ventral surface is less smooth and partially obscured by C1 lateral mass.

The transverse or vertebral artery foramina are stacked vertically from C7 to C3—in the spout of the transverse process and anterior to the contained cervical nerve—and they conduct the vertebral artery from C6 rostrally. At C2 the foramen curves dorsolaterally, and at C1 it is placed more laterally than the others, directing the vertebral artery dorsally onto the C1 lamina. The C2 foramen is poorly seen on lateral projection; the others are not seen. The vertebral artery curves medially dorsorostral to the lateral mass-laminar junction of C1, may groove the C1 lamina, and may be rostrodorsally enclosed (partially or totally) in a bony ring. Just medial to this the vertebral artery pierces the dura.

The occiput-C1 anatomy will be discussed superficially. A line dropped from the ventral lip of the foramen magnum (basion) in the spinal axis will encounter the mid tip of the dens; a line projected caudally down the slope of the clivus will provide a tangent to the dorsorostral dens.[1]

The separation from naso-oropharyngeal mucosa to ventral body surfaces, from anterior C1 to about C5, is 1 to 7 mm., or less than 25% of the ventrodorsal body dimension. The retrotracheal space (as the esophagus may be invisible) below caudal C5 is less than the body ventrodorsal dimension, decreases caudally, and measures 5 to 22 mm.

The alignment of the spine is evaluated by the dorsal body surfaces, by the dorsal pillar surfaces (to C6), or by the VLFs. Stress studies compare the same entities and note relative linear (rostrocaudal and ventrodorsal) and angulation movements. The VLF of C1 is a disturbing exception to continuous alignment; it may lie up to 5 mm. ventral to the VLF-opisthion curve.

FRONTAL PROJECTION (Figs. 5-3 and 5-4). In the cervical area the pedicles are directed from the vertebral body 45 to 50 degrees dorsolaterally. Therefore, the pillars are located entirely lateral to the body; in fact, the medial pillar margin and the lateral body margin overlap, so that neither is seen clearly or in its entirety. The projection is made postero-anterior (PA) with a 10- to 15-degree caudad angulation of the beam. This opens the mid-cervical intervertebral spaces, shows the rostral and caudal vertebral plates of the bodies, the dorsolateral uncinate processes, and the caudolateral notches (which receive the uncinate process, to form the uncovertebral or Luschka joints, from C2-3 to C7-T1). Increased caudal angulation is necessary to show more caudal intervertebral spaces, as a special projection for each patient. For the C1-2 area, an open-mouth projection is optimal, with the most caudal occipital bone (inferior retro-foraminal quadrant) and the tips of the incisor teeth (or gums if edentulous) superimposed.

The lateral pillar margins widen slightly in a caudal direction. The apophysial joints are seen in a frontal oblique projection, and can be identified poorly as transverse ovals (between the superior border of superior articular facet, and inferior border of inferior facet), and as small lateral bulges in the aligned pillar column. The C1 transverse process is lateral and wide. C2 to C6 transverse processes project only minimally

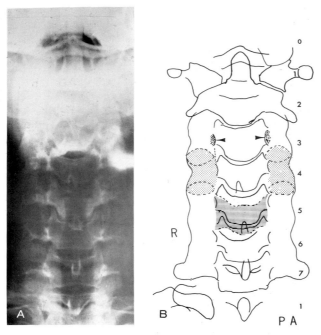

FIG. 5-3. *A*, PA view of cervical spine; *B*, shaded line drawing of *A*.

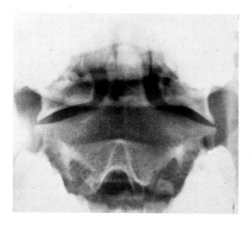

FIG. 5-4. Frontal view of C1 and C2.

lateral to the pillars (as the lateral tubercles). The medial aspects of the transverse process project over the pillars and are poorly seen. The C7 transverse process suddenly projects 5 mm. more laterally than C6, is slightly downturned, and nearly meets the slightly longer up-turned larger and more bulbous T1 transverse process. The pedicle is disappointingly difficult to see reliably on most frontal projections. The tangent seen is to its most dorsal-medial aspect, at the pillar. The laminar arch is even more discouraging; only the spinous processes are seen with any reliability, are bifid as an inverted-U from C2 to C6, project caudally over the next-lower body or interspace, and are frequently

asymmetric. The C3, C4, and C5 spinous processes may be difficult to define. The spinous processes referable to all other structures are the guide to circumaxial rotation, and this, therefore, may be difficult. Mandibular superimposition is best blurred in a cooperative patient, by filming during continuous wagging-jaw motion. The rostral and caudal laminar surfaces are seen but detail requires tomography.

The special C1-2 (dens) frontal projection clearly shows the near-triangular lateral masses of C1 with vertically tall concave lateral margins, and shorter convex doubled medial margins. The corresponding occipital condyle inclined joint surfaces are seen, not complete medially, and the C1-C2 lateral mass joints. The latter ends laterally with apposed beaks of C1 and C2, and ends medially at 1- to 3-mm. crevasses on C2. The dens has parallel or rostrally narrowing lateral cortices adjacent to C1, with the separation to C1 being symmetric or within 1 mm. of symmetric width. Asymmetry of this lateral dens-C1 space suggests pathologic subluxation, and must be evaluated by a true frontal film, in terms of deforming rotary scoliosis, and often by fluoroscopy. The dens above C1 (above the transverse ligament) has a bulbous or blunt-tapered tip.

OBLIQUE PROJECTION (Fig. 5-5). This projection serves to demonstrate vertebral arch anatomy on each side, and serves little use in body anatomy. The beam is projected PA, with a 10- to 15-degree caudal angulation, and as with all other cervical films, we use a 72-inch tube-film distance, and film with the patient erect. The body is rotated 60 degrees from the frontal projection, that is, the beam is 30 degrees off a lateral view. The projection is termed anterior-oblique; "right" or "left" defines the more anterior shoulder. Figure 5-5 illustrates an RAO view, and hence the right or ipsilateral intervertebral foramina are seen in axis. Less than 60-degree rotation results in inadequate demonstration of the intervertebral foramina, especially caudally, the side-to-side dimensions being reduced. Excess rotation toward a lateral projection has a similar disadvantage, with the pillars seen in a more lateral projection. An intentional 70- to 80-degree rotation will show pillar disease better than the 60-degree film.

The vertebral bodies and intervertebral spaces are seen obliquely and unsatisfactorily. The intervertebral foramina are seen in their axes. These foramina may be fairly uniform, though C3-4 is often small, C2-3 large, and C5-6 intermediate. The bony canal margins are pedicle rostrally and caudally (hence the vertical interpedicular distance is the intervertebral foramen), the body ventromedially, and the pillar and apophysial joint dorsolaterally.

The other important structures are the two pedicles and the ipsilateral lamina. Consider the RAO projection (right anterior oblique). The right (ipsilateral) pedicle is seen side-on, as two cortices and a lucent center directed dorsolaterally and slightly rostrally, from near

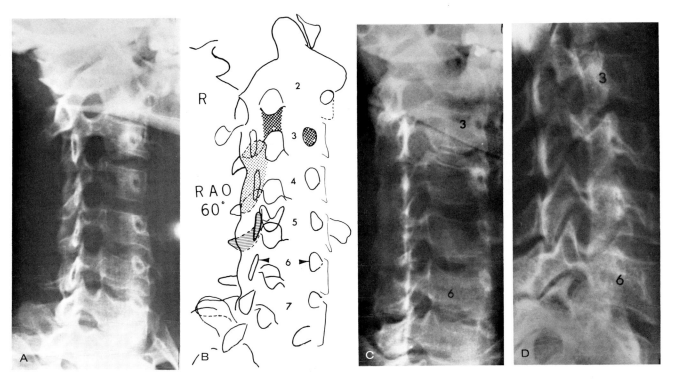

FIG. 5-5. *A*, Sixty-degree RAO view of cervical spine; *B*, shaded line drawing of *A*; *C*, 30-degree RAO view of cervical spine; *D*, 70-degree RAO view of cervical spine.

the rostral corner of the body to the mid ventromedial pillar. The left (contralateral) pedicle is seen end-on as a complete oval, projected over the body. The right lamina is projected end-on over the pillar as an elongated oval, with shingle-like relative inclination (not overlapping) to its fellows. The C2 lamina is large; the intermediate laminae are flattened, vertically oriented ovals. The left (contralateral) lamina is seen through the right intervertebral foramen, incompletely, especially its caudal margin. These structures must all be studied on the radiograph. The end-on laminae and pedicles are used as another method to assess vertebral alignment.

Each view has its own processes extending beyond the main mass of bone. In the RAO, the spinous process tips project to the right, and the left transverse processes project to the left. In C2 lateral mass, the transverse (arterial) foramen is seen.

The right transverse process projects over, and slightly caudal to, the right pedicle, and some appreciation of the tubercles and spout is possible.

The lateral masses of C1 and C2 are well identified, as are the occiput-C1 and C1-2 rotary joints, and the ipsilateral vertebral artery groove on C1.

SPECIAL PROJECTIONS. The C7-T1-T2 area is difficult or often impossible to evaluate well, especially in lateral projection. This is caused by radiodense shoulder structures and accentuated by a short stout neck, or by an athlete's physique. A slightly oblique view, termed a "swimmer's view," can be obtained, though with frequent difficulty. This obliquity can be obtained by circumaxially rotating the trunk about 15 degrees, keeping the cervical spine in true lateral projection, by retracting ventrally the more ventral shoulder, and by retracting dorsally the more dorsal shoulder. The latter upper extremity is best also raised overhead. The horizontal x-ray beam must be maximally confined or coned. This projection can be done with the patient erect or prone, less well with him supine, and is often used during myelography. It is essential to mark which shoulder is the more ventral, that is, to record the nature of the (small) spinal obliquity. This goal can be achieved in another way. That is, a "lateral" projection is made (no circumaxial rotation), with the beam angled from one axilla (arm raised overhead) obliquely toward the opposite supraclavicular fossa (shoulder retracted caudally), that is, in a small (15-degree) caudorostral angulation. Finally, true lateral, or slightly circumaxially rotated "lateral" (15-degree) tomograms can be made, and probably best define anatomy. The first two methods frequently are limited to assessment of vertebral alignment and integrity. Nevertheless I can readily recall several cases of dislocated C6-7 or C7-T1 spine, either missed completely or discovered only with diligent effort.

Pillar projections are preferred by some to view the pillar frontally, across or opening the apophysial joints. This requires a 37- to 45-degree frontal oblique projection, from ventrorostral to dorsocaudal (AP), or vice-versa (PA). These pillars are seen bilaterally down to mid cervical spine on a Towne skull projection, especially with waggling mandible. The more caudal pillar views may otherwise be made on the right, with mandibular symphysis slightly rotated to the left, and a left pillar view then added.

In closing this section, it must be emphasized that cervical spine roentgenography requires careful attention to fine skeletal (and soft tissue) detail. Stereoscopy and tomography are often employed to resolve problems. Fluoroscopy also may be used to evaluate the nature of the mobility, especially in acute trauma (with great caution) when instability is not otherwise evaluable or predictable, in trauma before or upon release from immobilization, and in spondylosis.

THORACIC SPINE

LATERAL PROJECTION (Fig. 5-6). The vertebral bodies are true rectangles, elongated ventrodorsally and aligned in a kyphotic curve.

The pedicles, which are tall and project backward from the total body base, terminate in the pars interarticularis as structures with a height one-half to two-thirds that of the body. The lateral mass, surprisingly, in all areas of the spine, is 50% (1.5×) higher than the rostrocaudal dimension of the body. In the cervical area this excess is distributed rostrally only; in the thoracic area the overlap is equal rostrally and caudally, the change occurring with C7. From T10 through the lumbar area the excess becomes more caudal. The lateral mass in the thoracolumbar area no longer resembles a pillar (as it does in the cervical area to C6), apparently because (1) in the thoracic and lumbar areas, the ventro-

dorsal dimension of the lateral mass is much smaller in relation to the rostrocaudal dimension than it is in the cervical area (cervical, 0.67; thoracic, 0.20; lumbar, 0.36 on one spine); (2) the thoracolumbar lamina blends smoothly into the dorsomedial lateral mass, whereas there is a definite dorsal differentiation in the cervical area; and (3) the transverse process (in the thoracolumbar area) is much larger, is based totally on the lateral mass, and at its base lies adjacent to the dorsal half of the vertebral canal and dorsal to it. Nevertheless, the facets are aligned in the long axis. In the thoracic area the inferior facets point almost ventrally and slightly (10 degrees) medially. The apophysial joint facet is angled 70 to 75 degrees from the transaxial plane (vs. 37 to 45 degrees in the cervical), that is, it is more nearly vertical. The intervertebral foramen is an oblique oval (from rostrodorsal to caudoventral). The ribs tend to obscure its caudodorsal aspect (for example, the 8th rib over the T8-9 foramen). This obscuration is accentuated when the patient is tilted; diminished if the radiograph is taken during respiration. However, lateral tomograms demonstrate the foramina more adequately. The apophysial joints are seen not in true open or side-on view—a slight oblique or a lateral tomogram is advised. The transverse process is invisible for practical purposes (obscured by rib). The VLF is usually reliably visible at several levels, in the line projected between the apophysial facets, from the middle of this line caudally. The transaxial plane (the closest approximation of VLF to body) is at the most rostral level of the caudal pedicle surface. These two guides will help to localize the VLF. The sagittal dimension of the thoracic spine increases only 1 to 3 mm. from top to bottom and, in the adult, is in the range of 15 to 22 mm. approximately, uncorrected for magnification (40-inch tube-film distance). The spinous processes are elongated thin blades with the greatest caudal angulation to be seen in the total spine; this is maximal at T5-T9 inclusive, and decreases above and below this area. Thus the spinous processes extend minimally to the rostral aspect of the next-caudal body, and maximally to the caudal aspect of the next-caudal body.

FRONTAL PROJECTION (Fig. 5-7). The projection is made anteroposterior (AP), usually with a vertical x-ray beam and the patient supine, thus opening several intervertebral spaces. Interest in focal areas, especially the more rostral or more caudal thoracic spine, will require tailored angled frontal projection. This requirement holds for the entire spine.

The body is wider caudally than rostrally by about 2 to 3 mm. The lateral body cortices vary from clear to unclear, the more visible being the more caudal; these cortices are concave into the body at its waist. *Caution:* The mediastinal soft tissues obscure (decrease the density and decrease the contrast) the left lateral thoracic spine more than the right—tending to cause osteolytic appearance of lateral cortex (or pedicle) more on the left.

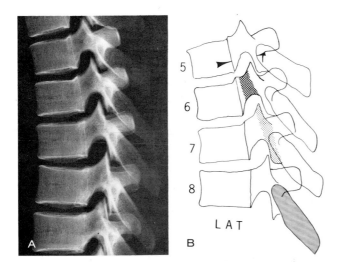

FIG. 5-6. *A,* Lateral view of thoracic spine; *B,* shaded line drawing of *A.*

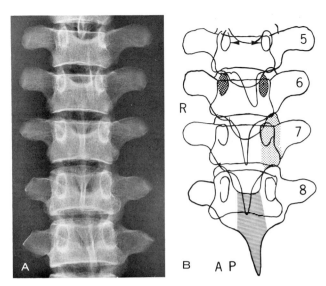

FIG. 5-7. *A*, AP view of thoracic spine; *B*, shaded line drawing of *A*.

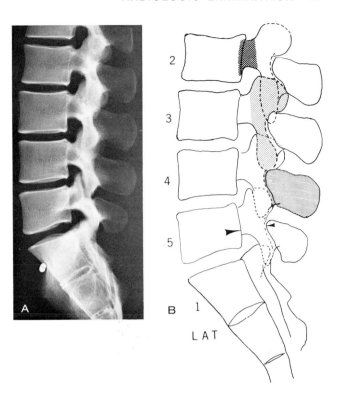

FIG. 5-8. *A*, Lateral view of lumbar spine; *B*, shaded line drawing of *A*.

The prominent body feature of the frontal projection is the vertically ovoid end-on pedicle. This is seen tangentially at its ventral aspect rostrally, and at its mid to dorsal aspect caudally. Thus this pedicle tangent is not truly parallel to the dorsal body surface, but is oblique, and about parallel to the apophysial facet plane. The pedicle tangent is seen behind the rostral one-half to two-thirds of the lateral one-fourth of the body, on each side. The horizontal interpedicular distance is the coronal width of the bony vertebral canal. The vertical interpedicular distance is the intervertebral foramen. The rostral and caudal laminar surfaces are visible inconstantly. The long blade-like spinous processes are seen at their bases, less clearly toward their tips. The ribs approach the body from rostro-laterally, obscuring the transverse process, and showing poorly a tangent to the costovertebral (body) and costo-transverse joint.

LUMBAR SPINE

LATERAL PROJECTION (Fig. 5-8). The projection is made preferably with the patient erect, or with the patient prone or supine and a horizontal beam, or with the patient on his side and a vertical beam. Centering is 1½ inches above the highest level of the iliac crest. The remarks about body, pedicle, intervertebral foramen, and lateral mass that appear in the discussion of the thoracic spine also pertain here. The VLF is even more difficult to see reliably, and often tomography in the midline is necessary. The same two localizing lines help to localize the VLF, though in the lumbar area it is 3 to 5 mm. dorsal to the axial interfacet line. The sagittal bony vertebral canal dimension (40-inch film, un-

corrected for magnification) is approximately 18 to 25 mm. (or greater), increasing from above downward, with L5 being either greater or narrower than L4. The entire spinous process is more lucent than the lateral mass, and the ventral contour of this is the VLF; this is not always helpful, however. The transverse process is projected over the pars interarticularis and is invisible. Unlike the thoracic area, a tangent to the dorsal surface of inferior articular process/lateral lamina may be visible, and this overlaps, resembles, and may confuse the VLF. The intervertebral foramen is seen well, though the two sides overlap.

FRONTAL PROJECTION (Fig. 5-9). The projection is made postero-anterior (PA), the patient erect or prone, with no tube angulation. An additional PA projection may be indicated to open and demonstrate the L5-S1 intervertebral space, and the relation of the L5 transverse process to the sacral ala. This latter is angled 20 to 35 degrees caudad. The vertebral bodies and pedicles resemble the thoracic model. The L5 pedicles are quite oblique and are more separated caudally than rostrally. The transverse processes are directed laterally from the lateral mass at pedicle level; usually L3 is the longest. The laminar arches are seen better in the lumbar area than elsewhere. The laminae blend into the pars inter-articularis and the inferior articular process in a widening pattern, to create a bi-winged shape. The L5 laminar arch is narrower and more transverse with less

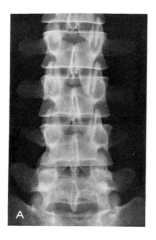 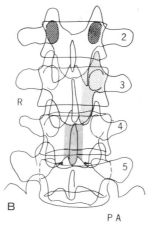

FIG. 5-9. A, PA view of lumbar spine; B, shaded line drawing of A.

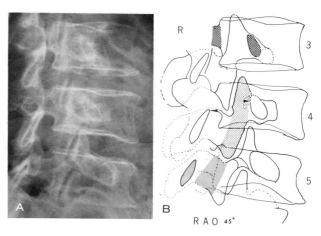

FIG. 5-10. A, RAO view (45-degree) of lumbar spine; B, shaded line drawing of A.

lateral flaring. The rostral aspect of the laminar arch is shallowly concave; the caudal aspect has deeper and narrower bilateral concavities beside the caudally directed spinous process. The lumbar apophysial joints are unique and quite different from above, the transition occurring sharply at T12. That is, the T11-12 apophysial joint is thoracic in type, the T12-L1 lumbar. The inferior (caudal) apophysial facet is convex from side to side and is directed 70 to 75 degrees (on the average) ventrolaterally. However, because of the convex inferior facet and concave superior facet surfaces, the lateral aspect of the joint is actually in the sagittal plane and the medial aspect in a vertical coronal plane. At L4 and L5 the inferior facet is less laterally inclined—45 to 50 degrees. These complex apophysial joints are slightly vertically elongated ovals at L1-L3 and circular or slightly horizontally elongated at L4 and L5. The surfaces are vertical, that is, there is no caudal or rostral angulation. The result of all this is that the apophysial joints are best seen in the oblique lumbar projection, but the lateral aspect may be seen in frontal view and the medial aspect in lateral view. Frequently, the apophysial joint character is quite different, right vs. left, at any one vertebra.

OBLIQUE PROJECTION (Fig. 5-10). This projection is made PA, with the patient's trunk rotated 45 degrees and no tube angulation. The RAO will be discussed (and compared to cervical RAO).

Direct observation of the intervertebral foramen occurs in the lateral projection, not in the oblique. As in the cervical area, the oblique projection is designed to demonstrate the vertebral arch—especially the right end-on lamina, the left end-on pedicle, and the left side-on lateral mass and lamina. The first and second resemble the cervical, the third is better in the lumbar area. In the lumbar area the right side-on pedicle is seen only ventrally, less completely than in the cervical area. The famous Scotty-dog outline refers to the left hemiarch, in the RAO. The eye is the left pedicle, the snout is the transverse process, the ear is the superior

articular process, the forepaw is the inferior articular process, the neck is the pars interarticularis, and the body is the laminar arch. The hindpaw could be the exception—the end-on right lamina. However, I rather consider the right laminae separately, and they align as in the cervical area. The right apophysial joint is not seen usefully. The spinous process projects to the right, as the dog's tail. The pars interarticularis appears narrower at L5, and a pseudo-collar may appear across the neck; actually the prominent dorsolateral projection of the inferior articular process superimposed on the pars interarticularis and the pedicle create this. Spondylolysis also appears as a dog collar, but distraction of elements at the collar allows focal approximation of adjacent inferior and superior facets (with spondylolisthesis, that is).

THE SACRUM (Figs. 5-11 and 5-12)

The sacrum is analyzed for fractures, osteolytic lesions, or vertebral canal lesions. The useful criteria on frontal projection are the alar and lateral body cortices, the fibrous dorsal and the synovial ventral sacroiliac joints, and the four pairs of ventral nerve foramina upon the pelvic face. The latter are seen as medially opened Us on frontal projection. The frontal projection is made AP, with 0 to 10 degrees caudal angulation, to avoid symphysis pubis superimposition, preferably in longitudinal stereoscopic filming. This is not a face-on projection, unfortunately, especially to the more rostral aspect.

In the lateral projection, the lumbosacral junction, the pelvic concave face, and the dorsal aspect of the vertebral canal should be seen well. The ventral aspect of the vertebral canal is usually not visible. Therefore, midline lateral tomography is justified when sacral area symptoms are being evaluated. Frontal projection is obviously the viewing of a curved surface; frontal

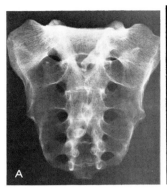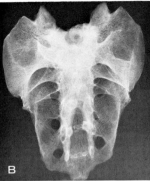

FIG. 5-11. *A*, AP view of sacrum, anatomic view; *B*, AP view of sacrum, radiologic view.

tomography, therefore, is the creating of a plane through a nonplanar object and is hence difficult and of limited value.

TOMOGRAPHY

The basic radiographic aims and principles outlined earlier apply also to tomography. Technical factors may complicate their realization more in tomography, however. The statements that follow deal with the problems and aims of tomography.

Lateral tomography can be arranged to satisfy one aim, that is, a plane is being extracted from a planar object. This fails in a scoliotic curve, or if the patient is tilted.

Frontal tomography is more complex because only short segments (if any) of the spine are planar here. Another complication is the technical difficulty or impossibility of aligning the x-ray beam in the pertinent transaxial plane (and further, the transaxial plane changes from vertebra to vertebra).

Tomography requires long exposures, and so patients must be cooperative or sedated.

Good tomography requires selection of the smallest port possible (coned field).

Lateral spine tomography should proceed stepwise from one lateral border to the other. Do not approach the midline from each side separately. The planes are then numbered carefully in terms of side and distance (in mm.) from the median sagittal plane; hopefully, symmetric cuts right and left result for comparison.

The procedure usually requires initial test films (for centering, etc.) and then the series. The patient ideally remains immobile from the time of the test film until the series has been evaluated, and then until needed additional cuts are made. This requires 14 to 18 minutes per projection. The patient needs to be informed of this, and made as comfortable as possible at the outset.

VERTEBRAL CANAL
(Figs. 5-13, 5-14, and 5-15)

The coronal aspect of the vertebral canal is satisfactorily and conveniently studied with the "age and height" charts of Haworth and Keillor.[2] These give an overall pattern, tend to underestimate some T11-T12-L1 distances, and are used rather loosely for small absolute variations. Standard deviations, unfor-

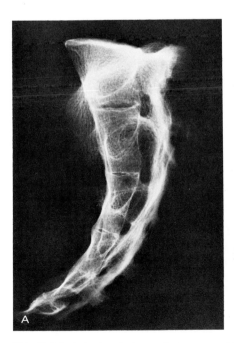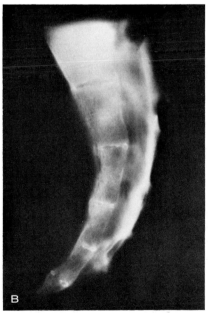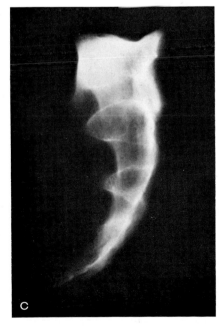

FIG. 5-12. *A*, Lateral view of sacrum, dried specimen; *B*, midline hypocycloidal tomogram of sacrum; *C*, lateralized hypocycloidal tomogram, through the sacral foramina.

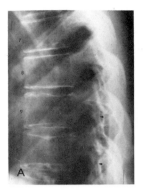
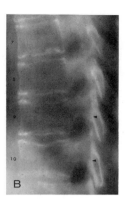

FIG. 5-13. *A*, Lateral view mid thoracic spine; *B*, midline hypocycloidal tomogram of *A*, to verify the nature of the sagittal vertebral canal.

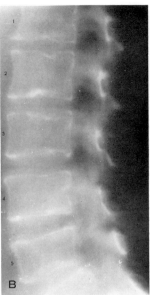
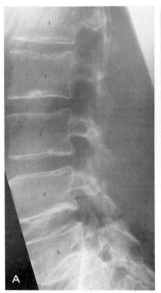

FIG. 5-15. *A*, Lateral view of lumbar spine in an adult, with difficult to impossible demonstration of VLFs; *B*, midline lateral hypocycloidal tomogram of *A*, to demonstrate two types of VLFs—the smooth sloping edge, and the notched double surface edge.

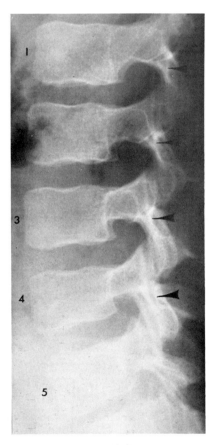

FIG. 5-14. Lateral view of lumbar spine in a child with arrows indicating the more clearly identified VLFs.

tunately, are not given. The cervical canal is wide, nearly uniform but maximal at C5 or C6. Rapid narrowing occurs C6 to T4 (60% of maximum cervical). The distance is constant to T8; then caudally gradual widening occurs to S1 (to equal or slightly greater than maximal cervical width). The largest single-segment enlargement occurs from L5 to S1. Tapering below S1 is more rapid.

The sagittal vertebral canal has been described in terms of landmarks already, and some casual measurements given in each section. I believe that good quantitation is still lacking here. Also, transaxial tomography, though still in a primitive technical state, indicates that significant canal stenosis is caused more by congenitally deformed canals than by small absolute measurements alone. At present this method is available in only a few areas, is in need of great technical improvement even there, and seems to be giving information that has not been correlated to conventional methods. Computerized Axial Tomography (CAT), now giving revolutionary information in the brain and elsewhere, undoubtedly will be applied to the spinal skeleton.

CASE REPORTS

Three cervical spine abnormalities will be described to illustrate the anatomic analytic concepts.

CASE REPORT 1. A 16-year-old girl complained of pain in the left rostral area of the neck after another girl landed on her neck during trampoline jumping. Five days later she noted a transient numbness and weakness in her left lower extremity. This recurred the following afternoon, and persisted as a severe left hemiparesis, left-facial sensory deficit, and pain in the left rostral area of her neck, precipitated by dancing. Radiographs taken within two hours in the emergency

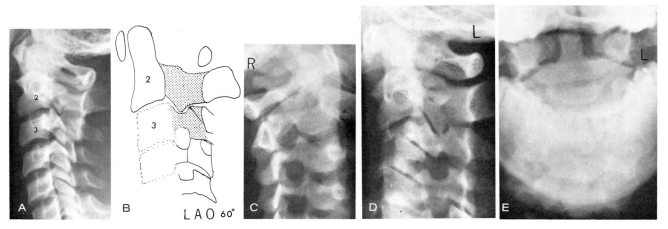

FIG. 5-16. Case report 1. *A*, Lateral view of cervical spine; *B*, shaded line drawing of *A*; *C*, RAO (60-degree) view of rostral cervical spine; *D*, LAO (60-degree) view of rostral cervical spine; *E*, PA view of rostral cervical spine.

room show a severe rotary focal C2-3 levoscoliosis (spinous processes to left maximal C2), a left C2 on C3 ventral apophysial dislocation, aligned bodies, and a suspected comminuted undisplaced left C2 lateral mass fracture (Fig. 5-16). She was placed in a felt collar, and hypocycloidal tomograms were performed two hours later. These were entirely normal, in frontal and lateral good quality projections. Repeated standard cervical spine films were normal (Fig. 5-17). The operating room reservation (for skull tong placement) was cancelled, the neck was immobilized in a plaster collar, and within

24 hours the hemiparesis cleared totally. The spontaneous apophysial reduction was attributed to a series of deep coughs. Note that this dislocation, apparently without earlier trauma, was probably without associated fracture. A most interesting feature of this patient is the spontaneous restoration of her radiographs to normal. I have seen many unstable cervical skeletal or fibrous injuries which had normal initial radiographs, but in whom chance or planned stress-motion films demonstrate instability. Thus, I believe strongly that fluoroscopic examination is necessary in

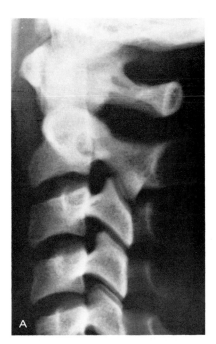

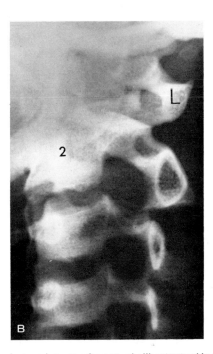

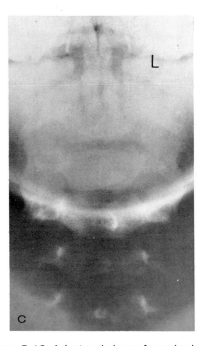

FIG. 5-17. Case report 1. Examination made two hours after study illustrated in Figure 5-16. *A*, Lateral view of cervical spine; *B*, LAO (60-degree) view of rostral cervical spine; *C*, PA view of rostral cervical spine.

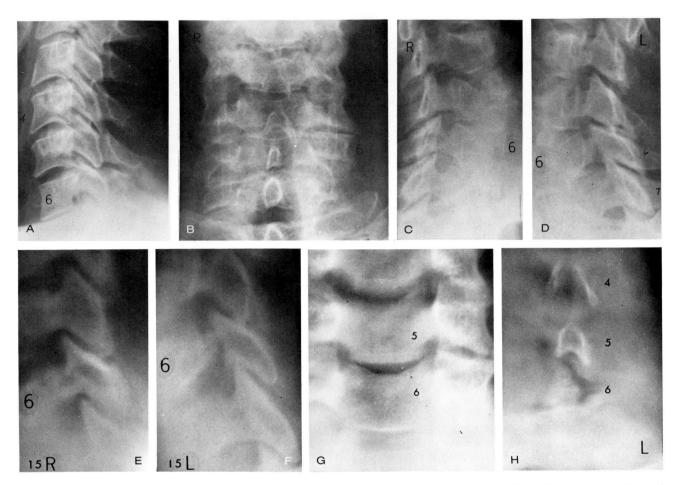

FIG. 5-18. Case report 2. *A*, Lateral view of cervical spine; *B*, frontal view of cervical spine; *C*, RAO (60-degree) view of cervical spine; *D*, LAO (60-degree) view of cervical spine; *E*, lateral hypocycloidal tomogram 15 mm. to right of midline, cervical spine; *F*, lateral hypocycloidal tomogram 15 mm. to left of midline, cervical spine; *G*, AP hypocycloidal tomogram through dorsal aspect of body and pillar; *H*, AP hypocycloidal tomogram through laminar arch.

the acute phase, before the patient is discharged (when the films are normal, but a definite injury, especially with neurologic deficit or focal sign, is present), and/or before immobilization is discontinued. In summary, this patient had a transient unilateral apophysial dislocation injury, an injury that is common at the mid to lower cervical area, but uncommon at C2-3.

CASE REPORT 2. A nondisclosed fracture of the left C6 hemi-arch was suffered by a 43-year-old professional football player in a forced-flexion playing injury (Fig. 5-18). Long-term radicular pain resulted, without signs, in the left C7 root. The initial cervical spine films were read by an astute, small-town radiologist who noted three abnormalities: a horizontal minimally displaced fracture through the C6 VLF; the left lamina in the LAO projection was displaced dorsolaterally and rotated slightly counter-clockwise; and in the frontal view, the left C5-6 apophysial joint was seen "opened" (in-line, rather than the usual oblique oval facet; always

normal and indicative of fracture deformity). Hypocycloidal tomograms were confirmatory of a vertical fracture through the dorsolateral aspect of the left C6 pedicle, a slightly comminuted fracture through lamina C6 slightly to the left of midline, and a counter-clockwise rotation of the hemi-arch fragment (when viewed in LAO projection). The C5-6 and C6-7 left apophysial joints were both abnormal (fibrous injury), but not subluxed. Injury to either C6 or C7 roots could be hypothesized; the latter was the fact, based on pain radiation. Union occurred in this position, and symptoms persist two years later. Hemi-arch fractures are not rare, are difficult to recognize, and perhaps are a variant sequela to the same mechanism that produces unilateral apophysial (fracture-) dislocations.

CASE REPORT 3. In a 10-year-old child who complained of unilateral neck pain, a pathologic focal C4 kyphosis was present, with absent right C4 hemiarch (Fig. 5-19). Hypocycloidal tomography showed incom-

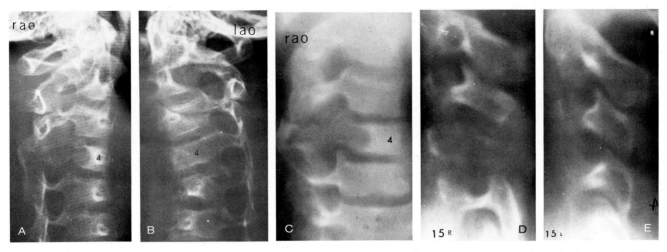

FIG. 5-19. Case report 3. *A*, RAO (60-degree) view of cervical spine; *B*, LAO (60-degree) view of cervical spine; *C*, RAO (60-degree) hypocycloidal tomogram of cervical spine through body and pillar; *D*, lateral hypocycloidal tomogram cervical spine 15 mm. to right of midline; *E*, Lateral hypocycloidal tomogram cervical spine 15 mm. to left of midline.

plete distended bony margins of the osteolytic lesion. A nearly complete resection of an osteoblastoma was performed and followed by radiation therapy.

References

1. Von Torklus D and Gehle W: The Upper Cervical Spine. Georg Thieme Verlag, Stuttgart, 1972.
2. Haworth JB, Keillor GW: Use of transparencies in evaluating the width of the spinal canal in infants, children, and adults. Radiology, *79:*109, 1962.
3. Grant JCB: Atlas of Anatomy. Williams & Wilkins Co., Baltimore, 1962.
4. Penning L: Functional Pathology of the Cervical Spine. Williams & Wilkins Co., Baltimore, and Excerpta Medica Foundation, 1968.
5. Kohler A, Zimmer EA, Case JT: Borderlands of the Normal and Early Pathologic in Skeletal Roentgenology. Grune & Stratton, New York, 1956.
6. Schmarl G, Junghanns H: The Human Spine in Health and Disease. Grune & Stratton, New York, 1959.
7. Acknowledgements to Dr. FJ Hodges III from whose teachings and encouragement developed my interest in the spine; and to Robert LG Stears, my son, for producing the artwork.

6

Electrodiagnosis of Neuromuscular Disease

J. M. MOSIER

Of the numerous electrical tests of neuromuscular function, electromyography is the most popular and the most informative. Nerve stimulation studies provide additional clinical information not obtainable from electromyography alone. Besides providing more clinical information, the use of both procedures allows each to serve as a reliability check upon the other. There is still a place for strength-duration curves in electrodiagnosis of neuromuscular disease. The faradic-galvanic test is too unreliable for clinical use, and along with most other electrical tests of neuromuscular function, it should best be remembered for historical reasons.

Electrodiagnostic testing, including electromyography, does not establish a clinical diagnosis. All are sensitive detectors of motor unit function and, in a sense, can be considered an extension of the clinical neurologic examination. Electromyography and related tests can detect disturbances of neuromuscular function that may not be evident upon clinical examination and often can distinguish between myopathy, neuropathy, and myoneural junction defect.

ELECTROMYOGRAPHY

Electromyography is a study of the action potentials of muscle fibers.

The electromyograph consists of a recording electrode system, high-gain amplifiers, a cathode-ray oscilloscope, and an audio system. All the commercial electromyographs are quite satisfactory for clinical electromyography. Two types of recording electrodes are in common use—monopolar (unipolar) and concentric (coaxial). The wave forms recorded from each are nearly

76

identical. Both types of electrodes come in size from about a 26-gauge needle to about an 18-gauge needle. Surface skin electrodes are unsatisfactory as they tend to integrate and summate the motor unit potentials, and the smallest diagnostic potentials (fibrillations) are not recordable.

The procedure consists of inserting the needle electrodes through the skin into varying depths of each particular muscle. Each muscle is usually examined at two or more different locations and at three or more directions at each location. Unless this minimum is carried out one cannot say there is no electromyographic abnormality in this particular muscle. The procedure is uncomfortable to painful, but sedation and analgesics usually are not required. The completeness of the examination depends largely on the cooperation of the patient.

Electromyographic Concepts

MOTOR UNIT. The motor unit is the anterior horn cell, its axon, terminal arborization, the myoneural junction, and all the individual muscle fibers innervated by that anterior horn cell.

MOTOR UNIT POTENTIAL. The motor unit potential is the summative action potential of all the individual muscle fibers of one motor unit.

The motor unit varies in size from the few muscle fibers in the eye muscles to the two thousand or more fibers comprising the large motor unit of a muscle in one of the limbs. The muscle fibers of a motor unit overlap and intermingle with those of adjacent motor units so that the territorial area a single motor unit occupies in a muscle is quite variable and may be as much as 3.4 sq. mm. in cross-sectional area. It follows then that the motor unit potential is variable in amplitude and duration. The normal motor unit potentials consist of two to four spikes, have an amplitude ranging from 0.2 millivolts to 2.0 millivolts, and sometimes ranging from 3.0 to 4.0 millivolts. Their duration varies from 3 to 15 milliseconds and they have a distinctive thumping sound. About 5% of the motor unit potentials from normal extremity and torso muscles are polyphasic, that is, the oscilloscope trace crosses the baseline four or more times.

INTERFERENCE. When a muscle contracts feebly only one or two motor unit potentials are recorded, and the details of each are easily displayed on the oscilloscope. As the muscle contracts more strongly more motor units are recruited, and their potentials tend to overlap each other on the oscilloscope screen, "interfering" with observations of details of an individual motor unit potential. As the muscle contraction becomes greater and greater, more and larger motor units are brought into the effort and the motor unit potentials overlap so much that at the baseline level only a blur is present. This is called "interference" and is normal.

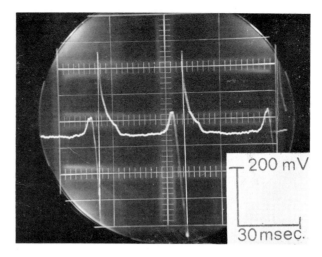

FIG. 6-1. Normal motor unit potentials. In this and subsequent figures positive EMG potentials are depicted as downward deflections, and negative EMG potentials are depicted as upward deflections.

POLYPHASIC MOTOR UNIT POTENTIALS. *Myopathies.* In myopathies, many motor units have a decrease in the number of muscle fibers; therefore the summative muscle fiber action potentials are of lower voltage and shorter duration than the average of normal motor unit potentials. The myopathic motor unit potentials are a series of spiky polyphasic patterns averaging less than 0.5 millivolts in amplitude and ranging from 3 to 7 milliseconds in duration. These are referred to as "myopathic" or "disintegrated" types of motor unit potentials as fewer than a normal number of muscle fibers comprise the motor unit. There is, however, an approximately normal number of motor units in the myopathic muscle. Interference is not significantly reduced in myopathies unless the myopathy is severe.

Neuropathics. In a denervated muscle the regenerating axons often innervate more of the denervated

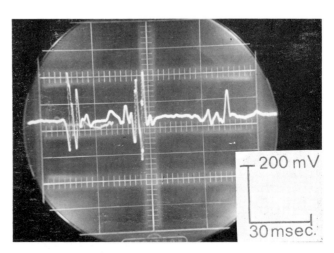

FIG. 6-2. Polyphasic activity.

muscle fibers than composed the original motor unit. In partially denervated muscle the terminal axonal sprouting of healthy nerve fibers increases the number of muscle fibers in the motor unit. The increase in the number of muscle fibers increases the territorial area of the motor units resulting in a longer time and a slightly asynchronous depolarization of the muscle fibers. This results in a motor unit potential of increased amplitude, because of more muscle fiber action potentials, and a longer duration, because of the larger territorial area (greater time for nerve impulses to reach the individual muscle fibers). The small terminal arborization conducts very slowly so that subunits of the motor unit fire at slightly different time intervals resulting in polyphasic motor unit potentials. Hence the polyphasic (complex) motor unit potentials of neuropathies tend to be of higher amplitude, of longer duration, and more complex than are normal motor unit potentials. The neuropathic polyphasic motor unit potential amplitude may vary from 1.0 to 10.0 millivolts or more and have a duration upward to 20 milliseconds or more.

"Giant" motor unit potentials are extremely high-voltage and long-duration motor unit potentials. These sometimes form from re-innervation. It has been suggested that sometimes two or more anterior horn cells may always fire synchronously and the summative motor unit activity results in a "giant" motor unit potential. This is seen especially in poliomyelitis. Or possibly some "giant" motor units are normally present but function only on maximal muscle contraction, and in poliomyelitis or other anterior horn cell disease the large motor units are from the remaining undamaged anterior horn cells.

In early nerve regeneration small low-voltage short-duration potentials that do not consistently appear are noted and represent the earliest stage of muscle fiber re-innervation. These motor units are sometimes referred to as "nascent" motor unit potentials and are detected sometimes a few weeks before there is any clinical indication of muscle contraction.

Though myopathic and neuropathic motor unit potentials as herein described are valid for most clinical patients, there are some contradictions. Low-voltage, short-duration motor unit potentials—so-called myopathic motor unit potentials—will occur if there is inexcitability of some muscle fibers, degeneration of some muscle fibers, defective neuromuscular transmission, or a degeneration of some of the nerve terminals. "Nascent" motor unit potentials are one example of "myopathic" motor unit potentials appearing in a neuropathy. In myasthenia, amyotrophic lateral sclerosis, and other neuropathies occasional areas of low-voltage short-duration "myopathic" motor unit potentials are noted. Strictly speaking, "neuropathic" or "myopathic" motor unit potentials are not diagnostic.

It is to be emphasized that the size range of normal motor unit potentials considerably overlaps those of myopathy and neuropathy. It is the relative proportion of small or large polyphasic motor unit potentials that favor an electromyographic impression of myopathy or neuropathy.

FIBRILLATION POTENTIALS. *Fibrillations of Neuropathy.* Fibrillations are the action potentials of individual or small clusters of denervated, healthy muscle fibers. The presence of fibrillations denotes healthy denervated muscle fibers awaiting re-innervation. Fibrillations of denervation, sometimes referred to as "true fibrillations," appear about 12 to 21 days after axonal separation or neuronal death, and somewhat sooner in trunk and facial muscles. Fibrillations do not appear unless there is axonotmesis; they are not found in disuse atrophy, neurapraxia, or hysteria. The electrical parameters of fibrillations are an amplitude of 20 to 200 microvolts and a duration of 0.5 to 1.5 milliseconds. They are diphasic or triphasic spikes with an initial positive deflection. They fire about 2 to 30 times per second and sound like relatively high-pitched clicks. When abundant their sound has been likened to "rain drops on a tin roof" or to the "crinkling of paper." Fibrillary twitching of muscle cannot be seen through the intact skin, but can sometimes be noted by reflected light from the moist surface of denervated tongue muscle.

Fibrillations of Myopathy. From the myopathies, especially polymyositis, repetitive spikes appear that are indistinguishable from the fibrillations of neuropathy. The origin of the fibrillary activity in myopathies is only speculative. Some may come from healthy denervated fibers because of terminal axonal damage due to scarring in some myopathic muscle. Possibly they originate from mildly diseased myopathic muscle fibers.

Significance of Fibrillations. The presence of fibrillation potentials almost always means the muscle is abnormal. One cannot distinguish neuropathy or myopathy because of fibrillations.

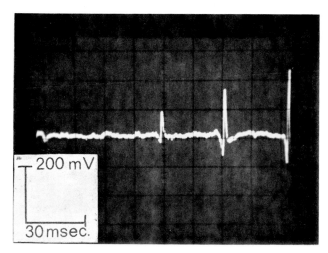

FIG. 6-3. Fibrillation potentials.

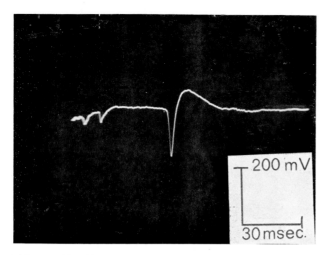

FIG. 6-4. Positive waves.

POSITIVE WAVES (positive sharp waves, V-waves, saw-tooth waves or positive potentials). Positive waves are of uncertain origin, but are thought to come from healthy denervated muscle fibers that are injured by the insertion of the needle recording electrode. Positive waves have an initial positive sharp deflection and a rather prolonged tail. Their size is variable, ranging in amplitude from 50 to 4000 microvolts and in duration to 100 milliseconds; their distinctive sound is between the "clicks" of fibrillation potentials and the "thumps" of motor unit potentials.

Positive waves are always abnormal and never appear from normal muscle. Positive waves are found in both neuropathic and myopathic muscle, as are fibrillations. Positive waves are sometimes found while fibrillations are few or absent. On the other hand, when fibrillations are present, positive waves are almost invariably present.

INSERTIONAL ACTIVITY. The recording electrode is large compared to the individual muscle fibers. Movement of the recording electrode compresses and irritates and even structurally damages a few muscle fibers. The electrical correlation of this movement in normal muscle is a series of spikes, possibly the summative activity of action potentials of many muscle fibers that ceases upon termination of movement. This is "normal insertional activity" and is present in all relaxed healthy muscle, but only during electrode movement.

In denervated or pathologic muscle the insertional activity persists with decreased intensity for a few seconds or longer after all needle electrode movement has ceased; this is termed "prolonged insertional activity." Often this merges into the spontaneous fibrillations of the pathologic muscle. Prolonged insertional activity may be the only indication of disease, especially in mild chronic neuropathy.

Insertional activity is absent from muscle whose fibers have largely been replaced with fat or from muscles with excessive collagen infiltrations that occur following crushing injuries to muscle.

FASCICULATIONS. Fasciculations are involuntary contractions of a motor unit or of a large number of adjacent muscle fibers, often producing a visible muscle twitch. When deep in the muscle they can be detected only by electromyography. Fasciculations have about the same electrical features as do the individual motor unit potentials. They appear randomly at a frequency of one to several per minute. The muscle must be completely relaxed and needle electrode movement must not occur if fasciculations are to be detected. Infrequent fasciculations often are not detected because the electromyographer does not take time to await their appearance.

Fasciculations are often present in the muscles of normal individuals. If a muscle exhibits only fasciculations, these are spoken of as "benign" fasciculations. When positive waves or fibrillations accompany fasciculations, the term "pathologic" is applied.

Sometimes fasciculations occur in clusters of two or three (doublets, triplets) or more (repetitive or grouped discharges). These clusters are occasionally seen in normal individuals, but are more frequently seen in metabolic disturbances such as tetany, uremia, or thyrotoxicosis. When fasciculations are numerous, producing undulations of the skin surface, the condition is referred to as myokymia.

HIGH-FREQUENCY DISCHARGES. *Myotonic Discharges.* Myotonic discharges are another form of prolonged insertional activity, occurring only in myotonic muscle, and consist of high-frequency repetitive spikes, sharp potentials, and other unusual wave forms having frequencies up to 150 per second, characterized by variable voltage and frequency. Their sound continuously waxes and wanes and has been likened to that of a dive bomber of the World War II era. The myotonic

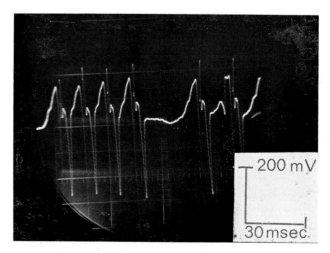

FIG. 6-5. High-frequency discharge.

discharge is thought to represent continuous repetitive firing of myotonic muscle fibers.

Myotonic discharges are found only in the myotonias, though myotonic discharges are reported to occur in the hyperkalemic form of periodic paralysis and in Pompe's disease, an amylo-1,4 glucosidase deficiency.

Bizarre High-Frequency Discharges (pseudo-myotonic discharges). Bizarre high-frequency discharges are rapidly firing repetitive discharges differing from myotonic discharges in their sudden changes in frequency and form as well as abrupt disappearance. They usually have a pleasant hum or musical sound. Like myotonic discharges they may be induced by needle electrode or muscle contraction or may just occur spontaneously. They may persist or be attenuated during muscle contraction. Their origin is unknown. Bizarre high-frequency discharges are sometimes abundant in the rapidly developing myopathies (acute polymyositis for example), but also are occasionally recorded from various neuropathies and unfortunately, though rarely, from normal muscle.

Various forms of high frequency discharges that are brief, often not repetitive, are noted from time to time in all muscles and are of unknown significance.

NERVE ACTION POTENTIALS. Nerve action potentials from small intramuscular nerve fibers may be confused with fibrillations in that both have about the same electromyographic parameters except that the initial deflection is negative for nerve action potentials. Nerve action potentials tend to fade away. The presence of nerve action potentials has no clinical significance.

END-PLATE NOISE. End-plate noise sounds much like normal background amplifier noise, but it has greater intensity and persists indefinitely as long as there is no muscle or needle electrode movement. Movement of the needle electrode by as little as 1 to 2 mm. leads to disappearance of the end-plate noise. It consists of rapid spikes, never exceeding 40 microvolts. The tiny spikes of end-plate noise are assumed to be the miniature end-plate potentials recorded by intracellular microelectrodes. End-plate potentials are the smallest potentials recorded electromyographically.

The Electromyogram

The electromyographer should examine each muscle in a completely relaxed state, as it is in this state that the spontaneous fibrillations are most easily demonstrated. During muscle contraction the small fibrillations and insertional activity are camouflaged by the large and numerous motor unit potentials.

In order to inspect the individual motor unit potentials, the muscle is examined during minimal voluntary contraction. In this state only one or two motor unit potentials appear from any one recording electrode position. The recording electrode is positioned to bring out the maximal amplitude and duration of the motor unit potentials. Several different motor unit potentials are examined from several different muscle sites to obtain a rough approximation of the average size and shape of the motor unit potentials in that particular muscle.

During stronger voluntary contractions more motor units are brought into action and the motor unit potentials overlap each other, thus interfering with detailed observation of individual motor unit potentials, and at maximal voluntary contraction the largest motor unit potentials emerge and interference is maximal (normal). All muscle contraction is against the resistance applied by the electromyographer. The electromyographer estimates the number of motor unit potentials (degree of interference) against the strength of voluntary muscle contraction, thus giving a crude estimate of severity of muscle disease.

ELECTROMYOGRAM, NORMAL MUSCLE FIBERS. With the muscle completely relaxed, insertion of the recording electrodes produces only normal insertional activity, meaning that the only electrical activity is during the electrode movement. Nerve action potentials, end-plate noise, and fasciculations may be present. No other electrical phenomena are noted during the period of complete muscle relaxation, and only background electronic noise appears on the oscilloscope tracing. This state is termed "electrical silence."

Motor unit potentials are normal in size, shape, and number. That the number of motor unit potentials is normal during maximal voluntary contraction is evidenced by the marked intensity of the interference pattern.

ELECTROMYOGRAM, DENERVATED MUSCLE FIBER. *Complete Nerve Severance.* If a peripheral nerve is completely severed, the muscles innervated distal to the separation exhibit no spontaneous activity. After a few days no insertional activity is induced. Only "electrical

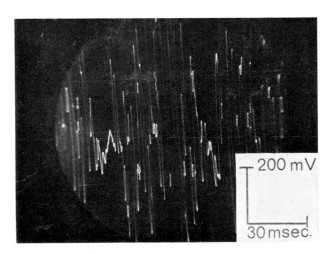

FIG. 6-6. Normal interference patterns. Maximal voluntary contraction.

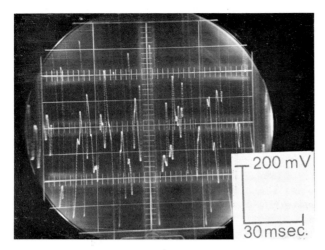

FIG. 6-7. Moderate interference patterns, reduced in number. Maximal voluntary contraction.

silence" shows on the oscilloscope screen. No motor unit potentials appear. In about 9 to 10 days, prolonged insertional activity in the form of abortive positive waves and fibrillations appear. In about 12 to 21 days, spontaneous fibrillations and insertionally induced positive waves are detected. After many weeks, as regeneration is progressing, there is a decrease in the abundance of spontaneous fibrillations and low-voltage "nascent" motor units are noted, even though there are still no voluntary muscle twitches. Slowly the duration of the polyphasic motor unit potentials increases and more appear. Finally the motor unit potentials become larger, so that perhaps the majority are of higher voltage and longer duration than normal. If all the muscle fibers have not been re-innervated, fibrillations may persist for months or years. If the denervated muscle fibers degenerate, there will be no fibrillations. This increased polyphasia, increased amplitude, and prolonged duration of the motor unit potentials is an electrical scar (permanent residuals) of the nerve damage. Regeneration is almost never complete and fewer motor unit potentials may be noted upon maximal voluntary contraction, as indicated by the less intense interference patterns, though sometimes this is difficult to detect.

Incomplete Nerve Severance. The only difference between complete and incomplete peripheral nerve severance is that in the latter some motor unit potentials can be voluntarily produced. The number of motor unit potentials appearing on maximal voluntary contraction depends on the severity of nerve injury—the less severe the injury the greater the number of motor unit potentials. In mild injuries, only a few fibrillation potentials and positive waves are present to indicate the neuropathy, and it becomes extremely difficult to estimate the decreased intensity of interference patterns. Later, with regeneration, the fibrillations disappear and one is hard pressed to demonstrate residuals of neuropathy.

Neuropathies. Unless extremely mild, the neuropathies show prolonged insertional activity, positive waves, spontaneous fibrillation potentials, and a definite decrease in the number of motor unit potentials upon maximal voluntary contraction. Recovery shows increased polyphasia, prolonged duration, and increased amplitude of the motor unit potentials. Chronic neuropathies may exhibit prolonged insertional activity only, often with normal size motor unit potentials but a decrease in number. Fibrillation potentials and positive waves often will not appear in longstanding neuropathies.

ELECTROMYOGRAM, MUSCLE FIBER DISEASE. In the degenerative myopathies, insertional activity, fibrillations, and positive waves may be prolonged in the myopathic muscle. There will be an approximately normal number of motor unit potentials. The individual motor unit potentials will be less than the average normal duration and will be mildly polyphasic. The average amplitude of the motor unit potentials will be reduced in voltage. In many of the slowly evolving dystrophies, the motor unit potentials are of normal amplitude and duration. There will be a mild increase in polyphasic motor unit potentials as the sole indication of pathology.

The reversible and metabolic myopathies also exhibit an increased proportion of shorter duration motor unit potentials and polyphasia. The different types usually cannot be identified electromyographically. In acute polymyositis the mean duration of motor unit potentials may be decreased by as much as 50 to 60%.

NERVE STIMULATION STUDIES

Studies of motor nerve conduction velocities and evoked sensory nerve responses are excellent tests of neuromuscular integrity. They are often more diagnostic than electromyography as in compressive syndromes, in identifying myasthenic states, or in detecting mild peripheral neuropathies.

MOTOR NERVE CONDUCTION VELOCITY. Motor nerve conduction velocity is usually determined for the ulnar, median, peroneal, and posterior tibial nerves. The motor nerve conduction velocity can be determined for other superficial peripheral nerves, but requires greater cooperation from the patient. The motor nerve conduction velocities for the larger motor nerves are in the range of 45 to 65 meters per second. Before the age of three years, the nerve velocities are about half that of a young adult, and by the age of five, approach the adult range. With increasing age the velocities slow almost imperceptibly, so that the average for the seventh decade is about 10 meters per second slower than for the third decade.

NORMAL

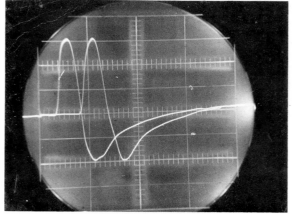

Latency   3 msec
Velocity   62 meters per second

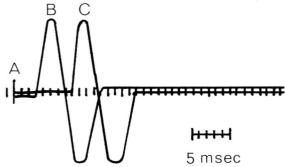

5 msec

A- Initial Shock Artefact
B- Response To Stimulus At Wrist
C- Response To Stimulus At Elbow

ABNORMAL

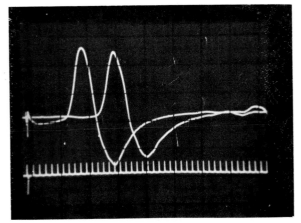

Latency   6 msec
Velocity   54 meters per second

FIG. 6-8. Median motor conduction studies.

A supramaximal percutaneous single electrical stimulus is applied at two different points over the skin along the course of the nerve. Recording electrodes from the monitoring muscle transfer the muscle action potentials to the electromyograph for oscilloscopic display. The muscle action potential (M-wave) is the summative action potential of all the muscle fibers of the monitor muscle. By measuring the distance between the two stimulus sites and the time interval between the two muscle action responses on the oscilloscope, one can calculate the motor nerve velocity for that portion of the nerve between the two stimulus sites. The amplitude response of the muscle action potential is measured in millivolts and the duration in milliseconds.

The motor nerve conduction velocity is slow only in conditions affecting the peripheral nerve. There will be normal or nearly normal velocities in myopathies and anterior horn cell disease. Slowing of motor nerve conduction velocity occurs in regenerating nerves, in some of the rare hereditary neuropathies, across nerve compressions, and in some chronic polyneuritis, as well as in some of the metabolic neuropathies (diabetes, for example).

The low-amplitude response from the monitor muscle means that there is a reduction in the number of muscle fibers contracting from the monitor muscle in response to the supramaximal nerve stimulation. This could be from primary disease of the muscle fibers (muscular dystrophy) or local trauma to the muscle fibers. It might be because all the nerve impulse is not reaching the muscle fibers, as in myasthenic states, or that some of the muscle fibers are denervated because of nerve trauma or neuritis.

EVOKED SENSORY RESPONSES. To determine conduction time in an afferent nerve, the cutaneous nerve endings are stimulated and the sensory nerve action potential at standard points along the nerve recorded. Only the large myelinated afferent nerve impulses are recorded because of their high nerve action potential voltage. The action potentials of the smaller myelinated and unmyelinated fibers are too low to be recorded.

Evoked sensory responses are easily obtained from the median and ulnar nerves at the wrist. They can be recorded from healthy radial and sural nerves. With neuropathy of any etiology the evoked sensory waves may be slowed or not obtainable, and often are a more sensitive indicator of neuropathy than are motor nerve conduction studies or electromyography. Various electronic averaging devices are needed to detect most other evoked afferent impulses, and these are not yet available to most electromyographers.

Clinically, the prolonged sensory conduction time of the distal median nerve is the most sensitive electrodiagnostic indicator of a carpal tunnel syndrome. In diabetes, uremia, and alcoholism there may be a prolonged sensory conduction time even without motor conduction velocity slowing.

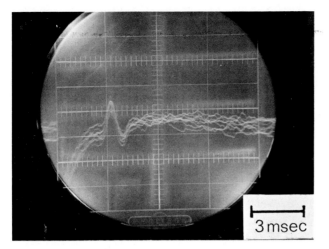

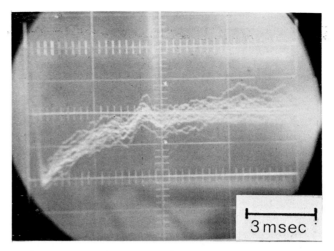

Normal   3.3 msec

Abnormal   5.2 msec

FIG. 6-9. Median sensory latencies.

STRENGTH-DURATION CURVES. In normal muscle, the intramuscular motor nerve fibers are more sensitive to electrical stimulation than are the muscle fibers. The motor terminal axons tend to concentrate at the motor points of the muscles.

A constant current or constant voltage stimulator produces a square wave stimulus. The smallest strength of stimulus applied for a prolonged period of time (300 to 1000 milliseconds) that will produce a barely detectable muscle twitch is called "the rheobase." The stimulus is applied at the motor point of the muscle. The

stimulus is repeated at shorter and shorter time intervals down to 0.01 millisecond. The strength of stimuli is plotted against the duration of the stimuli. The "chronaxie" is a point on the strength-duration curve where stimulus strength is twice that of the rheobase. In normal muscle this point is about 0.1 millisecond or less; with denervation it is closer to 1.0 millisecond or more. In normal muscle the strength-duration curve is nearly a horizontal line bending upward at about 1.0 millisecond or less, and represents the excitability of nerve tissue only. In completely denervated muscle the

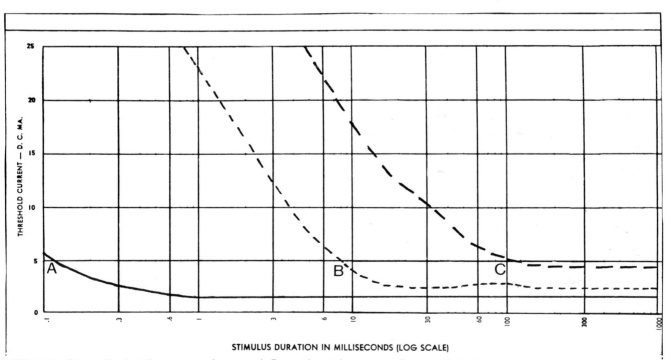

FIG. 6-10. Strength-duration curve: *A*, normal; *B*, moderately severe; *C*, complete denervation.

strength-duration curve slopes upward rather sharply to the left; this represents the electrical excitability of the denervated muscle only. From partially denervated muscle the excitable tissue is a mixture, which may consist of normally innervated muscle, re-innervated muscle fiber, normal nerve fibers, and regenerated nerve fibers. The resulting strength-duration curve is sloped between the normal and completely denervated curves. The different excitable tissues may evoke small kinks called "discontinuities" in the slope of the partially denervated strength-duration curve.

The strength-duration curves are limited to superficial muscles and the superficial layers of the large muscles. Nevertheless, the strength-duration curve is a more sensitive indicator of early denervation than is electromyography. In chronic neuropathies it may indicate mild denervation when fibrillation potentials are not found. It is a percutaneous stimulation procedure and is less distressing than electromyography. It is usually less sensitive in identifying the neuropathies than is electromyography. In selected cases, strength-duration curves are a more convenient method of following the progress of nerve fiber regeneration. It is useful to confirm results of other electrodiagnostic studies, especially in medicolegal cases.

APPRAISAL OF ELECTRODIAGNOSIS

The distribution of the denervation is the principal means the electromyographer uses in deciding whether a neuropathy is at the cord or root level, or involves the plexus or specific nerve or nerves. Mono-radiculopathies are confusing in that in many instances of nerve root syndromes, all the nerve root is not uniformly injured, but actually some of the nerve root fascicles are intact and function normally. The electromyogram may demonstrate denervation in all the muscles of that nerve root distribution if the nerve root is uniformly involved. Much more often only a few fascicles of the nerve root are injured, and as a result, only one or two muscles innervated by that particular nerve root will show evidence of denervation. Hence, the electromyogram in nerve root syndromes often suggests a mononeuropathy, thus the electromyogram must be correlated with clinical findings. In hysteria no abnormal electromyographic wave forms appear, and nerve stimulation studies indicate a normally functioning neuromuscular apparatus.

Nerve stimulation studies are more useful in detecting compressive neuropathies such as carpal tunnel syndromes than is electromyography.

The electromyographic report should state each muscle examined and the electromyographic findings in each muscle. The clinician can then better correlate the electromyographic findings with the clinical picture. The electromyographer should attempt to estimate the severity; this he does by estimating the amount of normal motor unit activity present in a muscle by observing the interference patterns. The amount of fibrillation activity present in a muscle is a poor guide to the severity of the neuropathy.

To provide the most electromyographic information for the clinician, clinician and electromyographer should keep each other apprised of clinical findings, other laboratory test procedures, and clinical impressions. Electromyography requires experience and patience. The electromyographer should be a person well versed in neuromuscular disease and not an occasional user of electromyographic equipment. The use of both electromyography and nerve stimulation studies gives the clinician considerably more diagnostic and prognostic information than either procedure alone in evaluating neuromuscular disease.

The old cliché that "EMG is to nerves and muscles what x-ray is to bone" is not completely true. Nevertheless, electromyography not only is helpful in establishing the diagnosis, but often provides the clinician with information that gives him a better understanding of the patient's symptoms. Weakness, myalgia, fasciculations, muscle spasms, dysthesias, reflex changes, fatiguability—these are symptoms and findings that electromyography may be of substantial assistance in explaining.

Section III

*Metabolic
and Infectious
Diseases*

7

Osteoporoses and Osteomalacias in Spinal Surgery

H. M. FROST

To MY KNOWLEDGE, no previous effort has been made to assemble and collate, in this particular way and for this particular purpose and audience, such material as is contained in this chapter. Consequently, if internists conversant on the subject of metabolic bone disease should find this a strange article, they might pause to recall that their own concerns differ greatly from a typical surgeon's and they (the former) have written almost all of the articles about metabolic bone diseases. Naturally such writings have been slanted toward the needs of the internist, while those of the surgeon have received short shrift.

Briefly, then, and in accordance with the particular needs of active surgeons, I will discuss here some features of osteoporoses and osteomalacias as they pertain to operative procedures on the spine in patients who also have such a disease. The medical and therapeutic aspects of these two groups of diseases are presented more appropriately and effectively elsewhere in the literature.[1-4,8,10]

OSTEOPOROSES

"Osteoporosis" means different things to different members of the medical community. For the purpose of our discussion we will elaborate on the *osteoporotic skeletal state* and on *osteoporosis the disease*.

OSTEOPOROTIC SKELETAL STATE. This designation connotes a condition in which the skeleton contains a smaller total quantity of bony tissue than normal for the sex, age, and culture of a particular patient. Normally the total quantity of bone tissue tends to accumulate during skeletal growth, to peak around age 20, and thereafter to decline gradually. By age 65 most people have lost 30% or so of the bony tissue they had accumulated by skeletal maturity.[3,8,9,12] Accordingly, it is a phenomenon rather than a disease or a pathologic condition (Fig. 7-1). Furthermore, in estimating the total quantity of skeletal tissue in adults by various means, one finds an essentially Gaussian distribution, that is, a mean skeletal bone mass characterizes a given age group, but individual variations on the high and low side extend over many standard deviations. Clinical observation leaves little doubt that at least a small majority of patients in whom we discover a subnormal bone mass incidental to their surgical problem do not in fact prove ultimately to have a skeletal disease that threatens their future, at least on that basis. Of course, in some of them a major problem can develop. Unfortunately we still have no reliable way to predict into which group a given individual with a substandard bone mass will fall; simple radiographic estimates of bone mass cannot do it. Figure 7-2 illustrates the major radiographic features of the typical osteoporotic skeleton.

OSTEOPOROSIS THE DISEASE. A patient with this disease has an osteoporotic skeleton—that is, a subnormal total quantity of bony tissue for the sex, age, and culture—*plus clinical disability associated with it*, usually in the form of vertebral compression fractures,

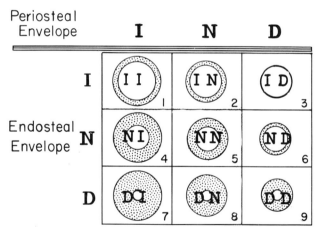

FIG. 7-1. The anatomic patterns of bone loss (or of inadequate or even supernormal accumulation during growth) can prove as distinctive as the quantities involved. Shown here are the patterns possible by conceiving the spaces circumscribed by the periosteum (the periosteal "envelope") and marrow cavity wall (the endosteal "envelope") as normal, increased, or decreased. Real examples of each (except possibly No. 7) are known to exist and all known pathologic states of systemic loss or accumulation errors fit within one of these nine squares. Thus PMO, SO, and CO belong in No. 2; postacromegaly OP in No. 1; children with frank osteogenesis imperfecta in No. 6. (From Frost HM: Orthopaedic Lectures. Vol. III, Springfield, Ill. Charles C Thomas, 1972.)

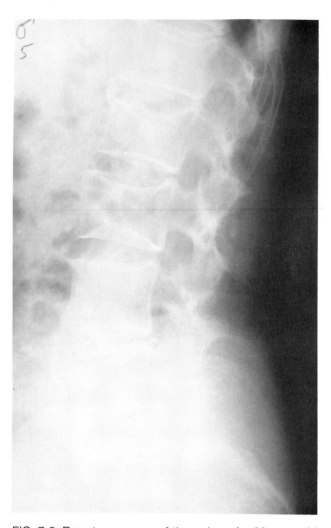

FIG. 7-2. Roentgenogram of the spine of a 60-year-old man with a low-turnover osteoporosis, probably of the "senile" type, but accentuated by a high ethanol intake. Note loss of radiographic density of the vertebral centra, end-plate collapses, and wedging. The latter arose some 10 years previously during his four years of symptoms and overt disability; he has had none attributable to this problem in the past six years.

which occur spontaneously or follow trivial incidents that would not harm normal people. Thus if an osteoporotic skeleton exists without its associated clinical disability, the patient may well have some other medical disease. The significance of the distinction is that the medical disease, *not the skeleton*, needs treatment.

The various kinds of osteoporosis are distinguished, one from the others, by such features as anatomic location of bone loss, age at onset, associated bone marrow and hematologic conditions, bone turnover speed, curability, and natural reversibility (Table 7-1).

RELATIONS TO SURGICAL MANAGEMENT. In planning a spinal operation and selecting an appropriate procedure for a patient with osteoporosis, the surgeon con-

TABLE 7-1. Osteoporoses: Clinical Features

Type of Osteoporosis (OP)	Frequency in U.S.	Typically causes clinical disability	Naturally reversible	Typical serum Ca, PO₄, alk. phosphatase	Typical urine chemistries	Typically true disease	Prone to spontaneous fracture	Special studies needed to make diagnosis	Bone tissue turnover speed (typical)
Physiologic OP of aging	C	O	O	N	N	O	O	O	N
Senile OP	C	+	O	N	N	+	+	O	D
Postmenopausal OP	C	+	O	N	N	+	+	O	D
Cushing's OP	C	+	O	N	N	+	+	+	D
OP of rheumatoid arthritis and Marie-Strumpell	C	O	O	N	N	O	O	O	D
Disuse (true) OP	C	O	O	N	N	O	O	P	D
Posttraumatic osteodystrophy	C	O	+	N	N	O	O	O	I
OP of Sudek's atrophy	C	O	+	N	N	O	O	O	I
OP of thyrotoxicosis	R	O	+	N	N	+	O	+	I
Migratory osteoporosis	R	+	+	N	N	+	O	+	I
OP of mast cell disease	R	+	O	N	N	O	O	+	N
OP of hyperparathyroidism	R	O	O	A	A	O	O	+	V
OP of osteogenesis imperfecta	U	+	O	N	N	+	+	+	I
Multiple myeloma	U	+	O	N	N	+	+	+	V
Hyperphosphatasia	R	+	O	A	A	+	+	+	I
OP of congenital biliary tract obstruction	R	O	O	A	A	O	O	+	V
OP of muscular dystrophy	C	O	O	N	N	O	O	O	D

Key: A = abnormal; C = common; R = rare; U = uncommon; N = normal; + = yes; O = no; D = decreased; I = increased; V = variable.

siders the following: (1) soft tissue and bone healing (the *probability* and the *speed* of healing) (Table 7-2); (2) whether some modification of the standard pre- or postoperative management will be necessary (Table 7-2); (3) the risk of anesthesia and surgery; and (4) whether, if untreated, the osteoporotic skeletal state itself threatens the patient with future problems not directly related to the operation. Problems peculiar to some specific conditions—posttraumatic osteodystrophy as opposed to true disuse osteoporosis, the phase lag pool loss, and biologic as opposed to technical failures in bone healing—are discussed on pages 94 and 95.

DIAGNOSIS. Ordinary x-ray views of the spine reveal its osteoporotic state as decreased radiographic density and thinning of its anterior and posterior cortices. The patient may give a history of fractures following trivial trauma or may complain of disability due to skeletal pain. Even in the presence of the osteoporotic skeletal state, a medical consultation may be necessary to rule out or ascertain osteoporosis the disease. Only in a few types of osteoporosis is the risk of anesthesia and operation increased (Table 7-2).

OSTEOMALACIAS

Different points of view exist which inflict communication with some serious semantic problems. To the internist "osteomalacia" suggests a variety of medical diseases plus pseudofractures, osteoid on rib biopsy, and potential good response to certain drugs; to another physician the same word signifies a specific adult vitamin D deficiency state; to a pathologist it implies a microscopic pattern seen occasionally in decalcified bone sections; and to a radiologist it connotes pseudofractures visible on plain x-ray films. The definitions offered here are intended simply to clarify our own meanings:

Osteoid—also termed *osteoid seam, osteoid border,* and *unmineralized newly formed, organic bone matrix*—is

TABLE 7-2. Osteoporoses: Prognosis and Therapy

Type	Progressive (without treatment)	Bed rest for two months is harmful	Curative therapy available	Bone embrittled	Bone fragility increased	Bone healing	Soft tissue healing	Surgical/anesthesia risk increased
Physiologic OP	+	O	O	O	O	N	N	O
Senile OP	+	O	O	+	+	N	N	O
Postmenopausal OP	+	O	O	+	+	N	N	O
Cushing's OP	+	O	O	+	+	N	N	O
OP of rheumatoid arthritis and Marie-Strumpell	O	O	O	O	O	N	N	O
Disuse OP (true)	O	O	O	O	+	N	N	O
Posttraumatic osteodystrophy	O	O	+	O	O	N	N	O
OP of Sudek's atrophy	V	O	+	O	O	N	N	O
OP of thyrotoxicosis	+	V	+	O	O	N	N	+
Migratory osteoporosis	O	O	+	O	O	N	N	O
OP of mast cell disease	+	V	O	O	O	N	N	+
OP of hyperparathyrodism	+	V	+	O	O	V	N	O
Op of osteogenesis imperfecta	O	V	O	+	+	N	N	O
Multiple myeloma	+	V	O	O	+	V	N	O
Hyperphosphatasia	+	V	O	O	+	N	N	+
OP of congenital biliary tract obstruction	+	O	+	+	O	V	N	+
OP of muscular dystrophy	+	O	O	+	+	N	N	O

Key: O = no; + = yes; N = normal; V = variable.

the organic material made by osteoblasts, and within which water is displaced by inorganic mineral salts, converting it thereby to bone. In life its deposition by a given "batch" of osteoblasts can proceed at a normal or subnormal pace, but no proven examples yet exist of supernormal deposition in that special context.

Pseudofracture is a transverse radiolucency across a bone which arises spontaneously and persists unhealed until the underlying metabolic and/or biochemical defects (an osteomalacia usually) have been identified and corrected.

Turnover is the special combination of bone resorptive and formative activities which replaces older with newer bone without changes of equal pace in its gross architecture or total quantity. Also termed *remodeling* by some.

OSTEOMALACIC STATE OF THE SKELETON. This pathologic state of bone tissue is characterized by great increases in the amount of unmineralized osteoid, decreases in the rates of both mineral deposition and elaboration of new osteoid in individual osteoid borders

or seams, and a disproportionately smaller but unmistakable increase in the number of resorption cavities in the bone (Fig. 7-3).

OSTEOMALACIA THE DISEASE. The patient is said to have osteomalacia when afflicted with an osteomalacic skeleton associated with impaired bone healing, pseudofractures (often), abnormalities in some serum chemical laboratory values, and abnormalities in the dynamics of net calcium absorption from the gut, of calcium transport in the blood, and of urinary calcium excretion. Many types of osteomalacia exist, and they may be classified according to etiology, pathophysiology, clinical features, or any mixture thereof.

DIAGNOSIS. Clinical features of osteomalacia include vague pains of bony origin, ready fatigue, muscle weakness, and sometimes muscle cramps, usually from hypocalcemia. The most significant radiographic findings are pseudofractures (Looser's zones of transformation), which are noted in approximately one-third of all patients with osteomalacia (in the United States), predominantly in the ribs and pelvic rami. Decreased

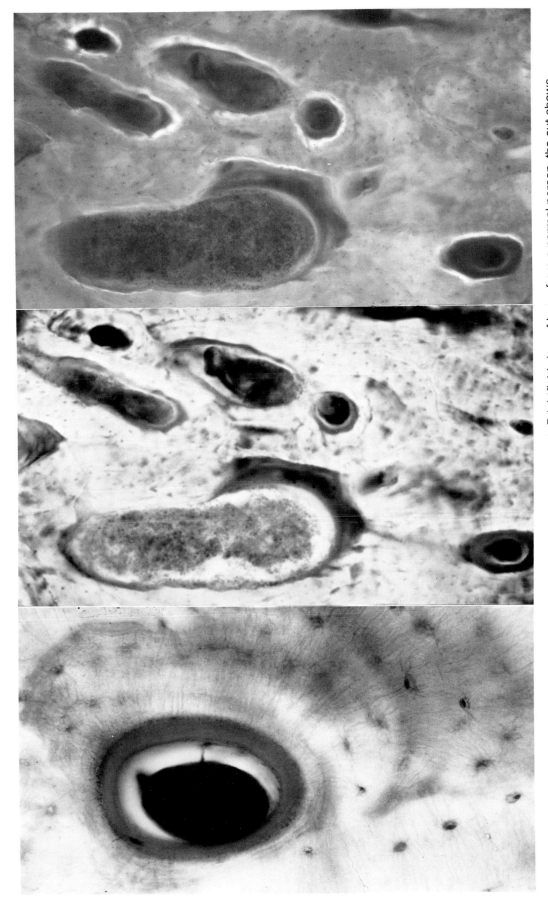

FIG. 7-3. Photomicrographs of stained undecalcified sections of human bone. *Left:* Brightfield view of bone from a normal person, the cut shows an osteoid seam (a "center of bone formation") at the upper left, in cross section (it is tubular like a piece of rubber tubing) and looking like a hyaline ring. The central oval hole (the haversian canal) contains a black plug—the shrunken and overstained vessels, osteoblasts, and soft tissues. New osteoid deposits on the inner side of the seam, while it mineralizes on the outer, so that the whole process moves centripetally. *Right:* Brightfield view of a rib biopsy of a girl with hypophosphatemic rickets. Abnormally large numbers of osteoid seams lie in evidence. *Middle:* An example of osteomalacic bone. Same field as above in the fluorescence microscope. The irregular bright rings represent tetracycline markers deposited a month before the biopsy (for details see the references). Measurements reveal greatly retarded deposition both of new mineral and of new osteoid in each bone-forming center plus a lesser but still great increase in their numbers.

bone density also is noted in about one-third of these patients but, uncommonly, it may even appear increased.

From the laboratory standpoint, a subnormal 24-hour urine calcium content (<75 mg./day) appears in more than 19 out of 20 cases of osteomalacia, and seldom occurs in patients without it. Consequently it provides an effective, simple, and economical screening test for outpatient clinic or office use.

Blood studies typically reveal a lowered serum calcium, often a depressed serum inorganic phosphate, and an elevated alkaline phosphatase. On occasion, however, florid osteomalacia can exist concurrently with persistently normal values of calcium, inorganic phosphate, and alkaline phosphatase.

The present ultimate in diagnostic accuracy, the court of last diagnostic resort, constitutes analysis of a rib biopsy done after double tetracycline bone labeling.[6,8,11] To make the point that increased osteoid alone does not identify or establish the diagnosis of osteomalacia, listed in Table 7-3 are some nonosteomalacic states in which great increases in the amount of osteoid regularly occur. In such patients the bony skeleton does not require any specific treatment. Tetracycline-based analysis of rib biopsies easily distinguishes these states, but microradiographic studies and conventional pathologic and histochemical studies seldom can, facts not yet widely appreciated in the community of internists in this country.

RELATION TO SURGICAL MANAGEMENT. Listed in Table 7-4 are some of the osteomalacias seen in North America, along with their identifying chemical and radiographic features. In Table 7-5 are some features of direct concern to a surgeon, such as whether bone healing proves impaired, and whether the treatments currently available to our internists effectively control the problem.

Whereas bone healing in osteoporoses usually proceeds quite normally, *bone healing in osteomalacias usually is impaired.* Pseudofractures usually specifically identify poor bone healing potential, and nonunions, delayed unions, and pseudoarthroses of bone grafting and fusion procedures skyrocket in incidence if done in such patients without prior identification and correction of their basic biochemical defect.

The impaired bone healing of osteomalacia tends to persist until the underlying metabolic defect has been corrected. Most osteomalacias characterized by hypocalcemia respond well to treatment with vitamin D in conservative doses, and bone healing is restored to normal in most cases after about two months of treatment. The chief exception is the patient with chronic renal failure, in whom vitamin D often has little effect. Hypocalcemia in patients with osteomalacia may cause carpopedal spasm or even tetany, particularly if the patients hyperventilate, or if hyperventilation inadvertently occurs during anesthesia. In such cases prompt correction can be effected with intravenous calcium gluconate.

In most *osteoporoses* bone healing proceeds normally; no unusual surgical or anesthetic risk arises; no pressing need exists to treat the osteoporotic state of the spine before, during, or immediately after operation; and the state usually is recognizable from simple history plus the findings on ordinary spinal x-ray films.

In most *osteomalacias* bone healing does not proceed normally, so that such procedures as spinal fusion should be deferred until the metabolic defect is corrected. Otherwise the risks attached to anesthesia and operation are increased because of possible tetany and/or electrolyte and acid-base imbalances, and prudence suggests that underlying metabolic problems be identified and corrected before elective procedures. Correct diagnosis often requires many laboratory tests, protracted study, and analysis of tetracycline-labeled rib biopsy.

SPECIFIC CONDITIONS

Herein we will briefly summarize some of the more common osteoporoses and osteomalacias a surgeon might encounter in his practice.

Osteoporoses

POSTMENOPAUSAL OSTEOPOROSIS (PMO). The basic cause of osteoporosis in postmenopausal women is unknown. In this condition bone loss affects all bones, *but* is confined to the surfaces in contact with marrow

TABLE 7-3. Conditions Typically Associated with Large Increases in Osteoid But not Osteomalacias in Any Medical Sense

Infancy and childhood	Thyrotoxicosis
Osteogenesis imperfecta	Active acromegaly
Posttraumatic osteodystrophy	Sudek's atrophy
Migratory osteoporosis	Some hyperparathyroid cases
Chronic osteomyelitis	Familial hypophosphatemic rickets
Axial osteomalacia	Any state of high bone tissue turnover
Hyperphosphatasia	

TABLE 7-4. Osteomalacias: Clinical Features

Type of Osteomalacia (OM)	Frequency in U.S.	Serum calcium	Serum PO$_4$	24 hr. urine calcium	Pseudofractures	Osteoporosis too	Has medical symptoms related to the disease	Typically causes back pain	Bone tissue turnover	Skeletal mineral turnover	Specific treatment	Curable by treatment available 1972
Nutritional rickets[a]	R	D	N-D	D	O	V	+	O	D	I	Vit. D	+
Nutritional osteomalacia	R	D	N-D	D	+	V	+	+	D	I	Vit. D	+
OM due to malabsorption of vit. D[b]	C	D	N-D	D	+	V	+	+	V	I	Vit. D	+
OM due to metabolic acidosis[c]	U	N-D	N-D	D	+	+	V	V	V	I	Alkalize	+
OM due to respiratory acidosis[c]	R	N-D	N-D	N-D	+	+	V	V	D	I	Alkalize	+
Familial hypophosphatemic rickets[d]	C	N	D	N	O	O	O	O	D	I	?	O
Renal rickets	U	D	I	D	+	V	V	O	V	I	Vit. D or[f]	O
OM due to chronic renal failure	C	N-D	I	D	V	O	V	O	D	V	Vit. D or[f]	V
Iatrogenic OM[e]	U	V	V	V	+	V	+	V	V	?	V	+
Adult hypophosphatemic OM	R	N	D	D	+	U	+	V	D	I	Suppl. PO$_4$	+
Fibrogenesis imperfecta ossium	R	N	N	D	+	+	+	+	N	I	?	O
Axial OM	R	N	N	N	O	O	O	O	N	N	None needed	NA

Key: D = decreased; C = common; N = normal; R = rare; U = uncommon; V = variable; I = increased; + = yes; O = no; ? = unknown; NA = not applicable–not a true disease

[a] Refers only to the osteomalacic element, not the rachitic component.

[b] Includes postgastrectomy, sprue, gluten enteropathy, short circuit procedures, milk-alkali syndrome.

[c] Includes ureterosigmoidostomy, chronic untreated diabetes mellitus.

[d] Seen in some cases of emphysema and chronic alveolar obstructive disease.

[e] Vitamin-D resistant rickets.

[f] Usually (at present) due to excessive use of fluoride or diphosphonates. Other forms may appear as biochemists find and use newer agents which interfere with those cell population dynamic and biochemical activities required to maintain a mechanically and histologically competent skeleton.

[g] 1-25 dihydroxycholecalciferol, when it becomes generally available.

tissue. It is a true disease but naturally self-limited in the disability it causes (i.e., typically one to four years). Spontaneous vertebral compression fractures usually occur. Occasionally fractures are seen in ribs, metatarsal bones, and hips, but it is the axial skeleton that is most affected. There is no cure or prevention of proved effectiveness. The skeleton is more fragile than normal. A greater fraction of spongy than of cortical bone is lost.

SENILE OSTEOPOROSIS (SO). Except for equal sex incidence, the features of this condition are exactly like those of postmenopausal osteoporosis.

CUSHING'S OSTEOPOROSIS (CO). The incidence is the same in both sexes. Usually the condition is iatrogenic, caused by prolonged treatment with corticosteroids. There exists no cure or prevention of proven effectiveness. Bone loss affects all bones, but is confined to

surfaces in contact with marrow tissue. A greater fraction of spongy than of compact bone is lost. The axial skeleton is most affected. Bone fragility and brittleness are increased, as in most other low bone turnover states (see Table 7-1). Spontaneous fractures occur, usually in vertebral bodies, but also in ribs and metatarsal bones. Aseptic necrosis may develop in femoral and humeral heads.

POSTTRAUMATIC OSTEODYSTROPHY (POD). This regional (as opposed to generalized) osteoporosis lacks sex preference and is directly due to tissue injury such as a burn, a fracture, or an injury to a major vessel or nerve or to the spinal cord. It affects extremities primarily, and takes at least two months to develop. The condition is inherently self-limited, but not in less than three months. All bony surfaces in the involved region are affected. It is related to Sudek's atrophy, which

TABLE 7-5. Osteomalacias: Features of Surgical Import

Type of Osteomalacia (OM)	Impaired Bone healing	Continued good health requires specific Rx.	Impaired soft tissue healing	Bone is brittle	Bed rest harmful	Preoperative correction necessary for safe anesthesia	Effective Rx available	A true disease
Nutritional rickets*	+	+	O	O	O	+	+	+
Nutritional OM	+	+	V	O	O	+	+	+
OM: Malabsorption of Vitamin D	+	+	O	O	O	+	+	+
OM: Metabolic acidosis	+	+	O	O	O	+	+	+
OM: Respiratory acidosis	+	+	O	O	O	+	+	+
Familial hypophosphatemic rickets	O	O	O	O	O	O	O	O*
Renal rickets	O	+	O	O	O	O	+f	+
OM of chronic renal failure	V	+	O	O	O	V	+f	+
Iatrogenic OM	+	+	O	O	O	V	+	+
Adult hypophosphatemic OM	+	+	O	O	O	O	+	+
Fibrogenesis imperfecta ossium	+	+	O	O	?	O	O	+
Axial osteomalacia	O	O	O	O	O	O	O	O

Key: + = yes; O = no; V = variable.

* Refers only to the osteomalacic skeleton, not the rachitic element.

f See footnote to Table 7-4.

probably simply represents a degree of it sufficiently extreme to make obvious the associated changes in the overlying soft tissues. When the tissue injury heals, so does the POD (spontaneously). No effective prevention is known. It is not a true disease, but just one sign of a more complex regional phenomenon which also affects sympathetics and regional blood flow patterns. Posttraumatic osteodystrophy is not directly responsible for any disability; fractures attributable to this condition are quite rare. Affected bone is *less* fragile than normal, as holds for most other high turnover states except osteogenesis imperfecta (see Table 7-1). Most modern articles about "disuse osteoporosis" in reality deal with posttraumatic osteodystrophy.

DISUSE OSTEOPOROSIS (DO). Associated with true and prolonged mechanical disuse, this condition shows no sex preference. It evolves in two stages: (1) a reversible phase, related to and deriving directly from the cause of the disuse, such as paralysis, and resolving in 4 to 18 months, and (2) a residual, gradually evolving, and irreversible marrow cavity expansion, with ultimate bone loss confined to the skeletal surfaces in physical contact with marrow tissue. There is no cure or prevention of proved effectiveness. The neuromotor disability deriving from the cause of the mechanical disuse far overshadows any deriving from the disuse osteoporosis itself.

LOW TURNOVER OSTEOPOROSES (see Table 7-1). Almost always irreversible, with or without attempts to treat, this condition usually is characterized by increased skeletal fragility and brittleness. (Note that these do not equate to bone strength.)

HIGH TURNOVER OSTEOPOROSES. Usually reversible, at least partially, this condition is characterized by decreased fragility and brittleness (except imperfecta).

PHASE LAG POOL LOSS. This phrase designates a condition commonly seen by surgeons who care for injured limbs (or spines). When bone turnover speed rises to high levels following some injury or operation (often $10\times$ normal in the bones surrounding a Colles' fracture or an L4–S1 fusion, for example), it does so not by "invigorating" the individual local osteoclasts and osteoblasts, but by increasing in direct proportion the total number of separate bone turnover centers or foci. And each such center represents a purely temporary "hole" or loss of $\approx .025$ mm.³ of bone. Particularly on trabecular surfaces, this can lead to an inherently temporary loss of more than 50% of the bone tissue originally there. We say "inherently temporary" because, when the cause of the increased turnover is removed, all of those holes become filled with new bone. And because no new ones replace them afterward, the bone loss "miraculously" heals. We call this phenomenon a "phase lag pool loss." It can distribute regionally (as is POD) or systemically (as in thyrotoxicosis).

BIOLOGIC FAILURE OF BONE HEALING. Some 50 years ago most cases (99%) of nonunion or bone graft failure were attributable to our technical inadequacies. With the present sophisticated techniques, such is not the case, and the blame for such failures has shifted to the *defective biologic responses* of the patient. I call these "biologic failures," and we currently do not understand them at all. Our best preventive measure at present consists in *fresh, autogenous* bone graft. These biologic failures do not represent osteomalacias (for which we have effective treatment) and so do not respond to treatment for the latter.

Osteomalacias

VITAMIN D-DEFICIENCY OSTEOMALACIA.[2] This condition shows no sex preference and involves all skeletal surfaces. Whether the cause is a deficient diet or deficient intestinal absorption, most of these patients have other but rather varied and sometimes complex nutritional deficiencies in addition to that related to vitamin D. Consequently, elective operations should be deferred until the condition is corrected, usually two to six months. Secondary hyperparathyroidism is common in these patients, although it seldom attains a magnitude leading to brown tumors, subperiosteal resorption, or concomitant osteoporosis. With only rare exceptions, this group of patients has a decreased 24-hour urine calcium excretion, even on an unprepared diet. Thus the test is valuable in the screening of outpatients.

HYPOPHOSPHATEMIC OSTEOMALACIAS.[2] Occurring in both acquired and congenital forms, this condition shows no sex predilection. Those affected lose phosphate through the urine and cannot maintain normal serum levels, yet they remain normocalcemic. Vitamin D alone does not control the defect, but can if supplemented by dietary phosphate, for example, as multiple small doses of Fleet's Phosphosoda. Diarrhea sets the limit on the dose. As a rule, these patients do not suffer from malnutrition or parathyroid malfunction; neither do they pose unusual anesthetic or surgical risks. Presenting symptoms are likely to include fatigue, bone pain, and symptoms of pseudofracture.

In vitamin-D resistant rickets an osteomalacic skeleton exists, but *bone healing proceeds normally,* and the bony part of the skeleton usually requires no active therapy, thus permitting osteotomy.

OSTEOMALACIA OF CHRONIC RENAL FAILURE. Thanks to recent studies of vitamin D physiology by DeLuca of Madison, we now understand some aspects of this problem much better than we did even three years ago. Briefly, dietary vitamin D itself does not promote calcium absorption by the gut; rather a chemically modified vitamin D molecule manufactured specifically in the kidney does so. When renal damage reaches the stage that this manufacture cannot keep up with the need, calcium absorption in the gut declines and the patient becomes hypocalcemic. That "turns on" the parathyroids, causing secondary hyperparathyroidism. But the patient remains hypocalcemic because (1) without that particular vitamin D-derived metabolite, parathyroid hormone cannot act to increase calcium absorption in the gut, and (2), the older idea that PTH primarily and normally acted to raise serum calcium by "invigorating" osteoclasts has proved mostly nonsense. When hyperparathyroidism is combined with hypocalcemia, osteomalacia can develop. A synthetically made metabolite (1, 25 dihydroxycholecalciferol) administered to such patients is likely to restore gut absorption and thus correct the problem. Lacking that, large doses of D may "load" the remaining functional renal tissue to the point that it produces enough metabolite to help the patient.

References

1. Aegerter E, Kirkpatrick JA: Orthopaedic Diseases. Philadelphia, WB Saunders, 1968, ed 3.
2. Arnstein AR, Frame B, Frost HM: Recent progress in osteomalacia and rickets. Ann Int Med. *67b:*1296-1330, 1967.
3. Barzel US: Osteoporosis. New York, Grune and Stratton, 1970.
4. Beeson PB, McDermott W (eds): Cecil's Textbook of Medicine. Philadelphia, WB Saunders, 1967.
4a. DeLuca HF: Vitamin D: new horizons. Clin Orthopaed Rel Res *78:*4-23, 1971.
5. Duncan H, Jaworski ZF: Osteoporosis. *In* Tice's Practice of Medicine, Vol. V. Maryland, Harper and Row, 1970, Ch. 52.
6. Frost HM: Tetracycline-based histological analysis of bone remodeling. Cal Tiss Res *3(3):*211-237, 1969.
7. Frost HM: Bone Dynamics in Osteoporosis and Osteomalacia. Springfield, Charles C Thomas, 1966.
8. Frost HM: Orthopaedic Lecture Series, Vol. III. Springfield, Charles C Thomas, 1970.
9. Garn S: The Earlier Gain and Later Loss of Cortical Bone. Springfield, Charles C Thomas, 1970.
10. Harris WH, Heaney RP: Skeletal renewal and metabolic bone disease. N Eng J Med *280:*193-202, 1969.
11. Sedlin ED, Frost HM, Villanueva AR: The eleventh rib biopsy in the study of metabolic bone disease. Henry Ford Hospital Med Bull *11:*217-219, 1963.
12. Trotter M, Broman GE, Peterson RR: Densities of bones of white and Negro skeletons. J Bone Jt Surg *42A:*50-58, 1960.

8

Infections of the Spine

PATRICK J. KELLY

INFECTIONS of the spinal column by organisms other than *Mycobacterium tuberculosis* are not common.[14] Nonetheless, they are important because of the difficulty of diagnosis and the serious consequences of delay in diagnosis. In spite of extensive studies, confusion still surrounds the classification of spinal infections and their diagnosis and treatment. Microbiologic diagnosis is not sought in every case, and for this reason, diagnosis often is presumptive. Some justification can be offered for this practice because obtaining tissue or aspirate for identification of the organism can be tedious if not difficult, and spinal infections often are self-limiting. On the other hand, failure to identify the organism precludes both accurate diagnosis and the choice of a truly specific antibacterial agent. It can also be argued that not all spinal infections are self-limiting.

DEFINITION OF TERMS

Hematogenous infections of the spine can be divided, according to site, into two large categories: vertebral osteomyelitis and disc space infections. The latter designation is controversial because it can be argued that, except in children, the disc space lacks a blood supply and therefore most infections involving the disc space are secondary to a primary vertebral body infection. Despite this difference of opinion, it seems clear that disc space infections do occur in two well-recognized groups—children[18] and patients who have undergone operations on the intervertebral disc.[23] Because vertebral osteomyelitis often involves the disc space and contiguous vertebrae, the disc space is the preferred area from which to obtain specimens for microbiologic studies.

96

HISTORY

The early clinical studies of Kulowski[15] and Wilensky[28] led to the establishment of certain clinical categories. A distinction between vertebral osteomyelitis and disc space infections was emphasized by Ghormley et al.[10] Infection of the disc space is clearly a separate entity, both in children and in certain postoperative patients.[7,] First described by Mayer in 1925,[16] the condition was given further importance by the clinical studies of Milone et al.[18] and by Rocco and Eyring.[21]

PATHOGENESIS

ANATOMIC CONSIDERATIONS. If one excludes postoperative disc space infection, one must conclude that infections of the spine are hematogenous. Studies by Coventry et al. indicate that there are vascular channels in the intervertebral disc with blood cells in their lumina during the first three decades.[5] These channels disappear after the third decade. Venous drainage of the vertebrae occurs via valveless veins. Three systems are interconnected: veins of the vertebral body, veins between the spinal canal and the dura, and veins running externally on the vertebral bodies. By injection studies, Batson has shown a connection between these vertebral veins and the veins of the body wall.[1] This subject has been extensively reviewed by Batson and summarized by Waldvogel et al.[27] On the other hand, Wiley and Trueta think that arterial spread is more important than spread through venous channels.[29] Suffice it to say that a blood-borne infection of the disc certainly is possible in children, and certainly in the adult, adequate vascular pathways exist for vertebral body infection.

Batson's observations offer an attractive theory to explain the association of urinary tract and pelvic infections with vertebral osteomyelitis. Reports of this relationship have appeared repeatedly in the literature.[9,12] Since bacteremia is so often noted in these patients, there seems to be little reason to question the connection. Also implicated as sources of vertebral infection are furunculosis,[8] infections of the female pelvic organs,[11] operations on bowel,[11] and even fractures of the mandible.[6]

MICROBIOLOGIC CONSIDERATIONS. Although *Staphylococcus aureus* remains the most common causative organism in vertebral osteomyelitis, gram-negative rods, principally *Escherichia coli* and *Pseudomonas aeruginosa*, and even *Klebsiella*[26] and *Salmonella*[22] have been implicated. Hematogenous disc space infections in children are most commonly due to *S. aureus*, although streptococci, and even pneumococci, have been found as well.

CLINICAL ASPECTS

DISC SPACE INFECTIONS IN CHILDREN. Synonyms for this condition are benign acute osteitis, spondylarthritis of children, nonspecific infections of the disc space, nonspecific spondylitis, and intervertebral disc infections in children.

Symptoms and Signs. An acute onset of back pain may be accompanied by hip or abdominal discomfort. Rocco and Eyring reported the major complaints to be back pain (40%), hip and leg distress (25%), irritability (19%), symptoms due to meningeal irritation (11%), and abdominal complaints (7%).[21] According to Bremner and Neligan,[2] the most constant clinical observation is the insidious onset of symptoms.

Limitation of back motion with lumbar lordosis secondary to muscle spasm can be a frequent physical sign. Fever occurs in about half the patients. On careful examination the child is found to have tenderness in the back with characteristic splinting.

Roentgenographic Changes. Disc space infections are more common in the lower thoracic and lumbar regions, although one case of infection in the cervical region has been reported.[17] Changes are not detectable roentgenographically for at least three to four weeks after onset of symptoms.

Vertebral end-plate irregularity is followed by disc space narrowing (Fig. 8-1). Rocco and Eyring noted herniation of disc material into the body.[21] Sclerosis and new bone formation are seen later, and even intervertebral fusion may occur in older children.

Laboratory Studies. Increased erythrocyte sedimentation rate is the most consistent abnormal observation. Leukocytosis is not a constant finding. The literature contains some evidence of hesitancy about obtaining microbiologic confirmation of infections. Milone, Bianco, and Ivins obtained specimens from six of their seven patients with disc space infection,[18] three by needle biopsy according to the method of Valls et al.[25] Since the disc level is predominately lumbar or thoracolumbar, areas safe for biopsy by needle technique, there is no reason not to pursue a microbiologic diagnosis. The past literature states that disc space infections are most commonly due to staphylococci; however, osteomyelitis due to gram-negative bacilli is on the increase in other anatomic areas, and staphylococci no longer dominate as the overwhelming cause of musculoskeletal infections.

Diagnosis. In any irritable, ill child with symptoms referable to the back, hip, or thigh, the diagnosis of disc space infection should be considered. An increased sedimentation rate and clinical signs of back tenderness lend further support, whereas roentgenographic changes such as disc space irregularity and narrowing are presumptive evidence. Finally, needle biopsy for microbiologic studies should confirm the diagnosis.

Treatment. Except for those complicated by paravertebral abscess, most cases do not require open surgi-

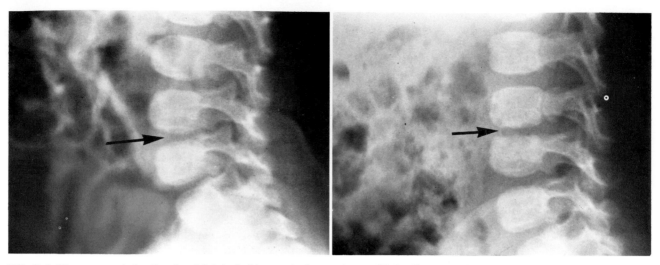

FIG. 8-1. Disc space infection in child. *Left,* At onset of symptoms. *Right,* One month later; narrowing is evident in L3 space.

cal treatment. Menelaus emphasized rest as the most important principle of treatment.[17] He required his patients to remain recumbent until there was no pain or limitation of motion, the sedimentation rate was normal, and roentgenograms indicated that erosion was no longer progressing. A body cast worn for three months and a supporting corset worn thereafter have replaced strict recumbency. Antibacterial agents are discussed on page 100.

VERTEBRAL OSTEOMYELITIS. Synonyms for this infection are pyogenic osteomyelitis, pyogenic infection of the spine, pyogenic vertebral osteomyelitis, and spinal osteomyelitis.

Symptoms and Signs. Back pain, the usual presenting complaint, is more often gradual than abrupt in onset. Nerve root referral is frequent and depends on the level of involvement. Fever is a frequent though elusive sign, often requiring hospitalization for detection. Muscle spasm, often extreme, is noted frequently, as is percussion tenderness over the area of infection.

Roentgenographic Changes. Early changes may be limited to mild narrowing of the disc space, but with time, bone destruction and even loss of vertebral height may occur (Fig. 8-2). Early in the course of the disease, laminograms may be helpful in localizing early destructive changes. Paravertebral swelling or masses can be demonstrated. The lumbar area of the spine is most commonly affected, the thoracic and cervical areas less often in that order.[8,11]

Laboratory Studies. An increased erythrocyte sedimentation rate is a basis for presumptive diagnosis. Since leukocytosis is not common, proof by microbiologic culture is to be encouraged. The lumbar vertebrae or thoracolumbar junctures can be approached safely by percutaneous techniques. Although the methods are time-consuming, they do facilitate bacteriologic diagnosis. In some instances the diagnosis

can be established by blood culture. Causative organisms are listed on page 97.

Diagnosis. In any patient past 50 years of age, back pain, of acute or insidious onset, which becomes constant, is present at night, and is associated with percussion tenderness over the spine, strongly suggests the diagnosis of vertebral osteomyelitis. Corroboration is provided by an increased sedimentation rate, roentgenographic localization, and bacteriologic confirmation. If needle biopsy is difficult or contraindicated (as in certain thoracic lesions), open biopsy may be necessary unless existing evidence is unequivocally diag-

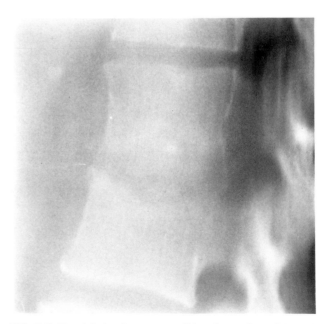

FIG. 8-2. Established osteomyelitis of vertebrae L1 and L2.

nostic (for example, positive blood cultures). The differential diagnosis often includes metastatic malignant disease.

Treatment. Rest is the essential treatment. Until the diagnosis has been established, restriction to bed is adequate therapy. Casts and braces, though condemned by some,[13] can be used effectively. A well-applied plaster cast or brace permits the patient to turn in bed and even to sit or stand for short periods beside the bed. Several months of rest in bed usually are required before signs of improvement—i.e., absence of pain, of fever, and of spasm and a sustained decrease in sedimentation rate—are noted. Operative treatment is reserved for the few instances in which an abscess has formed.[8,11] Antibacterial therapy is discussed on page 100.

POSTOPERATIVE DISC SPACE INFECTION IN ADULTS.

This condition is also known as closed space infection, discitis, and infection of vertebral interspaces.

Cause. Infection of the disc space in adults is almost uniformly secondary to surgical treatment for a protruded or ruptured intervertebral disc, although it can result from discography or inadvertent puncture of the disc during a spinal tap. In the early 1950s, this postoperative complication was not well recognized, but later studies by Ford and Key,[7] Sullivan and associates,[23] and Thibodeau[24] have clearly outlined the clinical picture. Pilgaard, in 1969, estimated the incidence to be 2.8%.

Symptoms and Signs. As early as four to five days or as late as 10 weeks postoperatively, the patient experiences severe pain which he describes as a "spasm in the back." The pain, which is indeed attributable to spasm of the erector spinae muscles, is typically lumbar, with referral to the lower abdomen, groin, or testes.

Fever is not a prominent sign and, in the postoperative patient, its absence may obscure the diagnosis. Neurologic abnormalities are not noted, although such an evaluation is difficult in a postoperative patient.

Roentgenographic Changes. Fuzziness of the epiphyseal plate adjacent to the involved disc is the earliest sign. With narrowing of the disc space, new bone proliferation occurs. These beaks of bone may coalesce as the disc space fills with bone. Fusion of the disc space was observed in 9 of the 11 patients studied by Sullivan et al.[23]

Laboratory Studies. The erythrocyte sedimentation is the most useful routine test, and the rate is uniformly increased. The most important information is obtained by needle biopsy of the involved space. While perhaps not mandatory, it is recommended because it provides microbiologic confirmation and data for proper selection of antibacterials. *S. aureus* is the most commonly found organism.

Treatment. Rest again is the keystone of treatment. Surgical drainage is not necessary unless abscesses develop in the paravertebral area. Antibacterial agents will be discussed on page 100.

PARAVERTEBRAL ABSCESS

It is possible for any of the previously discussed infections to be complicated by paravertebral abscess. An abscess may extend from the retroperitoneal space; this is not uncommon with *Bacteroides* infections.[19] The genesis of most nontuberculous paravertebral abscesses is an infection after an operation for protruded disc or spinal fusion.

Unexplained fever or pain after an interval of relative subsidence of pain postoperatively should alert the clinician to the possibility of a deep-seated infection. A fluctuant mass may be noted in the area of the wound. At this point it is appropriate to aspirate the wound under aseptic conditions and to culture the aspirate. The wisest course is to proceed with the exploration of the wound and evacuation of an infected hematoma. In some instances it is possible to close the wound after four to five days, even in cases of bone graft, and to institute closed suction irrigation of the infected area, especially if the bone is autogenous iliac bone. Although no statistical data are available to support this approach, if done in the early postoperative period it could prevent a serious postoperative complication. Removal of a few sutures and antibacterial treatment are not adequate measures to prevent the worst complication possible—chronic vertebral osteomyelitis complicated by paravertebral abscess.

Once sinus formation occurs, only extensive surgical treatment can correct the problem. Sinograms obtained with radiopaque dye under image intensification are useful in identifying the course of the sinus (Fig. 8-3). Clawson and Dunn advised injection of methylene blue on the day before operation,[4] to guide the surgeon in his dissection. It may be necessary to utilize an anterior approach by exposing the retroperitoneal space. Such an approach has been described by Thibodeau,[24] and

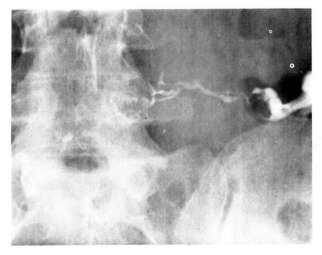

FIG. 8-3. Sinogram of postoperative infection, after spinal fusion, in lumbosacral region.

requires preliminary sinograms and special roentgenographic views including planograms, so that the surgeon can provide adequate drainage. In some instances, closure of the extensive wounds can be accomplished and suction irrigation can be used to prevent re-accumulation of drainage with recurrent sepsis.

ANTIBACTERIAL AGENTS

There has been a significant shift toward an increase in gram-negative bacilli as a cause of osteomyelitis. It is not known whether cell wall-defective bacterial variants, as defined by Charache,[3] play a significant role in the cause of infection or the outcome of therapy.

Because antibacterial agents are so important in treatment, every effort should be made to establish a microbiologic diagnosis. For staphylococcal infections, penicillin remains the treatment of choice for penicillin-sensitive organisms. In penicillin G-resistant infections, a semisynthetic penicillinase-resistant penicillin is preferred. In patients allergic to penicillin, lincomycin, kanamycin, or gentamicin may be considered. Treatment of gram-negative bacilli cannot be standardized because antibiotic susceptibilities of the organisms vary greatly. If the organism is susceptible to ampicillin, carbenicillin, or cephalosporin and the patient is not allergic to these drugs, one of these should be used. Many gram-negative rods, such as *P. aeruginosa*, are not susceptible, and in these cases treatment with kanamycin or gentamicin may be indicated. Brucella infections of the spine are best treated by a combination of streptomycin and tetracycline. Salmonella infections are best treated by either chloramphenicol or ampicillin.

Nephrotoxicity, ototoxicity, and superinfection represent hazards with the use of aminoglycoside drugs. Renal function should be checked twice weekly by measurement of serum creatinine levels. Treatment is continued for a minimum of three to four weeks for any deep-seated bone infection. In many instances, no suitable drug for oral administration is available for long-term treatment. The final guiding concept should be microbiologic identification of the infecting agent and suitable in vitro susceptibility studies.

References

1. Batson OV: The vertebral vein system: Caldwell lecture, 1956. Am J Roentgenol Radium Ther Nucl Med 78:195-212, 1957.
2. Bremner AE, Neligan GA: Benign form of acute osteitis of the spine in young children. Br Med J 1:856-860, 1953.
3. Charache P: Cell wall-defective bacterial variants in human disease. Ann NY Acad Sci 174:903-911, 1970.
4. Clawson DK, Dunn AW: Management of common bacterial infections of bones and joints. J Bone Joint Surg [Am] 49:164-182, 1967.
5. Coventry MB, Ghormley RK, Kernohan JW: The intervertebral disc: its microscopic anatomy and pathology. Part I. Anatomy, development, and physiology. J Bone Joint Surg 27:105-112, 1945.
6. Fein SJ, Torg JS, Mohnac AM, et al: Infection of the cervical spine associated with a fracture of the mandible. J Oral Surg 27:145-149, 1969.
7. Ford LT, Key JA: Postoperative infection of intervertebral disc space. South Med J 48:1295-1302, 1955.
8. Garcia A Jr, Grantham SA: Hematogenous pyogenic vertebral osteomyelitis. J Bone Joint Surg [Am] 42:429-436, 1960.
9. Genster HG, Andersen MJF: Spinal osteomyelitis complicating urinary tract infection. J Urol 107:109-111, 1972.
10. Ghormley RK, Bickel WH, Dickson DD: A study of acute infectious lesions of the intervertebral disks. South Med J 33:347-352, 1940.
11. Griffiths HED, Jones DM: Pyogenic infection of the spine: a review of twenty-eight cases. J Bone Joint Surg [Br] 53:383-391, 1971.
12. Henson SW Jr, Coventry MB: Osteomyelitis of the vertebrae as the result of infection of the urinary tract. Surg Gynecol Obstet 102:207-214, 1956.
13. Jordan MC, Kirby WMM: Pyogenic vertebral osteomyelitis. Arch Intern Med 128:405-410, 1971.
14. Kelly PJ, Weed LA, Lipscomb PR: Infection of tendon sheaths, bursae, joints, and soft tissues by acid-fast bacilli other than tubercle bacilli. J Bone Joint Surg [Am] 45:327-336; 386, 1963.
15. Kulowski J: Pyogenic osteomyelitis of the spine: an analysis and discussion of 102 cases. J Bone Joint Surg 18:343-364, 1936.
16. Mayer L: An unusual case of infection of the spine. J Bone Joint Surg 7:957-967, 1925.
17. Menelaus MB: Discitis: an inflammation affecting the intervertebral discs in children. J Bone Joint Surg [Br] 46:16-23, 1964.
18. Milone FP, Bianco AJ Jr, Ivins JC: Infections of the intervertebral disc in children. JAMA 181:1029-1033, 1962.
19. Nettles JL, Kelly PJ, Martin WJ, et al: Musculoskeletal infections due to bacteroides: a study of eleven cases. J Bone Joint Surg [Am] 51:230-238, 1969.
20. Pilgaard S: Discitis (closed space infection) following removal of lumbar intervertebral disc. J Bone Joint Surg [Am] 51:713-716, 1969.
21. Rocco HD, Eyring EJ: Intervertebral disk infections in children. Am J Dis Child 123:448-451, 1972.
22. Schweitzer G, Hoosen GM, Dunbar JM: Salmonella typhi spondylitis: an unusual presentation. S Afr Med J 45:126-128, 1971.
23. Sullivan CR, Bickel WH, Svien HJ: Infections of vertebral interspaces after operations on intervertebral disks. JAMA 166:1973-1977, 1958.
24. Thibodeau AA: Closed space infection following removal of lumbar intervertebral disc. J Bone Joint Surg [Am] 50:400-410, 1968.
25. Valls J, Ottolenghi CE, Schajowicz F: Aspiration biopsy in diagnosis of lesions of vertebral bodies. JAMA 136:376-382, 1948.
26. Van Wel HJB, Zwijsen HJC: A patient with klebsiella

osteomyelitis of the cervical spine. Arch Chir Neerl *24*:37–42, 1972.

27. Waldvogel FA, Medoff G, Swartz MN: Osteomyelitis: a review of clinical features, therapeutic considerations and unusual aspects. N Engl J Med *282*:316–322, 1970.

28. Wilensky AO: Osteomyelitis of the vertebrae. Ann Surg *89*:561–570; 731–747, 1929.

29. Wiley AM, Trueta J: The vascular anatomy of the spine and its relationship to pyogenic vertebral osteomyelitis. J Bone Joint Surg [Br] *41*:796–809, 1959.

9

Tuberculosis of the Spine

A. R. HODGSON

Tuberculosis of the spine is becoming a rarity in Europe and North America,[11] but it is still a common disease in many parts of the world. This is especially so in Asia and Africa, where the incidence is so great that in many places facilities are inadequate for the treatment of the case load. Despite improved diagnostic procedures, it is sometimes difficult to isolate the organism, and hence to make a diagnosis. It may be necessary to approach the lesion directly, to perform a biopsy and take pus for culture and guinea pig inoculation, in order to make or confirm the diagnosis. Koch's postulates still hold. The earlier the diagnosis is made, the better the prognosis.

Adequate treatment is most important, as inadequate treatment leads to deformity and to paraplegia, both of which have a grave prognosis and lower life expectancy.

PATHOGENESIS

Tuberculosis of the spine is always secondary to an active primary focus elsewhere in the body. This fact dictates that the patient must be examined as a whole and treated as a whole, and not only as a "case of spinal tuberculosis." To find the primary site, orthopaedic surgeons often find it necessary to consult specialists in the treatment of tuberculosis.

The tubercle bacillus that causes skeletal tuberculosis may be one of two types: the human and the bovine varieties. Many years ago, skeletal tuberculosis was attributed to the bovine bacillus in a high proportion of cases in some parts of the world. In 1914, in Edinburgh, Fraser reported that 60% of cases were infected with the bovine form of the bacillus.[9] At that time, public health measures had not been introduced to ensure a supply of clean milk. In 1955, Campos reported that not one case of bovine type bacillus was found in 1,000 cases of bone and joint tuberculosis,[6] and our experience has been the same. In some parts of the world, tuberculosis-like organisms can produce spinal lesions that are clinically tuberculous.

The most common primary focus in tuberculous infection is in the lung and it is called the primary complex. Many authors, including Key,[20] consider that the tubercle bacillus spreads from the lung to the spine by way of the arterial blood supply exactly as the staphylococcus may spread to give rise to osteomyelitis.

Wilkinson[35] has postulated that the paravertebral plexus of veins described by Batson[2] may serve as a pathway of spread to the spine. He says it would also account for the frequency (10%) with which tuberculous lesions in the spine are found to be multiple.

Although some cases of spinal tuberculosis undoubtedly result from arterial hematogenous spread, this route is probably the least common. Without going into this subject too deeply, I have produced experimental spinal tuberculosis in monkeys, guinea pigs, and rats by injecting the kidney and other abdominal or pelvic organs. The animals were sacrificed at 2, 4, 6, 8, 10, and 12 weeks. Serial histologic sections enabled us to trace the spread of the infection to the spine by way of Batson's venous plexus, usually from a focus in the kidney (Fig. 9-1 A and B). It would seem that this is the more usual course of spinal infection, as hematogenous osteomyelitis of the spine occurs in less than 5% of all cases of osteomyelitis, whereas tuberculosis of the spine has occurred in 58.7% of a consecutive series of 1,000 cases of bone and joint tuberculosis seen here in Hong Kong from 1957 to 1958. The only way that this great difference in frequency of spinal involvement in osteomyelitis and tuberculosis can be explained is to postulate another method of spread, which we believe to be by way of Batson's venous plexus (Fig. 9-2).

STATISTICS

In 2,000 consecutive cases of bone and joint tuberculosis seen at the special clinic in Hong Kong between

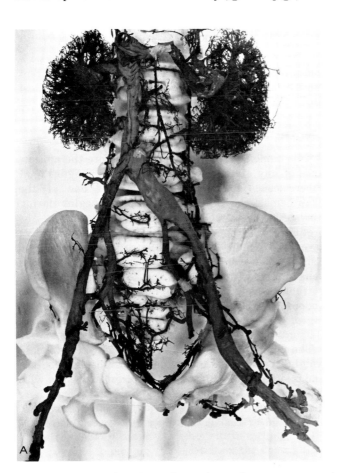 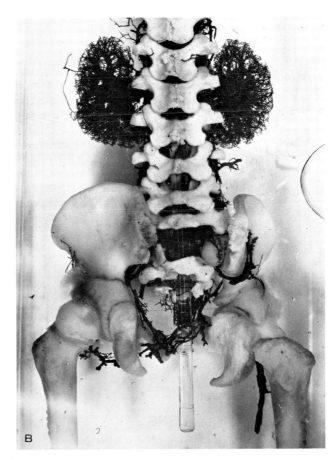

FIG. 9-1. *A*, Anterior view of specimen from one-year-old child in which vena cava has been ligated above renal veins and left renal vein injected with latex. *B*, Posterior view of specimen in *A*. Note rich vertebral venous plexus. (From Hodgson et al.[15])

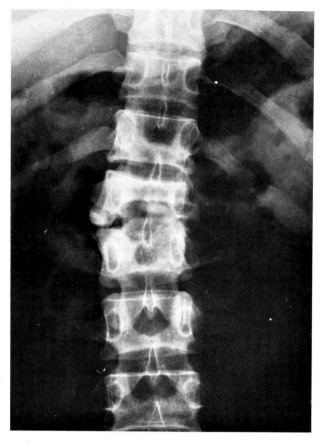

FIG. 9-5. Lateral deviation of spine in tuberculosis of lumbar spine.

bodies and also to the intervertebral discs which become wedged, apex posterior and base anterior (Fig. 9-6).

ATTITUDE. There are various characteristic attitudes at various levels of spinal involvement.

In *cervical disease* there is a lateral inclination of the head so that the ear becomes close to the shoulder, somewhat similar to a congenital torticollis without the rotation. In some cases, the head is extended and in others flexed, where it may be held in the hands. These attitudes are found only in extensive disease.

In *cervicothoracic disease*, the head and neck appear to sink into the thorax, so that the shoulders appear raised and the shoulders and arms are thrown backward. The upper chest is flattened and lower chest and sternum flare outward (Fig. 9-7).

In *thoracic disease*, kyphosis occurs. The ribs become more horizontal and the sternum is displaced forward to give a globular shape to the thorax. The trunk is shortened and the arms appear longer than normal (Fig. 9-8).

In *thoracolumbar and upper lumbar disease*, the abdomen is prominent and the patient stands with legs placed apart. The head and upper part of the body are thrown backward for balance.

In *lumbar disease* slight kyphosis is present with approximation of the ribs to the iliac crests. The abdomen is prominent.

In *lower lumbar disease*, destruction of the fifth lumbar vertebra may produce spondylolisthesis.

Sinus Formation

A sinus may form if the paravertebral abscess ruptures through the skin to discharge its contents. A sinogram is a useful investigation in these cases. The sinus may become secondarily infected, and in the pre-antibiotic era this often led to septicemia and amyloidosis, complications now rarely seen. The discharge from a sinus should always be cultured and sensitivity tests performed.

In some cases the contents of the abscess penetrate an organ and are discharged by way of that organ. By far the most important and most likely organ to be penetrated is the lung. This condition was described in detail in 1968 by Yau and Hodgson,[36] who found 32 cases of lung penetration in 327 consecutive cases of tuberculosis of the thoracic spine.

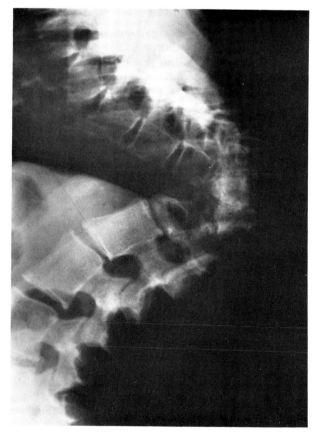

FIG. 9-6. Tuberculosis of spine with kyphosis. Note reversal of height/width ratio of vertebral bodies and wedging of intervertebral discs.

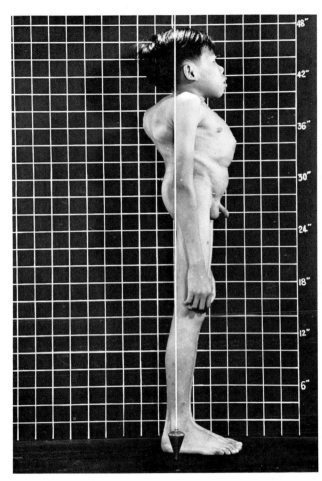

FIG. 9-7. Marked kyphosis with tuberculosis of mid-thoracic spine.

Clinical Tests

YIELDING OF THE SPINE UPON PRESSURE. In the destructive stage of the disease, the palm of the hand is placed upon the apex of the kyphosis and, upon firm pressure, the spine may be felt to spring and give under the examiner's hand. The more vertebral bodies involved in the disease process the greater the degree of yielding. As healing and repair occur, a definite feeling of resistance may be felt, which becomes complete when bony healing has occurred.

TEST FOR HEALING OR BONY UNION. Lippmann, in 1932, introduced a test for the degree of union in a fracture.[21] He showed that a stethoscope placed over the superficial surface of one end of a long bone receives the sound of a finger tap at the other end. In a fracture of the bone this sound is interrupted, giving a sound similar to that effected by percussion of a cracked pot. As healing progresses, the transmitted sounds approach the normal pitch and amplitude.

We have used this test as an indication of healing of tuberculosis of the spine and after incorporation of an anterior graft. We place the stethoscope upon the spinous process of the vertebrae at one end of the diseased area and percuss the spinous process at the other end. We find, with experience, that this is a useful indication of the state of healing of graft or disease.

"LIVING PATHOLOGY"

The term "living pathology," as applied to spinal tuberculosis, refers to the pathologic features noted at operation, which differ greatly from the postmortem appearance. In the latter, disease is usually terminal and the role of the blood supply and of body stresses cannot be appreciated. "Living pathology" is concerned mainly with the abscess and its contents, although other secondary changes may occur in advanced disease.

Granuloma

Granulation tissue forms in an early stage of tuberculous infection and is found to be closely associated with veins. As the vertebral bodies have a much larger

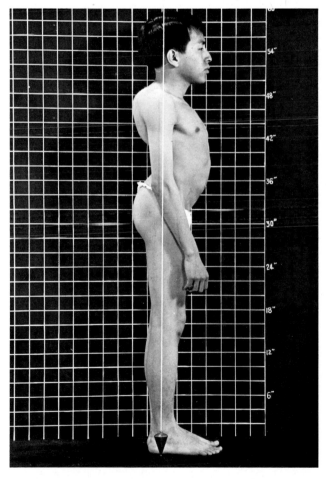

FIG. 9-8. Marked kyphosis with tuberculosis of high thoracic spine.

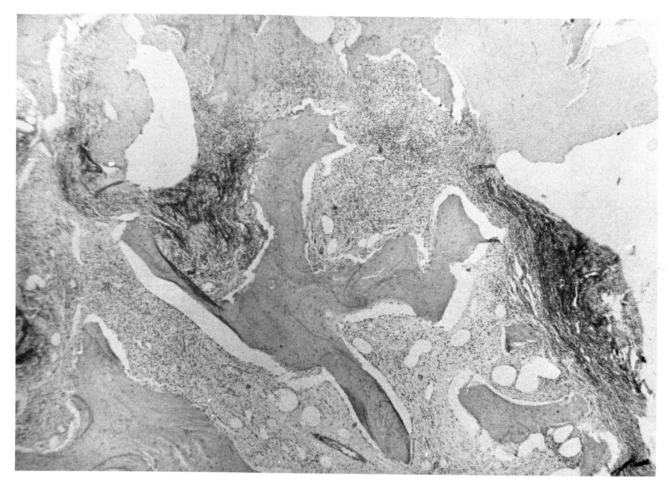

FIG. 9-9. Granulation tissue permeates this vertebral body.

venous than arterial circulation, the vertebral body may be permeated by tuberculous granulation tissue (Fig. 9-9) and form a vertebral granuloma. This granuloma may weaken the vertebral body to such an extent that it will collapse in a manner similar to the collapse associated with neoplasia, a condition we have named "concertina collapse"[15] (Fig. 9-10 A, B). Granulation tissue also is found lining the abscess wall and around the vertebral veins in the spinal canal, and this has been called "pachymeningitis externe" by Michaud.[23] This granulation tissue may involve the dura and cord to produce a tuberculous myelitis and is a cause of Pott's paraplegia.

Pus

Pus is formed by the breakdown of granulation tissue and, in the early stages of the disease, it is found within the granulation tissue. It is fluid in the early stages, solid and caseous later. It may be copious, and quantities over 1,000 cc. are not uncommon. In the thoracic region, the paravertebral pus strips up the paraverte-

bral ligaments and deprives the vertebral body of its peripheral blood supply, causing the extensive disease so often found in this region, and also the aneurysmal syndrome. This pus may track in various directions and ultimately be discharged through the skin, at which time other organisms may invade the sinus tract and the lesion. Sloughs may be contained within the pus.

Sequestra

We have found sequestra in the diseased focus, except in cases of granuloma. They are usually large in adults, measuring up to 1½ to 2 inches (Fig. 9-11), but tend to be small in children, and easy to overlook. As in osteomyelitis, their presence leads to chronicity.

Sequestrated Discs

The intervertebral disc, being avascular, tends to resist the disease, and involvement is peripheral. Therefore the disc easily becomes sequestrated, and often is retropulsed onto the spinal cord, with bony sequestra, to

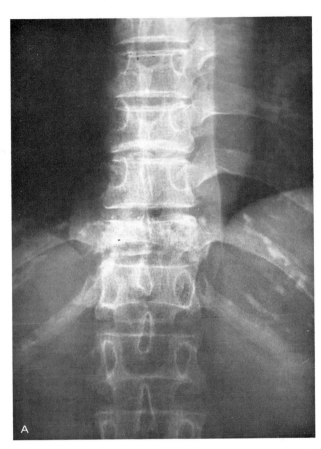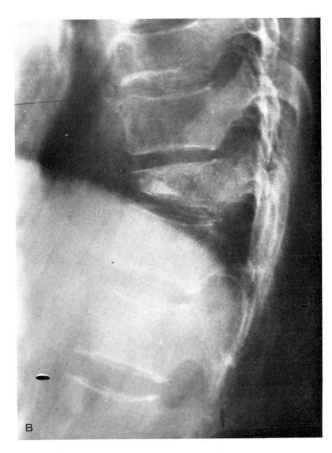

FIG. 9-10. Concertina collapse. *A,* Anteroposterior view; *B,* lateral view.

produce pressure upon the spinal cord and paraplegia. Narrowing of the intervertebral joint, as noted on x-ray examination, is an early sign of tuberculosis; this narrowing is not due to involvement of the disc by the disease, but to interference with the nutrition of the disc owing to involvement of the vertebral bodies on either side of the disc. Calcification of the nucleus pulposus of the intervertebral disc may occur either above or below the lesion.

Increased Bony Density of the Vertebral Body (Revascular Phenomenon)

This can be seen radiographically, particularly in the lumbar region, as marked increased density (Fig. 9-12). This increase in density is due to a great increase in width of the bony trabeculae in the vertebral bodies. In the active stage of the disease, the trabeculae are surrounded by granulation tissue and pus and lose their blood supply. If the disease heals, new bone grows or flows along these avascular trabeculae, thickening the trabeculae with accumulation of new bone on either side of dead bone, a state of affairs that we have named "revascular phenomenon."

Abscess Wall

In the active stage, the abscess wall is vascular and is lined with granulation tissue; in the healed phase it is composed of fibrous tissue, which may be as much as an inch in thickness.

Secondary Changes

COMPENSATORY LORDOSIS. As a result of the destruction of the vertebral bodies, a kyphotic deformity usually develops, although in the lower thoracic and lumbar vertebrae a lateral tilt may occur as a result of unilateral destruction of the vertebral body.

If kyphosis occurs in a growing child, a compensatory lordosis occurs above and below, the deformity owing to changes in the vertebral bodies and in the intervertebral discs. The vertebral bodies reverse their height/width ratio; normally the vertebra has a greater width than height, but this is reversed. The nucleus pulposus of the intervertebral disc becomes displaced anteriorly, and the disc is wedged from before back, with the base of the wedge anterior.

CHANGES IN THE RIBS. In the presence of a severe kyphosis in the thoracic area, with destruction of

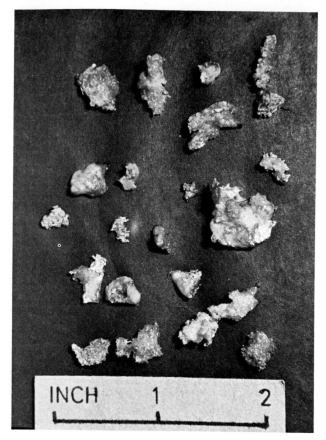

FIG. 9-11. Collection of sequestra removed from patient with tuberculosis of spine.

several vertebral bodies, the posterior portions of the ribs approximate and become exposed to pressure, which changes their shape.

It will be appreciated from the "living pathology" that there is an avascular lesion within the abscess wall. The abscess wall is vascular and the antibiotics pen-

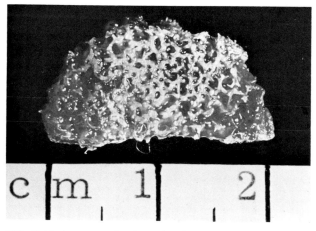

FIG. 9-12. Increase in size of trabeculae here indicates revascular phenomenon.

etrate in adequate concentrations up to the wall, but they have to diffuse into the avascular contents of the abscess, which we have described.

RADIOGRAPHIC APPEARANCE

Space precludes detailed description of the many radiographic appearances that this disease may produce. Those interested in such a description should consult Hodgson et al.[15]

The Abscess and Its Contents

The paravertebral abscess has a different appearance, according to the site involved. It is best seen in the thoracic region, which is fortunate, since in most cases this site is involved. Here it may be pyramidal, globular, unilateral, fusiform (pointed on one side, indicating lung penetration), or double.

The contents of the abscess seen on x-ray examination are sequestra, pus, and increased vertebral density, indicating revascular phenomena.

Changes in the Spine Itself

These changes include demonstration of the site of the disease (tomography is useful); concertina collapse of the vertebral body; aneurysmal syndrome; lateral deviation; bony bridging; reversal of the height/width ratio of the vertebral bodies and wedging of the intervertebral disc; calcification of the intervertebral disc; and changes in the ribs.

Special radiographic investigations which are useful include tomography, myelography, venography, lymphangiography, and arteriography.

DIFFERENTIAL DIAGNOSIS

Usually there is little difficulty in diagnosing tuberculosis of the spine. However, with a decreasing frequency of the disease in certain countries, the disease is unfamiliar and this makes diagnosis more difficult. Conditions that may cause confusion with Pott's disease are: low-grade pyogenic infection, acute hematogenous osteomyelitis, brucellosis and typhoid fever, eosinophilic granuloma, congenital anomalies, Schmorl's nodes, Scheuermann's disease, kyphoscoliosis and scoliosis, intervertebral disc lesion, retrospondylolisthesis, spondylosis, neoplasms, primary and secondary, multiple myeloma, hemangioma, Hodgkin's disease, leukemia, and infection by other organisms resembling the tubercle bacillus (Batty strain).

Space precludes details of how to make the diagnosis. However, if this list of conditions is borne in mind and considered carefully, most of them can be excluded by careful examination of the patient and, when necessary, biopsy, or by carrying out Koch's postulates in the case of infections. The best way is to diagnose the tuberculosis of the spine bacteriologically and pathologically.

TREATMENT

In the last 20 years or so the approach to treatment of tuberculosis of the spine has changed greatly. Although there is no agreement at present, there are two main schools: those who treat the condition conservatively throughout, and those who combine removal of the abscess with conservative treatment, usually including anterior interbody fusion. Whatever the treatment, it should not be instituted until the diagnosis is made by pathologic and bacteriologic means, including guinea pig inoculation and sensitivity tests.

Conservative Treatment

Conservative treatment consists in hospitalization and application of the principles of HO Thomas: rest —*enforced, uninterrupted, and prolonged.*[11] The principles of the sanatorium regime, including adequate nutrition with a high protein diet, adequate fresh air, and exposure to sunlight, are important. To this classic treatment may be added the antituberculosis drugs: the first-line drugs—streptomycin, para-aminosalicylic acid, and isoniazid—and the second-line drugs, which are used to replace the first-line drugs in cases of drug resistance. There is no doubt that healing may take place with conservative treatment alone; I have even seen healing without any treatment at all. The point is—what percentage will heal on conservative treatment alone. Reliable figures are unobtainable at this time, and it is hoped that they will be available soon.

Chemotherapy, combined with ambulation and the wearing of a plaster jacket, has produced poor results in our hands. For this reason we have adopted a radical surgical approach to the problem.

Costotransversectomy

It appears that this operation was first suggested by Boekel in 1882,[3] and used by Vincent[33] and by Auffet[1] in 1892, and by others later.

In 1888, Nasilov described an approach to the esophagus which was similar,[24] and this was quoted by Quénu and Hartman in 1891.[28] It appears that this approach was carried out at postmortem examination in all these cases.

Schaeffer described two cases of lumbar spinal tuberculosis. In one of these cases the procedure extended to the tenth dorsal vertebra, at which point dead bone was removed and the abscess drained.[29] In still another case the lesion was in the cervical region. These procedures were not true costotransversectomies.

Vincent, in an excellent paper, reported his efforts to remove the tuberculous disease of the spine in cases of Pott's paraplegia.[33] He used a bilateral costotransversectomy on either side of the kyphosis and a through-and-through drain, which passed through the diseased area. This procedure became popular in the following decade.

Bryant, in 1895, gave a good account of the surgical anatomy,[5] and Stoyanov, in 1899, collected 15 cases.[31] Menard and many others performed this procedure,[22] but the operation was discarded because of the high mortality rates from secondary infection. A further argument against operative treatment was the necessity to segregate patients with tuberculosis in sanatoria, a measure that usually separated them, geographically, from surgeons. From the early years of this century until the 1940s, only the exceptional surgeon attacked the focus in a tuberculous spine. Ito et al. and members of the Vienna school were among these exceptions.[18]

In 1933, Capener introduced what he called lateral rhachiotomy,[7] and others, particularly Griffiths, Seddon, and Roaf, used a similar approach and called it anterolateral approach in the treatment of Pott's paraplegia.[10] With the introduction of antibiotics in the late forties and early fifties, a direct surgical approach on the lesion in spinal tuberculosis became commonplace, and Wilkinson,[34] Kastert,[19] and Orell[25] became the leaders in the use of the costovertebral approach as a means of eradicating the tuberculous focus.

Transthoracic Approach

Hodgson and Stock introduced this approach to the spine in 1956 to enable them to perform a radical clearance of the abscess and its contents in the extensive lesions seen in tuberculous spines at that time.[14] The average number of vertebrae involved in the first 100 cases operated upon was 3.4, and as many as eight thoracic vertebrae were removed. Not only was the transthoracic approach used, but when necessary it was extended into the lumbar region by detaching the diaphragm. The cervical spine was approached by the lateral route. The lumbar spine was approached by the retroperitoneal route and, in some cases of disease in the lower lumbar and upper sacral regions, by a transperitoneal route.

Fang and Ong introduced a transoral approach to C1-C2 and a transthyrohyoid approach to C2-C4.[8] This region can be reached from a lateral approach.

Technique of Anterior Fusion

Anterior fusion was described in 1956[14] and we should like to give a short description here. An anterior approach is used, using one of the approaches to the spine described in previous articles[8a]

There are two principles prescribed in present day treatment of spinal tuberculosis; the first is to eradicate all the avascular contents of the abscess, which are pus (may be fluid or caseous), sequestrated intervertebral discs, bony sequestra, sloughs, and granulation tissue, particularly lying on the dura mater and also lining the abscess. Avascular bone should also be removed so as to leave a raw, bleeding bed into which the antibiotics can reach in adequate concentration to sterilize the abscess (Fig. 9-13). This is the most important part of the operation and it is useful, in many instances, to irrigate the abscess with sterile saline, as this demonstrates pockets of disease and itself has a cleaning action on the abscess. It is very important that this portion of the operation be carefully performed and completed, great care being taken to make sure that disease is not left behind.

The next portion of the operation is the anterior fusion. Any autogenous bone transplant may be used, but we have found it most convenient to use the rib which had been removed in the cases with thoracic disease when the anterior approach was performed. The rib is a good graft, but it has to be carefully placed. It is usual to mortice the first rib graft carefully into the bone of the vertebral body above and the vertebral body below, and it is usually possible to spring the kyphotic deformity open so that this graft is under compression. In addition, springing the kyphotic deformity open reduces the kyphotic deformity. Then at least four, and possibly more, other rib grafts are placed around this first key graft to bridge the gap between the healthy vertebra on the upper side of the lesion and the healthy vertebra on the lower side of the lesion. As these grafts cannot be firmly fixed in the manner of the key graft, it is usual to lock them to the key graft by means of two double catgut sutures, one at the top end and one at the bottom end of the graft, so as to make them rather like a faggot of wood.

The wound is now closed and adequate underwater drainage performed, especially in cases which have a thoracotomy performed. If the anterior graft bridges two vertebral bodies or more, it is usual to supplement this procedure with a posterior fusion.

The surprising results of this procedure in the first 300 cases were reported in 1964 (Tables 9-1 to 9-6).

It was concluded that this procedure produced the greatest percentage of cures in the shortest time.

Laminectomy

Griffiths et al. emphasized that this is a dangerous operation to perform in cases of Pott's paraplegia.[10] They stated "It is impossible to expose and to remove an anterior extradural compressing agent by a posterior extradural approach. In addition, it destroys the stability of the posterior elements, further kyphosis occurs, and further extradural pressure is exerted upon the anterior surface of the dura and cord. This may convert a simple Pott's disease into a Pott's paraplegia,

TABLE 9-1. Results in 300 Cases of Anterior Fusion

	Number	%
Lost to follow-up	15	5
Not grafted	9	3
Recurrence of disease	10	3.3
Non-union	12	4
Died	14	4.7
Fused on radiologic examination	240	80
Total cases	300	

From Hodgson AR.[14]

TABLE 9-2. Fusion Time as Determined by Radiographic Findings

Average	22.2 months
Shortest	7 months
Longest	42 months

TABLE 9-3. End Results in 125 Cases of Paraplegia

Complete recovery	89
Partial recovery	20
No recovery	4
Died	8
No follow-up	4
Total	125

TABLE 9-4. Causes of Death

	Number
Poor risk, extensive pulmonary and spinal tbc	9
Pulmonary edema due to over-transfusion of saline	1
Hepatic failure seven days after cholecystectomy (after recovery from spinal fusion)	1
Bilateral pneumonia	2
Lung collapse and bronchopneumonia (second postoperative day)	1
Total	14 (4.7%)

TABLE 9-5. Segmental Distribution of Lesions in 300 Cases of Pott's Disease

5	Cervical
4	Cervicothoracic
77	Lumbar
4	Double lesions
181	Entire thoracic
29	Thoracolumbar

TABLE 9-6. Age Incidence of 300 Cases

Up to 5 years	129 cases	43%
6 to 10 years	80 cases	27%
11 to 70 years	91 cases	30%

and a partial Pott's paraplegia into a complete one. It is only in the occasional case, when either tuberculosis of the posterior elements exists or tuberculous granulation tissue presses upon the posterior columns, that this approach is indicated and only in the presence of an intact and stable anterior body."

POTT'S PARAPLEGIA

This condition occasionally may be a presenting sign in tuberculosis of the spine. Despite its classic description by Pott in 1779 and again in 1782,[26,27] the cause of the paraplegia has usually been poorly understood. An exception to this was Michaud,[23] who described the condition well and in great detail. On the basis of our observations during operation, we suggest the following classification.[13]

Classification

It is easy to determine at operation whether the disease is active or healed, and we have divided the causes into two main groups: group A, or paraplegia of active disease, and group B, paraplegia of healed disease.[16,17]

GROUP A. The causes of group A may be subdivided into three main subgroups: (1) external pressure on the spinal cord; (2) tuberculous infection penetrating the dura and involving the spinal cord; and (3) thrombosis of the arterial supply to the spinal cord (only one report exists in the literature, Seddon's in 1935).[30]

External Pressure on the Spinal Cord. Pressure on the spinal cord that could ultimately result in paraplegia can be attributed to one or several of the following conditions:

1. *Pressure of the pus within the abscess.* Of necessity the pus must be fluid to exert pressure, though caseous pus may be pressed back upon the cord in some cases. We have attempted to measure the pressure exerted by fluid pus and we have obtained readings of 15 to 20 mm. of mercury in the thoracic paravertebral abscess.

2. *Bone Sequestra.* It is common to find bony sequestra in the contents of the abscess. In some cases of paraplegia they are retropulsed or squeezed onto the cord and cause pressure on it. When they are removed they leave an imprint on the cord.

3. *Sequestrated Intervertebral Disc.* We have found the intervertebral disc resistant to the tuberculous infection. When vertebral bodies on either side of the disc are destroyed, the disc becomes loose and, like the

bony sequestrum, may be retropulsed upon the spinal cord.

4. *Granulation Tissue.* As we have seen, tuberculous granulation tissue forms in the spinal canal extradurally. Its bulk may press upon the cord and distort it (Fig. 9-2).

5. *Concertina Collapse.* This occurs when a single vertebral body is permeated by granulation tissue; it may be weakened to such an extent that it collapses in a fashion similar to the collapse of a vertebral body involved by a neoplasm.

6. *Subluxations and Dislocations.* These occur where there has been destruction of two or more vertebral bodies, and they are most common at the cervicothoracic and thoracolumbar parts of the spine. The cord is subjected to pressure in these cases.

7. *Tuberculosis of the Neural Arch.* This rare cause of paraplegia is characterized by predominance of sensory impairment as opposed to the more usual motor impairment.

Penetration of the Dura Mater. Penetration of the dura mater as a cause of paraplegia was described by Michaud.[23] In 1967, my colleagues and I described nine consecutive cases of tuberculosis of the spine without paraplegia in which routine dural biopsies were performed. In two of these cases, complete dural penetration had occurred.

When the cord becomes involved in the tuberculous infection, tuberculous meningomyelitis occurs. This condition may be differentiated clinically from a pure pressure paraplegia by the much greater spasticity exhibited. Spasticity in pressure paraplegia is usually mild. Examination of the spinal fluid may show increase in cells and protein, and a myelogram can be diagnostic. Meningomyelitis also may be associated with a pure pressure paraplegia. The prognosis in paraplegia secondary to meningomyelitis is poor in either case.

GROUP B. The causes of group B may be subdivided into two main subgroups.

Transection of the spinal cord by a bony bridge. As described by Bouvier in 1958,[4] and by Griffiths, Seddon and Roaf in 1956,[10] this bony bridge is produced in the healing phase. In the presence of an increasing kyphosis, the soft new bone is retropulsed into the spinal canal where it transects the spinal cord. Prognosis is poor.

Constriction of the cord by the surrounding granulation tissue. As healing takes place, the granulation tissue surrounding the cord becomes fibrous tissue and this constricts the cord. Prognosis is poor.

Frequency and Prognosis

The group in which penetration of the dura mater is the cause forms about 75% of cases of Pott's paraplegia, and it has a good prognosis. The others form the remaining 25% of cases and have a poor prognosis. The prognosis is better in children than in adults, and even in adults some recovery may be expected over the years.

Treatment

It may be a cliché to state that the proper treatment of Pott's paraplegia is the proper treatment of Pott's disease. In other words, if Pott's disease were treated according to accepted principles, fewer cases of paraplegia would develop. However, when the latter does develop, the classic principles of treatment of tuberculosis of the spine should still be applied, but with a few additions.

It is most important to expose the cord for the entire diseased area and to remove the granulation tissue from the dura. If the dura is seen to pulsate, all is well; if it does not pulsate, aspiration of cerebrospinal fluid through a small needle should be attempted. If this fails, we do not hesitate to open the dura and examine the cord. We have found small tuberculous abscesses (tuberculoma) within the substance of the cord, but it is more usual to find an inflammatory meningomyelitis with adhesion between the meninges and the cord, and loculation of the cerebrospinal fluid.

References

1. Auffet: De l'intervention chirurgicale dans les affections du rachis. Arch Med Nav *57:*379-399, 1892.
2. Batson DV: The function of the vertebral veins and their role in the spread of metastasis. Ann Surg *112:*138, 1940.
3. Boeckel J: Fragments de Chirurgie Antiseptique. Paris, 1882, p. 462.
4. Bouvier H: Leçons Cliniques sur les Maladies Chroniques de l'Appareil Locomoteur. Paris, 1858.
5. Bryant JD: The surgical technique of entry to the posterior mediastinum. Trans Am Surg Assn *XIII:*443-445, Philadelphia, 1895.
6. Campos OP: Bone and joint tuberculosis and its treatment. A general review, clinical and statistical, of tuberculosis in Brazil. J Bone Jt Surg *37A:*937-966, 1955.
7. Capener N: The evolution of lateral rhachiotomy. J Bone Jt Surg *36B:*173, 1954.
8. Fang HSY, Ong GB: Direct approach to the upper cervical spine. J Bone Jt Surg *44A:*1588, 1962.
8a. Fang HSY, Ong GB, Hodgson AR: Anterior spinal fusion. The operative approaches. Clin Orthop *35:*16-33, 1964.
9. Fraser J: Tuberculosis of the Bones and Joints in Children. London, Black, 1914.
10. Griffiths DL, Seddon HJ, Roaf R: Pott's Paraplegia. London, Oxford University Press, 1956.
11. Hasche-Klünder R, Schwab R: Zum tuberkulosisschicksal von knochen—und gelenktuberkulose—kranken. Tuberkulosearzt *8:*308, 1954.
12. Hodgson AR: Report of the findings and results in 300 cases of Pott's disease treated by anterior fusion. J Western Pacific Orth Assn *1:*3-7, March, 1964.
13. Hodgson AR, Skinsnes OK, Leong CY: The pathogenesis of Pott's Paraplegia. J Bone Jt Surg *49A:*1147-1156, 1967.
14. Hodgson AR, Stock FE: Anterior spinal fusion. A preliminary communication on the radical treatment of Pott's disease and Pott's paraplegia. Brit J Surg *185:*266-276, 1956.
15. Hodgson AR, Wong W, Yau A: X-ray Appearances of Tuberculosis of the Spine. Springfield, Charles C Thomas, 1969.
16. Hodgson AR, Yau A: Pott's paraplegia: A classification based upon the living pathology. Paraplegia *51:*1-16, 1967.
17. Hodgson AR, Yau A, Kwon JS, Kim D: A clinical study of 100 consecutive cases of Pott's paraplegia. Clin Orthop *36:*128-150, 1964.
18. Ito H, Tsuchiya Y, Asami G: A new radical operation for Pott's disease. J Bone Jt Surg *16:*499, 1934.
19. Kastert J: Eine neue chirurgische methode zur behandlung der wirbelsäulen-tuberkulose. Chirurg *21:*691, 1950.
20. Key JA: The pathology of tuberculosis of the spine. J Bone Jt Surg *22:*799-806, 1940.
21. Lippmann RK: The use of auscultatory percussion for the examination of fractures. J Bone Jt Surg *14:*118, 1932.
22. Menard V: Etude Practique sur le Mal de Pott. Paris, Masson et Cie, 1900.
23. Michaud JA: Sur le Meningite de la Myelite dans la Mal Vertebrale. Thèse de Paris, 1871.
24. Nasilov II: Oesophagotomia et resectio oesophagi endothoracica. Vrach *9:*481-482, 1888. (Abstracted in Am Surg *8:*308, 1888.)
25. Orell S: The radical treatment of bone and joint tuberculosis. Acta Ortho Scand *21:*189, 1951.
26. Pott P: Remarks on that Kind of Palsy of the Lower Limbs Which is Frequently Found to Accompany a Curvature of the Spine and is Supposed to be Caused by it, Together with its Method of Cure. London, 1779.
27. Pott P: Further Remarks on the Useless State of the Lower Limbs in Consequence of a Curvature of the Spine. London, 1782.
28. Quénu, H: Des voies de pénétration chirurgicale dans le médiastin postereur. Bull Soc Chirurgie *17:*82-85, Paris, 1891.
29. Schaeffer FC: Vertebral surgery with a report of three cases and a new method of operating in the dorsal region. JAMA *17:*943-946, 1891.
30. Seddon HJ: Pott's paraplegia: prognosis and treatment. Brit J Surg *22:*769-799, 1935.
31. Stoyanov PN: Les interventions chirurgicales sur le médiastin posterior et les organes y contenus; état actuel de la québstion. Rev Chir *19:*388-404, 1899.
32. Thomas HO: Diseases of the Hip, Knee and Ankle Joints. 2nd ed. Liverpool, T Dobb and Company, 1876.
33. Vincent E: Contribution à la chirurgie rachidienne du drainage vertébral dans le mal de Pott. Rev Chir *12:*273-294, 1892.
34. Wilkinson MC: Curretage of tuberculous vertebral disease in the treatment of spinal caries. Proc Roy Soc Med *43:*114, 1950.
35. Wilkinson MC: Non-respiratory tuberculosis. Symposium of Tuberculosis. Edited by FRG Heaf. London, Cassell and Company, 1957, p. 537.
36. Yau A, Hodgson AR: Penetration of the lung by the paravertebral abscess in tuberculosis of the spine. J Bone Jt Surg *50A:*243-254, 1968.

Section IV

Operative Approaches

Introduction

DANIEL RUGE

THE SEARCH for the perfect approach to the spine has been intensive and often innovative.

The posterior approach is not the most direct approach to every lesion of the spine, spinal cord, and cauda equina, but will probably continue to be the most frequently employed because of its applicability from the foramen magnum to the sacrum. Other advantages are the absence of major vessels, nerves, and viscera on the posterior aspect of the spine and the possibility of extending incisions without adversely affecting vertebral stability. The technique of laminectomy is presented in Chapter 10. The same approach gives access for the standard lumbar spinal fusion described in Chapter 15, and for the operation of osteotomy described in Chapter 18.

The head and upper neck are major obstacles to the ventral approach of the upper cervical vertebrae. Chapter 11 gives descriptions of ventral transoral and anterior neck approaches. The applicability for definitive operation on the spine and spinal cord is rare, and the distance restricts the surgeon considerably. It is, however, an avenue which may be useful for biopsy and stabilization procedures.

The lower cervical spine has escaped the impediment of the mandible but the rather fixed trachea, esophagus, and thyroid force modification of an anterior approach to the side—hence the anterolateral approach serves access to the lower cervical vertebrae. Chapter 12 contains descriptions of this approach which is medial to the sternomastoid muscle, the carotid artery, interval jugular vein, and vagus nerve and lateral to the trachea, esophagus, and thyroid.

The so-called lateral approach to the cervical spine adapted by Verbiest begins as an anterolateral approach, but access to the lateral aspect of the cervical spine is possible if the sternocleidomastoid muscle and the carotid sheath with its contents are mobilized adequately to retract them far laterally. Chapter 13 contains steps which permit one to enlarge the scope of the popular anterolateral approach to include otherwise inaccessible lateral structures.

In Chapter 14, Larson has depicted operations which expose lateral and anterior spinal structures in the thoracic and lumbar areas. Even though the initial approach is from the posterior aspect, he has outlined procedures which give access to lateral and ventral areas of the spine. He has not recommended this exposure for dealing with intradural problems.

Chapters 15, 16, and 17 deal with stabilization operations for the lumbar spine. The exposures for the paraspinal fusion and anterior body fusion are unique, and the writers have given detailed instructions for access to the spine.

Chapter 18 provides a detailed description of the osteotomy designed to correct flexion deformities.

10

Laminectomy

DANIEL RUGE

A SURGICAL procedure on the dorsal aspect of the spine is a major operation and generally requires that the patient be given inhalation anesthesia. In the planning of such a procedure, the needs of the patient and the anesthesiologist, as well as those of the surgeon, must be considered.

The patient's needs include matters of safety related to respiration, circulation, and protection of the eyes and skin, to name only a few. The anesthesiologist is responsible for meeting some of these needs, and therefore requires easy access to the patient.

POSITION

A frame used for traction occasionally doubles as an operating table for the patient with an unstable or fractured spine. Traction actually facilitates proper positioning and alignment, removes some of the awkwardness of the patient's prone position, and permits operation without unusual movement of the spine.

Although some surgeons prefer their patients to be prone for all posterior spinal operations, the sitting position is gaining acceptance for procedures on the cervical and upper thoracic spine. Forward flexion facilitates interlaminar exposure and removal or decompression of a lateral mass, but should be avoided if there is a midline lesion, either ventral or dorsal to the spinal cord.

Elevation and wrapping of the lower extremities reduces the danger of air emboli, but constant awareness of this complication is important.

Thoracic, lumbar, and sacral operations may be performed with the

117

patient lying on his side; however, frames that support the anterior torso and thighs also permit the patient to lie prone. They permit good respiratory excursion and reduce venous pressure. The lumbar lordosis is also removed, and this facilitates dissection of soft tissue and laminae.

Operation

The skin of the back is coarse and thick and contains many sebaceous glands and hair follicles, making thorough cleansing essential. The cleansing procedure used depends on the preference of the individual surgeon, but we employ the same technique for cleansing the patient's skin as the surgeon uses for his own hands. Draping covers all but the area to be incised.

A vertical incision placed accurately over the spinous processes permits modification in either direction should the need arise. Occasionally, a transverse incision may be preferred to avoid excessive scarring.

Since there are not many satisfactory superficial landmarks, it might be helpful, at the time of myelography or other radiologic examination, to indicate on the skin the precise site for incision.

The dorsal configuration of atlas and axis is distinct and quite invariable, and serves as a point of reference in the upper cervical spine. We have not found the presence of bifid spines to be consistent enough to serve as a reliable landmark. Unless there is a developmental anomaly, one can use the dorsal shape of the laminae of C7 and T1 as landmarks. When viewed or palpated, the laminae of C7 are convex, whereas the laminae of T1 are concave. It is essential to see *both* C7 and T1 to appreciate this anatomic aid; the configuration of one alone cannot serve as a guide, because the adjacent cervical laminae resemble C7 and the adjacent thoracic laminae resemble T1. This anatomic feature has proved to be so reliable that radiologic verification, procedures for which are awkward at best, has not been necessary.

Unfortunately, there is no satisfactory anatomic landmark in the remainder of the thoracic and lumbar spine except for the lumbosacral junction. The mobility

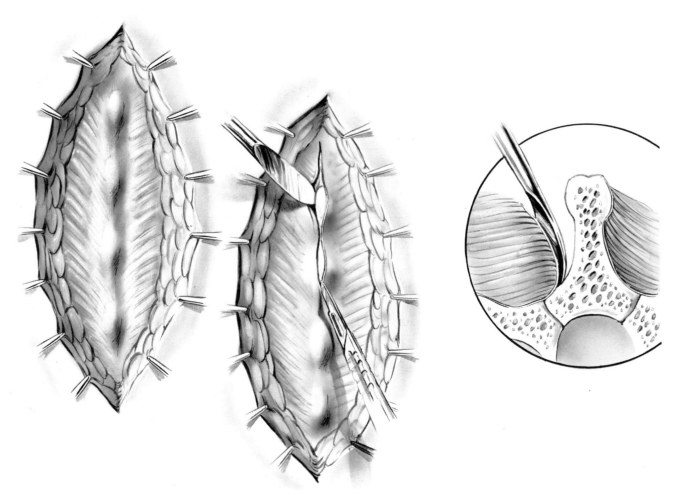

FIG. 10-1. Incision of skin, subcutaneous tissue and fascia is followed by subperiosteal separation of muscles from spinous processes and laminae.

of the lumbar spinous process adjacent to the immobile sacrum and the presence of intervening ligamentum flavum characterize the junction of L5 and S1 (or the inferior lumbar spine and the sacrum).

After the vertical incision has been carried to the fascia, rows of hemostats placed in the adipose fibrous tissue, when turned back, provide hemostasis and separate the skin from contact with the deep tissues. Further incision is made directly over the spinous processes through the periosteum to expose bone.

Subperiosteal Dissection

When the demarcation between periosteum and bone is visible, a periosteal elevator is used to separate the muscles from the spinous processes and laminae without producing hemorrhage or injury to the muscles. Cutting is against the bone—not the soft tissues. Inserting sponges with the elevator aids in retraction and hemostasis.

Exposure

Self-retaining retractors are placed to ensure good exposure and continued hemostasis.

Removal of Spinous Process and Laminae

The spinous processes and interspinous ligaments are easily removed with rongeurs, and the lamina is removed prior to removal of ligamentum flavum. This is a crucial point in the performance of laminectomy; one should remove the lamina from below upward and try to develop a satisfactory cleavage between the undersurface of the lamina and the ligamentum flavum attached to it.

Completion of laminectomy includes removal of the exposed ligamentum flavum, but preservation of extradural fat, particularly around nerve roots, will lessen formation of adhesions. One should observe for paucity

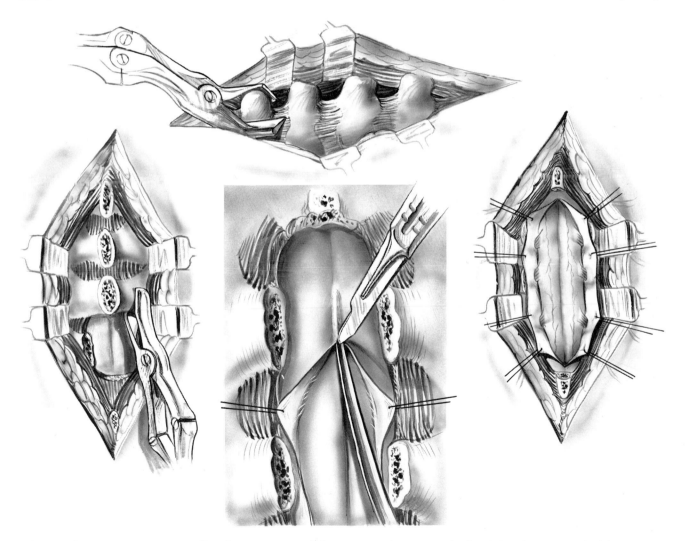

FIG. 10-2. Spinous processes and laminae are removed to expose dura mater. Incised dura is retracted with sutures.

of fat, a possible clue to the location of the neoplasm or mass. In the lower thoracic and lumbar region, there is usually no visible pulsation of the dura mater, and so the absence of pulsation has little import in indicating the presence of space-taking mass.

When feasible, effort should be made to avoid entering facets; occasionally, however, adequate exposure demands that this be done. It is certainly more important to have adequate exposure than to risk neural injury because of restricted operative field.

Bone wax is unsurpassed in controlling bleeding from cut bone, but it is better to apply it sparingly and with pressure against the cut surface, not against the dura mater or lateral gutter. Irrigation with warm (not hot) saline aids hemostasis, removes bone and wax fragments, and moistens the soft tissues. If it is necessary to coagulate vessels lying outside the dura mater, one may retract them away from the dura and its contents with a ball-point hook.

Opening of the Dura Mater

A superficial incision into the midline of the presenting dura mater permits one to place a sharp hook into it, and then to incise carefully down to the arachnoid membrane. A groove director placed just under the dura mater facilitates further incision and aids in protection of the spinal cord. Dural retraction sutures are applied as soon as expedient and before the dural incision is complete. Initial sparing of the arachnoid is a further safeguard, and permits a degree of inspection.

Modification of the standard laminectomy and technical matters dealing with specific operations are described in other portions of the text.

In all operations upon the spine, hemostatic, layer-to-layer closure of the deep muscles, fascia, subcutaneous tissue, and skin are required. In patients in whom the dura mater has been left open, tight closure of muscle and fascia is essential.

11

Transoral and Transinfrahyoid Cervical Operations

GEORGE A. SISSON

THE MOST direct surgical approach to the upper cervical spine is via the mouth by retracting the palate. In difficult situations, a midline palatal split may be required to ensure good exposure. The transoral approach to the cervical spine is not new and has been previously described by Southwick, Robinson, Mosbert and Lipman.[1,2] In 1962, Fang and Ong reported six cases in which they had successfully reduced and fused atlanto-axial dislocations.[3] Mullan et al., in 1966, reported eight patients on whom they had used an anterior approach.[4] The anterior lateral neck approach was used on four, the thoracic anterior lateral approach was used on one, and the transoral approach was used on three.

Although surgeons continue to favor the anterior lateral neck approach, as advocated by Cloward,[5] the need for adequate exposure may cause problems when operating on the atlas, the axis and in some instances the C3 vertebra. The preferred route for lesions involving C4 through C7 is through the neck, but this may be difficult to perform on patients who have had a tracheostomy. In these latter cases, the transoral approach should be considered, particularly if the lesion is at the level of C2 through C4. If a tracheostomy is present and the lesion involves C4 through C6, the transthyrohyoid route is preferable to the lateral neck approach.

Even though good results have been reported using the transoral approach, surgeons hesitate to use it because of their fear of infection and inadequate exposure. Infection should not occur if appropriate preoperative measures are instigated. It is most important that all teeth be examined by an oral surgeon prior to operation. Infected teeth should be removed. It is equally important to culture the oral cavity, and initiate an appropriate antibiotic regimen until cultures are negative. For many years, head and neck surgeons have grafted the mandible using the intraoral approach without fear of infection from intraoral contaminants.

Adequate exposure is obtained if the surgeon is trained in the use of high speed drills and is comfortable operating with the microscope. Proper instrumentation to facilitate dissection under magnification is essential.

INDICATIONS FOR TRANSORAL APPROACH

The Negus transoral approach to evacuate a retro-pharyngeal abscess involving the space between the prevertebral bodies from C1 to C3 is the procedure of choice.[6] Congenital or traumatic abnormalities of the atlas or axis and primary or metastatic tumors of vertebral bodies from C1 to C3 are also best managed by a transoral operation. Reduction of dislocations of the atlas and axis, removal of clivus chordomas, removal of metastasis, and exenteration of an osteogenic sarcoma or multiple myeloma are all examples of procedures that lend themselves to this approach.[2]

TECHNIQUE

After the aforementioned measures against infection are taken, a preliminary tracheostomy is performed under local anesthesia five days prior to operation. Once the tracheostomy is tolerated and the initial secretions abate, the patient is ready for the definitive procedure. He is placed on a broad-spectrum antibiotic and given a general anesthetic via the tracheostomy tube.

The patient is positioned so that the head is hyper-extended and a Davis-Crowe retractor is inserted. The palate is retracted by means of two No. 14 nasal catheters. If more cephalad exposure is required, the palate is divided in the midline and retracted. The Davis-Crowe mouth gag is readjusted for maximum caudal exposure by depressing the tongue.

First the operating microscope is positioned and adjusted to 6× power (Fig. 11-1); then the pharyngeal

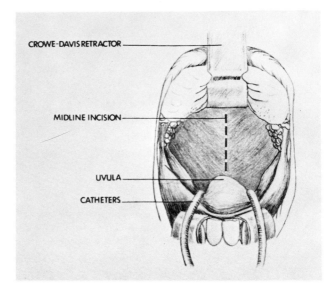

FIG. 11-2. Midline incision on post-laryngeal wall.

mucous membrane and muscles, together with the prevertebral fascia, are divided in the midline, from the posterior border of the nasal septum to C3 or C4 depending on the location of the lesion (Fig. 11-2). The most prominent bony protuberance is C1, and C2 is identified at just above the plane in line with the posterior palate (Fig. 11-3). Stay sutures (No. 1 silk) are placed in the edges of the incision to facilitate retraction of the fascia and muscles. A firm tough ligamentous structure, the anterior longitudinal ligament, is incised in the midline over the vertebral body to be explored (Fig. 11-4). This incision is carried 1 cm. above and 1 cm. below the vertebral body. The ligament is elevated to both lateral aspects and retracted by means of fine hooks or stay sutures.

If one is still uncertain as to the site of the lesion, a No. 25 spinal needle is inserted in the area of disease and its precise location is confirmed by a lateral portable roentgenogram. Once localization is exact and both

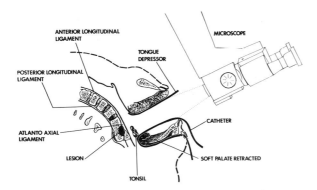

FIG. 11-1. Relationship of microscope to oral pharynx at operation.

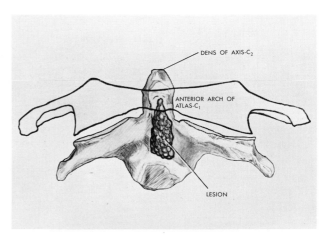

FIG. 11-3. Anatomic relationship of C1 to C2.

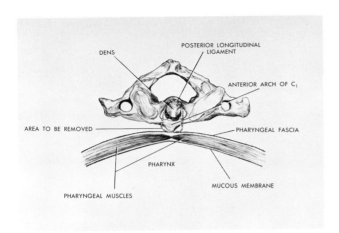

FIG. 11-4. Relationship of dens C2 to atlas C1 (transverse-superior view).

superior and inferior landmarks are identified, the operating microscope, with a 400-mm. lens and vertical viewing head, is brought into the operating area for better visualization. A 6× or 10× power objective is used when the operative field is limited.

An air drill (Hall) with a small cutting burr is used to rapidly exenterate the vertebral process involved and suction facilitates removal of the bone dust. If it is necessary to exenterate bone laterally the microscope makes early identification of the vertebral arteries possible and reduces the possibility of hemorrhage. Since the posterior longitudinal ligament is the last protecting structure anterior to the spinal cord, should it be exposed, drilling should cease. Roentgenograms and operative conditions at this time dictate which portions of the vertebral bodies should be removed, i.e., part or all.

If a bone graft is to replace diseased bone, a dowel of bone from the iliac crest is fashioned. The cortical bone is removed because cancellous bone is resilient and permits rapid healing (Figs. 11-5 and 11-6). The incision in the anterior longitudinal ligament is approximated

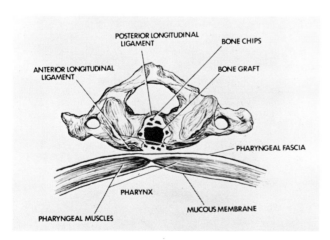

FIG. 11-5. Bone dowel in place (transverse view).

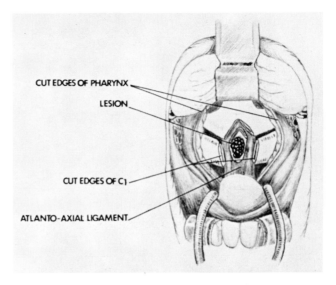

FIG. 11-6. Lesion exposed after bone cuts.

with an interrupted 4-0 monofilament suture. The pharyngeal fascia is closed as a second layer. The final layer of the pharyngeal muscles and mucous membrane are similarly sutured.

Postoperatively the patient lies flat. The head must be hyperextended by placing adequate support under the shoulders. A small pillow may be used under the head to stabilize it. The patient is fed intravenously and given therapeutic dosages of a broad-spectrum antibiotic for at least one week. If a graft has been placed into the vertebral defect, it is necessary to maintain hyperextension with a cast or halo brace for two months. Thereafter, the patient is advised to wear a head and neck brace for at least six months. The tracheostomy tube is removed on the fourteenth postoperative day.

TRANSINFRAHYOID APPROACH

Precautions to avoid postoperative infection are instituted before operation, and it is imperative that a tracheostomy be performed prior to operation. After an anesthetic has been administered, the head is hyperextended and a transverse incision is made equidistant between the inferior border of the hyoid bone and the superior border of the thyroid cartilage. The incision may be extended laterally as far as the medial border of the sternocleidomastoid muscles. It is then carried down through the subcutaneous tissues and on through the investing fascial layer of the neck and the platysma muscle. The medial borders of the superior bundles of the omohyoid muscle are identified on each side. Care is taken to avoid or to identify the external laryngeal nerves and the superior laryngeal arteries which are located along the medial aspects of the omohyoid muscle. The incision is carried down through the strap muscles. It is meticulously continued through the thyrohyoid membrane, and since fibers of this thin but strong ligament are separated, one can usually palpate and visually identify the epiglottis. Care is taken not to cut into the epiglottis, which is best avoided by carefully cutting through the thyrohyoid membrane in one small section of the incision, entering the pharynx and then elevating the thyrohyoid membrane away from the epiglottis. This part of the thyrohyoid incision can be completed with scissors.

Retractors are placed to separate the thyrohyoid membrane widely, permitting visualization of the posterior pharyngeal wall and the vertebral bodies of C2 through C4. A midline incision is now made over the appropriate vertebrae, and the dissection is carried down and closed as in the transoral approach.

The operation is completed by suturing the thyrohyoid membrane as a separate layer using 4-0 atraumatic needles, suturing the thyrohyoid and sternohyoid muscles as a separate layer, and finally suturing the platysma and skin. It is important to drain the wound with a small penrose drain or small Hemovac.

Postoperative management is essentially the same as for the transoral procedure. A cast or halo brace is worn for a period of three months, after which the patient should have a form-fitting collar to continue this support for at least six months.

When either the transoral or infrahyoid approach is used for children under five years of age, decannulation is not recommended for at least four weeks after healing is complete and the child's deglutition has returned to normal, so as to prevent complications from the early removal of a tracheostomy tube.

References

1. Southwick WO and Robinson RA: Surgical approaches to the vertebral bodies in the cervical and lumbar regions. J Bone Jt Surg *39A*:631–644, 1957.
2. Mosbert WH and Lipman EM: Anterior approach to the cervical bodies. Bull Med Univ Sch Med *45*:10–17, 1960.
3. Fang HSY and Ong GB: Direct anterior approach to the upper cervical spine. J Bone Jt Surg *44A*:1588–1604, 1962.
4. Mullan S, Nauton R, Hekmatpanah J and Vailati G: The use of an inferior approach to vertically placed tumors in the foramen magnum and vertebral column. J Neurosurg *24*:536–543, 1966.
5. Cloward RB: The anterior approach for removal of ruptured cervical disks. J Neurosurg *15*:602–617, 1958.
6. Thomson, St. Clair and Negus VE: Diseases of the Nose and Throat. A Textbook for Students and Practitioners. Ed. 5, London, Cassell & Co., Ltd., 1947, pp. 489–509.

12

Anterolateral Approaches to the Cervical Spine

HENRY H. BOHLMAN, LEE H. RILEY, JR.,
AND ROBERT A. ROBINSON

ANTERIOR surgical approaches to the cervical spine are several, and the choice of exposure depends on the level at which the spine is involved and the nature of the disease. A great proportion of spinal diseases, such as tumors, infections, degenerative disc disease, and traumatic osseous and disc protrusions, occur in the anterior and lateral aspects of the cervical spine.

DIRECT EXPOSURE OF THE ANTERIOR VERTEBRAL BODIES AND DISC SPACES FROM C3 THROUGH C7 LEVELS

The original work on anterior approaches to the cervical spine was begun by Robinson in the early 1950s on animals and cadavers and then applied to living man. The results were first reported in 1955.[10] Since that time various detailed reports have described the technique.[1,6,12,13] The following is a summary of the salient points of the Robinson approach.

With the patient supine on a standard operating table, a folded sheet is placed under the shoulders which are pulled distally by three-inch adhesive tapes attached to the operating table. This position allows for intraoperative lateral x-ray films of the lower cervical spine. A thyroid bag is placed under the neck for support. If discograms are to be performed, a padded cassette is placed under the cervical spine for the anteroposterior view. Five pounds of cervical traction are applied by a head halter following endotracheal anesthesia. The skin is "prepped" from the chin to the nipple line, including both sides of the neck. Either iliac crest can be prepared and draped as the graft site. The cervical area is draped with towels, which are sewn in place so that the customary towel clips will not obstruct the lateral x-ray view. The incision is made on the left side to avoid damage to the recurrent laryngeal nerve. A transverse incision is made two to three finger-breadths above the clavicle, beginning in the midline and extending laterally to the sternomastoid muscle (Fig. 12-1).

If the upper cervical area is to be approached, the transverse incision is made four finger-breadths above the clavicle. A longitudinal incision is used if the entire cervical spine is to be exposed, and extends along the anterior border of the sternomastoid muscle (Fig. 12-2). Following the skin incision, the platysma muscle is identified and bluntly elevated from the underlying structures with Metzenbaum scissors, then transversely incised. Next the superficial layer of deep cervical fascia is incised along the anterior border of the sternomastoid muscle.[7] This is an important step which allows for adequate retraction later. The omohyoid muscle is seen as it passes across the field and may be retracted or divided. The carotid sheath is identified by its pulsation. The next important structure is the middle layer of deep cervical fascia, which is divided vertically, medial to the carotid sheath, as the surgeon's fingers retract the carotid artery laterally for protection.

Blunt dissection is carried out through the loose areolar tissues toward the midline of the neck and vertebral bodies. The esophagus is identified and retracted medially with the trachea, by means of a medium-sized Richardson retractor. The carotid sheath and sternomastoid muscles are retracted laterally with a thyroid retractor. The recurrent laryngeal nerve descends along the carotid sheath and ascends between the trachea and esophagus. Care must be taken not to damage these structures by sharp-pointed retractors or prolonged pressure.

The midline of the vertebral bodies is palpated, and the prominent anterior tubercle of the sixth vertebra aids in the identification of a particular spinal level. The alar and prevertebral fascias are next incised vertically in the midline, revealing the shiny white anterior longitudinal ligament. Laterally, to either side of the anterior longitudinal ligament, the longus colli muscles are seen, and care must be taken not to damage the cervical sympathetic chain of nerves lying superficial to these muscles.

At this point in the operation, the disc or discs to be excised are identified by means of a 22-gauge spinal needle placed into the disc space. The needle is guarded by a clamp placed 8 mm. proximal to the tip. A lateral roentgenogram is obtained. If discography is to be performed, care must be taken to place the needle tip in the central nucleus pulposus and not against the cartilage or bony end plate; the latter position would result in a false-negative study. An anteroposterior film also is obtained for the discogram.

Excision of the diseased disc should be complete and is begun by the excising of a rectangular window in the

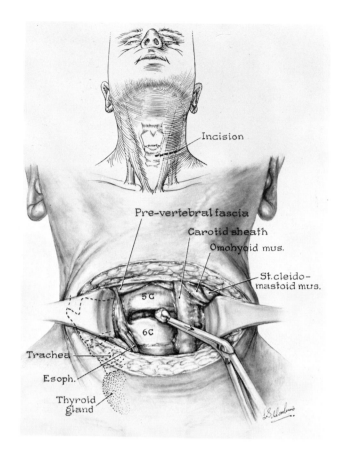

FIG. 12-1. Exposure of fifth and sixth cervical segments after prevertebral fascia has been incised and carotid sheath retracted laterally and trachea and esophagus medially. (From Robinson RA, Riley LH: Anterior interbody fusion of the cervical spine. *In* The Craft of Surgery. Edited by P Cooper. Boston, Little, Brown & Co., Vol. III, 2nd Ed., 1973.)

anterior longitudinal ligament with a small scalpel. The disc material is loosened with a curet and removed with pituitary forceps. The entire disc is removed as far laterally as the vertebral body extends and posteriorly to the posterior longitudinal ligament. Fragments of disc may protrude through rents in the posterior longitudinal ligament centrally or laterally. These fragments can be removed with the aid of a blunt nerve root hook, small curet, and small pituitary forceps. Visualization is aided here by distracting the vertebral bodies with a spreader, or added traction of 20 pounds, and a high-intensity head light. The hyaline cartilage plates are removed entirely from the superior and inferior vertebrae, and care is taken not to remove the subchondral bone. If too much subchondral bone is removed, the bone graft will sink into the vertebral body substance postoperatively. The subchondral bone, if sclerotic, is perforated in several places with a small-angled curet to aid the blood supply to the healing graft. The height, depth, and width of the disc space are

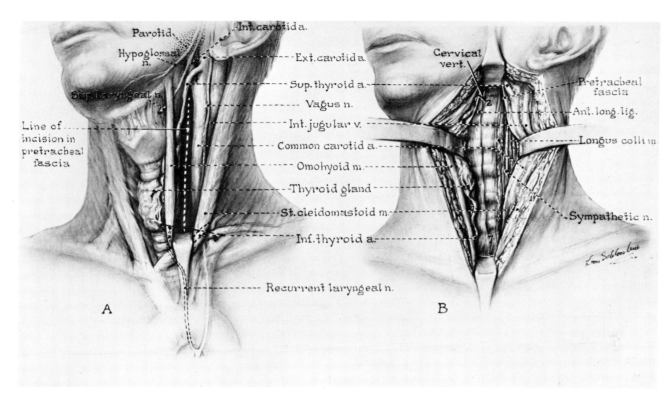

FIG. 12-2. *A,* Line of incision in pretracheal fascia between carotid sheath and omohyoid muscle; *B,* exposure obtained after retraction and incision of prevertebral fascia. (From Smith GW, Robinson RA: J Bone Jt Surg *40A.*613, 1958.)

measured with the aid of a metallic malleable probe, and recorded.

The bone graft is obtained from either iliac crest, and cutting is confined well posterior to the anterior superior iliac spine, so that the lateral femoral cutaneous nerve is protected. Both sides of the iliac crest are exposed subperiosteally, and a one-inch block of ilium is removed, including the inner, outer, and superior cortices. The bone graft is fashioned with a saw according to the dimensions of the disc space (Fig. 12-3). The graft includes three cortical surfaces, which become the anterior and lateral margins, and the cancellous bone represents the superior and inferior surfaces (Fig. 12-4).

Two millimeters are subtracted from the recorded depth of the disc space to allow the graft to be countersunk. The iliac wound is then closed by approximation of periosteum, subcutaneous tissue, and skin in separate layers.

After the bone graft has been trimmed to size and 20 pounds of traction has been applied, it is ready to be placed in the disc space. The bone graft is tapped into place by means of a wide tamper, which is curved on its tip to conform to the shape of the superior iliac crest (Fig. 12-5). It is important not to use small punches that may fracture the cortex of the graft, bringing about rapid collapse of the graft postoperatively. The graft is countersunk beneath the lips of the anterior vertebral body and another lateral roentgenogram is obtained to

check its final position. Stability of the graft is immediately checked by release of traction, deflation of the thyroid bag, and gentle flexion of the neck by the anesthesiologist. Drainage of the wound is left to the

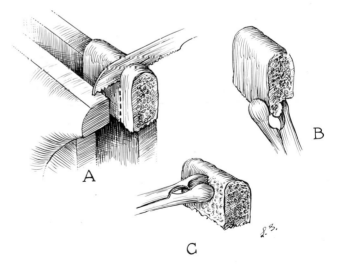

FIG. 12-3. Shaping iliac bone graft: *A,* cutting height of graft; *B,* trimming depth; *C,* trimming width. (From Robinson RA, Riley LH: Anterior interbody fusion of the cervical spine. *In* The Craft of Surgery. Edited by P Cooper. Boston, Little, Brown & Co., Vol. III, 2nd Ed., 1973.)

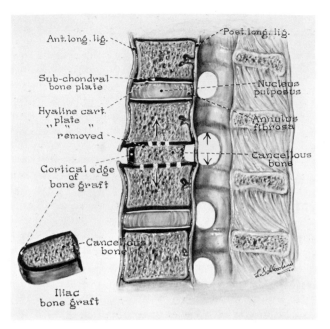

FIG. 12-4. Positioning of bone graft in prepared disc space. Note distraction of foramen and small perforations of bony end plates. (From Robinson RA et al.: The results of anterior interbody fusion of the cervical spine. J Bone Jt Surg 44A:1569, 1962.)

surgeon's discretion. The wound is closed by approximation of the platysma muscle first, then the subcutaneous layer and skin.

Ambulation may be permitted on the evening of the operative day, at which time a soft collar is worn by the patient. He is then fitted with a brace which he wears eight weeks.

In our opinion, removal of posterior or foraminal

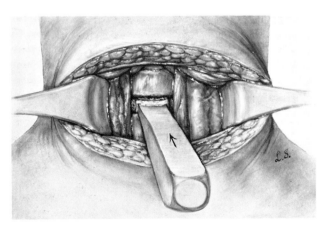

FIG. 12-5. Technique of tapping bone graft in place using broad impactor which conforms to shape of graft cortex. (From Robinson RA, Riley LH: Anterior interbody fusion of the cervical spine. In The Craft of Surgery. Edited by P Cooper. Boston, Little, Brown & Co., Vol. III, 2nd Ed., 1973.)

osteophytes, as advocated by the Cloward technique, rarely is necessary. Cervical spondylosis may cause spinal cord impingement by soft disc protrusion, bony osteophytes, and buckling of the ligamentum flavum. A congenitally narrow spinal canal may further compromise space for the cervical cord. Anterior fusion by the Robinson technique removes the soft disc and prevents ligamentum flavum impingement by immobilization of the cervical segment with the fusion. Distraction of the segment opens the foramina to relieve nerve root compression. Large posterior osteophytes, when anterior spinal cord compression symptoms are present, can be removed with an angled curet. Finally, osseous spurs resorb within nine to eighteen months by the process of normal bone remodeling.

A block-type graft has distinct advantages over the dowel-type graft. The capacity of the block-type graft to withstand immediate vertical compressive loads is greater than that of the dowel-type graft.[16] The danger of retropulsion of cortical fragment into the spinal canal is greater in the dowel-type graft.[4] Also, when the trephined hole technique of Cloward is used, a large area of bleeding bone is exposed which can cause hematoma formation and secondary cord compression postoperatively. In the three large reported series of Robinson-type fusions used for cervical spondylosis, there has been no case of postoperative increase in neural deficit.[6,9,12] Finally, in our opinion, the dowel-type graft for acute cervical fracture-dislocations results in poor immediate stability.[2]

EXPOSURE OF THE ANTERIOR ARCH OF THE ATLAS, DENS, AND BODY OF THE AXIS

The atlas and axis may be exposed through a longitudinal, transpharyngeal incision as described by Fang and his associates,[5] and by Robinson and Southwick.[11] An anterolateral approach has been reported by Stevenson.[14] The above techniques are useful for open biopsy, tumor excision, abscess drainage, odontoid osteotomy, or anterior fusion of the atlas and axis. When more extensive exposure is required—to include the base of the skull, atlas, axis, and lower cervical spine—the following technique as described by Riley[8] or Robinson and Smith[10] is used.

A tracheostomy is performed first, through which anesthesia is given. A submandibular skin incision is made transversely, extending from the midline to the left, through the submandibular area, and toward the angle of the mandible posteriorly. The incision is then curved distally to follow the posterior border of the sternomastoid muscle down to the fifth cervical vertebra, where it is curved toward the midline anteriorly. The incision then crosses the clavicle toward the suprasternal space, and is deepened through the sub-cutaneous fascia and platysma muscle to form a flap which is reflected medially (Fig. 12-6). Following retraction of the skin flap, exposure of the sternomastoid, strap muscles, trachea, thyroid, and submaxillary fossa is accomplished. Care must be taken to identify and protect the mandibular branch of the facial nerve, at the angle of the mandible. The superficial layer of deep cervical fascia is split along the anterior border of the sternomastoid muscle, and this allows its lateral retraction. The omohyoid muscle is identified and transected. The middle layer of cervical fascia is incised medial to and parallel to the carotid sheath. The strap muscles, thyroid, trachea, and esophagus are then retracted medially, exposing the anterior surface of the vertebral bodies.

The superior thyroid artery is identified next as it passes from the external carotid artery laterally to the thyroid medially. The superior thyroid artery is ligated and transected to allow for dissection in a cephalic direction. The superior laryngeal and hypoglossal nerves should then be identified and retracted superiorly. The hypoglossal nerve can be located inferior to the origin of the stylohyoid muscle laterally and crosses superficial to the external carotid artery medially. The digastric and stylohyoid muscles are then divided and retracted. The superior laryngeal nerve accompanies the superior laryngeal artery, inferior to the hyoid bone. Both pierce the hypothyroid membrane.

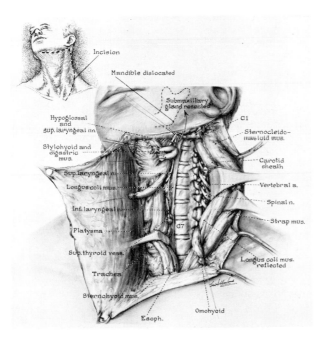

FIG. 12-6. Exposure of entire anterior cervical spine including base of skull. Temporomandibular joint is dislocated, and submaxillary gland resected. (From Riley, LH: Surgical approaches to the anterior structures of the cervical spine. Clin Ortho 91:16, 1973.)

If the superior laryngeal artery originates from the external carotid artery and not from the superior thyroid artery, it is ligated. The larynx and pharynx are retracted medially, the external carotid artery laterally, and the floor of the submaxillary triangle superiorly, exposing the base of the skull and anterior arch of the atlas. Wider visualization is accomplished if the temporomandibular joint is dislocated anteriorly and the submaxillary gland excised. The mandible is rotated superiorly and to the right side of the patient. Access is now gained to the atlas, axis, vertebral arteries, and base of the skull. To close the wound, the temporomandibular joint is reduced, the digastric, stylohyoid, and platysma muscles reapproximated, and the subcutaneous layer and skin closed. Suction drainage is used because the wide dissection predisposes to dangerous hematoma formation.

EXPOSURE OF THE TRANSVERSE PROCESS AND PEDICLES OF THE C3 THROUGH C7 SEGMENTS

Tumors and osteophytes may involve the transverse processes, pedicles, and vertebral arteries of the third through seventh cervical vertebrae, and exposure of these structures is best accomplished as described by Riley. However, the lateral approach of Verbiest also can be used.[15] Riley's anterolateral approach begins with a transverse skin incision, which extends in a gentle curve laterally and superiorly to the posterior border of the sternomastoid muscle (Fig. 12-7). The incision is deepened through the platysma muscle. The anterior and posterior aspects of the sternomastoid muscle are delineated, and the muscle is transected after its deep portion is freed. The omohyoid muscle is also divided and retracted superiorly and inferiorly, while the carotid sheath is retracted medially. The anterior scalene muscle and phrenic nerve are thus exposed, and the brachial plexus cords can be seen exiting from beneath the anterior scalene muscle. The phrenic nerve is mobilized and retracted laterally. After careful delineation of the anterior scalene muscle and underlying brachial plexus, the muscle is divided and the superior portion excised.

It is extremely important to protect the vertebral artery as it passes through the vertebral foramen. To gain access to the pedicles, the vertebral artery is controlled with tapes superiorly and inferiorly, and the longus colli muscle is reflected medially. The remaining origins of anterior scalene muscles may be reflected distally. One can now identify the nerve roots, transverse processes, pedicles, and neural foramina (Fig. 12-8). Verbiest removes the anterior tubercles and retracts the vertebral artery medially; however, this may endanger major radicular artery branches, which supply the anterior spinal artery. The wound is closed by reapproximation of the omohyoid, the sternomastoid, and the platysma muscles. A drain is used, and the skin is closed with fine sutures, which are removed the third postoperative day.

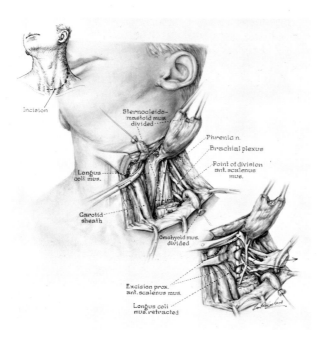

FIG. 12-7. Exposure of transverse processes of cervical spine after resection of proximal portion of anterior scalene muscle. (From Riley LH: Surgical approaches to the anterior structures of the cervical spine. Clin Ortho *91:*16, 1973.)

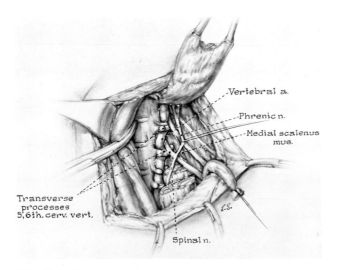

FIG. 12-8. Exposure of transverse processes, pedicles, and neural foramen after reflection of anterior scalene and longus colli muscles. (From Riley LH: Surgical approaches to the anterior structures of the cervical spine. Clin Ortho *91:*16, 1973.)

BONE GRAFT FOR ACUTE OR DELAYED ANTERIOR DECOMPRESSION AND STABILIZATION OF CERVICAL VERTEBRAL BODY FRACTURES

The method of discectomy and small osseous fragment removal has been described. Vertical compression fracture of the cervical spine frequently causes a kyphotic deformity, with osseous and disc protrusion against the anterior surface of the cervical spinal cord. In the case of an incomplete cord lesion, the offending elements should be removed.[2,3] We both use the following technique at our respective institutions (Fig. 12-9).

The vertebral bodies are exposed through the anterolateral approach. The discs superior and inferior to the crushed vertebral body are localized by x-ray examination and partially excised as described in the Robinson technique. Partial removal of the anterior portion of crushed vertebra is accomplished with a bone rongeur. Each disc space and its adjoining normal vertebral surface is used as a landmark to approach the posterior longitudinal ligament. All disc material is removed from the spaces superior and inferior to the crushed vertebra, including the cartilage end plates. The midportion of crushed vertebral body is removed by careful use of a dental burr until the posterior longitudinal ligament is approached. The deep posterior portion of fractured vertebra is picked away from the posterior longitudinal ligament with a small angled curet, with care taken to avoid penetrating the ligament or entering the spinal canal. In most cases of trauma the fracture and disc fragments remain anterior to the posterior longitudinal ligament.[2,3] Once all of the compressive elements have been removed, the surgeon can visualize a convexity of the posterior ligament, and thus decompression is complete. At this point an appropriate-sized rectangular iliac crest graft is taken and fashioned so that the posterior height is slightly greater than the anterior cortical height. This shape locks the graft in place and conforms to the vertebral body surfaces superiorly and inferiorly. The graft consists of three cortical surfaces of the superior iliac crest. Prior to placing the graft, oblique holes are drilled through the anterior lips of the vertebral bodies above and below the graft and through the anterior cortical edges of the graft itself. A heavy silk suture is threaded through the holes at either end of the graft and through the vertebral bodies. After maximal distraction of the cervical vertebrae by skull traction, the graft is gently tapped into place with a wide tamper and is slightly countersunk. Position of the graft is checked by lateral roentgenogram, and the silk sutures are then tied.

If the spine is unstable posteriorly as a result of injury or laminectomy the patient must be strictly

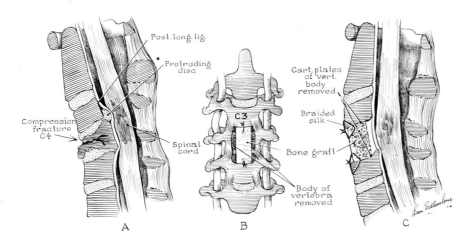

FIG. 12-9. *A*, Pathologic features of vertical compression fractures in incomplete cord lesion. *B* and *C*, Technique of vertebral corpectomy and iliac graft replacement to remove disc and osseous fragments and to correct kyphotic deformity. (From Bohlman HH: Pathology and current treatment of cervical spine injuries. *In* American Academy of Orthopedic Surgeons: Instructional Course Lectures. Vol XXI, St. Louis, The CV Mosby Co., 1972.)

immobilized until fusion is solid. If posterior stability exists the patient may be ambulatory in a halo cast or sturdy brace.

References

1. Bailey RW, Badgley CE: Stabilization of the cervical spine by anterior fusion. J Bone Jt Surg *42A:*565, 1960.
2. Bohlman HH: Cervical spine injuries: a critical review of 300 cases. Submitted for publication in J Bone Jt Surg.
3. Bohlman HH: Pathology and Current Treatment Concepts of Cervical Spine Injuries. American Academy of Orthopaedic Surgeons, Instructional Course Lectures, Vol. XXI, St. Louis, CV Mosby, p. 108, 1972.
4. Cloward RB: Complications of anterior cervical disc operation and their treatment. Surgery *69:*175–182, 1971.
5. Fang HSY and Ong GB: Direct anterior approach to the upper cervical spine. J Bone Jt Surg *44A:*1588, 1962.
6. Filtzer DL and Aronson N: The Management of Soft Cervical Disc Herniation. American Academy of Orthopaedic Surgeons, Instructional Course Lectures, Vol. XXI, St. Louis, CV Mosby, p. 122, 1972.
7. Grodinsky M, Holyoke EA: The fasciae and fascial spaces of the head, neck and adjacent regions. Amer J Anat *63:*367–408, 1938.
8. Riley, LH: Surgical approaches to the anterior structures of the cervical spine. Clin Orthopaed *91:*16, 1973.
9. Riley LH, Robinson RA, Johnson KA, Walker AE: The results of anterior interbody fusion of the cervical spine. J Neurosurg *30:*127–133, 1969.
10. Robinson RA, Smith GW: Anterolateral cervical disc removal and interbody fusion for cervical disc syndrome. Bull Johns Hopkins Hosp *96:*223, 1955.
11. Robinson RA, Southwick WO: Surgical approaches to the cervical spine. American Academy of Orthopaedic Surgeons, Instructional Course Lectures, Vol. XVII, St. Louis, CV Mosby, pp. 299–330, 1960.
12. Robinson RA, Walker AE, Ferlic DC, Wieching DK: The results of anterior interbody fusion of the cervical spine. J Bone Jt Surg *44A:*1569, 1962.
13. Robinson RA, Riley LH: Anterior interbody fusion of the cervical spine. *In* The Craft of Surgery. Edited by P Cooper. Vol. III, 2nd ed., 1973.
14. Stevenson GG, Stoney RJ, Perkins RK, Adams JE: A transcervical approach to the ventral surface of the brain stem for removal of a Clivus chordoma. J Neurosurg *24:*544, 1966.
15. Verbiest H: A lateral approach to the cervical spine: technique and indications. J Neurosurg *28:*191, 1968.
16. White AA, Jupiter J, Southwick WO, Panjabi MM: An experimental study of the immediate load-bearing capacity of three surgical constructions for anterior spine fusions. Clin Orthopaed *91:*21, 1973.

13

Lateral Approach to the Cervical Spine

ERIC K. LOUIE AND DANIEL RUGE

HENRY[3] AND KAPLAN,[5] in their discussions of surgical approaches to the neck, credit Fiolle and Delmas for devising the basic dissection involved in the lateral approach to the cervical spine.[2] This operation offers an optimal exposure to the contents of the carotid sheath, the brachial plexus, and the lateral and anterolateral aspects of the cervical spine. Despite its theoretic beauty and simplicity, the greater technical difficulty of the lateral exposure, as compared to a posterior exposure, necessitates a judicious analysis of the diseased structures to be treated before a decision regarding approach can be made. One clear indication for the lateral approach is a procedure on the vertebral artery as it passes through the foramina transversaria. This approach permits the vertebral artery to be ligated between the atlas and the axis, facilitates repair of vertebral arteriovenous fistulas, and allows removal of spondylotic outgrowths compressing the vertebral artery. Another possible use for this approach is the treatment of postganglionic upper brachial plexus traction injuries. The use of the lateral approach in the surgical treatment of narrowing of the intervertebral foramen due to hypertrophic bony development at the zygapophyseal joints, or for the removal of laterally protruding intervertebral discs, must be considered against the alternative, posterior foramenectomy. The latter operation has the disadvantage, avoided by the lateral approach, of requiring sacrifice of the posterior articulations that bear the majority of the stress in the cervical lordosis. Verbiest[7] has also suggested that in those cases of lateral intervertebral disc protrusion complicated by the scalenus anticus syndrome, the lateral approach allows access for removal of the protruding disc and section of the anterior scalene muscle which may provide relief from both conditions.[6]

THE OPERATION

Whereas Fiolle and Delmas obtained optimal exposure by positioning the patient's head turned away from the side of the incision,[2] Verbiest cautions that in patients with bony compression of the vertebral artery, this positioning may aggravate the condition, and thus he prefers to maintain the patient's head in a neutral midposition.[7] Choice of incision depends on the anticipated extent of the operative field required and the level of the approach. Generally, a longitudinal incision along the medial border of the sternocleidomastoid muscle provides optimal exposure of the middle and lower cervical spine, and permits extension of the incision as may later be required. Operations on the upper cervical spine, as in vertebral artery ligation, require the eversion of the mastoid origin of the sternocleidomastoid muscle to permit mobilization of this muscle. To effect this, the longitudinal incision must be extended inferiorly to the sternal head of the sternocleidomastoid and extended superiorly until the mastoid process is reached, at which point the incision passes posteriorly across the mastoid head. In rare instances, when the disease is localized with certainty to a given level, a transverse incision at that level may be employed. Despite the better cosmetic effect obtained with transverse incisions, the reduced operative field and the difficulty in extending the incision to include higher or lower levels militate against the use of transverse incisions.

After the initial skin incision is made, the platysma and underlying fascia also should be incised to allow definition of the medial border of the sternocleidomastoid muscle. Gentle blunt dissection of the underside of the sternocleidomastoid will allow it to be retracted laterally. In operations on the upper cervical spine, during which the sternocleidomastoid muscle is separated from its attachment to the mastoid process, division of the investing deep fascia could result in section of the anterior cervical and great auricular nerves. Since the latter serves sensation to areas in front of the angle of the mandible where men shave, it may be desirable to attempt to spare this nerve. Care must also be taken to preserve the spinal accessory nerve (XI) as it leaves the deep fascia and penetrates the underside of the sternocleidomastoid one-third the length of the muscle from the mastoid process.

Division of the omohyoid muscle as it lies in the anterior triangle deep to the sternocleidomastoid and clearing of the surrounding fascia is recommended by Henry[3] and by Kaplan.[5] Division of the omohyoid muscle may not be absolutely required for proper access to the cervical spine at more superior levels.

Further blunt dissection reveals the carotid sheath lying parallel and deep to the medial border of the sternocleidomastoid muscle. From lateral to medial the contents of the carotid sheath include the internal jugular vein, the vagus nerve, and the common carotid artery, each of which should be identified. The approach to the cervical spine is now facilitated by lateral retraction of the carotid sheath and its contents along with the sternocleidomastoid muscle and by medial retraction of the trachea, esophagus, and anterior strap muscles.[7] The recurrent laryngeal nerves running in the fascia between the esophagus and the trachea are not injured with gentle retraction of these midline structures. In the case of complete sternocleidomastoid eversion Henry suggests that the carotid sheath and its contents be retracted medially with the trachea, esophagus, and anterior strap muscles rather than laterally.[3] In either case, care must be taken not to damage the cervical sympathetic chain, which is embedded in the posterior wall of the carotid sheath. Retraction of the carotid sheath may be restricted by the many large veins that anastomose with the internal jugular vein, either singly or via the thyro-linguo-facial venous trunk. The latter may be safely ligated and divided if necessary.[2]

At this stage of the operation, the surgeon must palpate the anterior tubercles of the transverse processes of the cervical vertebrae and identify the level of his dissection precisely with radiograms. We shall discuss here the further dissection required to expose vertebrae C3-C6. The atlas and axis have their own peculiar anatomic configuration, the surgery of which is set forth in depth by Henry.[3] To gain access to the transverse processes of the cervical vertebrae, the longus colli and longus capitis muscles must be detached from the anterior tubercles of the transverse processes and retracted medially. Henry notes that when the longus colli muscle is being stripped at levels above the C4-C5 intervertebral disc, a superiorly directed motion should be used, but at levels below this disc an inferiorly directed motion is indicated. Finally, the anterior intertransverse muscles, which extend between the anterior roots of the transverse processes, are removed. In some cases, when the anterior scalene muscle has attachments to the nerves of the brachial plexus, these should be delicately disrupted, and if the surgeon desires to remove the anterior tubercle, attachments of the anterior scalene muscle to the anterior tubercle must be sectioned.

The exposure is now adequate for surgical intervention at the foramina transversaria or at the intervertebral foraminae. Resection of the anterior root of the transverse process and the costotransverse lamella, with precautions against injuring the nerve roots as they emerge above or below, allows the vertebral artery to be retracted laterally. Lateral retraction of the vertebral artery may proceed for at most a few millimeters, while care is taken not to injure the radicular arteries leaving the vertebral artery some 0.1 to 1.0 centimeters inferior to a given nerve root.[7] Care must also be taken to minimize venous bleeding from the vertebral vein and its associated plexus about the vertebral artery. In the intertransverse space the verte-

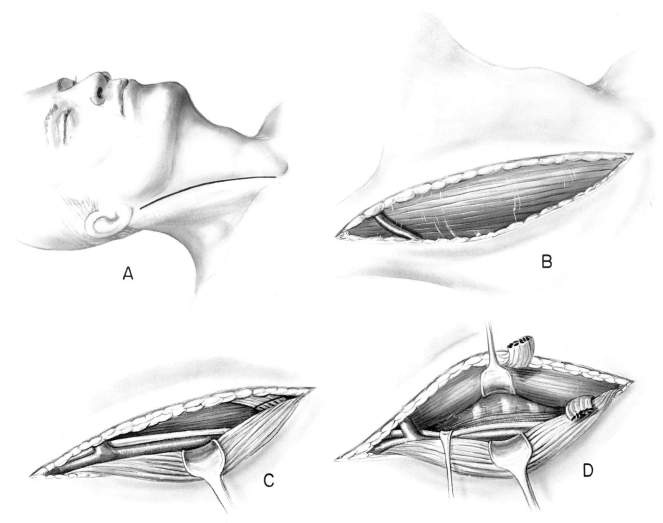

FIG. 13-1. Lateral approach to cervical spine. *A,* Superficial landmarks such as thyroid and cricoid cartilages are palpated to obtain approximate localization of vertebral levels. Belly of sternocleidomastoid muscle is palpated and cutaneous incision is made along its medial border. *B,* Carrying incision through platysma and gently retracting skin flaps permits visualization of medial border of sternocleidomastoid muscle. Care must be taken not to inadvertently tear external jugular vein as it courses superficial to muscle. *C,* Lateral retraction of sternocleidomastoid and blunt dissection of deep fascia reveals contents of carotid sheath and omohyoid muscle as they lie in anterior triangle deep to medial border of sternocleidomastoid. *D,* Division of omohyoid muscle, accompanied by retraction of trachea, esophagus, and anterior strap muscles medially, and retraction of contents of carotid sheath and sternocleidomastoid laterally, provides exposure of anterolateral aspect of spine depicted here, with longus colli and longus capitis muscles stripped from their more lateral insertions and retracted medially. Ligation and division of inconstant thyro-linguo-facial trunk arising from internal jugular vein may be necessary in order to obtain adequate retraction of carotid sheath.

bral venous plexus may receive anywhere from 20 to 60 feeder veins, which course along with the nerve root.[3] Within the foramen transversarium, the vertebral venous plexus is made tightly adherent to the bony channel by fibrous tissue, further complicating the task of hemostasis when bony elements are resected.[3] Verbiest suggests that the vertebral venous plexus should be stripped from the vertebral artery and the lateral branches should be occluded.[7] Further venous bleeding can be arrested by application of Surgicel.

With retraction of the vertebral artery, a rongeur may be used to remove lateral spurs which compress the artery. Delicate dissection of the connective tissue posterior to the vertebral artery and investing the anterior ramus of the nerve root will reveal the intervertebral foramen. Then under clear visualization of the nerve roots and the retracted vertebral artery, small osteotomes or a guarded drill may be used to remove osteophytes encroaching on an intervertebral foramen. Similarly, pituitary forceps may be employed

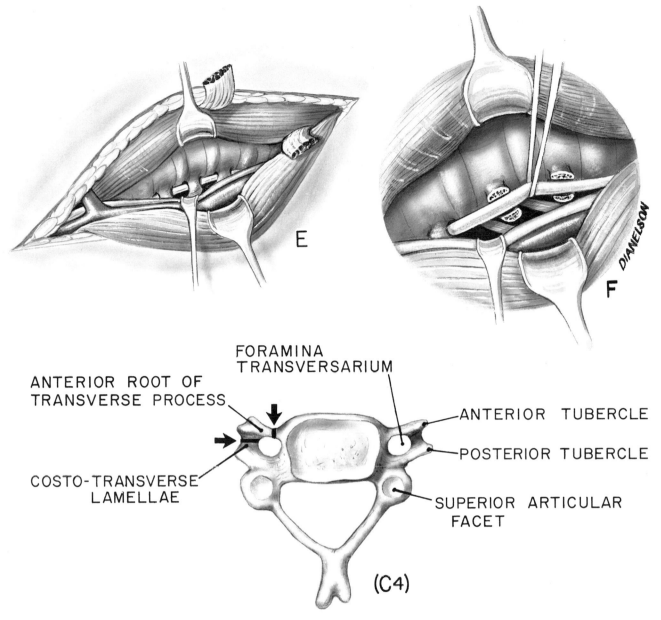

FIG. 13-1. Lateral approach to cervical spine (continued). *E*, Further medial retraction of paravertebral muscles and clearing of anterior intertransverse muscles allows visualization of vertebral artery. *F*, Resection of anterior tubercles and costotransverse lamellae at two levels permits gentle mobilization of vertebral artery. Extreme care must be taken to avoid damage to nearby emerging nerve roots. *G*, This view of superior surface of C4 vertebra indicates relations of various bony elements. Arrows indicate points of resection.

to excise the uncinate process and the disc, allowing further removal of transverse ridges as the surgeon proceeds inward from the intervertebral foramen. This exposure also allows removal of laterally protruding intervertebral discs. At all times curetting should proceed in the direction of the posterolateral aspect of the vertebral body, hence avoiding the dural sac or the nerve roots.

References

1. Elkin DC, Harris MH: Arteriovenous aneurysm of the vertebral vessels. Ann Surg *124*:934–951, 1946.
2. Fiolle J, Delmas J: The Surgical Exposure of the Deep Seated Blood Vessels. Trans by CG Cumstron, London, William Heineman, 1921, pp. 68–82.
3. Henry AK: Extensile Exposure. Baltimore, Williams and Wilkins, 1959, pp. 53–72.

4. Jefferson G, Bailey RA, Kerr AS: Suboccipital arteriovenous aneurysms of the vertebral artery. General discussion with detail of three cases. J Bone Jt Surg *38B:*114-127, 1956.

5. Kaplan EB: Surgical Approaches to the Neck, Cervical Spine and Upper Extremity. Philadelphia, Saunders, 1966, pp. 6-40.

6. Kirgis HD, Reed AF: Anatomical relations of possible significance in the production of the scalenus anticus syndrome. Anat Rec *97:*348, 1947.

7. Verbiest H: A lateral approach to the cervical spine: technique and indications. J Neurosurg *28:*191-203, 1968.

14

The Lateral Extrapleural and Extraperitoneal Approaches to the Thoracic and Lumbar Spine

SANFORD J. LARSON

THE PROCEDURE is similar to that described by Alexander[1] and by Capener.[2] Initially designed for the treatment of tuberculous spondylitis, the method is useful in any case in which the pathologic process is extradural and anterior to the thoracic spinal cord or cauda equina.

LATERAL EXTRAPLEURAL APPROACH

The patient is placed on the operating table in the prone position. A midline skin incision is made from well above the lesion to well below it and then curved laterally for about 12 cm. (Fig. 14-1 A). The subcutaneous fat is separated from the investing fascia of the muscles and the skin flap retracted laterally. In the thoracic region, depending upon which vertebrae are to be exposed, the trapezius, the latissimus, and the rhomboids are either retracted or split. The iliocostalis, the longissimus, and other deep muscles of the back are separated from the ribs (Fig. 14-1 B). The number of vertebral levels to be approached determines the number of ribs to be resected, but usually it is desirable to remove at least two. The rib is transected 8 cm. lateral to the costotransverse joint and removed with rongeurs. The pleura is separated from the endothoracic fascia by finger dissection. The neurovascular bundle is identified and the intercostal nerve separated from the vessels. The costotransverse joint is incised and the remainder of the rib removed including the costovertebral articulation (Fig. 14-1 C, D). This is necessary because throughout most of the extent of the thoracic spine, the terminal portion of the rib and the radiate ligament are attached across the intervertebral disc. The transverse processes and associated intertransversarii

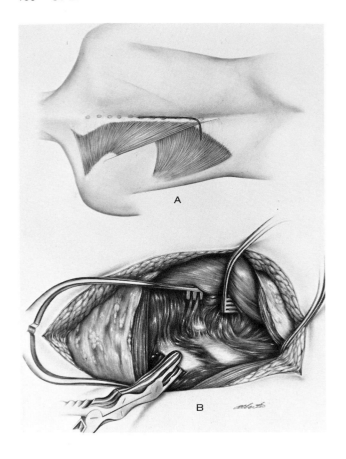

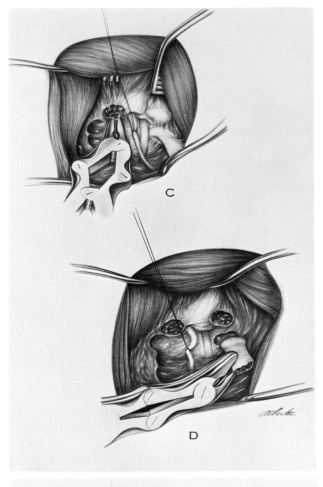

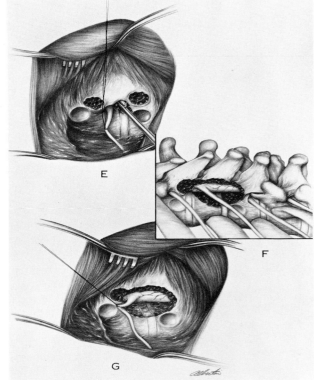

FIG. 14-1. Lateral retropleural approach: *A,* skin incision is midline and curved laterally; *B,* muscles are retracted to expose ribs; *C,* rib is resected; *D,* rib, including costovertebral articulation, is removed; *E,* anulus is incised and disc is removed; *F, G,* contiguous portions of bone are removed from dorsal portions of vertebral bodies.

muscles are removed. The intercostal nerve is traced to its foramen. At this time it is usually desirable to clip and cut the segmental artery and vein. The intercostal nerve is divided between ligatures leaving a central stump of 2 to 3 cm. The ligature on the central stump is not cut and can be used to retract the central segment of the nerve in various directions (Fig. 14-1 *E*). A blunt hook is used to dissect the soft tissue from the bony margins of the intervertebral foramen. The pedicle is resected with punch and rongeurs. It is sometimes advantageous to begin by resecting a pedicle above or below the lesion, where the anatomic relationships are more likely to be normal. This is particularly true if the operation is done for tuberculous spondylitis with extradural granuloma. The operating table is now tilted laterally, so that the spinal canal and related structures can be more fully seen. The anulus is incised below the floor of the spinal canal, and by curettage the intervertebral disc and contiguous portions of bone are removed as far as the opposite side of the vertebral bodies. This resection involves only the more dorsal portion of the vertebral body and is facilitated by use of a brace and bit. The floor of the spinal canal is preserved to avoid the epidural veins for as long as possible. The dura is identified and separated from the floor of the spinal canal. Sharp curets are introduced between the dura and the floor of the canal, and the disc material and attached portions of bone are broken downward into the previously created cavity (Fig. 14-1 *F, G*). Bleeding from the epidural veins can be brisk, but packing with cottonoids is avoided to decrease the possibility of injury to the cord. Adequacy of resection can be determined by means of a dental mirror placed anterior to the dura. Fusion or application of Harrington rods also can be done as part of the same procedure. The bone graft can be placed into the defect in the vertebral body, or over the lamina, or at both places.

If the pleura has been lacerated, a bronchopleural fistula may result. To test for this injury, the pleural cavity is filled with saline and the lungs expanded. If the lungs are intact, the pleural laceration is closed around a small catheter which is led out through the wound. The wound is closed in layers. A syringe is attached to the catheter for aspiration while the lungs are expanded and the catheter withdrawn. If a bronchopleural fistula exists, a chest tube connected to a closed drainage system is, of course, required.

LATERAL EXTRAPERITONEAL APPROACH

In the lumbar region, a similar incision is used (Fig. 14-2 *A*). The lumbodorsal fascia is incised and the latissimus split (Fig. 14-2 *B*). Depending on the patient's build, the erector spinae muscle is either retracted medially or split. In the lower lumbar region it is usually necessary to incise the erector spinae from its

attachment to the ilium and sometimes from the superior surface of the sacrum. Usually at least two transverse processes are identified, and their superior surfaces cleared of the erector spinae muscle and inferior surfaces of the quadratus lumborum. The transverse processes and associated intertransversarii muscles are resected (Fig. 14-2 *C*). While a stick sponge or other instrument is used to depress the quadratus lumborum and retroperitoneal fat, the elements of the lumbar plexus are identified. These tend to be mingled with the fibers of the psoas but can be separated without difficulty. The first nerve seen is that which has exited through the foramen immediately above. Further resection of transverse processes and soft tissue permits identification of the nerve at the level of the pathologic process. The nerve is traced to the foramen and sufficient bone is removed from the pedicles above and below to provide adequate exposure of the spinal canal and contents. Division of connecting rami to the sympathetic chain allows sufficient mobility of the nerves to permit excision of the intervertebral disc and adjacent bone (Fig. 14-2 *D*). The remainder of the procedure is much the same as in the thoracic

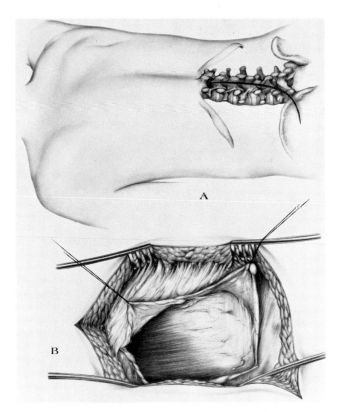

FIG. 14-2. Lateral retroperitoneal approach: *A*, lumbar incision is comparable to that used in thoracic area; *B*, lumbar fascia is incised; *C*, transverse processes and associated intertransversarii muscles are resected; *D*, disc is removed; *E, F, G*, bone is removed from vertebral body and fusion is achieved with iliac bone graft.

(*Figure continued on page 140.*)

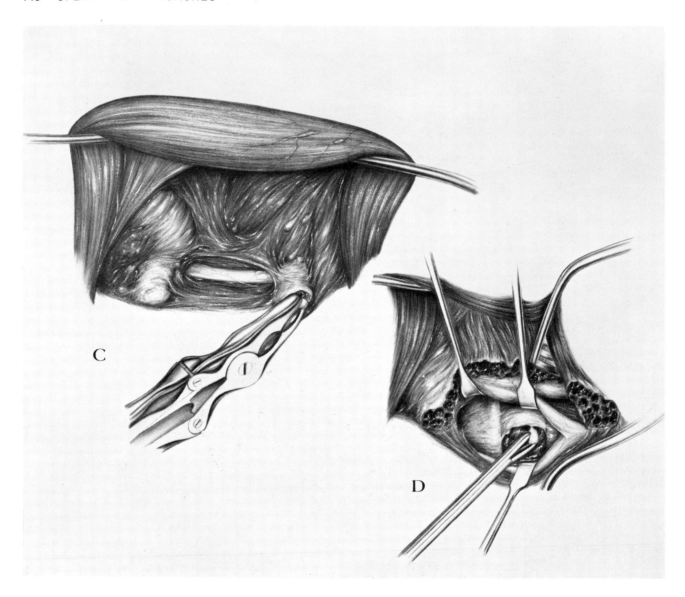

FIG. 14-2 (*Continued*)

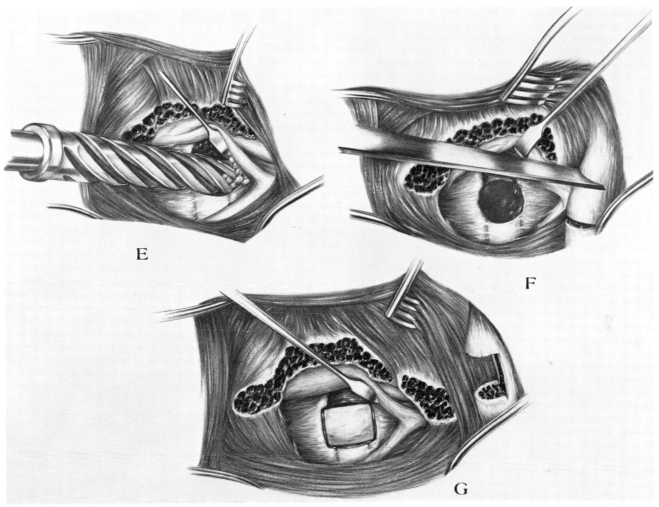

FIG. 14-2 (*Continued*)

region, except that cottonoids can be used more freely. If desired, interbody fusion can be done with bone from the conveniently located iliac crest (Fig. 14-2 *E, F, G*). If the L5–S1 level is to be approached, it is necessary to resect the superior portion of the sacrum.

The lateral approach makes possible the removal of lesions that cannot be safely reached by laminectomy or costotransversectomy. With the extrapleural or extraperitoneal route, the morbidity and complications of thoracotomy or laparotomy are avoided. Also, in the lumbar region it is sometimes difficult at laparotomy to

mobilize the iliac arteries and veins sufficiently to achieve adequate exposure. The major disadvantage of the procedure is difficulty in controlling bleeding, which can be profuse.

References

1. Alexander GL: Neurological complications of spinal tuberculosis. Proc Roy Soc Med *39*:730–734, 1946.
2. Capener N: The evolution of lateral rhachotomy. J Bone Joint Surg *36B*:173–179, 1954.

15

Lumbar Spinal Fusion

LEON L. WILTSE

THE PLACE of spinal fusion in the treatment of lumbar disc disease has been the subject of some critical re-examination during the past ten years.

It was believed at one time that a solid fusion assured a painless low back. If pain persisted, the fusion was thought to be a failure, and an exploration had to be done to find the pseudarthrosis and repeat the arthrodesis procedure. In the light of present information, it would appear that this attitude is not justified. We are seeing many cases in which the fusion is unquestionably solid, yet severe pain persists.

The work of DePalma and Rothman, in which they reviewed 448 spinal fusions (39 had definite pseudarthrosis), presents a comparison of the pseudarthrosis cases with a matched group having solid fusion, chosen from the remaining 409.[4] They found that the group with pseudarthrosis were as free of pain as those with solid fusions; this finding has tended to jar the faith of many of us who viewed the spinal fusion as a nearly infallible means of relieving discogenic back pain.

There is no doubt that the child or young adult with spondylolisthesis responds well to fusion,[9] as do patients with instability due to fracture or dislocation. However, when pain alone is the problem, the value of the spinal fusion must be re-examined.

Heretofore, spinal fusion has been added in cases of laminectomy when narrowed disc space is noted. Yet, following laminectomy, disc spaces narrow markedly over a period of years in 79% of cases. With the advent of chymopapain, significant narrowing of the disc space has been noted in most cases, yet most have not required spinal fusion to date.

Many of the common anomalies of the low back, either congenital or acquired, which we once considered indications for spinal fusion, are no longer thought to be. These include cases of transitional vertebrae, tropism, degenerative spondylolisthesis, instability noted on flexion-extension roentgenograms,[8] increased lumbar lordosis, lumbosacral tilt, and others.

In the past, a patient who failed to obtain relief from laminectomy was further treated by decompression of the (apparently) offending nerve root and by fusion from L4 to sacrum. Before 1952 it was our practice to fuse L5 to sacrum—one level in other words. Because many of these patients continued to have trouble, usually requiring further treatment by laminectomy of L4 and an extension of the fusion to L4, the one-level fusion has been abandoned in the treatment of patients with discogenic pain.

We now often inject chymopapain into the spine of the patient who has not obtained relief from laminectomy. If the injection fails to relieve pain we then perform a wide decompression, and only if this fails do we perform a spinal fusion. As a result of these practices, we find ourselves performing far fewer fusions than previously.

When a fusion is necessary, we usually proceed through a paraspinal approach (see Chap. 16),[9] but through a midline skin incision, since most of these patients have already had a midline skin incision. With the paraspinal approach, circulation to the spinous processes is not curtailed, which is not the case when muscles are stripped bilaterally.[3]

Crock has reported that in fusing a spine through the midline approach, he often fuses only one side from the tips of the transverse processes to the tips of the spinous processes.[3] Six weeks later he returns and fuses the other side. He claims, having made an extensive study of the problem, that when both sides are opened at the same time, virtually no circulation remains in the laminae or spinous processes, and chances for successful arthrodesis are reduced.

Three level fusions are almost a thing of the past in

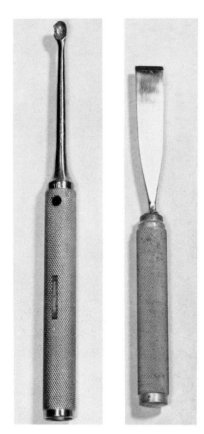

FIG. 15-2. *A,* Large curette designed by McElroy is excellent. *B,* One-inch wide, long-handled chisel of type shown here is useful as periosteal elevator.

our practice, because of the low rate of solid fusion that results. In the last 14 years we have used the paraspinal approach in most cases, but for the occasional case when a spinal fusion is done through the midline, the technique is described here.

MIDLINE APPROACH (FIG. 15-1)

The patient is positioned on the operating table, either prone with pads under his iliac crests or, if preferred, in the kneeling position as described by Hastings and others. A midline skin incision is made, starting at the spinous process of the vertebra above the level to be fused and extending distally to the spinous process of S2.

With a one-inch wide, long-handled chisel (Fig. 15-2), the muscles are stripped subperiosteally from the sides of the spinous processes and the laminae. Care is taken not to extend the stripping higher than the vertebra that is to be fused. The facets are denuded of capsule.

As the stripping proceeds laterally over the facet, bleeding is likely to occur. This can be controlled by cautery, or a square of Surgicel, about 3 × 3 cm., can be wadded and tamped into the bleeding hole. It is our

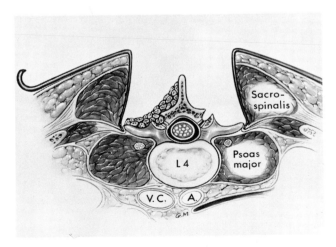

FIG. 15-1. Skin incision is midline and all tissues are stripped from spinous processes, laminae, and transverse processes. Anterior two-thirds of facets are excised.

practice to remove the Surgicel before closing, but no ill effects are noted if it is accidentally left in the wound.

At this stage the transverse processes can be felt with the finger. The transverse process lies at a level between the two articular processes. For example, the transverse process of L5 lies just caudad to the superior articular process of L5.

Once the transverse process has been located with the finger, it is denuded of soft tissue with a sharp chisel. Care must be taken not to break it. Once the tip is reached we usually cut partially, with a small scalpel, the ligament that attaches to the tip, and hook a special retractor over the end (Fig. 15-3). A heavy self-retaining retractor, such as the one designed by McElroy, is of value. Until the tip is reached, however, we find it easier to work on one side at a time without the large self-retaining retractor in place.

The posterior primary divisions of the lumbar nerves, along with the posterior extensions of the lumbar arteries and veins, extend posteriorly just above the bases of the transverse process, and also at the cephalo-medial corner of the ala of the sacrum. There is no way to avoid cutting these (Fig. 15-4), causing a segment of muscle to be denervated. Fortunately it is going to be fused, and so this denervation is of no great concern.

The posterior primary divisions of the L4 and L5 nerve roots have no sensory component to the skin; therefore hypesthesia of the skin does not occur here (Fig. 15-5). However, if the fusion is extended to L3, an area of hypesthesia, about 5 cm. wide, results over the region of the greater sciatic notch, since the L3 lumbar nerve root has a sensory component to the skin.

We normally excise the posterior two-thirds of the

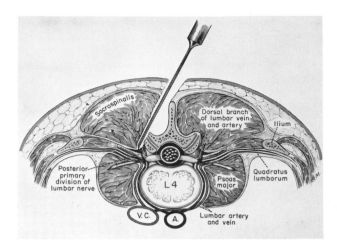

FIG. 15-4. As chisel or other periosteal elevator is passed out over facets and onto transverse processes, there is no way to avoid cutting posterior primary division as it comes posteriorly just above base of transverse process.

facet and tamp bone into this space. We also excise the ligament between the spinous processes because we believe it to be weakened and of little value (Fig. 15-6). The facet of the lamina of the segment above the area to be fused should not be exposed except for the outer

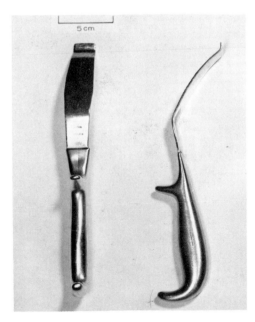

FIG. 15-3. Retractor shown is effective when slipped over tip of transverse process. Very little pressure should be exerted or transverse process will be fractured.

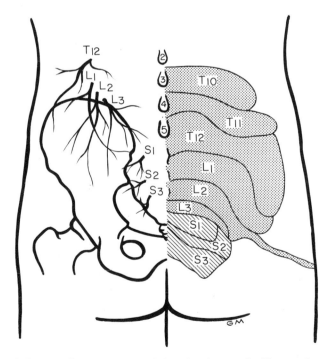

FIG. 15-5. Sensory areas in low back supplied by posterior primary divisions. Note that L4 and L5 lumbar nerves supply no skin area. This is important since these posterior primary divisions are cut in doing transverse process fusion of L4 and L5 to sacrum. (From Wiltse LL, Hutchinson RH: The surgical treatment of spondylolisthesis. CORR 35:126, 1964.)

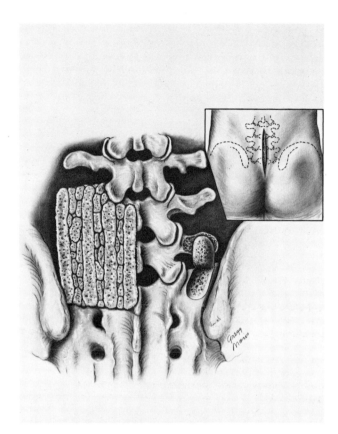

FIG. 15-6. Fusion of L4 to sacrum through midline approach. Strips of graft from posterior ilium are laid from sacrum to transverse process of L4. Care is taken to denude outer face of superior articular process of L4, but not to damage facet between L4 and L3.

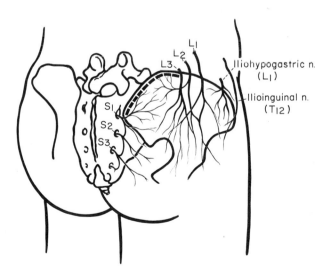

FIG. 15-7. Note that cluneal nerves come across iliac crest about handbreadth from posterior superior iliac spine. If incision is kept well posterior and area in front undermined, one can avoid cutting these. (From Wiltse LL, Hutchinson RH: The surgical treatment of spondylolisthesis. CORR 35:126, 1964.)

face of the superior articular process of the uppermost vertebra to be fused.

The same incision can be used to obtain bone from the posterior ilium. It is not necessary to extend the incision or to angle it off laterally toward the iliac crest (Fig. 15-7). The skin can be undermined as far as the posterior superior iliac spine without difficulty. Then, with a sharp scalpel, the tough ligament on top of the posterior spine can be cut, and with the wide chisel, a periosteal dissection can be done on the outer face of the ilium. A special retractor can be slipped into place and bone removed from the outer face (Fig. 15-8).

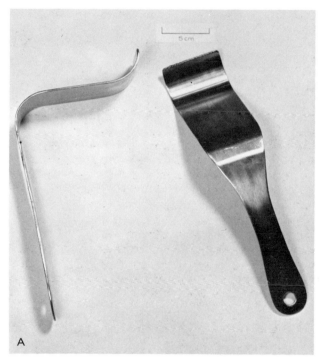

A

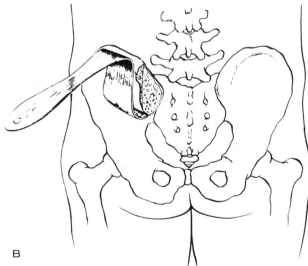

B

FIG. 15-8. A, Midline incision will serve to get bone from outer face of ilium. Then this special retractor can be slipped down outer side of ilium. B, Retractor in place.

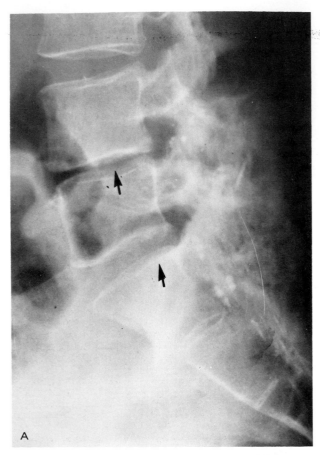

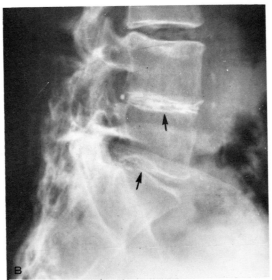

FIG. 15-9. *A,* Fusion from L4 to S1 done in 1957 in Caucasian woman aged 46. Discectomies were done at both L4 and L5. *B,* Observe marked narrowing and calcification of disc at L4, and narrowing, but with less calcification, at L5, in roentgenogram taken 13 years after fusion.

If an area has been decompressed, and it is believed that bone might fall into the opening and compress the cauda equina, we often cover this area with a flake of bone taken from the ilium. This flake is placed smooth-side down in the hope that bone will not grow inward. The nerve that has been exposed is then carefully covered with Gelfoam.

One iliac crest nearly always supplies enough bone to fuse both sides. Closure is routine. We do put in medium-sized siliconized drains, which can be attached to a suction apparatus, though we simply allow them to drain into a voluminous dressing. The drains are removed 48 hours after operation. We have seen great advantage in draining these wounds, and no disadvantage except that sometimes bleeding can be quite profuse, and it can be difficult to obtain enough pressure to stop the bleeding as long as the drains are in place. In our experience, however, this problem has not been insurmountable.

These patients are allowed to be up as soon as they are able and are started on a routine of isometric abdominal setting exercises in a few days. These abdominal setting exercises are continued indefinitely and are an integral part of routine low back care, both before and after operation.

An interesting phenomenon has been noted in the intervertebral discs of patients who have had a solid posterior lateral fusion for several years. The disc spaces tend to become much narrower. It is not known whether this happens when no discectomy has been done, but it has occurred in all cases I have subjected to x-ray examination years later (Fig. 15-9 *A, B*). This phenomenon seems not to occur in cases fused posteriorly only, perhaps because enough spring remains to keep the disc more nearly normal.

INTERBODY FUSION OF THE LUMBAR SPINE

Discussion of anterior interbody fusion in this chapter will be principally directed toward its use in the treatment of discogenic disease and spondylolisthesis, in which cases the procedure is done for the relief of pain. However, anterior fusion is also used in the treatment of other conditions of the lumbar spine. Tuberculosis of the spine, as well as other infections, is probably best treated by excision of the tuberculous mass and fusion (see Chap. 9).

Anterior decompression of the spinal cord by removal of the infected mass has been known to reverse progressive paraplegia (see Chap. 9). In cases of fracture dislocation of the spine, anterior fusion may be necessary to remove masses of bone or intervertebral disc to decompress the cord (see Chap. 9). Severe congenital kyphosis in children often requires removal of all or part of a vertebral body from an anterior approach and fusion of the two remaining adjacent vertebral bodies.

Interbody fusion has been in use for many years in the treatment of the painful low back, but never widely. The following reasons can be cited:

1. The success rate for obtaining good solid fusion is low. In the hands of a few surgeons, those who have had much experience and have almost made a hobby of interbody fusions, the success rate is satisfactorily high. I would warn, however, that the surgeon who does only an occasional interbody fusion is likely to be disappointed.

2. Often interbody fusion does not relieve the patient's pain. This is not entirely the fault of the fusion, which is often performed as a salvage procedure after previous posterior fusions have failed. We are all well aware that heroic attempts to get a solid fusion are usually disappointing because pain continues.

3. Interbody fusions through the anterior approach result in considerably more complications than do posterior or posterior-lateral fusions. Because of their proximity, every so often one of the great vessels is torn and requires repair. For this reason, no one should embark on an anterior interbody fusion unless he feels capable of repairing a large vessel or has a vascular surgeon in attendance (see Chap. 17).

4. The incidence of sexual dysfunction in the male is a definite factor to consider. Any of the larger reported series have cases of retrograde ejaculation. These seem to involve about two cases in 50, on the average. Although impotence is commonly complained of, this is not secondary to the operation but is a psychologic phenomenon. We have always used a special waiver form, which both husband and wife are asked to sign. This sets forth all of the possible dangers to sexual function. Even this is not complete legal protection.

Problems with anesthesia or infection have not been any greater with the anterior approach than with the posterior or posterolateral approach. Also, such technical errors as driving a plug back into the cauda equina can occur, but in our experience fortunately have not.

In discogenic disease we use the anterior interbody fusion only after at least two attempts at posterior spinal fusion have failed. We prefer to perform the anterior interbody fusion at one level only. The posterior fusion from L4 to the sacrum often has succeeded at the L5 to S1 level and failed at the L4 to L5 level. In the patient with favorable psychometric studies, we occasionally perform an anterior interbody fusion, especially if preoperative relief has been afforded by a cast or brace.

Patients with spondylolisthesis when first seen by us have had the posterior elements removed and a transverse process fusion performed, either from L5 to the sacrum or from L4 to the sacrum. Frequently these spines are quite unstable and the L5 vertebra actually slips backward and forward on S1 when the patient stands or lies down (Fig. 15-10). These are candidates for anterior interbody fusion. In these cases when the fusion desired is only from L5 to S1, we perform a Freebody procedure between L5 and S1. If it is believed necessary to include L4, it has been our custom to fuse the L4 level with blocks of ilium as noted in Figure 15-10. Here we see the blocks of ilium in place shaped like little horseshoes. We block the spine as far apart as possible before inserting these; then between L5 and S1, we use the Freebody technique.

TECHNIQUE FOR ANTERIOR LUMBAR SPINE FUSION

Raney Technique

Frank Raney of San Francisco has developed a technique for fusion of the lumbar spine. The details of this technique are given in Chapter 17.

Freebody Technique

Mr. Douglas Freebody of London has developed a technique that now bears his name.[5] The details are as follows: A midline incision is made in the lower abdomen, and the abdominal contents are moved out of the way. A catheter should be placed in the urinary bladder preoperatively to keep it as small as possible. A longitudinal incision is made in the posterior peritoneum overlying the vertebrae to be fused. Before this is done, the tissues overlying the bodies of L4-L5 to S1 are infiltrated with saline and epinephrine. This maneuver facilitates the identification of structures, permitting the presacral nerve and vessels to be pushed laterally with a "pusher," as they pass over the sacral promontory. Bleeding also is diminished by the epinephrine. Electrocoagulation should never be used here. If the bifurcation of the great vessels is high the fifth disc can be approached between them. If the bifurcation is low, the vessels can be retracted to the right after ligation of the left lumbar vessels, which pass laterally around the vertebral bodies (Fig. 15-11). The large vessels are carefully pushed over as far as possible to expose the disc and retractors are driven into place. A flap of anulus based to the right is then freed, and the disc is completely excised. A portion of the end plates is removed to raw bone.

A trap door is removed from the front of the body of L5, as seen in Figure 15-12. Through this trap door access is gained to the top of S1. With a curette (or if the bone is too hard, a large drill) a hole is made through S1 to about the center of S2, perhaps 4 cm. in depth into the sacrum.

An osteoperiosteal flap is then lifted off the crest of the ilium and a full-thickness bone graft is removed from the top of the iliac crest at its thickest point. This graft is about 2.5×6 cm. and is about the shape and size of a man's thumb. It is driven into the prepared slot across L5 into S1. The trap door is impacted back into the body of L5. The spaces on either side of the graft,

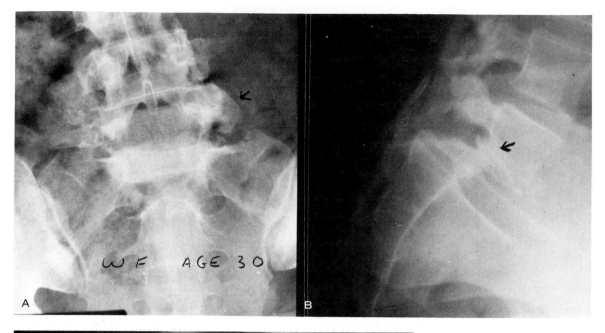

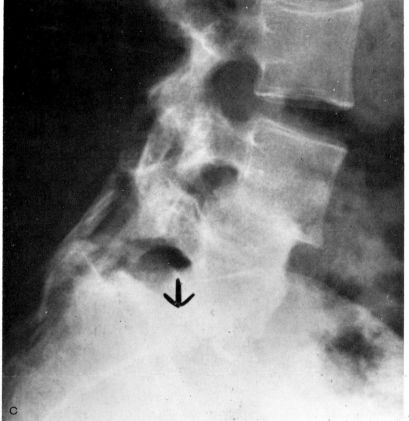

FIG. 15-10. *A* and *B,* This 30-year-old Caucasian woman had removal of loose element plus two previous attempts to get fusion posteriorly between L4 and sacrum. Failure of fusion occurred at both levels, and L5 remained especially unstable, slip actually increasing by standing. *C,* Blocks of ilium were used to fuse L4 to L5 anteriorly and Freebody grafting was done between L5 and S1.

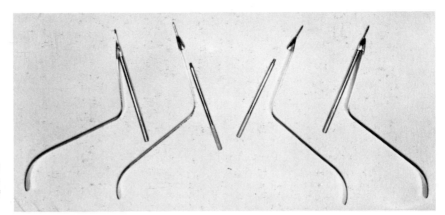

FIG. 15-11. These retractors used for anterior interbody fusion were designed by Dr. Frank Raney of San Francisco.

which had been occupied by disc tissue, are curetted to bleeding bone and tamped full of cancellous bone. The prepared flap of anulus is sutured back into place, and the wound is closed. The patient is kept in a plaster bed for six weeks before ambulation is permitted, and then only in a molded plastic jacket, which he wears until the fusion appears solid (Fig. 15-13).

Our results with the Freebody arthrodesis have been only fair. In several of our cases, non-union resulted even though the procedure seemed to have been performed well technically, and the patients were kept immobilized postoperatively as recommended.

It is not necessary to fuse two levels in most patients with spondylolisthesis but many have already undergone extensive surgery posteriorly, and the fourth disc space has been cureted. Under these circumstances we feel it advisable to stabilize the L4 space also. We do not use the Freebody technique to stabilize this space, but prefer to use multiple horseshoe-shaped blocks of ilium cut from the top of the iliac crest (Fig. 15-14).

We prefer the transperitoneal approach when we must do an anterior fusion between L5 and S1, especially if there is high-grade slip in spondylolisthesis. In such cases it is virtually impossible to perform a satisfactory fusion of the L5–S1 interspace through a retroperitoneal approach.

LEFT FLANK APPROACH

Abdominal hernia occurs occasionally in the line of incision with both of the above approaches. For this reason we have adopted a left flank incision, similar to that used for nephrectomy or sympathectomy, when we intend to fuse the L3 or L4, but not the L5 level. This approach is easily closed and is free of complications. The incision is an oblique one, halfway between the lower rib cage and iliac crest. It is usually necessary to extend the incision an inch or two more medially

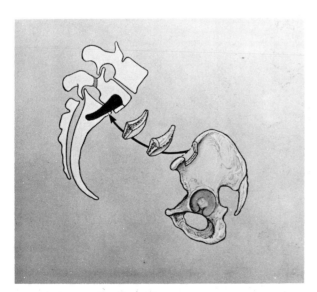

FIG. 15-12. Drawing of technique of Freebody fusion.

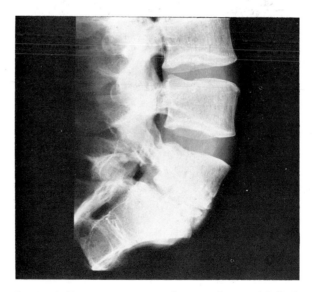

FIG. 15-13. Roentgenogram of case of spondylolisthesis at L5, for which arthrodesis was done by Freebody technique one year ago.

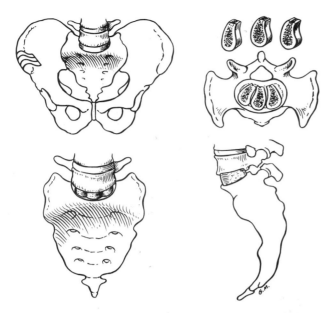

FIG. 15-14. Type of graft shown here fuses well in our experience only if there has been an attempt or two at posterior fusion, so that stability has already been obtained.

than is required for sympathectomy. The incision is then carried through the external oblique, internal oblique, and transverse abdominal muscles. The vertical muscle bundles encountered generally have to be divided to obtain adequate exposure. To enter the retroperitoneal space, the posterior peritoneum is gently and bluntly dissected medially, a maneuver that exposes the anterior surface of the psoas muscle. The ureter has to be carefully mobilized so that it is not damaged. Exposure is continued, by blunt dissection primarily, but it is a matter of mobilizing the vascular structures proximally and distally enough to expose the appropriate lumbar intervertebral space. Surgical hemoclips are helpful in the control of small bleeders, but one troublesome problem is fragile lumbar veins, which can bleed profusely if torn.[7] Another real advantage of this approach is that bone for the fusion can easily be removed without a separate skin incision.

OTHER TECHNIQUES FOR INTERBODY FUSION

Using Fibula Only

To fuse just one level we use fibula alone (Fig. 15-15). We specify one level because enough fibula to fuse two levels is difficult to obtain from one leg. It is not advisable to remove fibula below the junction of its middle and lower thirds or less than two inches from its top. When fibular struts are used the vertebral end plates are excised, and the bodies spread severely. The segments of fibula are sawed with a reciprocating saw and impacted into place securely. They are stood on end between the bodies. It is mandatory that these fibular grafts be held in place securely, and that they be in a straight up and down position between the vertebral bodies. If they tip over, fusion will not occur.

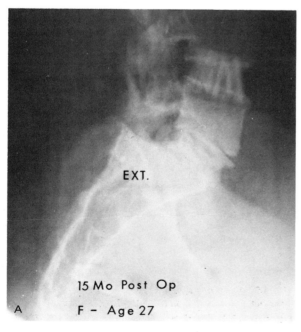
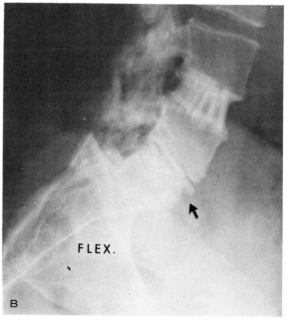

FIG. 15-15. *A* and *B*, Fibular graft was used at both L4 and L5 spaces. At L4 fusion succeeded but at L5 it failed because fibular grafts tipped over. Fibular grafts in lower lumbar spine in adult must stand squarely on end and bodies must be wedged severely apart with much pressure put on grafts or fusion will not occur.

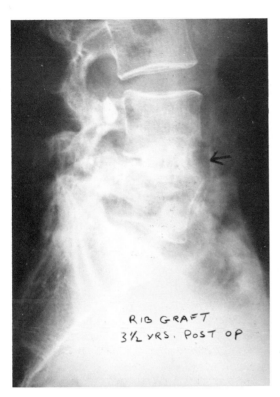

FIG. 15-16. L4 space was fused with segments of rib made to stand on end. Rib is rather soft but has good osteogenic potential and fuses better than ilium.

Rib Grafts

Rib grafts are satisfactory in some situations (Fig. 15-16). The rib grafts are cut to approximate length, the vertebral bodies are spread, and the segments are stood on end between the bodies. Rib is much weaker than fibula, but has good osteogenic potential. It works well in the occasional child who needs an interbody fusion. Also it is used to good advantage in cases of tuberculosis when cavities in the vertebral bodies must be filled with bone. Often some rib has been removed in the approach in these cases.

"Horseshoe" Iliac Grafts (see Fig. 15-14)

When an interbody fusion of the L4 space is combined with a Freebody graft at the L5 space, the type of graft shown in Figure 15-16 is satisfactory. In these cases, one or two attempts at posterior fusion have usually been made, and so some stability is already present.

All interbody grafts, no matter what type, should be so placed that the entire space, front to back, is filled.

Dowel Grafts (Fig. 15-17)

Dowel grafts have been used extensively by Harmon[6] and by others. We have had some experience with these,

but have found that unless considerable stability is already present from attempts at posterior fusion, pseudarthrosis is the rule.

Lumbar Interbody Fusion by the Posterior Route

Cloward has described a method of interbody fusion through a posterior midline approach.[2] In this operation the laminae are approached as for a classic laminectomy. The interspinous ligament and the margins of the adjacent spinous processes are removed to permit insertion of a special vertebral spreader. About half of the adjacent laminal edge is removed along with the articular facets. The cauda equina is retracted to one side. The posterior anulus is excised, along with the nucleus pulposus. The cortical surfaces of the adjacent vertebral bodies are removed as far as raw bleeding bone.[1]

Full-thickness autogenous iliac grafts are then driven into the space, two on each side, making a total of four to completely fill the disc space. The wound is closed routinely, and the patient is permitted out of bed when able.

We have used this fusion on a number of occasions, but have found that failure of fusion was the rule. We then added a posterior fusion to the procedure, and found that with this combination solid fusion nearly always occurred. However, solid fusion usually occurs with one-level posterior fusions without the anterior component. We now use the Cloward interbody fusion in the occasional case of L4 spondylolisthesis in the adult in which the posterior element must be removed

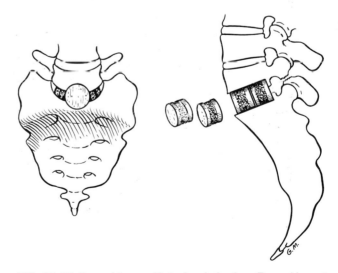

FIG. 15-17. Dowel type of interbody fusion. Dowel is cut from ilium by special plug cutters. Hole cut between vertebral bodies must be made with smaller plug-cutter than one used to cut dowel from ilium in order to make it fit snugly. As usual, bodies should be spread severely before hole is cut to obtain maximum compression of graft. Even then failure of fusion is the rule.

as part of the decompression procedure. The combination of the interbody and an intertransverse process fusion will succeed in cases in which either alone would fail.

A note of caution should be sounded: if the procedure extends above the area where the conus of the spinal cord ends, great care should be used in retracting the dura and its contents in getting the plugs in. Several cases of partial paralysis have been reported.

POSTOPERATIVE CARE

Except in the case of the Freebody operation, we permit ambulation just a few days after operation. A brace is worn during ambulation, more as a reminder to avoid bending than as an actual immobilizer of the lumbar area.

TESTING THE SOLIDITY OF THE FUSION

The question whether the fusion is or is not solid is always troublesome.

In cases of anterior interbody fusion, one must see trabeculae crossing the interspace to be sure of fusion.

We use bending films on all fusion cases, whether anterior interbody or posterior, and feel strongly that they are valuable. Figure 15-18 *A* illustrates the clamp we use to prevent the pelvis from rolling when taking anterior-posterior bending films. The patient pulls himself into right and left lateral flexion as much as possible. Intravenous Demerol is given if pain is a limiting factor. The films are simply superimposed over a bright light. Figure 15-19 *B* shows the lateral view being taken. A simple square is laid against the bony prominences to be sure that the patient is not twisting while exposures are made during flexion and extension.

Unfortunately, in the patient who has had multiple back operations and still has pain and pseudarthrosis, even a solid fusion often does not relieve the pain. What then is the place of lumbar interbody fusion in the treatment of low back pain? We still use it in the patient who fulfills the following criteria: (1) non-union at one level instead of two; (2) evidence that the levels above the area of contemplated fusion are reasonably normal; (3) partial relief from a brace or corset; (4) favorable psychometric studies; and (5) good general health and under 55 years of age. I limit the age, because older people are probably best advised to limit their activities.

No one should attempt an anterior interbody fusion of the lumbar spine without special retractors. Several types have been designed, but all work on the same basic principle, that is, once the large veins and arteries

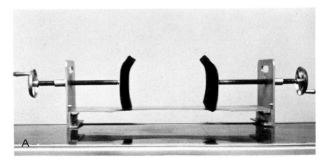

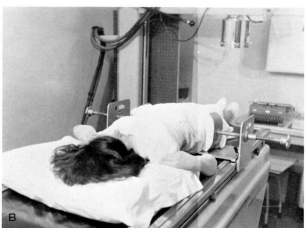

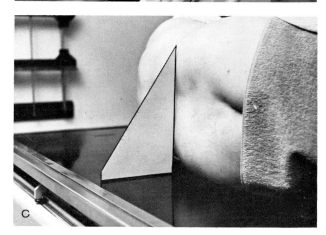

FIG. 15-18. *A,* This apparatus fits on top of most x-ray tables. Pelvis is held between padded arms of clamp so that, when patient bends, pelvis does not roll. *B,* Patient is shown in apparatus. She takes hold of knob on side and pulls herself into lateral flexion. *C,* Square is used to ensure that patient does not roll as flexion and extension are performed.

have been mobilized, a spike-type retractor is driven into the vertebral body. We have used a type designed by Frank Raney (see Fig. 15-11).

Finally I would warn that the surgeon who only occasionally does an anterior lumbar fusion is likely to find that his nonunion rate is unacceptably high.

References

1. Cloward RB: Lesion of the intervertebral discs and their treatment by interbody fusion methods. Clin Orthop *27*:51-77, 1963.
2. Cloward RB: The treatment of ruptured intervertebral discs by vertebral body fusion. Ann. Surg. *136*:987-992, 1952.
3. Crock H: Personal communication, 1971.
4. DePalma A, Rothman R: The nature of pseudoarthrosis. Clin Orthop Rel Research *59*:113-118, 1968.
5. Freebody D, Bedall R, Taylor RD: Anterior transperitoneal lumbar fusion. J Bone Joint Surg *53B*:617-627, 1971.
6. Harmon PH: Anterior disc excision and fusion of the lumbar vertebral bodies: a review of diagnostic testing with operative results in more than 700 cases. J Inter Coll Surg *40*:572-586, 1963.
7. Hickman E: Personal communication, 1973.
8. Wiltse LL: The effect of the common anomalies of the lumbar spine upon disc degeneration of low back pain. Orth Clin N Amer *2*:569-582, 1971.
9. Wiltse LL: The paraspinal sacrospinalis-splitting approach to the lumbar spine. J Bone Joint Surg *50A*:569-582, 1971.

16

Paraspinal Approach to the Lumbar Spine

LEON L. WILTSE

THE PARASPINAL approach to the lumbar spine is one that passes through the sacrospinalis muscle about two fingerbreadths lateral to the midline,[10] providing better access to the transverse processes and lateral masses of the vertebrae.

OPERATIVE TECHNIQUE

The patient is placed on the operating table either prone or in a modified knee-chest position.

If there has been no previous operation on the lower spine, two skin incisions may be made, each about 4.5 cm. lateral to the midline and just medial to the posterior superior iliac spines (Fig. 16-1). The incisions curve slightly medialward caudally. If, on the other hand, the patient has undergone operation, one may be reluctant to add further scars and may thus use the usual midline incision, extending it a bit on each end to permit retraction first to one side and then to the other, in order to make the paraspinal approach through the muscle (Fig. 16-2). We have also used transverse skin incisions in young women in whom cosmetic appearance was very important.

After the skin and subcutaneous tissues are incised, the lumbodorsal fascia is seen (Fig. 16-3). It is cut longitudinally 4.5 cm. lateral to the midline, bringing the sacrospinalis muscle into view. This muscle has a thick fascial layer as it approaches its caudal end. A longitudinal incision is made in the fascia of the sacrospinalis about three-fourths of the way toward its lateral border. The incision swings medially at its caudal end in the shape of a hockey stick, thus cutting the heavy conjoined fascia transversely for about

154

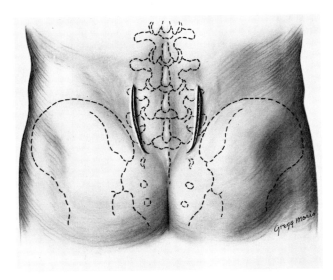

FIG. 16-1. Incisions as pictured are long enough to expose transverse processes of L4, L5, and the sacral ala.

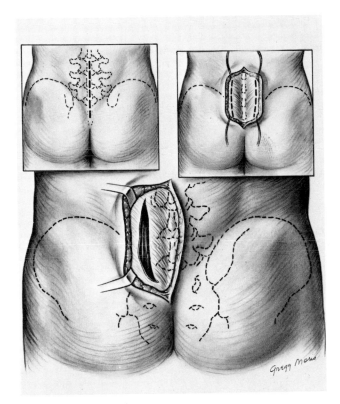

FIG. 16-2. If preferred, single midline incision may be used. This incision must be slightly longer than usual and skin must be undermined sufficiently to allow it to be retracted two fingerbreadths lateral to midline, so that fascial incisions can be made in their proper places. Upper left insert shows extent of skin incision. If single midline incision is used, skin is undermined and retracted, first to one side and then to the other, to make fascial incision.

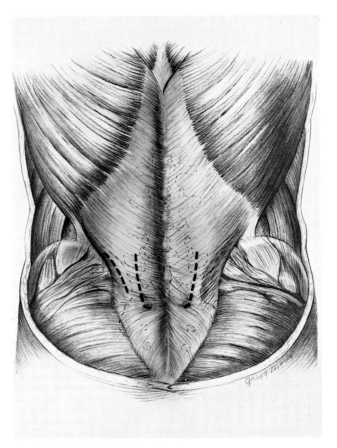

FIG. 16-3. Broken lines show where incisions in fascia are made. Broken line over posterior superior iliac spine indicates line of incision in fascia where bone graft is to be taken. One iliac crest will supply enough bone for both sides in most cases. (From Wiltse LL, Bateman JG, Nelson WE: Paraspinal sacrospinalis-splitting approach to the lumbar spine. J Bone Joint Surg 50-A:920, 1968.)

1 cm. to allow for retraction. The index finger can then be used to dissect through the muscle mass down to the sacrum and can be slipped down the back of the sacrum to the articular processes of the fifth lumbar and the first sacral vertebrae, as well as to the space between the transverse processes of L5 and the sacral ala.

It should be noted that the muscle fibers do not split cleanly, since at this level they run in various directions. They *can* be separated, however, and any tag ends of loose muscle are removed before the wound is sutured. Since this muscle will be denervated, only enough muscle need be left for adequate closure.

If a lumbosacral fusion is to be done, care is taken to avoid the natural tendency to dissect too far cephalad, or one will inadvertently expose the fourth lumbar vertebra. Two Gelpi retractors, bent to a right angle at a point two inches from their tips, are excellent for retracting the muscle. The sacrospinalis is then split only enough to expose the vertebra to be fused. On the sacrum the top of the ala should be denuded of soft tissue, but its posterior surface should not be denuded more than necessary to get exposure because bone grafts will be placed in contact with the top of the ala primarily. The laminae of the vertebra to be fused are exposed as far as, and well onto, the sloping bases of the spinous processes. The lumbar transverse processes should be denuded of soft tissue completely out to their tips and well around their superior and inferior borders. One may use a No. 15 blade scalpel to cut around the transverse processes, but it is wise not to dissect far anteriorly so that injury to a spinal nerve can be avoided (Fig. 16-4).

The lumbar arteries and veins pass just above the bases of the transverse processes and also at the angle of the medial point of the sacral ala.[5] They often bleed freely and may be difficult to electrocoagulate. These bleeding "holes" may be plugged with Surgicel. Vessels exiting from the superior sacral foramen also may bleed profusely and also can be plugged with Surgicel.

The operation may then proceed, and Surgicel may be removed once the bleeding has stopped.

Only the lateral surface of the superior articular processes of the topmost vertebra to be included in the fusion should be denuded, care being taken not to remove the capsule or to damage the adjacent joint. One should not expose any part of the vertebra immediately above the fusion area. If these precautions are observed, any tendency for the fusion to extend upward will be avoided. Within the fusion area, the lateral surface of the superior articular process, as well as the pars interarticularis and lamina, is meticulously denuded of soft tissue as far medially as the base of the spinous processes. The spinous processes are not exposed, and their ligamentous attachments and some of their blood supply are thereby preserved. The intervertebral joints within the fusion area are carefully exposed, and the articular cartilage in the posterior two-thirds of each joint is removed.

The graft bed is prepared as in a classic Hibbs fusion. A flap of bone from the top of the ala of the sacrum,

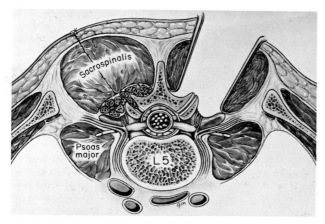

FIG. 16-4. Two bent Gelpi retractors seem to be best instruments for retraction of muscle. Note location of bone grafts after closure of wound (left).

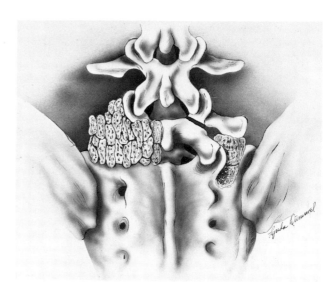

FIG. 16-5. Extent of bone graft. Note that graft covers lateral surface of superior articular process of fifth lumbar vertebra and joint between fifth lumbar and first sacral vertebrae is fused. Joint between L4 and L5 is not injured, but graft extends onto lateral aspect of superior articular process of fifth lumbar. Identical area is fused on opposite side also. *Note:* On right in picture, flap of bone has been turned upward from ala of sacrum, so that it bridges gap between ala and transverse process. (From Wiltse LL, Bateman JG, Hutchinson RH, Nelson WE: Paraspinal sacrospinalis-splitting approach to the lumbar spine. J Bone Joint Surg *50-A:*921, 1968.)

based anteriorly, is turned forward and cephalad to form a bridge to the transverse processes of the fifth lumbar vertebra (Fig. 16-5). Iliac grafts can be obtained from one or both sides of the pelvis through the same skin incisions, depending on the amount of bone needed. To obtain the graft, an incision is made through the fascia over the posterior superior iliac spine and extended along the iliac crest. The incision should not extend more than a hand's breadth forward on the crest in order to avoid injuring the cluneal nerves (see Fig. 15-7).[9] Bone for the graft is taken from the outer face of the posterior ilium, leaving the inner cortex intact. Cancellous bone is impacted between the denuded articular process and strips of cancellous iliac and cortical bone are tamped securely around the transverse processes, care being taken not to break them. The softer, pure cancellous bone is packed in first because it stays down well against the host bone.

The wound is then closed. The muscle is sutured loosely with a fine, chromatized catgut suture. The heavy fascia should be sutured securely.

POSTOPERATIVE MANAGEMENT

The patient is encouraged to get out of bed when he feels able, which is usually in a few days, and he is permitted to walk freely. It is better if he sits in a straight-backed chair and avoids deep, overstuffed sofas for two months. A routine of exercises, consisting of isometric abdominal and gluteal setting exercises, is started two or three days after the operation. All patients are trained to avoid motion of the low back by rolling like a log instead of twisting, and by squatting instead of stooping. Corsets or braces are not used unless the patient prefers to wear one, because neither enhances fusion.

In the past we have felt that, if there were more than 50% slip, the child must be kept recumbent for eight weeks or there would be an increase in slip during the healing phase following fusion.[3] This was definitely true when we were doing midline approaches.

Figure 16-6 shows a patient on whom a classic Hibbs spinal fusion was performed for spondylolisthesis in 1951, when he was ten years old. Note that in the lateral view on the left, there is 50% slip before the fusion. On the right, ten years after operation (via midline approach), the fusion is completely solid, the young man is well, and back doing heavy work, but note how markedly the L5 vertebra has slipped. It ended up clear

around in front of the sacrum. This is because most of the posterior ligaments that support the vertebra are cut (particularly the interspinous and the supraspinous ligaments) when a midline approach is made. By contrast in the paraspinal approach, relatively few of the supporting ligaments are cut, and consequently there is no further slip during the healing phase.

Recently we have been permitting the children to get out of bed immediately, no matter how much slip is present. A standing spot lateral of the lumbosacral joint is made preoperatively to be used as a baseline. Then, after the child has been ambulatory for three or four days, another single spot lateral is made, and it is repeated a week later. If there is any sign of slip, the child is put to bed until the fusion becomes solid, in about two months. If not, weekly x-ray examinations are continued for another two weeks and then at two-week intervals for one month. The gonads should be shielded with lead, but the total radiation received during the entire healing phase is equivalent to the radiation exposure of a standard low back series, since only single spot standing laterals are taken.

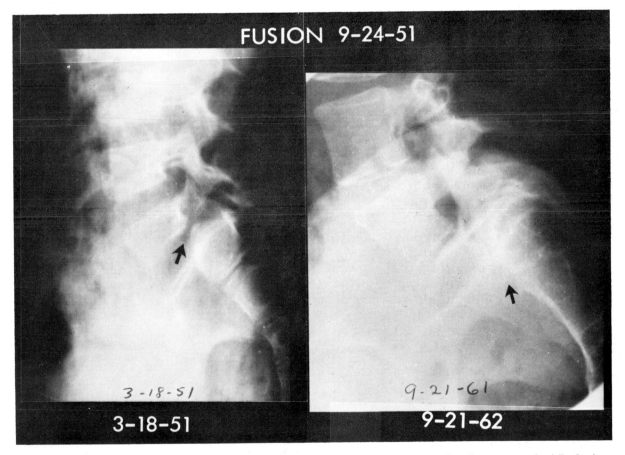

FIG. 16-6. This case had Hibbs type fusion of posterior elements only. Increase in slip occurred while fusion was becoming solid. Once fusion was solid, no further slip occurred. Note in above case that fifth lumbar vertebra slipped from third degree to complete spondyloptosis. This boy had no symptoms when last seen. Slipping has not occurred after operation in any of our cases in which we used paraspinal approach. (Courtesy Dr. Vernon Nickel, Downey, Calif.)

If the loose posterior element has been removed in a case of spondylolisthesis, there is an increased likelihood that slipping will occur, and if the anulus has been incised for the removal of a ruptured disc at the same level, in addition to removal of the loose element, progression is virtually certain if the patient is allowed to be ambulatory before the fusion is solidified.

When decompression of the cauda equina and nerve roots is indicated, it may be accomplished easily through the lateral route because it is centered almost directly over the region where the nerve root compression occurs, particularly in spondylolisthesis (Fig. 16-7). It is not necessary to perform a complete hemilaminectomy. With only a portion of the lamina removed, it is possible to trace the nerve root laterally and decompress it completely (Fig. 16-8). If a fibrocartilaginous mass is associated with spondylolisthesis, it lies in the direct line of approach and can be removed. In this connection it is worth noting that, except in cases of high-grade slip, it is the fifth lumbar root that is compressed in the presence of spondylolisthesis of the fifth lumbar vertebra. This may give the clinical picture of a ruptured disc at the interspace between the fourth and fifth lumbar vertebrae because an L4 disc usually compresses the L5 nerve root. In the rare cases in which it is felt that the posterior superior border of the sacrum must be removed, a midline approach is better.

If posterior rhizotomy is indicated because of intract-

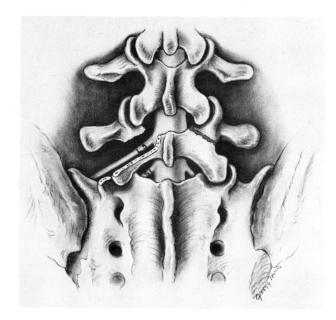

FIG. 16-8. It is advantageous to leave part of lamina, as shown here. Remaining portion of loose lamina is fused to sacrum, and thus rocking of this loose fragment, which may produce pain, is prevented. (From Wiltse LL, Bateman JG, Hutchinson RH, Nelson WE: Paraspinal sacrospinalis-splitting approach to the lumbar spine. J Bone Joint Surg 50-A:923, 1968.)

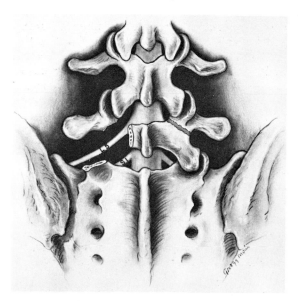

FIG. 16-7. Identifying and decompressing nerve root is more easily done through this approach than through midline approach. Here entire lateral half of lamina, including articular process and part of defective pars interarticularis, have been removed. (From Wiltse LL, Bateman JG, Hutchinson RG and Nelson WE: Paraspinal sacrospinalis-splitting approach to the lumbar spine. J Bone Joint Surg 50-A:923, 1968.)

able pain, this procedure can also be performed through this approach.

If there is a great deal of scarring from previous operations through a midline approach, or if there has been an infection on one side and the area can be bypassed, the approach described here might well be considered. When this approach is used for operations at higher levels, where the sacrum cannot be used as a guide, roentgenography with some type of marker should be used to ensure accurate localization.

An approach starting lateral to the sacrospinalis has been used by several surgeons.[2,4,6-9,11] The technique described here differs in that the muscle is split instead of being undermined from the lateral side. The laminae are also included in the fusion, but the spinous processes are avoided.

Through this approach either a one-level or a multilevel fusion can be done, leaving the supraspinous and interspinous ligaments intact, so that there is less instability postoperatively and hence less pain.

The anatomy of this approach is somewhat more complicated than that of the midline approach, since one does not have the spinous processes exposed to serve as a guide.

The question has arisen: can this approach be used with a very high-grade slip? Figure 16-9 shows roentgenograms of a child with an extremely high-grade slip who was operated upon through this approach. It is noted that this child has almost a vertical sacrum, with

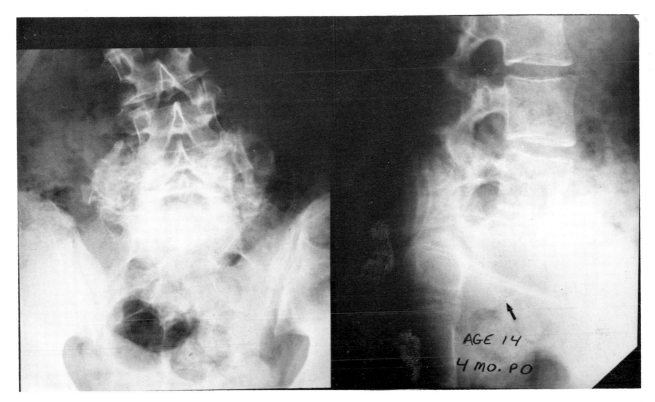

FIG. 16-9. This 14-year-old girl had high-grade slip and tight hamstrings. We found it technically advantageous to include L4 in fusion. Solid fusion occurred, and by end of year after operation tight hamstrings had disappeared.

the body of L5 around in front of S1. In this instance L4 was included, but it is preferable not to include it in most instances because one-level fusions succeed more frequently than do two-level fusions.

The question is often asked, "If one simply performs a fusion in the child with tight hamstrings, will the tightness of the hamstrings disappear?" In our experience, it always has. In a child with tight hamstrings who does not have severe sciatica, it is recommended that one perform a fusion and leave the loose element in place. This causes complete stability of the area and prevents rocking of the loose element. We believe that tight hamstrings are secondary to irritation of the cauda equina, one cause of which is the rocking of the loose element with each muscle contraction. Once this is completely stopped, the nerves adjust to their cramped quarters, and the tight hamstrings disappear over a period of several months.

The posterior primary divisions of the spinal nerves arising in the segment operated on are always cut whether one approaches the transverse process from the midline or by the route described here. Since the muscle is to be denervated anyway, it makes little difference whether it is undermined or split. The sacrospinalis is segmentally enervated, so that paralyzing a segment or two where the spine is to be fused does little harm. Fortunately the posterior primary divisions of the fourth and fifth lumbar nerves have no sensory

component to the skin, and so numbness does not result. The posterior primary division of the first sacral nerve does have a sensory component to the skin, but in our experience this nerve was injured just as frequently when we were making a midline approach and not extending the fusion out onto the transverse processes, as it is now with our present approach. Fortunately the area of hypoesthesia is quite small and seems to cause little trouble.

The advantages of the paraspinal sacrospinalis-splitting approach, and indications for its use are:

1. It is a good approach for patients in whom there is already solid fusion, but it is necessary to expose the nerves to decompress them.

2. It is useful for spinal fusion in patients who have had a wide midline laminectomy and there is some danger associated with a midline approach (Fig. 16-10).

3. In cases of spondylolisthesis the loose element is included in the fusion mass, so that it will not rock back and forth with each muscle contraction and possibly traumatize the cauda equina, causing pain and tight hamstrings. Ideally it simply elevates the sacrum one segment. It does not, however, produce interbody fusion (Fig. 16-11).

4. Because there is a layer of muscle between the fusion mass and the ilium, the fusion does not tend to extend to the ilium (Fig. 16-12). In children, if a sacroiliac joint is fused, the pelvis does not grow normally

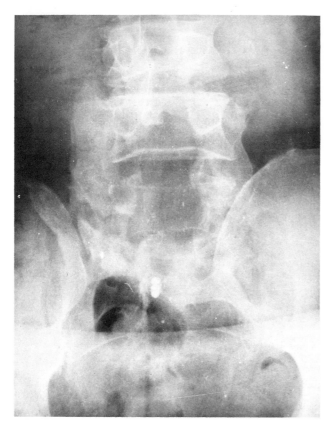

FIG. 16-10. This patient had had four previous laminectomies. By approaching spine more laterally, we were in safer, relatively unscarred area.

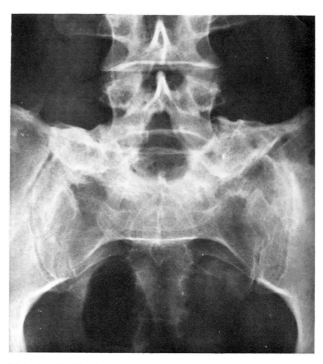

FIG. 16-12. If all soft tissue is removed from between ilium and fusion mass, direct bridge of bone may grow from ilium to L5 and to sacrum. This is undesirable in children. (From Wiltse LL, Hutchinson RH: Surgical treatment of spondylolisthesis. Clin Ortho Rel Res 35:128, 1964.)

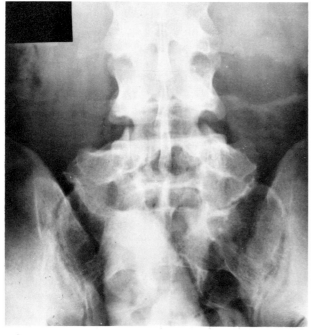

FIG. 16-11. A 19-year-old man two years after one-level fusion for spondylolisthesis. Note sacrum appears to be elevated one segment.

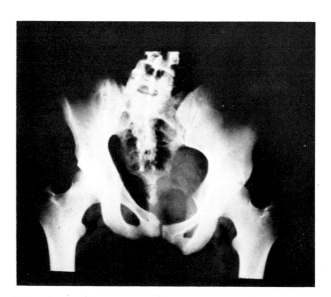

FIG. 16-13. This patient had fusion of right sacroiliac joint at age 11 because of tuberculosis. Note asymmetry of pelvis. For this reason we believe it wise to avoid allowing graft to bridge from ilium to L5 and sacral ala.

(Fig. 16-13). This complication is avoided by this approach.

5. No special instruments are necessary. Bone can easily be obtained from either ilium.

6. There is less pain postoperatively because the supraspinous and interspinous ligaments are left intact.

7. For the same reason increased slip during the healing phase does not occur in spondylolisthesis.

8. Through this approach, the surgeon has freer access to laterally placed structures and hence can decompress the nerves more easily than he can through the midline approach.

9. A herniated disc can be removed with ease through this approach.

10. Since the spinous processes are left intact, the graft may be covered by better-vascularized tissue than is the case when the spinous processes are denuded bilaterally, as in the midline approach. Crock believes this to be a matter of such importance that, if he performs a midline approach, he fuses only one side at a time, waiting a few weeks before doing the other side.[1] In carefully executed vascular studies of the vertebra, he has shown that, when a bilateral midline approach is made, the spinous processes and part of the laminae are rendered virtually avascular.

11. Vigorous retraction is not necessary and hence there is less muscle ischemia.

12. This is an especially good approach in salvage operations of the spine, in which it is necessary to get out into virgin territory.

References

1. Crock HV: The anatomical basis of spinal surgery. Paper read at the combined meeting of English-speaking Orthopaedic Surgeons, April, 1970, Sydney, Australia.
2. Davis JB: Posterior lateral lumbosacral fusion for spondylolisthesis. Paper presented at meeting of Western Orthopaedic Association, Oct. 18, 1961, Dallas, Texas.
3. Friberg S: Studies in spondylolisthesis. Acta Chir Scand 82(Supp. 55):1–40, 1939.
4. Mathieu P, Demirleau J: Surgical therapy in painful spondylolisthesis. Rev D'Orthop 23:352–363, 1936.
5. MacNab I, Dall O: The blood supply of the lumbar spine and its application to the technique of intertransverse lumbar fusion. J Bone Joint Surg 53-B:628–638, 1971.
6. Truckley G, Thompson WA: Posteriolateral fusion of the lumbar and lumbosacral spine. J Bone Joint Surg 35-A:505–512, 1962.
7. Watkins MB: Posteriolateral fusion of the lumbar and lumbosacral spine. J Bone Joint Surg 35-A:1014–1018, 1953.
8. Watkins MB: Posteriolateral bone grafting for fusion of the lumbar and lumbosacral spine. J Bone Joint Surg 41-A:388–396, 1959.
9. Watkins MB: Posteriolateral fusions in pseudarthrosis and posterior element defects of the lumbar spine. Clin Ortho Rel Res 35:80–85, 1964.
10. Wiltse LL, Hutchinson RH: The surgical treatment of spondylolisthesis. Clin Orth Rel Res 35:116–135, 1964.
11. Wiltse LL, Bateman JG, Hutchinson RH, Nelson WE: The paraspinal sacrospinalis-splitting approach to the lumbar spine. J Bone Joint Surg 50-A:919, 1968.

17

Anterior Lumbar Interbody Fusion

FRANK L. RANEY, JR.

ANTERIOR lumbar interbody fusion is a logical and satisfactory method of fusing the lumbar spine. With careful attention to the details of the method herein described, fusion can be accomplished regularly and well, and major disabling complications become a rarity. The many possible complications should deter the occasional surgeon from undertaking the method without first having had additional instruction in the surgical problems of the anterior vertebral column, retroperitoneal space, and great vessels. Anterior lumbar interbody fusion has a number of advantages over other methods of fusion:

1. Greater mechanical stability is accomplished by production of larger and more strategically placed bone struts, and this often results in appreciable immediate back and leg pain relief.

2. Disc space can be elevated to its original height, thereby tightening the entire disc anulus and the anterior and posterior longitudinal ligaments. This correction also realigns the facet joints and the facet joint capsules, and separates the floor and roof of the intervertebral foramen with a resultant enlargement of the foramen and nerve root decompression. Actually, as far as the involved segments are concerned, this movement accomplishes mechanical results similar to those accomplished by a lumbar flexion jacket (Fig. 17-1).

3. Bone grafts are placed in immediate contact with cancellous bone of the vertebral body above and below, and an environment where blood supply is fresh and abundant.

4. Grafts are under compression, not tension, which favors healing (bone is least strong in tension).

5. Bone grafts are at the center of rotation (which is in the disc space with anterior-posterior and lateral bending).

162

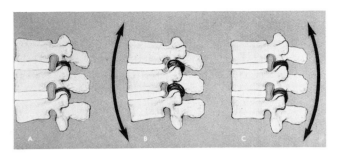

FIG. 17-1. Mechanical effects of flexion on disc and size of intervertebral foramen: *A*, neutral; *B*, extended; *C*, flexed.

6. Bone grafts are locked by flexion of the spine rather than being subjected to bending moment or tension, as when placed posteriorly.

7. If posterior pseudoarthrosis exists, bone grafts gain more mechanical advantage in blocking motion the further forward anteriorly they are located (Fig. 17-2).

8. No new scar is added in the neural canal around nerve roots, or in the back musculature, and the back muscles are not denervated by the fusion procedure.

9. A much larger opening in the disc anulus can be made allowing better visualization and improved access to the disc space and thus more thorough excision of the disc material.

The possible disadvantages of the fusion method described herein are: (1) detailed exploration of the neural canal is not feasible; (2) operative procedure is more difficult technically and is more time-consuming; (2) two types of bone, iliac and fibular, are required, necessitating two sites, and hence a greater area of postoperative pain; (4) more, different, and potentially more serious complications can occur requiring the operating surgeon to have wider and more diverse surgical knowledge if these complications are to be avoided. Postoperative infection is particularly of more serious consequence after anterior approach.

Anterior lumbar fusion by the method described herein has application under the following circumstances:

1. As a salvage procedure for repair of a posterior fusion pseudarthrosis.

2. As a salvage procedure after an unsuccessful laminectomy to correct settling of the space, or for a fusion when most of the lamina is gone.

3. As a primary procedure in the large, heavy patient with a long torso, in whom the bending moment and weight-bearing load on the disc space is great. In such cases stability is obtained, and yet height of the disc space is regained which is most important when pain apparently is related to settling of a soft, degenerated disc.

4. As a primary procedure in the patient with L3–L4 disc protrusion, especially if the patient has a long torso and the L3–L4 disc space is expected to be included in a fusion to be done at the time of the disc excision.

5. As the method to accomplish posterior spinal stability anteriorly, so that the interbody neural arch elements can be completely excised to allow for maximum decompression of the neural canal and intervertebral foramen when persistent neural element compression is thought to be the cause of pain.

TECHNIQUE

Bone grafts are obtained both from the ilium, as full thickness blocks from the right anterior iliac crest, care being taken to protect the lateral branch of the iliohypogastric nerve where it crosses the crest; and from the fibula, by removal of a section of the entire shaft five or six inches in length through the interval between the soleus and the peroneus longus muscles, care being taken to leave a section four inches in length distally, and to protect the superficial peroneal nerve (Fig. 17-3).

The lumbar spine is approached extraperitoneally on the left through a left paramedian incision medial to the rectus muscle (Fig. 17-4). The peritoneal contents and greater vessels are displaced to the right, the anulus fibrosis is opened as a flap turned toward the

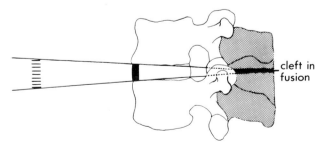

FIG. 17-2. Effect of extending lever arm anteriorly.

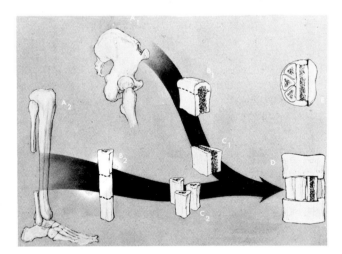

FIG. 17-3. Donor sites and method of graft placement: A_1, B_1, C_1, iliac grafts; A_2, B_2, C_2, fibular grafts; *D*, *E*, final position.

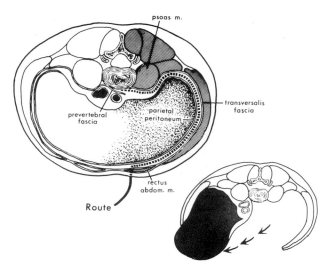

FIG. 17-4. Surgical approach in anterior lumbar fusion; route and handling of peritoneal contents.

right side, and the intervertebral disc material is excised back to the posterior anulus (Fig. 17-5). Cortical plates are then excised back to within one centimeter of the posterior margin of the disc space to provide a posterior ledge, thus to prevent bone grafts from being driven into the neural canal (see Fig. 17-3). A kidney rest on the operating table is then elevated to hyperextend the lumbar spine. Resultant hyperextension first tightens the disc anulus, and the anterior longitudinal ligament, and then spreads the vertebral bodies, thus tightening all ligamentous structures and elevating the disc to its maximal height. To secure blocking in this position, a tightly fitting combination of cancellous and

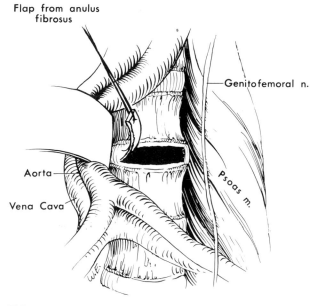

FIG. 17-5. Surgical approach in anterior lumbar fusion; handling of great vessels and disc.

cortical bone grafts (iliac crest and fibula) is placed into the disc space. The cortical bone maintains disc space height while the cancellous bone is incorporated, and the incorporated cancellous bone continues to support the cortical graft as it is softened during its incorporation. The iliac crest graft is fashioned to a 3×1 to 1.5 cm. rectangular section of full-thickness anterior iliac crest bone (two cortical plates with cancellous bone sandwiched between them), measured to fit exactly between margins of the prepared disc space, with the space elevated to its maximal height. The cortical plates are oriented vertically and the long axis of the graft transversely, and the graft thus measured is driven back against the previously formed ledges posteriorly (see Fig. 17-3). Thus both above and below, the cancellous bone of the graft is in contact with the cancellous bone of the opposing vertebral bodies, and the bodies are kept the maximal distance apart by the vertical position of the cortices of this graft. Vertical fibular struts are then measured to again just barely fit between the anterior margins of the prepared disc space, and are driven into place just anterior to the iliac graft (see Fig. 17-3). An attempt is made to place three such fibular grafts, two with their triangular bases facing posteriorly, and a third with its base faced anteriorly, to act as a keystone graft. All fibular struts must be entirely within the disc space and impacted inside the anterior cortices of the vertebral bodies. Only as many fibular grafts as can be placed anteriorly within the disc space are used. The anular flap formed initially is then closed back over the front of the space over Surgicel strips to establish hemostasis in the disc space. Each level to be fused is dealt with in essentially the same manner, except that L5–S1 is done in the bifurcation between the iliac vessels, whereas the spaces above this level are exposed by displacement of the great vessels to the right. Self-retaining retractors that are driven into the vertebral bodies are used to maintain exposure while the disc spaces are being fused. When all levels to be fused have been completed, closure of the abdominal wound is effected in layers.

Postoperatively, lost blood is replaced until preoperative hematocrit and hemoglobin levels are restored. The patient is fed orally as soon as peristalsis has been re-established. Ambulation and weight-bearing (within tolerance of pain), with a scultetus binder in place, is permitted on the first or second postoperative day. Initially this activity usually consists of just standing at the bedside, to be increased gradually to walking as pain in the donor sites and abdominal wound will allow.

As soon as tenderness of the abdominal wound subsides, the patient is placed in a previously prepared plastic bivalved removable, and adjustable, lumbar spinal jacket. The patient wears this jacket at all times when he is ambulatory, except in the shower, during which time he must remain upright. The jacket is to be replaced immediately after he dries, even before he steps out of the shower. Physical activities are limited

have been
one year c
all levels
arthrosis (
16 cases, ã
Pseudarth
primary :
arthroses
operation
arthroses
occurred i
and only
viously fã
arthrosis.
bone were
in 125 cas
rior fusio
before th
done. Fo1

primarily to walking, sitting for meals, and the use of the toilet. Ambulation is encouraged only to the point of fulfilling daily needs, and the patient otherwise is encouraged to remain lying down with lumbar spine flexed, either in a contour position or on his side in bed with his hips and knees flexed. Hyperextension of the lumbar spine is carefully avoided. The patient may continue to wear his plastic spinal jacket while lying down at any time, but he is not required to sleep in it. He continues to wear the jacket until there is radiologic evidence of incorporation of the bone grafts, at which time a gradual "weaning" begins, to progressively reduce his dependency on the support. If the change from full support to no support is not tolerated easily, an intermediate lesser support in the form of a corset reinforced with paraspinal steels is then used, with the patient alternating between the jacket and corset, progressively increasing the use of the corset until he can graduate to it entirely. The corset is then progressively discontinued by the method recommended for withdrawal of the jacket. An exercise program, other than walking, is not started until the grafts are radiologically incorporated, but then is increased progressively in the form of postural exercises, walking, swimming, bicycle riding, and eventually to the limits of the patient's tolerance, or willingness, to exercise to strengthen the back, trunk, abdominal, and lower extremity muscles.

In our series of 160 cases,* complications were as follows:

1. Death nine months postoperatively due to deep infection with abscess formation and rupture of the aorta (1 case).
2. Interbody disc space infection (2 cases; one responded to antibiotics and cast).
3. Soft tissue infection in fibular site (1 case).
4. Superficial abscess, or subcutaneous infection in abdominal wall (3 cases; all responded to local drainage).
5. Major arterial damage requiring prosthetic graft replacement (1 case).
6. Major venous damage requiring vascular surgical repair (2 cases).
7. Postoperative ankle instability associated with removal of fibula too far distally (2 cases; both responding to stabilization of the fibula to tibia).
8. Dehiscence of abdominal wound with ventral hernia formation (1 case).
9. Snapping iliotibial band after excessive plication in the iliac crest wound (1 case).
10. Persistent sympathectomy in the left leg from division of sympathetic chain (almost consistent after procedure, but rarely persistent, and never disabling).

11. Postoperative difficulty in maintaining erection after anterior fusion (3 cases; two had had some previous trouble after posterior fusion).
12. Postoperative ejaculation into bladder (2 cases; one persistent).
13. Persistent lateral thigh numbness from division of lateral branch of iliohypogastric nerve, or injury to lateral femoral cutaneous nerve. Exact number not known, but estimated at 0.5 to 1% of total cases.
14. Pseudoarthrosis (present at one level in 27 cases).
15. Retroperitoneal hematoma (1 case).
16. Thrombophlebitis (3 cases).

The most serious complications of anterior fusion are rupture of aorta from mycotic abscess, postoperative ejaculation into the bladder, difficulty in maintaining erection, left leg sympathectomy, or ankle instability from removal of too much of the distal portion of the fibula. Rupture of the aorta can be avoided if abscess is prevented by early use of antibiotics and by cast immobilization and/or removal of bone grafts early if the infection does not respond to antibiotic treatment. Ejaculation into the bladder postoperatively has been persistent in only one case, and can be avoided if care is taken not to strip off the prevertebral sympathetic fibers bilaterally. The same precaution can prevent difficulty in maintaining erection. This condition was present to some extent in only three patients, and was present in two of these prior to the anterior fusion but worsened postoperatively. Some difficulty persisted in two cases.

Postoperative left leg sympathectomy, an early complication in most cases, usually does not persist if the sympathetic chain is not divided. Since a warm, dry leg more often than not is preferred by the patient, the complaint is usually that the right leg is cold, not that the left leg is warm. Ankle instability has occurred in only two cases; in both instances the distal four inches of fibula had not been left in place. Both patients obtained relief when the fibula was stabilized to the tibia. Thrombophlebitis has occurred postoperatively in only three cases in our series, with pulmonary embolism in two. On one occasion vena caval ligation was necessary when anticoagulant therapy failed to control the embolism.

With care, most complications can be avoided. In the last 75 patients on whom I have operated, complications have consisted of two superficial wound infections, one retroperitoneal hematoma, one interbody infection which responded by fusing after the use of antibiotics and cast immobilization, one thrombophlebitis with embolism, and three pseudarthroses.

RESULTS

Results in 139 of the 160 patients subjected to anterior lumbar interbody fusion between 1957 and 1969

---

*Neurosurgeon John E Adams was my co-surgeon in at least two thirds of the cases.

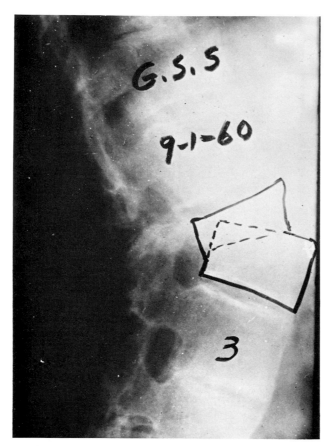

FIG. 18-10. Transverse separation through vertebral body.

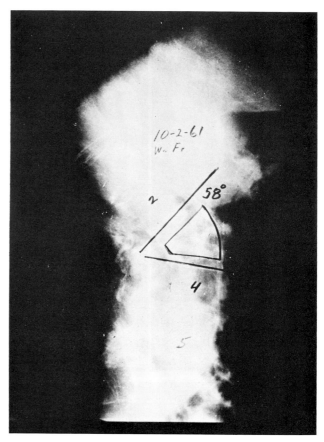

FIG. 18-12. A 58-degree correction with crushing down of posterior vertebral body and some increased anterior body height.

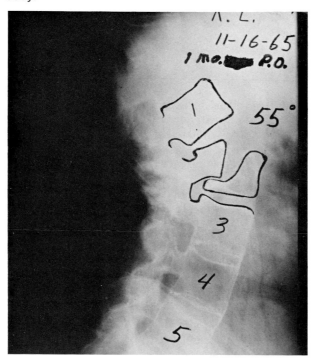

FIG. 18-11. Anterior separation through vertebral body from anterior superior to posterior inferior.

correction of 60 degrees, partial paraplegia developed, requiring laminectomy within 24 hours. Incomplete recovery followed. Two patients developed cardiac arrest; one recovered, but one in his middle fifties did not. Another patient, a woman in her late sixties, operated upon only after she pleaded for a long time, expired within 24 hours, probably from cerebral anoxia resulting from the prolonged dependent position of her head (see Fig. 18-4).

The procedure of spinal osteotomy, in summary, can be successful if adequate care is given to (1) proper selection of patients; (2) careful preoperative precautions; (3) meticulous attention to operative technique and details; and (4) adequate attention to the immediate postoperative management and careful supervision during the prolonged follow-up, requiring at least a year.

Section V

Deformities

19

Scoliosis

THEODORE R. WAUGH AND EDWARD J. RISEBOROUGH

THE TERM "scoliosis" is usually credited to Hippocrates; however, it is apparent from the treatments advocated that neither Hippocrates nor his contemporaries separated anteroposterior from lateral curvatures of the spine.[29] During the sixteenth century, Paré described the deformity that we recognize today,[48] and in the eighteenth century, Andry, in his textbook of orthopaedics, further defined the deformity and postulated on its pathogenesis.[2]

During the nineteenth century, great interest was generated in the pathogenesis of scoliosis, and each theory was propounded to justify its author's form of therapy. These theories included Stromeyer's inequality of the ribs,[61] Guérin's contractural theory,[25] and Meyer's mechanistic approach.[40] As the nineteenth century drew to a close, the great interest in morphologic pathology resulted in precise descriptions of the disease, as seen at autopsy.[63,64]

The modern era in the treatment of scoliosis began with Hibbs' publication of his initial experience in the treatment of severe structural scoliosis by spinal fusion,[28] although the first actual spinal fusion procedure for this disease had been performed in 1911 by Forbes. To the present day, while techniques of correction vary and include various plaster jackets, braces, and both anterior and posterior spinal instrumentation, there remains only one generally accepted method of maintaining correction in severe spinal curvature, and that is fusion.

PATHOGENESIS

MUSCLE PARALYSIS. In 1941, Colonna and Vom Saal attempted to correlate muscle paralysis with type of curvature.[8] James subsequently reported that leg and arm muscle paralyses were not related to the production of scoliosis, nor were paralyses of the midline muscles, such as the erector spinae and the anterior abdominals. In a significant number of cases, however, he found that the intercostals, the lateral abdominals, and the latissimus dorsi were weak on the convexity. With regard to specific curve patterns, James found that intercostal muscle weakness was associated with thoracic scoliosis, and weakness of the quadratus lumborum, the lateral portion of the anterior abdominal muscles, and possibly the latissimus dorsi with lumbar curves.[32]

Gruca[22,23] and Risser[54] have advanced muscle weakness theories for the pathogenesis of idiopathic scoliosis. It was Gruca's belief that idiopathic scoliosis was caused by impaired equilibrium at the level of the initial curvature. Yamada and associates have produced scoliosis experimentally by destroying the equilibrium center in the brain stem of bipedal rats,[72] and Liszka produced the condition by unilateral transection of multiple spinal roots.[37] Similarly, MacEwen was able to produce scoliosis by dividing the dorsal sensory nerve roots adjacent to the spinal cord.[38] In a series of experiments on bipedal monkeys, we were unable to produce scoliosis by sectioning intercostal nerves immediately adjacent to the vertebral column.

The literature implies that damage to the neuromuscular unit may be responsible for some types of scoliosis, but existing evidence does not support this contention.

COSTOTRANSVERSE LIGAMENTS. In 1951, Wenger observed that the development of scoliosis following thoracoplasty depended on whether the transverse processes and related ligaments had been injured.[70] Langenskiöld and Michelsson attempted to produce in animals spinal deformities comparable to scoliosis in man, and found that the significant common factor among the effective thoracic operative procedures was section of the posterior costotransverse ligaments.[36,41] Many surgeons sought to produce a counterscoliosis in adolescents by either sectioning the concave costotransverse ligaments, resecting the medial portion of the posterior concave ribs, or resecting the concave transverse processes. Unfortunately, procedures performed on the concave side of scoliosis in man do not appear to have produced lasting benefit. Many authors, however, have noted improvement in the convex rib hump after sectioning the base of the transverse processes or partially resecting segments of ribs.

VERTEBRAE. In 1941, a majority of members of the Research Committe of the American Orthopaedic Association believed that scoliosis was the result of a disturbance in the growth plate.[14] Bick, in 1961, cited the Heuter-von Vokmann law, the effect of pressure and traction on growth plates producing asymmetric expansion, as a basis for the changes that develop in scoliosis.[3] Others subscribed to the theory that unilateral growth disturbances were either totally responsible or at least contributory, and that wedge-shaped vertebrae did not develop as a result of compression but of interference with unilateral growth. Some substantiation for the development of scoliosis as a result of unilateral damage to the vertebral growth plate resulted from a careful follow-up of children treated for tumors by radiation therapy.[34] Also, unilateral damage to the growth plates induced surgically in animals has resulted in the development of scoliosis. However, the therapeutic application of the principle of compensatory growth arrest, by stapling either the growth plates or the transverse processes, or by surgical epiphyseal arrest with inlaid bond grafts, has generally been unsuccessful.

Although unilateral epiphyseal injury may produce a deformity in many respects resembling idiopathic scoliosis, it seems more likely that the pathologic changes in the vertebrae are not the primary cause of the deformity, but rather the result of abnormal pressure from outside the vertebral column.

METABOLISM. Results of biochemical studies on children with idiopathic scoliosis have proved statistically insignificant. Stearns et al., in investigating the metabolism of protein, found a clear negative balance.[60] Scoliotic children required high protein diets in order to retain sufficient nitrogen for normal growth, and normal diets of children generally do not contain this amount of protein. It was noted that scoliotic children had an increased excretion of taurine and cysteic acid and/or methionine sulfoxide, representing a significantly high loss of sulfur-containing amino acid derivatives.[60] Glauber and associates found increased alpha 1 globulin and total protein-bound hexose and alpha 1 glycoprotein in the serum, changes which were assumed to be a consequence of a disturbance in the metabolism of mucoprotein.[19] Ponseti believed that the increased excretion of sulfur-containing amino acid derivatives suggests an abnormality of mucopolysaccharide metabolism.[51] The exact mechanism of action for such an abnormality remains undefined.

HEREDITY. According to the literature, similar curves have been noted in identical twins.[43] Many authors have found a significantly increased incidence of idiopathic scoliosis in close relatives, indicating a dominant form of inheritance.[18,71] Cowell, Hall, and MacEwen developed considerable evidence, based on radiographic examination of entire families, that idiopathic thoracic scoliosis was inherited as a sex-linked dominant trait, although the characteristic had variable expressivity and limited penetrance.[10]

PATHOLOGY. Information regarding the pathologic features of idiopathic scoliosis has been derived from two main sources: Classic autopsy descriptions and serial roentgenographic examinations by orthopaedists and radiologists. The pathologists described distorted vertebrae with the body shifted toward the convex side of the thorax, the spinous process deviated to the concave side, and thick wide laminae on the concave aspect as compared with thinner elongated laminae on the convex side. The entire thorax is significantly altered, the convex side being markedly decreased in size by an acutely angular deformity of the rib with a correspondingly opposite change on the concave side, resulting in a net decrease in the entire volume of the thorax. Unfortunately, this source of information, although interesting, sheds little light on the more dynamic aspects of the development of the deformity. Recent studies have tended to concern themselves more with the presence or absence of changes during the active phase of curve development and progression. James reported autopsy material from an 11-month-old child with infantile idiopathic scoliosis in whom microscopic evaluation of vertebral epiphyses was normal.[31] Examination of a 15-year-old girl with actively progressing right thoracic scoliosis, comparing the convex and concave sides of the curvature, revealed thinning of the end plates on the concave side with horizontal flattening of the cartilage cells. On the convex side, these changes were much less evident, the cartilage columns approaching that seen in a normal child of the same age. Concave compression of the disc with displacement of the nucleus to the convex side of the intervertebral space has also been reported.[49,50]

TERMINOLOGY AND CLASSIFICATION

Scoliosis is defined as a lateral curvature of the spine, the term usually being applied to curves in excess of 10 degrees. Scoliotic curves may be either structural (i.e., fixed), characterized by fixed rotation on forward bending, or compensatory, tending to maintain body alignment of the head over the pelvis. In the latter type, fixed rotation and permanent deformation of the vertebrae are generally absent. The terms "major" and "primary" have in the past been used synonymously with "structural." "Minor" and "secondary" have been used in place of "compensatory." However, it has become increasingly obvious that structural curves may not be either major or primary; hence the use of these terms is considered undesirable. When two curves, in the same spine, each meet the requirements of a structural curve, the resultant curve is described as a double structural curve. Curves are described according to the location of the apical vertebra. When the apex is from C1 to C6, the curve is termed cervical; at C7 or T1, cervicothoracic; from T2 to T11, thoracic; T12 or L1, thoracolumbar; from L2 to L4, lumbar; and at L5 or the sacrum, lumbosacral. Kyphoscoliosis is lateral curvature of the spine associated with either increased posterior or decreased anterior angulation in the sagittal plane in excess of the accepted normal for that area. In the thoracic region, 25 to 45 degrees of kyphosis is considered normal. Similarly, lordoscoliosis is lateral curvature of the spine associated with an increase of anterior or a decrease of posterior angulation in the sagittal plane. In the scoliotic thoracic spine, where posterior angulation is normally present, a loss of posterior angulation below 25 degrees would represent lordoscoliosis.[68]

In 1948, Cobb developed an etiologic classification of scoliosis in which approximately 90% of cases fell within the idiopathic category.[6] In 1973, the Scoliosis Research Society adopted the following classification of structural spine deformity:

Classification of Spine Deformity

I. Idiopathic Conditions
   A. Infantile
      1. Resolving
      2. Progressive
   B. Juvenile
   C. Adolescent

II. Neuromuscular Disorders
   A. Neuropathic
      1. Upper motor neuron lesion
         a. Cerebral palsy
         b. Spinocerebellar degeneration
            i. Friedreich's ataxia
            ii. Charcot-Marie-Tooth disease
            iii. Roussy-Lévy syndrome
         c. Syringomyelia
         d. Spinal cord tumor
         e. Spinal cord trauma
         f. Other
      2. Lower motor neuron lesion
         a. Poliomyelitis
         b. Other viral myelitides
         c. Traumatic
         d. Spinal muscular atrophy
             i. Werdnig-Hoffmann syndrome
            ii. Kugelberg-Welander disease
         e. Myelomeningocele (paralytic)
      3. Dysautonomia (Riley-Day syndrome)
      4. Other
   B. Myopathic Disorders
      1. Arthrogryposis
      2. Muscular dystrophy
         a. Duchenne (pseudohypertrophic)
         b. Limb-girdle
         c. Facial-scapulo-humeral
      3. Fiber type disproportion
      4. Congenital hypotonia
      5. Myotonia dystrophica
      6. Other

III. Congenital Disorders
   A. Congenital scoliosis

1. Failure of formation
   a. Wedge
   b. Hemivertebra
2. Failure of segmentation
   a. Unilateral bar
   b. Bilateral (fusion)
3. Mixed
B. Congenital Kyphosis
   1. Failure of formation
   2. Failure of segmentation
   3. Mixed
C. Congenital lordosis
D. Associated with neural tissue defect
   1. Myelomeningocele
   2. Meningocele
   3. Spinal dysraphism
      a. Diastematomyelia
      b. Other
IV. Neurofibromatosis
V. Mesenchymal Diseases
   A. Marfan's syndrome
   B. Homocystinuria
   C. Ehlers-Danlos syndrome
   D. Other
VI. Traumatic Disorders
   A. Fracture or dislocation (nonparalytic)
   B. Post-irradiation
   C. Post-laminectomy
   D. Other
VII. Soft Tissue Contractures
   A. Post-empyema
   B. Burns
   C. Other
VIII. Osteochondrodystrophies
   A. Achondroplasia
   B. Spondyloepiphyseal dysplasia
   C. Diastrophic dwarfism
   D. Mucopolysaccharidoses
IX. Scheuermann's Disease
X. Infection
   A. Tuberculosis
   B. Bacterial
   C. Fungal
   D. Parasitic
   E. Other
XI. Tumor
   A. Benign
   B. Malignant
XII. Rheumatoid Disease
   A. Juvenile rheumatoid
   B. Adult rheumatoid
   C. Marie-Strümpell disease
XIII. Metabolic Disorders
   A. Rickets
   B. Juvenile osteoporosis
   C. Osteogenesis imperfecta
XIV. Conditions Related to Lumbosacral Area

   A. Spondylolisthesis
   B. Spondylolysis
   C. Other congenital anomalies
   D. Other
XV. Thoracogenic Conditions
   A. Post thoracoplasty
   B. Post thoracotomy
   C. Other
XVI. Hysteria
XVII. Functional Disorders
   A. Postural
   B. Secondary to short leg
   C. Other

IDIOPATHIC SCOLIOSIS. This type of scoliosis is classified according to both age at onset and location of the structural curve. In general, the earlier the onset, the worse the prognosis; yet approximately 50% of cases of the infantile variety resolve spontaneously and may be related to position in utero.[30,31] The curves are named by the location of the apical vertebra, the vertebra most rotated in a structural curve and most deviated from the vertical axis of the patient. Peculiarly, according to James, the direction of the convexity varies with age of onset and location of the curve; thus, infantile thoracic scoliosis is to the left in 90% of cases and is as common in boys as in girls. Juvenile thoracic scoliosis is directed to the right and left in equal proportions. However, in the adolescent form of thoracic scoliosis, 90% of patients are girls and 90% of the curves are to the right. It is this variety that appears most likely to have a genetic basis. Lumbar curves also tend to be directed to the right and left equally.[33]

NEUROMUSCULAR SCOLIOSIS. Neuropathic and myopathic scolioses are spinal curvatures caused by disease or anomalous function or development of nerve tissue or muscle. Characteristically, neuromuscular scoliosis is associated with some unusual features, which facilitate identification of such curves. Usually, paralytic scoliosis is a long C-type curve that tends, in its early stages, to be mobile and associated with less rotation.

CONGENITAL SCOLIOSIS. Congenital scoliosis reflects anomalous development in utero. This group of skeletal abnormalities has been subdivided by Goldstein into extravertebral (e.g., rib fusion) and vertebral, which can be further subdivided into open and closed.[20] The open varieties may occur with neurologic deficit, as in meningomyelocele, or without, as in spina bifida occulta; the closed type also can be associated with neurologic deficit (diastematomyelia), and without (hemivertebra and unilateral unsegmented bars). It has been found that anomalies of the vertebral column are frequently associated with congenital anomalies of the urinary tract.[39] Accordingly, studies of the genitourinary system are indicated. Although most congenital curvatures do not progress to a significant degree, many become extremely severe, particularly a curvature associated with a unilateral bar. Because correction of congenital scoliosis is frequently unsatisfactory, early spinal fusion often is advocated to prevent the development of this deformity.

NEUROFIBROMATOSIS. In 1882, von Recklinghausen described the relationship between peripheral nerves and the subcutaneous nodules that are typical of the disease in its severe adult form.[52] In children, café-au-lait skin pigmentation, limb hypertrophy, and palpable nodules are frequently seen, and sarcomatous degeneration has been reported. A severe scoliosis frequently develops, and is characterized by a short acute curve, which is frequently immobile. In many cases the contour of the vertebrae is altered to some extent, although such changes need not necessarily be associated with tumors in the neural canal or protrusion through the neural foramina. Because of the relentless course of this form of scoliosis, careful early treatment is indicated.

MISCELLANEOUS. Various tissue disorders, such as Marfan's syndrome, a mendelian-dominant disorder affecting the bones, eyes, ligaments, tendons, and cardiovascular system, and Ehlers-Danlos disease or hyperelastosis, may be associated with scoliosis. Trauma, such as spinal fracture, may result in scoliosis, as may radiation for the malignant tumors of childhood, such as Wilms' tumor and neuroblastoma. Resultant damage to the growth plates is more severe on the side of the tumor, with inequality of vertebral growth causing deformed wedge-shaped vertebrae.[23] Postradiation scarring, also, undoubtedly contributes to the concave contracture of these curves.

Empyema may be present, producing a degree of fibrous contracture, the scoliosis being concave to the side of the infection. Many osteochondrodystrophies are accompanied by severe forms of scoliosis, which are difficult to treat because of the dwarfism; fabrication of a suitable brace will test the skill of the orthotist. Osteogenesis imperfecta is classically considered to affect the extremities; however, severe degrees of spinal curvature frequently develop and are extremely difficult to treat. Despite weakened bone, surgical intervention may be successfully carried out and a solid spinal fusion will maintain correction.

CLINICAL EVALUATION

The family of a child with scoliosis is prompted to seek medical advice by a variety of observations: the child has unequal shoulder height, unilateral prominence of the hip, posterior protrusion of a scapula, or unilateral prominence of one breast. During adolescence, modesty may cause the trunk of the child to be hidden from the parents, resulting in considerable progression of the deformity before it is discovered. Commonly, spinal curvature is noticed during the summer months when children are at the beach and their backs are exposed.

The incidence of scoliosis was found by Shands and Eisberg in 1955 to be 1.9%, based on a review of 50,000 chest films in the State of Delaware. Of this total number, only 0.5% of the curves exceeded 20 degrees in individuals over 14 years of age.[58] Similar data have been reported by others.

It is important to recognize that scoliosis is often a symptom of another and frequently more serious disease. To this end, it is mandatory that the patient be subjected to a thorough general history and physical examination.

PATIENT'S HISTORY. Most adolescents with scoliosis, particularly milder forms, have few symptoms. However, it is not uncommon, as the end of the school day approaches, for children to complain of an occasional feeling of tiredness in the lumbar area. With advancing age the pain of osteoarthritis is common and, in the more severe varieties, radiculitis as well as the pain of impingement of the ribs on the iliac crest may be severe.

In severe scoliosis, shortness of breath may occur, though it is frequently denied by a child.

A history of febrile illness may suggest a subclinical attack of poliomyelitis, but with vaccination becoming increasingly common, this diagnosis is now less likely. Questioning regarding other members of the family may bring to light some of the hereditary degenerative CNS diseases that often result in scoliosis. The age at menarche and a comparison of the child's height with that of the parents may provide the examiner with some idea of the child's growth potential.

The parents' impression of the rate at which the deformity has developed may be of some value, particularly if the child has been seen by others and merely observed rather than treated. Unfortunately, it is still common for physicians to observe children with spinal curvature for prolonged periods until they feel the deformity has reached a stage for which operation may be necessary. This type of careful neglect may result in loss of the golden period for nonoperative treatment.

PHYSICAL EXAMINATION. With the child completely disrobed, an examination is made of his general appearance and development, and for skin pigmentation such as cafe-au-lait markings and hairy patches. Specific examination of the spinal deformity requires a definition of shoulder heights, prominence of posterior ribs with overlying scapula, prominence of a flank, and apparent protrusion of a specific hip. Trunk alignment is important as a dimension of the present problem and is of prognostic significance inasmuch as the body attempts to place the skull over the middle of the sacrum, and the fact that this is not being accomplished can indicate weakening paraspinal musculature. The simplest method of determining balance is to drop a plumb line from the occiput and determine the relationship of this line to the natal cleft. Measurement is made in centimeters to the right or left. It is frequently found that balance of the trunk is lost as the day progresses and may be associated with the sense of tiredness in the lumbar area.

Measurements of height (standing and sitting) are important in the evaluation of trunk growth. The arm span should be measured and used as a method of estimating vital capacity, because of the decreased height of patients with scoliosis.

Side bending is the method of assessing flexibility, and forward bending not only provides an indicator of structural deformity, but also permits evaluation of the thoracic cage deformity. The concave side of a thoracic curve will be depressed and the convex side elevated. In the past, it was customary to use a spirit level and measure the difference between the convex rib hump and concave rib depression in centimeters. However, the angle of inclination which is the angle in degrees by which a plane across the posterior rib cage at the apex of a structural curve deviates from the transverse or horizontal plane, is easier to measure (Fig. 19-1).

Pelvic obliquity, the deviation of the plane of the pelvis from the transverse, may be fixed or unfixed, and if fixed may be attributable to contractures either above or below the pelvis. Leg length discrepancies produce unfixed pelvic obliquity and cause spinal curvatures convex to the shorter side. Length of the lower extremities is customarily measured from the anterior

superior spine to the medial malleolus when these structures are palpable.

Complete examination of the central nervous system is particularly important in scoliosis, as both the neuromuscular and congenital categories of structural spine deformity are often associated with abnormalities of this system. In congenital scoliosis, spinal dysrhaphism may result in varying degrees of loss of function distal to the lesion.

Clinical photographs are an important part of the long-term evaluation of a patient and provide an objective method of assessing the success of treatment. A minimal photographic examination should include the

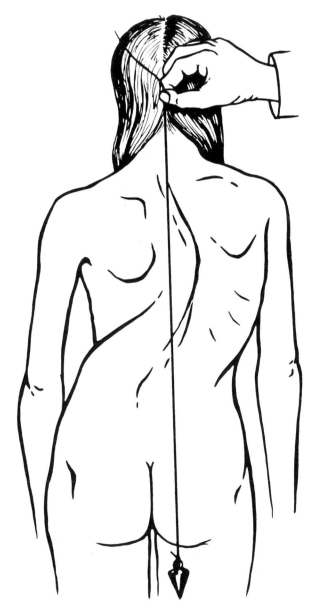

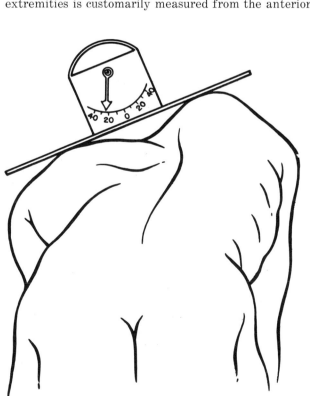

FIG. 19-1. *A,* Measurement of rib hump and rotation of thorax with inclinometer. Angle of inclination is recorded with patient flexed forward 90 degrees. *B,* Alignment of trunk is demonstrated by use of plumb line.

back with the patient erect and with forward bending, to define the profile of the rib deformity.

RADIOGRAPHS. In order to obtain the basic information required for proper evaluation, while minimizing radiographic exposure, it is essential that the child have a complete scoliosis series. This includes an erect anteroposterior and lateral view of the entire spine, preferably on a 36-inch cassette. If such is not available, two 17-inch cassettes will suffice, depending on the age and size of the patient. Additional recumbent films should include an anteroposterior view and right and left side-bending films. A lateral view of the lumbosacral region is desirable to rule out spondylolisthesis.

An anteroposterior view of the left hand and wrist is useful for comparison with a standard atlas, such as that of Gruelich and Pyle, in order to establish bone age.[21] Since one of the most important determinants of treatment is the potential for further spinal growth, it is essential that the bone age be established with relative certainty.

Lateral side-bending films are valuable to determine flexibility, which also can be estimated by comparison of the erect and recumbent anteroposterior views. The lateral-bending films are more informative than the latter.

The frequency of radiographic re-examination is dictated by clinical progress rather than by specific time intervals; however, re-examination is frequently carried out every three to six months.

All radiographs should be measured carefully and the angular scoliosis deformity recorded. The popular methods available for this determination include the Lipman-Cobb and Ferguson techniques. The former is carried out by (1) selecting the upper end vertebra, that is, the most cephalad whose superior surface tilts maximally to the concavity of the curve; (2) erecting a perpendicular to the superior surface; (3) selecting the lower end vertebra, that is, the most caudad whose inferior surface tilts maximally to the concavity of the curve; (4) erecting a perpendicular to the inferior surface; and (5) measuring the angle between the two perpendiculars[6] (Fig. 19-2). In extremely acute curves, a line through the superior surface of the upper end vertebra may intersect the line through the inferior surface of the lower end vertebra on the x-ray film. In such circumstances, it is not necessary to erect intersecting perpendiculars. If the vertebral end plates are poorly visualized, in the interest of accuracy, a line through the bottom or top of the pedicles may be used.

The Ferguson method of measurement requires identification of the center of the vertebral bodies of the apical and end vertebrae. The end vertebrae are usually in neutral rotation, whereas the apical vertebra is maximally rotated. The center points are then joined by a straight line and the angle of intersection measured.[15]

The Scoliosis Research Society has agreed to standardize their reporting of curves by adopting the Cobb

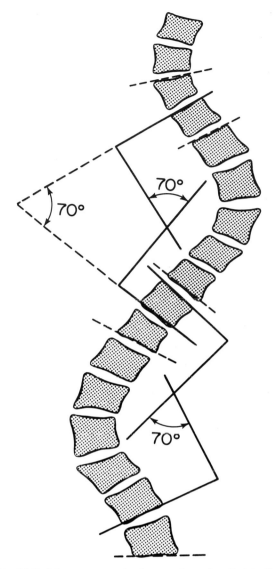

FIG. 19-2. Measurement of curvature by Cobb Technique. Perpendiculars are erected to lines through upper and lower endplates and angle of intersection measured. End vertebrae are those maximally tilted to concavity of curve.

method. George and Rippstein compared the two methods in 27 curves and calculated the average difference to be 25%. Contrasting the correction achieved, these authors found 16% greater correction when the Cobb technique was used for measurement. This is undoubtedly due to the increased correctability of the end vertebrae. These authors also suggested, as still another method of measurement, the joining of the two end vertebrae with measurement of the distance of the apex from that line.[17]

Assuming the scoliosis patient is in balance, with the head centered over the sacrum, the sum total of curves to the right will equal curves to the left. If this situation does not exist, it is apparent that the spine is not in balance.

In defining the structural curve or curves, the permanent deformation of the vertebrae will serve as a valuable clue. Such curves usually are less flexible on side bending with significant residual uncorrectable deformity.

During the course of clinical examination, by either measuring the rib hump or the inclination, an assessment of the degree of rotation is possible. While lateral bending is inextricably linked to rotation of the vertebral spine, it is the rotation that produces the more significant clinical deformity. Using the relationship of the pedicle or the spinous process to the body of the vertebra, it is possible radiographically to assess the degree of rotation. The technique advocated by Nash and Moe includes four grades based on the position of the pedicles. Thus, as examples, in grade 1 rotation, the convex pedicle is moved slightly toward the midline, and the concave pedicle is overlapping the vertebral edge; with Grade 3 rotation, the convex pedicle occupies a middle position in the vertebral body, and the concave pedicle is not visualized. Because spinous processes are so frequently removed during operative treatment of scoliosis, the use of the pedicle is preferable (Fig. 19-3).[45]

The anteroposterior roentgenographic examination provides information with regard to the further growth potential of the vertebrae. According to Risser and Ferguson, when the excursion of the ossification in the iliac epiphysis (apophysis) from the anterolateral margin of each ilium to the junction of the ilium is completed (as seen in the anteroposterior roentgenogram of the spine), vertebral growth is completed.[56] It is commonly believed that an additional six-month period is desirable in the interest of safety. A further radiographic sign, which is more accurate than Risser's and Ferguson's but not visualized as easily, is the closure of the vertebral ring apophyses. These are traction apophyses lying at the superior and inferior peripheral margins of the vertebral body and do not contribute to the longitudinal growth of the vertebrae. Their closure is closely related to the termination of vertebral end-plate growth.

PULMONARY EVALUATION. The deformity of scoliosis results in the rotation of the vertebral bodies into the convex thorax, which probably, of itself, results in relatively little alteration in the general volume. However, with rotation of the attached ribs, the convex thorax becomes markedly diminished, and although the concave thorax appears to be enlarged, the net effect is a decrease in overall volume. Additionally, the curvature shortens the length of the thorax, resulting in further decrease in total volume. These changes are reflected in the alterations of vital capacity that are commonly seen with thoracic scoliosis. In a study of patients with scoliosis of many years duration, Nachemson found that after 40 years of age pulmonary

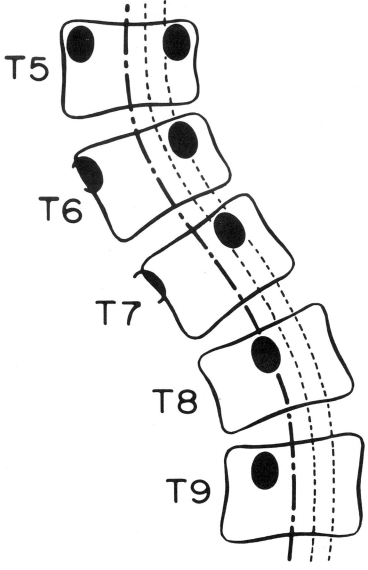

FIG. 19-3. Pedicle method of measuring vertebral rotation radiographically. T5 is neutral; T6, grade 1; T7, grade 2; T8, grade 3; and T9, grade 4. Gradation is determined by location of concave pedicle. In grades 3 and 4 convex pedicle is not seen.

disability became evident, and patients with severe curvature had significantly increased disability and shortened life expectancy.[44]

Although diminished vital capacity is the rule, based on expected vital capacity predicted by arm span, it is not until the thoracic scoliosis exceeds 50 degrees that altered blood gases are anticipated. The oxygen tension is generally reduced, carbon dioxide tension increased, and oxygen saturation diminished. With respect to lung volume—vital capacity, residual volume, and total lung capacity are all significantly reduced in severe cases. Similarly, the functional residual capacity is also reduced.

More sophisticated methods of measuring pulmonary function, particularly the use of Xenon, reveals the lack of utilization of significant areas of the lung in thoracic scoliosis, with resultant pulmonary arteriovenous shunting, causing impaired gaseous exchange.

It is customary to investigate thoroughly the pulmonary status of all patients with thoracic scoliosis, except those in whom the curvature is minimal. According to most studies, pulmonary function may not be appreciably altered.[24,73] It may well be that a prolonged period of cast immobilization and fusion of the costo-transverse joints during the course of the spinal fusion procedure prevent the logically anticipated increase in respiratory function.

TREATMENT

Historically, one of the most popular forms of prescribed treatment has been the various stretching exercises for children with scoliosis. Unfortunately, no one has proved that such exercises affect the natural history of the curvature, but they may be of value in improving pulmonary function. Certainly exercise has become an important adjunct to treatment with the Milwaukee brace. Whether exercises are of value in increasing the flexibility of the spine prior to a surgical corrective procedure seems doubtful.

MILWAUKEE BRACE

In 1945, Blount, Schmidt, and Bidwell developed an axial distraction brace with traction pads, which has proved to be the first orthotic device that can effectively control the scoliosis deformity (Fig. 19-4).[5]

Blount has repeatedly stressed there are two important aspects to correction by the Milwaukee brace. The first of these is the distraction component, which is probably very small, and the other, the active correction by the patient. This is the area in which improvement may be achieved through a good exercise program.

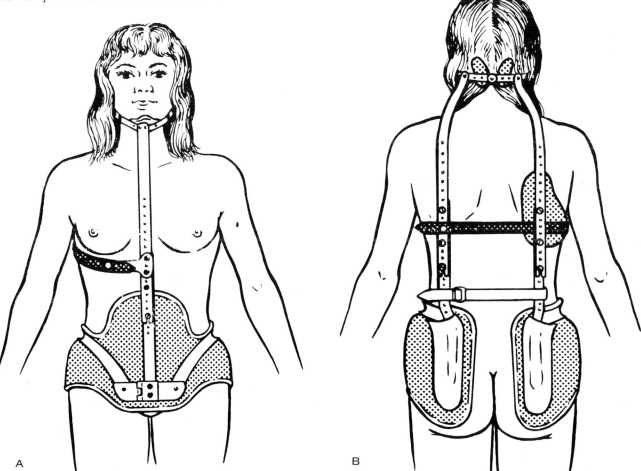

FIG. 19-4. *A*, Front view of patient in Milwaukee brace. Throat mold does not apply pressure to mandible. *B*, Back view of patient in Milwaukee brace. Pad lies over hump in right thoracic curve. Occiput pads are continued to back of skull.

Actual measurements of the mean total distraction force, in a series of ten children undergoing active treatment in the brace, indicated a mean force of 5.7 pounds. This was contrasted with the traction applied to the apex of right thoracic curves, in which case a mean force of 5.5 pounds was measured.[7]

According to some reports, the median final correction effected by the Milwaukee brace is approximately 20 to 25%,[42] of which lumbar and thoracolumbar curves are most successfully treated.[47] For many mild curves, the prevention of progression added to the limited correction are adequate. In a few cases, however, it is not possible to prevent further deterioration of the curve. Apparently, the forces at play in the development of the scoliosis exceed those produced by the brace. In such cases, a spinal fusion must be performed early, before the curvature worsens.

Treatment with a Milwaukee brace requires the services of a team: the orthopaedic surgeon, an orthotist, and a physiotherapist. (Prior to the substitution of the throat mold for the chin piece, it was customary to include an orthodontist.)

Following an initial period of adjustment, the child is encouraged to wear the brace for 23 hours a day. Few restrictions are imposed, and in fact, one is encouraged to participate fully in all activities. In the early period following application of the brace, treatment must be carefully supervised and frequent adjustments made. When satisfactory correction is achieved and maintained, visits to the doctor may be less frequent.

The mechanism of correction with the Milwaukee brace is to relieve pressure on the concave side of the vertebral growth plate. When radiographs indicate that growth of the vertebrae is complete, and removal of the brace for increasing periods demonstrates retention of correction, the patient is gradually weaned from the brace. Because of the tendency of children to assume a position of scoliotic deformity during sleep, it is customary to retain the brace, for a year or two, at night.

PLASTER AND PLASTIC JACKETS

Hibbs, at the New York Orthopaedic Hospital, developed the first turnbuckle cast. Initially, the hinge was placed on the convex side of the curvature and the turnbuckle on the concave, thereby providing both a bending moment and traction. Because of difficulty with pressure areas, Risser modified the turnbuckle jacket and placed the hinges anteriorly and posteriorly over the apex of the curvature.[57] This technique of correction has been shown through the decades to be extremely effective, probably as much so as the Harrington instruments. Unfortunately, hospitalization was prolonged and pressure areas common, despite preventive measures.

Subsequently, Risser[55] and Von Lackum[65] incorporated in jackets some correctional principles that can be traced to the nineteenth century.[4] Their application made possible acceptable levels of correction in patients with moderate curvature, at the same time claiming the advantages of simple application and instantaneous correction.

The Risser "localizer" employs cephalopelvic traction in addition to "localizer" pressure pads. By means of this technique, it is possible not only to correct the spinal curvature, but also to derotate the spine and reduce the prominence of the rib hump.

Von Lackum developed a three-point traction system with circumferential straps, which he termed surcingle correction. The name is derived from the strap that is used to encircle the trunk of a horse. The major surcingle strap is placed over a bony prominence in relation to the apex of the curve, with countertraction applied above and below. When the procedure was introduced by Von Lackum, axial traction was not considered necessary, and the patient lay on the table in a prone position. The technique has since been modified to increase the derotation and reduce the rib hump by fixing the dorsal end of the apical surcingle. Thus with tightening of the unfixed ventral end, significant derotation is achieved. Keim has recently further modified this technique by applying the cast with the patient supine.[35]

The Von Lackum surcingle system of contralateral pressures provides both lateral correction and derotation and almost complete absence of pressure sores. This is true because of the use of wide muslin bandages for the apical surcingle. The force is applied over such a large area that the actual skin pressure is relatively low. Naturally, the overcorrection of secondary curves, which was seen with hinge turnbuckle jackets, is avoided.

Plaster jackets have been used both as a method of achieving correction and as a means of sustaining it in the postoperative period while the fusion solidifies. However, plaster casts have also been used as a method of achieving correction and preventing progression of the scoliosis deformity without fusion. In such cases, the plaster jackets have been hinged and made removable for skin care. The use of plastic materials in place of plaster has the advantage of water resistance. Some plastics also permit local changes in the shell after initial fitting.

PREOPERATIVE TRACTION

During the nineteenth century, axial traction was used as a form of treatment, but its effect was only temporary.[4] Hibbs used axial traction to correct curvature prior to his fusions for scoliosis. When it became evident that greater correction could be achieved with the turnbuckle cast, axial traction was discontinued.[27] Today, axial traction is used both with the localizer correction and with Keim's modification of the surcingle technique. Cotrel has developed a leather head halter and padded pelvic straps which are controlled by the patient.[9] These are applied preoperatively to soften contracted soft tissue.

The halo was initially developed as a method of precisely controlling the skull by attachment to a plaster body cast. Later, it became apparent the halo could be used with countertraction provided by pins inserted in the distal femora. The four pins used with the halo distribute the weight more satisfactorily than do tongs, and are less likely to be dislodged. Weights are gradually added to the system until a maximum of 30 pounds traction is applied to the skull and 15 pounds to each femur. Correction with this technique is significant and apparently greater than by either the turnbuckle jacket or Harrington instrumentation; correction is maintained by a posterior bilateral spinal fusion. Following wound healing, the patient is placed in a body jacket, incorporating the halo. When upper limits of acceptable weight are applied attention must be directed to the hips to prevent dislocation, a complication more frequent in patients with neurologic scoliosis.

DeWald has developed a pelvic halo to avoid the possibility of damage to the hip joints.[11] Two transfixion rods are inserted through the wings of the ilium and attached to a regular halo applied to the skull in the customary manner.[46] The scoliosis is then corrected by turnbuckle distraction. An additional advantage of this technique is that it permits the patient to be ambulatory.

SPINAL INSTRUMENTATION

In 1955, Allan reported a series of eleven severe cases of scoliosis in which he had inserted a metal jack into the base of the transverse processes on the concave side of idiopathic curves.[1] In 1958, Gruca described his technique of anterior and posterior alloplasty, which depended on the attachment of springs to the transverse processes in the so-called posterior alloplasty or the pedicles in the anterior alloplasty.[23] For more severe degrees of scoliosis, alloplasty was combined with a distraction device on the concave side, which was also springloaded. In 1961, Wenger reported 36 cases treated by the insertion of a turnbuckle jack through a direct intrathoracic paravertebral approach to the concave side of the curve.[69] In 1962, Harrington reported a decade of experience with compression and distraction devices of his design.[26] The major correction is achieved by the distraction device, which is inserted superiorly into the articular facet or lamina and inferiorly into the superior surface of the lamina. The compression system for the convex side of the curve consists of a series of hooks applied to the transverse processes. As the amount of force applicable by the convex compression system is of a low order of magnitude, the greatest part

of the correction probably is achieved by the convexed distraction system, the benefit of the convex system being largely one of stabilization.[67] Harrington instruments are inserted through a midline posterior approach to the spine as used for posterior spinal fusion (Fig. 19-5).

In 1965, Dwyer and associates developed a system of correction by which (1) a plate or staple is driven to span the vertebral body; (2) a screw is inserted through the plate into the vertebra; (3) a cable is then positioned, and correction is achieved; (4) the head of the screw is then swaged to the cable. To achieve better correction, the intervertebral discs are thoroughly excised and bone is added between the vertebral endplates to complete an interbody fusion. This technique is particularly valuable when posterior elements are deficient, as following extensive laminectomy, or congenitally absent, as in meningomyeloceles. This technique has the further advantage of correcting lordosis (Fig. 19-6).[13,59]

It should be apparent that spinal instrumentation provides methods of achieving additional correction. Because of the forces generated, Harrington instruments allow an average of 10 degrees more correction than can be secured by the localizer or surcingle cast alone, and probably comparable correction to that achievable by a turnbuckle jacket.[62] Dwyer instruments, from preliminary results available, provide somewhat more correction than that obtained by posterior instrumentation. Ultimately, however, the maintenance of any correction depends on an intact spinal fusion.

SPINAL FUSION

POSTERIOR APPROACH. Since the performance of the first posterior spinal fusions by Hibbs and Albee, and the subsequent application of this technique to the treatment of scoliosis by Forbes and Hibbs, the technique has changed to some extent during the intervening six decades.

It is customary to approach the spine posteriorly through a straight vertical incision, which provides the additional illusion of spinal straightness, following correction of scoliosis. Deep to the skin the loose subcutaneous tissue permits retraction to the midline, and further dissection is carefully maintained in this area to eliminate bleeding. The spinous processes are used as a guide, and the overlying cartilage caps and interspinous ligaments are split. Dissection is then carried deeply beneath the periosteum, which is generally left intact. It is then possible to remove the tissue between the spinous processes and lamina in a clean layer out onto the transverse processes in the thoracic region. By attention to these details, considerable blood loss is avoided and a minimal amount of soft tissue is left in position to be removed subsequently. It is customary to

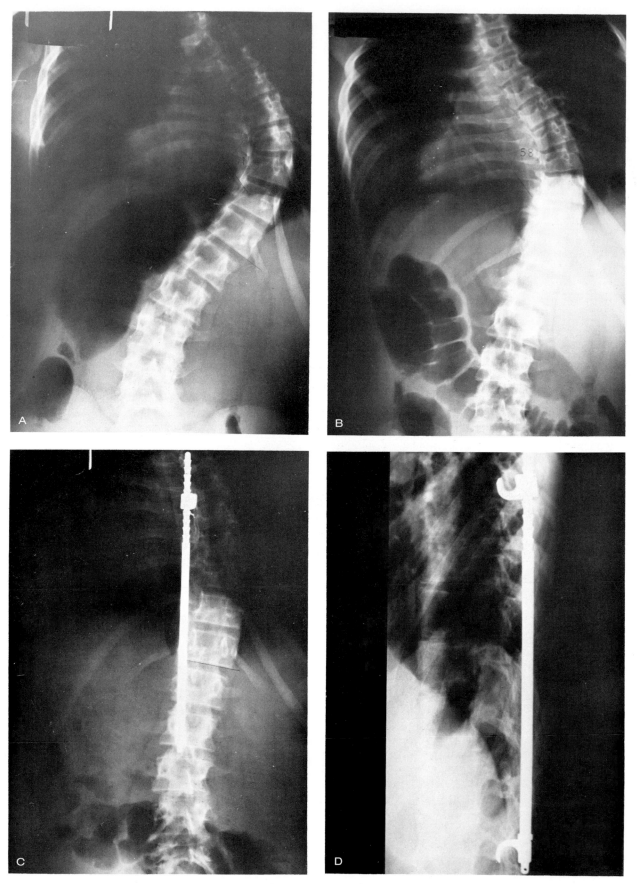

FIG. 19-5. *A,* Erect roentgenogram of 16-year-old girl with thoracic structural curve measuring 71 degrees erect, using T7 and T12 vertebrae; *B,* recumbent film measured 58 degrees; *C,* Correction was possible to 33 degrees using a Harrington distraction rod; *D,* Rod is seen to be well seated in laminae.

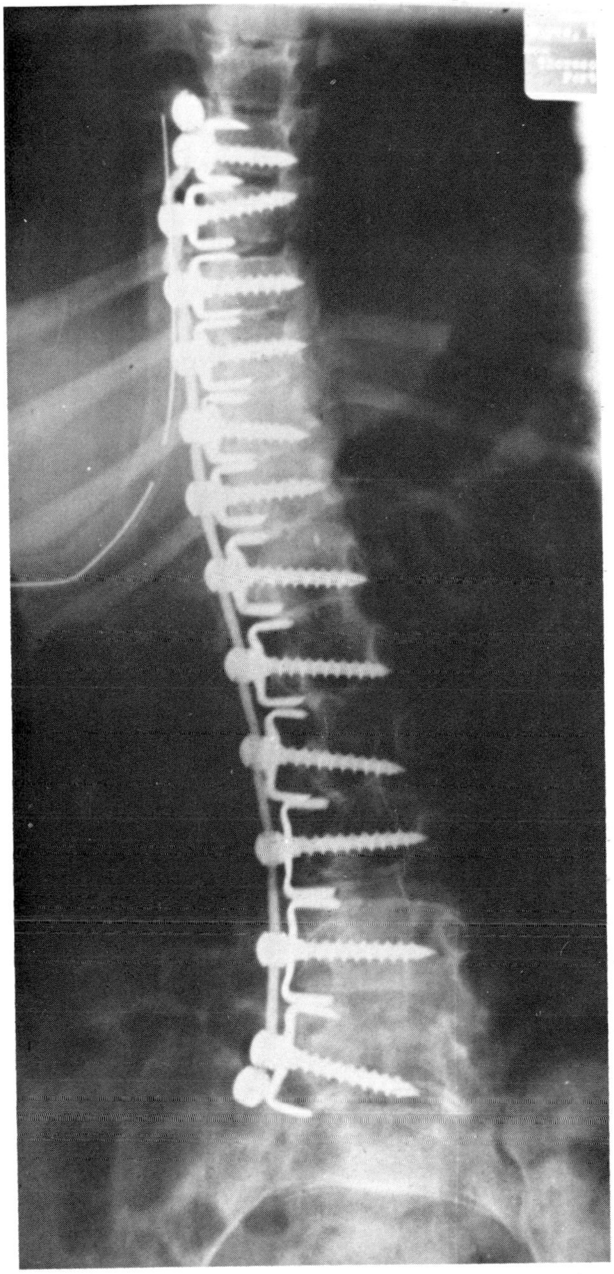

FIG. 19-6. Postoperative roentgenogram of 11-year-old boy with T7 paraplegia secondary to rhabdomyo-sarcoma. Irradiation and antimetabolites were used successfully. T6 to L3 curve of 47 degrees developed and was unstable. Following Dwyer correction and stabilization from T6 to L5, curve measures 6 degrees.

remove the superficial layer of the ligamentum flavum with a sharp curette. This is expedited by appreciation of its position running from the deep surface of the lamina above to the superficial surface of the lamina below.

If it is desired to insert a Harrington rod, sites should be selected for the superior and inferior distraction hooks, the superior being put into the facet joint or lamina and the inferior into a notch in the superior surface of a lumbar lamina. Similarly, if the compression system is desired, the transverse processes for the application of hooks must be protected. If a considerable rib hump is present, correction of this deformity may be enhanced by osteotomy of the transverse processes or ribs on the convex side of the curvature. Harrington has devised an outrigger, which permits the application of the distraction force during decortication and removal of the bone for graft. It has been found that the initial force applied to achieve correction slowly falls as tissue relaxation occurs, and use may be made of this fact to achieve a greater degree of correction.[67] The decortication procedure consists of removing the outer cortical layer of the laminae and interarticularis. The spinous processes may be removed and cut up into bone grafts or turned as chips into the general fusion bed in the method originally described by Hibbs.[27] Various surgeons have approached the facet area in different ways. The majority believe it is desirable to remove the cartilaginous surfaces, and this may be done either with a curette or by a facet-destruction technique.

Most surgeons performing a posterior spinal fusion believe that the addition of autogenous bone, either from the posterior iliac crest or elsewhere, materially reduces the incidence of pseudarthrosis. In our own studies, the pseudarthrosis rate with copious autogenous bone was 3% whereas with bank bone the rate was 50%. For the purposes of this study, pseudarthrosis was defined as a loss of correction of 8 degrees or more.[16] If it is desired to add bone from the posterior iliac crest, this may be secured either through an extension of the midline incision or through a separate incision over the iliac crest. In all probability, to ensure increased survival of the osteocytes, bone chips no more than 3 mm. in thickness should be taken. This grafting material is then laid longitudinally over the prepared bed after the instruments have been inserted.

There is some controversy regarding when operation should be performed and nonsurgical treatment abandoned. However, it is generally agreed that the nonoperative treatment, primarily the use of a Milwaukee brace, should be used on the mild curves in children with growth remaining. If the degree of curvature is such that brace treatment cannot be expected to produce a satisfactory result, for example, a thoracic curve greater than 40 degrees, surgical treatment should be considered. Correction after the termination of growth can only be achieved through surgical means. Adjunctive spinal instrumentation is probably unnecessary in the treatment of lesser curvatures if, by plaster correction alone, the curvature can be reduced to a level that is both functionally and cosmetically satisfactory. However, not only does the instrumentation permit a greater degree of correction, but it also reduces the incidence of pseudarthrosis.

If surgical treatment is contemplated the extent of the fusion should be the least necessary to achieve a satisfactory result. Whereas it was once customary to fuse between parallel vertebrae, it is now more common, in the mature spine, to fuse only the structural curve. In children, it is preferable to add one vertebra above and one or two below to allow for inclusion of additional vertebrae in the curve with growth. If Harrington instrumentation is to be employed, it is generally safer to place the inferior hook in the lamina of L1 or below, because of the termination of the spinal cord.

Postoperatively we frequently apply a posterior molded splint, which is worn until a plaster jacket can be applied. Although not essential if the hooks are well placed, the splint facilitates nursing care and provides general comfort to the patient, particularly when he is rolled from side to side.

A plaster jacket has been found to be necessary to prevent loss of the correction effected by instrumentation, apparently from erosion of the hooks. The jacket is applied in such a manner as to relieve the pressure on the compression system and, in certain cases, actually may provide additional correction. However, no matter how snugly the plaster jacket is applied, it loosens within a period of two or three days.

The postoperative routine is variable. Immediate ambulation is our policy for slim children, provided the jacket is snug; the jacket is worn for seven months. However, if some question exists regarding the firmness of the attachment of the distraction hooks, the strength of the bone, or the fit of the jacket, correctional loss can be avoided if the child is kept recumbent for as long as three months after operation. Harrington has shown that several years are required for the spinal fusion to mature, hence sports and other strenuous activities are restricted for the first two years after operation.

Although the Harrington instrumentation technique is suitable for correction of most types of scoliosis, fixation of the cord in the congenital form may result in damage, even when myelographic studies have failed to demonstrate an intradural abnormality. For this reason most surgeons prefer an early prophylactic fusion in congenital scoliosis to a major late correctional attempt.

ANTERIOR APPROACH. The anterior approach to the vertebral spine has been used for as long as four decades in the treatment of vertebral tuberculosis, and attempts to correct scoliotic and kyphotic deformities through an anterior approach have been described.[66]

With the development of the Dwyer instruments for the correction of scoliotic and lordotic deformities, familiarity with the anterior approach to the spinal column has become essential.

Vertebrae, from T5 to L5, can be approached by means of two individual incisions. If a large segment of the spinal column is to be exposed, two incisions may be necessary. The vertebrae in the lumbar region can be exposed by a simple flank incision. If vertebrae in the lower thoracic and lumbar region need to be exposed, an approach removing the tenth rib and dividing the diaphragm to enter the abdominal cavity will give exposure from the pelvis to T9. Removal of a rib more proximally will increase the exposure into the upper thoracic region.

According to Riseborough, the rib selected for removal should be one above the highest vertebra requiring exposure. If a lower rib is removed, the exposure is inadequate and the operation more difficult, because ribs passing over the vertebral body limit access.[53] Dwyer varies his selection of the rib to be removed according to the vertebral level, but also according to the slope of the ribs, a higher rib removal being necessary with a more vertical orientation.[12]

A retropleural approach should be avoided, as such exposure is limited, making the operation within a confined space more involved and the control of hemorrhage, should it occur, extremely difficult.

Excision of the tenth rib allows an adequate intrathoracic and retroperitoneal exposure, through which most deformities of the lower axial skeleton can be corrected.

The patient should be placed in the lateral position usually with the convexity of the curve uppermost. The incision follows the line of the tenth rib, extending forward across the abdomen to the lateral edge of the rectus sheath and then turning down toward the symphysis pubis, the distance of the abdominal incision depending on the number of lumbar vertebrae to be exposed. The tenth rib is removed from its costal angle to the costochondral junction and the costal cartilage split longitudinally, allowing entrance to the abdominal cavity. Separately the edges of the divided costal cartilage are cut. The peritoneum can be freed from the undersurface of the diaphragm and from the bodies of the lumbar vertebrae. The diaphragm may be detached from its costal insertion circumferentially, posteriorly to the vertebral body, leaving only enough attachment to the rib for resuturing. The pleura over the vertebral bodies is divided to expose the number of thoracic vertebrae required. Further stripping of the peritoneum from the vertebral column will expose the lumbar vertebrae to be included in the correction.

The crura of the diaphragm should be removed from the bodies of L1 and L2 on the left, and L1, L2, and L3 on the right. The sympathetic chain should be isolated, but not divided, and in the abdomen the psoas muscle can be freed from its attachment to the intervertebral disc and upper and lower edges of the vertebral bodies and retracted posteriorly.

The bodies of the vertebrae appear as depressions and the discs as prominences. The tissue over the intervertebral disc is relatively avascular, but segmental vessels and nerves pass around the vertebral body. These should be isolated and tied, but vessels too close to the intervertebral foramen should not be tied, as this may destroy an anastamosing plexus passing up and down between the segmental vessels close to the intervertebral foramina. The tissue over the discs is avascular, and dissection should begin over the disc and extend onto the body. All areolar tissue and pleura should be freed from the body in the relatively avascular plane over the disc, and with the tying and dividing of the segmental vessels and freeing of the areolar tissue over the vertebral body, it should be possible to pass a finger around each body exposed to reach the angle between the transverse process and the body on the opposite side.

If it is necessary to expose vertebrae above T9, it will be necessary to remove the sixth rib as well as the tenth; for even wider exposure, the sixth rib is excised and the incision extended distally by the freeing of remaining costal cartilages from the sternum.

In the more distal lumbar regions at the level of the fourth and fifth lumbar vertebrae, the approach is complicated by the bifurcation of the aorta and the junction of the common iliac veins to form the vena cava, but with care these can usually be freed and lifted forward, exposing the bodies of L4 and L5.

Osteotomies, hemivertebra excisions, and interbody fusions with Dwyer instrumentation can easily be performed through these incisions. Wound closure requires pleural repair and reattachment of the diaphragm with underwater drainage of the thoracic cavity.

The anterior thoracoabdominal approach provides specific advantages. Extravital studies with static testing of vertebral elements show the limiting factor on the achievement of correction to be largely the anulus fibrosis. Accordingly, a surgical approach that permits excision of the intervertebral disc should provide better correction. It is important to recognize, however, that the anterior approach, while usually associated with significantly less blood loss and morbidity than the posterior approach, should not be performed without an intensive care unit where the patient can be adequately cared for postoperatively.

The thoracoabdominal approach with Dwyer instrumentation is proving to be the procedure of choice when posterior elements are deficient and when it is desired to correct a significant degree of lordosis. It is probably contraindicated in kyphosis and in high thoracic curves, and probably less applicable in very long curves.

THE FUTURE

It is apparent to anyone studying scoliosis that a great deal remains to be learned. Many theories of pathogenesis exist, but the mechanism of production of the spinal curvature remains unclear.

It is hoped that further investigation into the genetic aspects of the disease and possible biochemical aberrations may clarify the matter, so that in the future the disease may be prevented rather than treated by cumbersome braces or extensive surgery.

References

1. Allan FG: Scoliosis: operative correction of fixed curves. J Bone Jt Surg 37B:92, 1955.
2. Andry N: Orthopaedia. London, A. Millar, 1743.
3. Bick EM: Vertebral growth: its relation to spinal abnormalities in children. Clin Orthop 21:43, 1961.
4. Bigg HH: Orthopraxy, the Mechanical Treatment of Deformities, Debilities and Deficiencies of the Human Frame. J. Churchhill and Sons, London, 1865.
5. Blount WP, Schmidt AC, Keever ED, Leonard ET: The Milwaukee brace in the operative treatment of scoliosis. J bone Jt Surg 40A:511, 1958.
6. Cobb JR: Outline for the study of scoliosis. Am Acad Orthop Surgeons Lect 5:261, 1948.
7. Cochran GVB, Waugh TR: The external forces in correction of idiopathic scoliosis. J Bone Jt Surg 51A:201, 1969.
8. Colonna PC, Vom Saal F: A study of paralytic scoliosis based on 500 cases of poliomyelitis. J Bone Jt Surg 23:335, 1941.
9. Cotrel Y, Morel G: La technique de L'E.D.F. dans la correction des scoliosis. Rev Chir Orthop 50:59, 1964.
10. Cowell HR, Hall JN, MacEwen GD: Genetic Aspects of Scoliosis. A Nicholas Andry Award Essay, 1970. Clin Orthop 86:121, 1972.
11. De Wald R, Ray RD: Skeletal traction for the treatment of severe scoliosis. J Bone Jt Surg 52A:233, 1970.
12. Dwyer AF: Experience of anterior correction of scoliosis. Clin Orthop 93:191, 1973.
13. Dwyer AF, Newton NC, Sherwood AA: An anterior approach to scoliosis. Clin Orthop 62:192, 1969.
14. End-result Study of the Treatment of Idiopathic Scoliosis. Report of the Research Committee of the American Orthopaedic Association. J Bone Jt Surg 23:963, 1941.
15. Ferguson AB: Roentgen Diagnosis of the Extremities and Spine. New York, Paul B Hoeber, 1939.
16. Fielding JW, Waugh TR: Postoperative correction of scoliosis. JAMA 182:541, 1962.
17. George K, Rippstein J: A comparative study of the two popular methods of measuring scoliotic deformity of the spine. J Bone Jt Surg 43A:809, 1961.
18. Gilly R, Stagnara P, Frederich A, Dalloz C, Robert JM, Goldblatt B: Medical aspects of essential structural scoliosis in children. Lyon Med. 95:79, 1963.
19. Glauber A, Fernbach J, Massanyi L, Medgyesi G: Protein metabolism in idiopathic scoliosis. J Bone Jt Surg 44A:1553, 1962.
20. Goldstein LA: Report of the Terminology Committee of the Scoliosis Research Society. 2nd Annual Meeting, Houston, Texas, 1967.
21. Greulich WW, Pyle SL: Radiographic Atlas of Skeletal Development of the Hand and Wrist. Stanford Univ. Press, Calif., 1950.
22. Gruca A: Pathologenesis of idiopathic scoliosis. Acta Chir Orthop Traum Cech 29:65, 1962.
23. Gruca A: The pathogenesis and treatment of idiopathic scoliosis. A preliminary report. J Bone Jt Surg 40A:570, 1958.
24. Gucker T, III: Changes in vital capacity in scoliosis. Preliminary report on effect of treatment. J Bone Jt Surg 44A:469, 1962.

25. Guérin J: Premier Memoine sur le Traitement des Deviations de l'Epine par la Section des Muscles du Dos. Douzieme Memoine sur les Difformities. Ed. 2. Paris, au buneau de la Gaz. med., 1843.

26. Harrington PR: Treatment of scoliosis. Correction and internal fixation by spine instrumentation. J Bone Jt Surg 44A:591, 1962.

27. Hibbs RA: A report of 59 cases of scoliosis treated by the fusion operation. J Bone Jt Surg 6:3, 1924.

28. Hibbs RA: An operation for progressive spinal deformities. A preliminary report of three cases from the service of the New York Orthopaedic Hospital. New York Med J 93:1013, 1911.

29. Hippocrates: The Genuine Works of Hippocrates. London, F. Adams, 1849.

30. James JIP: Infantile idiopathic scoliosis. Clin Orthop 21:106, 1961.

31. James JIP, Lloyd-Roberts GC, Pilcher MF: Infantile structural scoliosis. J Bone Jt Surg 41B:719, 1958.

32. James JIP: Paralytic scoliosis. J Bone Jt Surg 38B:660, 1956.

33. James JIP: Scoliosis. Edinburgh and London, E. and S. Livingstone, Ltd., 1967.

34. Katzman HM, Waugh TR, Berdon WE: Skeletal changes following irradiation for childhood malignancy. J Bone Jt Surg 51A:825, 1969.

35. Keim HA, Waugh TR: The surcingle cast in scoliosis treatment. Clin Orthop 86:154, 1972.

36. Langenskiöld A, Michelsson J: Experimental progressive scoliosis in the rabbit. J Bone Jt Surg 43B:116, 1961.

37. Liszka OP: Spinal cord mechanisms leading to scoliosis in animal experiments. Acta Med Pol 2:45, 1961.

38. MacEwen GD: Experimental scoliosis. Clin Orthop 93:69, 1973.

39. MacEwen GD, Winter RB, Hardy JH: Evaluation of kidney anomalies in congenital scoliosis. J Bone Jt Surg 54A:1451, 1972.

40. Meyer GH: Die mechanik de skoliose. Arch Path Anat 35:225, 1866.

41. Michelsson J: The development of spinal deformity in experimental scoliosis. Acta Orthop Scand, Suppl 81, 1965.

42. Moe JH, Kettleson DN: Idiopathic scoliosis analysis of curve patterns and preliminary results of Milwaukee brace treatment in 169 patients. J Bone Jt Surg 52A:1509, 1970.

43. Murdoch G: Scoliosis in twins. J Bone Jt Surg 41B:736, 1959.

44. Nachemson A: A long-term follow-up study of non treated scoliosis. Acta Orthop Scand 39:466, 1968.

45. Nash CL Jr, Moe JH: A study of vertebrae rotation. J Bone Jt Surg 50A:223, 1968.

46. Nickel VL, Perry J, Garrett A, Heppenstall M: The halo—a spinal skeletal traction fixation device. J Bone Jt Surg 50A:1400, 1968.

47. Nordwall A: Strides in idiopathic scoliosis. Acta Orthop Scand, Suppl 150, 1973.

48. Packard FR: Life and Times of Ambroise Pare. Ed 2. New York, Paul B. Hoeber, 1926.

49. Perey O: Discography in early cases of idiopathic scoliosis. Acta Orthop Scand 33:392, 1963.

50. Perey O, Rydman T: Idiopathic scoliosis, a preliminary report. Acta Orthop Scand 32:39, 1962.

51. Ponseti IV: Personal Communication, 1966.

52. Recklinghausen FD von: Uber die Multiplen Fibrome der Haut und ihre Bezrehungen zu den Neuromen. Festschr R. Virchow, 1882.

53. Riseborough EJ: The anterior approach to the spine for the correction of deformities of the axial skeleton. Clin Orthop 93:207, 1973.

54. Risser JC: Scoliosis: past and present. J Bone Jt Surg 46A:167, 1964.

55. Risser JC: The application of body casts for the correction of scoliosis. Am Acad Orthop Surgeons Lect 12:255, 1955.

56. Risser JC, Ferguson AB: Scoliosis: its prognosis. J Bone Jt Surg 18:667, 1936.

57. Risser JC, Lauder CH Jr, Norquist DM, Craig WA: Three types of body casts. Am Acad Orthop Surgeons Lect 10:131, 1953.

58. Shands AR Jr, Eisberg HB: The incidence of scoliosis in the state of Delaware. A Study of 50,000 minifilms of the chest made during a survey for tuberculosis. J Bone Jt Surg 37A:1243, 1955.

59. Sherwood AA: The engineering problems involved in the design of a device for the correction of spinal curvature. Engineering Year Book 101, 1965.

60. Stearns G, Chen JY, McKinley JB, Ponseti IV: Metabolic studies of children with idiopathic scoliosis. J Bone Jt Surg 37A:1028, 1955.

61. Stromeyer, GF: Beitrage zur Operativen Orthopaedik. Hannover, 1838.

62. Tamborino JM, Ambrust EN, Moe JH: Harrington instrumentation in the correction of scoliosis: a comparison with cast correction. J Bone Jt Surg 46A:313, 1964.

63. Virchow H: Der zustand der ruckenmuskulatur bei skoliose und kyphoskoliose. Z Orthop Chir 34:1, 1914.

64. Virchow H: Uber drei nach form zusammengesetzte skoliotische rumpfe. Z Orthop Chir 29:263, 1911.

65. Von Lackum WH: The surgical treatment of scoliosis. Am Acad Orthop Surgeons Lect 5:236, 1948.

66. Von Lackum HL, Smith AD: Removal of vertebral bodies in the treatment of scoliosis. Surg Gynec Obstet 57:250, 1933.

67. Waugh TR: Intravital measurements during instrumental correction of scoliosis. Acta Orthop Scand 39:136, 1968.

68. Waugh TR: Report of the Terminology Committee of the Scoliosis Research Society, 8th Annual Meeting, Gothenburg, Sweden, 1973.

69. Wenger HL: Spine jack operation in the correction of scoliotic deformity. Arch Surg 83:901, 1961.

70. Wenger HL: Transversectomy for scoliosis. J Bone Jt Surg 33A:253, 1951.

71. Wynne-Davies R: Familial scoliosis. Proceedings of a Symposium on Scoliosis. Action for the Crippled Child Monograph, London, 36, 1965.

72. Yamada K, Yamamato H, Ikada T, Nakagawa Y, Kinoshita I, Tezuka A, Tamura T: A neurological approach to the etiology and therapy of scoliosis. J Bone Jt Surg 53A:197, 1971.

73. Zorab PA: Pulmonary function in spinal deformity. Clin Orthop 93:33, 1973.

20

Spondylolisthesis and Its Treatment: ConservativeTreatment; Fusion, with and without Reduction

LEON L. WILTSE

HERBINAUX, a Belgian obstetrician, noted in 1782 that there were times when a bony prominence in front of the sacrum caused problems in delivery. He is generally credited with having first described spondylolisthesis, probably the complete type, in which the body of L5 is actually lying in front of the sacrum—in other words, "spondyloptosis".[18]

Spondylolisthesis is the slipping of all or part of one vertebra forward on another. The term was coined by Kilian in 1854,[22] and is derived from the Greek *spondylo*, meaning vertebra, and *olisthesis*, meaning to slip or slide down a slippery path. Kilian did not recognize the fundamental defect in the pars, but believed the lesion to be caused by a slow subluxation of the lumbosacral facets. One year later Robert of Koblenz established the location of the fundamental lesion to be in the pars interarticularis, but did not recognize the nature of the defect.[36] Lambl demonstrated the lesion in the pars in 1855.[25] Naugebauer, in 1881, made an extensive study of anatomic specimens throughout Europe and was the first to recognize that slip can occur by elongation of the pars without their coming apart.[29]

The types of this condition are as varied as its causes. The type of most clinical importance in people under age 50 is the one in which the lesion is in the isthmus or pars interarticularis. However, there are several other conditions that permit this forward slip of one vertebra on another. The discussion in this chapter will be limited to the lumbar spine, except to note that the disease does occur in the cervical spine, and a few cases of pars defects in the thoracic spine have been reported. These are so rare as to be of little importance. The classification of spondylolisthesis presented here combines an anatomic with an etiologic classification.

TABLE 20-1. Classification of Spondylolisthesis

TYPE I. *Isthmic type.* Lesion in pars interarticularis (Fig. 20-1), and can appear as any of the following subtypes:

> *Subtype A. Lytic type.* Due to separation or dissolution of pars. Most common type afflicting persons under 50 years of age, and type of most concern to orthopaedists. Newman has called this type "spondylolytic."[30]

> *Subtype B. Elongation of pars without separation* (*Fig. 20-2*). Fundamentally same disease as subtype A.

> *Subtype C. Spondylolisthesis acquisita.* Occurs at the uppermost vertebra of a spinal fusion.[2,12,44]

> *Subtype D. Pathologic type.* Secondary to either localized or generalized bone disease.

> *Subtype E. Acute pars fracture.* Usually the result of severe trauma, although this is not always obvious (Fig. 20-3).

TYPE II. *Dysplastic type.* Failure of supporting structures allows vertebra above to slip forward on one below.[30] No separation of pars at first and no pars defect; pars is not elongated. Superior sacral facets have failed to hold.

TYPE III. *Degenerative type.* Due to giving-way at anulus and remodeling of articular processes at level of involvement.

TYPE IV. *Peduncular type.* Characterized by loss of continuity of pedicles due to fracture or, in some cases, to elongation of pedicles from generalized bone disease.

ETIOLOGY

Type I. Isthmic Spondylolisthesis

SUBTYPE A. LYTIC TYPE. The pars interarticularis, that is, the part of the vertebra that lies between the articular facets, is the site of this defect. To demonstrate this condition radiographically, oblique and Ferguson views are added to the routine anterior-posterior and lateral views. The 45-degree lateral oblique views are the most informative, but the 30-degree caudocephalad view (Ferguson view) also gives good confirmatory evidence. If there is still doubt, 30- and 60-degree lateral oblique views often confirm the diagnosis. Also, a lateral view with the patient standing with weights on his shoulders may cause the pars to separate more and demonstrate the lesion, especially in young people. Planigrams have been of little value.

The lytic type of spondylolisthesis occurs only in man and man alone has a true upright stance. Defects do not occur in other primates.[41] Rosenberg reviewed roentgenograms of 125 patients in an institution, none of whom had ever assumed the standing position, and found not a single pars defect.[38] Man alone has the bipedal gait and only in this species does true lumbar lordosis occur.

There is no evidence that the defect is present at birth.[5,40] The most common age of onset is between five and seven years.[4,40] The incidence increases until adulthood,[40,43,50] but does not increase significantly thereafter in Caucasians.[40]

In patients under 50, this type is by far the most significant from a clinical standpoint. After this age, degenerative spondylolisthesis becomes more important.

A familial tendency exists.[54] In the 36 families I studied in 1952,[54] no defects were found in members under the age of five years, yet the incidence was 40% in members over the age of ten. Defects do occur, though rarely, before the age of five years.[54] In one reported case, spondylolisthesis of L5 with a high degree of slip was discovered in a 3-month-old infant.[23] After being observed for about eight years, the child was treated surgically. A definite pars defect was found. Since this was an infant, the patient had never assumed the standing position when the defect was discovered, and this fact may seem to conflict with Rosenberg's findings.[39] However, the defect could be attributed to birth trauma or to such injuries as are seen in the "battered child."

Slipping rarely occurs after the age of 20, unless there has been surgical intervention or severe injury. The period of most rapid slipping is between the ages of nine and fifteen (Fig. 20-4 A, B).[54]

Unilateral defects can affect an otherwise normal-appearing lumbar vertebra.[50] A few cases with unilateral defects have undergone actual forward slip. The one intact pars is elongated and is usually twisted in these cases. In some bilateral cases the defects are much narrower than the amount of forward slipping of the body, suggesting that the pars interarticularis had lengthened before coming apart.[44]

There are well-documented cases of young children and adolescents with normal roentgenographic findings in whom full-blown spondylolisthesis has later developed.[53] We are also seeing teen-aged boys with several pars fractures in the lumbar spine, all having been engaged in vigorous athletics such as football or pole-vaulting.[53]

Baker has found the incidence of the defect in adult Caucasian Americans to be 5.8%.[5] Roche and Rowe, from a study of 4,200 adult skeletons, found a smaller incidence of 4.2%.[37] They found in their studies that the incidence in the Caucasian male was 6.4%, in the Negro male 2.8%, in the Caucasian female 2.3%, and in the Negro female 1.1% Hasbe found the incidence among

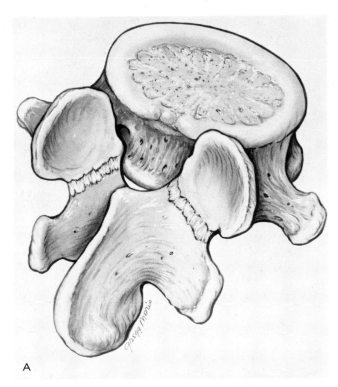

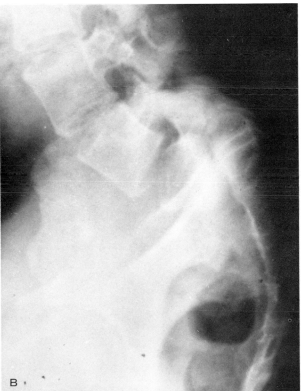

FIG. 20-1. *A,* Drawing of lateral aspect of lower lumbar vertebra showing spondylolysis defect in pars. *B,* Lateral roentgenogram of 15-year-old girl with pars defects and high-grade spondylolisthesis.

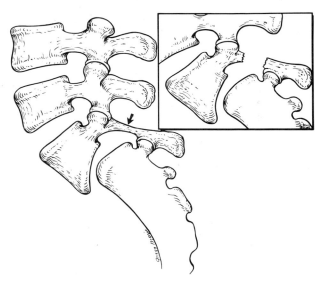

FIG. 20-2. Intact but elongated pars which is stretched by cracking and healing. Insert shows separation of pars.

Japanese to be 5.5% in 125 skeletons studied.[17] Stewart found Eskimos to have by far the highest incidence, as high as 50% in isolated communities north of the Yukon.[43] This study was carried out on skeletons found in Eskimo graveyards.

According to our studies of 1,134 consecutive roentgenograms of the spine,[50] spina bifida is 13 times more common when it is associated with a defect in the pars interarticularis than in the normal spine. A wide open sacrum was found to be four times as common in the presence of pars defects. Also the incidence of severe scoliosis of the lumbar and lower thoracic spine is four times as frequent among patients with pars defects.[50] In at least some of these cases, the scoliosis was originally "sciatic scoliosis," which later became structural.

The vertebral segment showing a defective pars varies within the same family (Fig. 20-5),[50] and several vertebrae may be affected in the same individual. In a pair of identical twins with spondylolisthesis, the twenty-fourth segment was involved in one and the twenty-fifth segment in the other. In the twin with the twenty-fourth segment involved, the twenty-fifth segment was fused to the sacrum; in the other twin the twenty-fifth segment was free. Another set of identical twin girls showed L3 to be affected in one twin and L5 in the other (Fig. 20-6). We have seen many families in which several members had spondylolisthesis, but at different levels.[50]

Transitional vertebrae, which are rather stable, are virtually immune to the defect.[40]

In 1969 Steele reported to me in a personal communication that athetoid patients have an increased in-

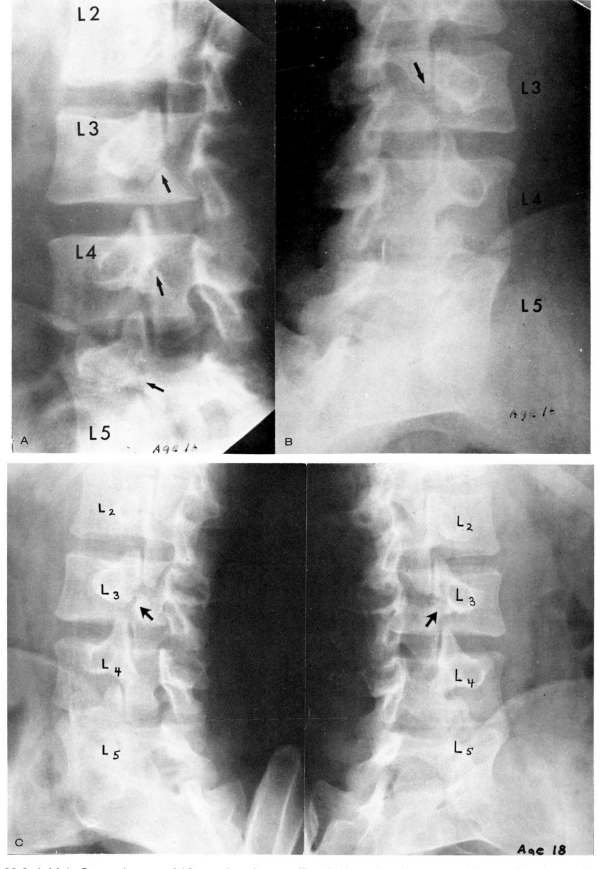

FIG. 20-3. *A*, Male Caucasian, aged 16, was hurt in a scuffle with juveniles: Note pars defects of L3, L4, and L5 (at arrows); *B*, defect of L3 is indicated; *C*, the pars of L4 and L5 have healed. Both pars of L3 remain defective (arrows). (From Wiltse LL.: Spondylolisthesis: classification and etiology. Symposium on the Spine, American Academy of Orthopaedic Surgeons. St. Louis, CV Mosby Co., 1969. Courtesy Dr. J. B. Josephson.)

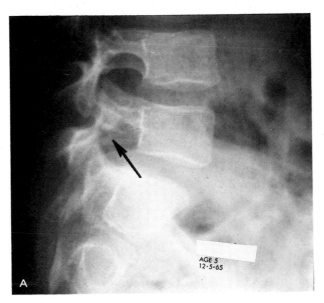
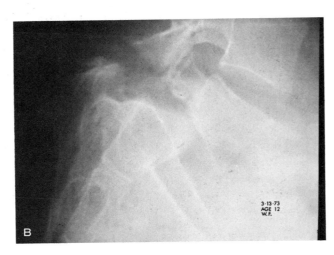

FIG. 20-4. This child had mild back pain at age 5 which prompted the taking of the first roentgenogram: *A,* the line defect was missed by a good radiologist; *B,* at age 12, note the high grade slip. The child was referred to an orthopaedist when his gymnasium teacher noticed that "something didn't appear just right" about the child's back.

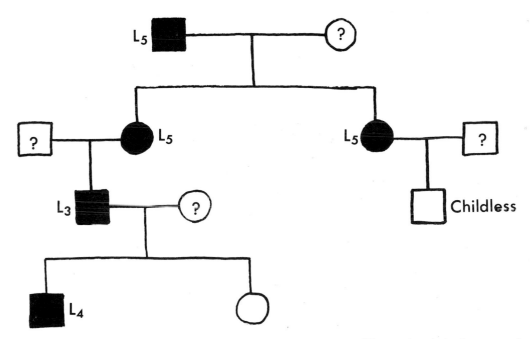

FIG. 20-5. Four generations of one family. Note that the defect occurs at different levels in the same family. (From Wiltse LL: Spondylolisthesis: classification and etiology. Symposium on the Spine, American Academy of Orthopaedic Surgeons. St. Louis, CV Mosby Co., 1969. Courtesy Dr. I. Markowitz.)

cidence of the disease, owing presumably to the characteristic frequent twisting motions.[42] Morisaki in 1972 also reported an increased incidence of 9.8%.[28]

We have shown by tetracycline uptake studies that the bone in the pars is similar to normal bone and is not bone of low vitality (as has been suspected.) It func-

tions as other bone does and contributes to the body's pool of bone metabolites.[47]

SUBTYPE B. ELONGATION OF THE PARS WITHOUT SEPARATION (FIG. 20-2). Fundamentally the same disease as the lytic type, this classification embraces those cases that show a minimal-to-high degree of slip

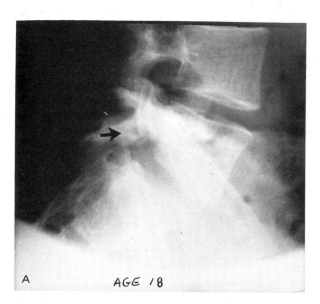

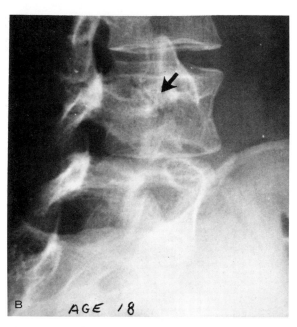

FIG. 20-6. Pars lesions, but involving different levels, in identical twin girls: *A,* lesion in the pars of L5; and *B,* lesion in the pars of L3.

with an intact pars. A high grade of slip is more likely to be associated with the syndrome of tight hamstrings[34] and peculiar "spastic" gait. Often there is change in the angle of the facets at the top of the sacrum[30] and wide spina bifida in L5 or S1 and S2. Wide open sacrum is four times more frequent than in normal spines[50] and, along with spina bifida, is noted almost invariably in cases of intact but elongated pars. Five of our patients with elongated but intact pars have parents and siblings with typical pars defects. This would indicate that this type and subtype A are the same basic disease, but with different manifestations (Figs. 20-7 and 20-8). We believe that the elongation occurs because of repeated cracking and healing of

the pars, which permits successive lengthening. These fractures may be microfractures. In some cases the elongated pars finally separates, leaving thin, elongated stumps of pars.[8,19]

SUBTYPE C. SPONDYLOLISTHESIS ACQUISITA.[2,14,46] This type of spondylolisthesis is believed to be a fatigue fracture resulting from the increased strain and stress on the pars at the upper end of a fused segment of spine. Injury to the pars at the time of operation may play a part.[53] Most patients affected have undergone fusion for spondylolisthesis, and so the basic underlying predisposition must be a factor in the occurrence of this subtype. Sullivan and Bickel reported three such cases.[45] In two, the lesion healed when the patient was immobilized in a cast.

Dissection of the muscle masses away from the area may produce a predisposition to the development of the fracture. Such a dissection would interfere with the venous drainage of the lamina and pars, giving rise to partial death of bone in the area.[26] Also, when the fusion becomes solid, extra stresses are placed on the pars. Another possibility is that the pars is partially cut through during the feathering of the lamina in preparation for the bone graft.

Since we began performing transverse process and lateral mass fusions, we have not seen any cases of spondylolisthesis acquisita, presumably because the site where the lesion develops is supported by the graft.

Spondylolisthesis occasionally results from removal of the supporting structures by an extensive operative procedure, as in radical laminectomy with removal of the facets (Fig. 20-9). This has been called iatrogenic spondylolisthesis.

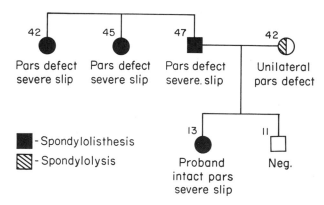

FIG. 20-7. The 13-year-old girl in the second generation is the proband. She had elongated but intact pars. Other affected members had typical pars defect. (Courtesy Dr. Louis Valli, Carmichal Calif.)

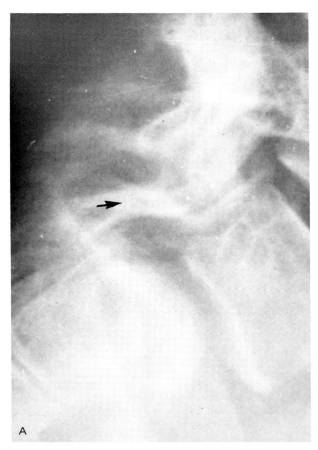

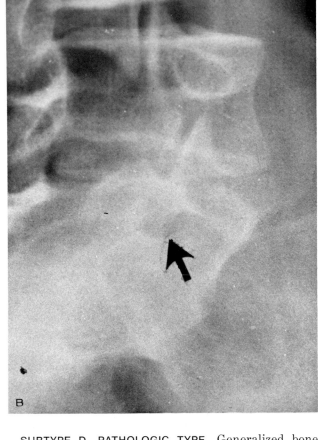

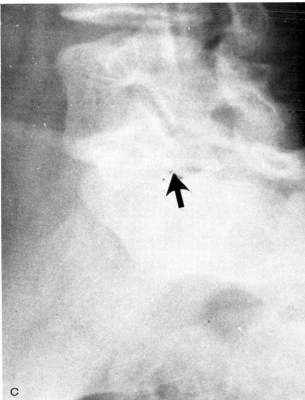

SUBTYPE D. PATHOLOGIC TYPE. Generalized bone disease is another cause of spondylolisthesis. We have seen fractures of the pars in three children with Albers-Schoenberg disease, too high an incidence to be due to simple chance. Also, defects in the pars in children with osteogenesis imperfecta seem to occur too frequently, but we have no statistics to prove this assumption. The cause would appear to be tension and torsional stresses on the pathologic bone with resultant fatigue and separation (Fig. 20-10).

SUBTYPE E. ACUTE PARS FRACTURE. Fractures of the pars, which result from acute severe trauma, are considerably more common than has been believed heretofore. They are fairly common in teen-age boys who are playing sand-lot football and receiving repeated injuries. In actuality, these are probably fatigue fractures.

We have seen cases in which several pars fractures occurred along the spine following one injury (see Fig. 20-3). These were examples of acute pars fractures rather than fatigue fractures, but the dividing line often is indistinct.

FIG. 20-8. Roentgenographic examination of the 13-year-old proband identified in Figure 20-7. Note the intact but elongated pars in the lateral view, *A*, and in the two oblique views, *B* and *C*, of L5.

L5 are permitted to slide forward without either a break or an elongation of the pars of L5.

This type is more common than has been previously believed.

Type III. Degenerative Spondylolisthesis

This type is common, possibly the most common type of spondylolisthesis. None of those affected are younger than 40 and very few are under 50. Most are much older when first seen by the orthopaedist. This type occurs four to five times as frequently in the female as in the male.

Junghanns first described this condition in 1929.[20] Macnab published the clinical description in 1950 and gave it the name of "pseudospondylolisthesis."[27] Newman, in 1963, first gave it the more descriptive title of "degenerative spondylolisthesis."[30] There is no pars defect and the slip is never great, but may reach 30% of the width of the vertebral body in the most extreme cases. Advanced degenerative disease of the zygapophyseal joints is the exclusive finding that separates this condition from all other types of spondylolisthesis (Fig. 20-12 A, B). The facets at the level of slip show severe degeneration, having an appearance somewhat similar to that of a knee with advanced degenerative arthritis. The anulus fibrosis is degenerated in every case. The normal anulus fibrosis does not permit this type of tilting motion, but the degenerated anulus does.

The L4 space is six to nine times more commonly affected than any other level, with the L3 and L5 spaces following in that order. When this occurs at L4, the L5 vertebra has been observed to be more stable than average,[38] thus causing an increased amount of motion to occur at the L4 space (Fig. 20-13A). Often the body of L5 is block-shaped and a higher percentage than average show sacralization of L5. The incidence increases as age increases.

Degenerative spondylolisthesis is rarely seen in association with isthmic spondylolisthesis, probably because in the presence of defects at the isthmus the L5 level is unstable and takes the stress off L4 (Table 20-2).

Erosion of the subchordal bone of the facets takes place at the level of slip, and forward slip occurs not because the facets above slip between the ones below, but rather because the articular processes actually remodel so that the longitudinal plane inclines forward.

Sacralization of L5 is associated with degenerative spondylolisthesis four times as frequently as in the general population.

Spina bifida is virtually never seen below the level of

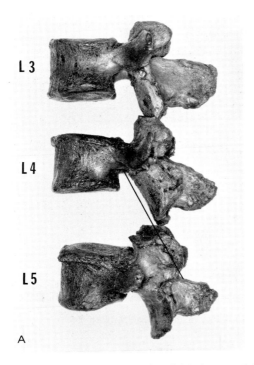

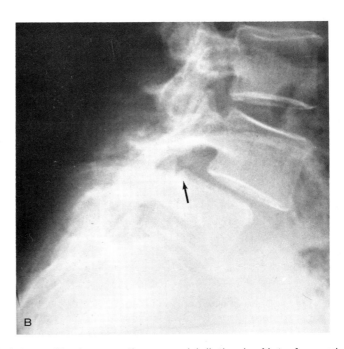

FIG. 20-12. *A,* Photograph of L3, L4, and L5 from skeleton with degenerative spondylolisthesis. Note forward angulation of inferior articular process of L4 and posterior angulation of superior articular process of L5. (From Norman Rosenberg's paper presented at the meeting of the American Orthopaedic Association, Hot Springs, Virginia, 1973.) *B,* Lateral roentgenogram of 56-year-old Caucasian woman with degenerative spondylolisthesis of L4 on L5. Note that angle of facets has changed and there is posterior angulation of inferior articular processes of L4 and forward angulation of superior articular processes of L5. Inferior articular processes of L4 do not slip between superior processes of L5 as has been thought in the past.

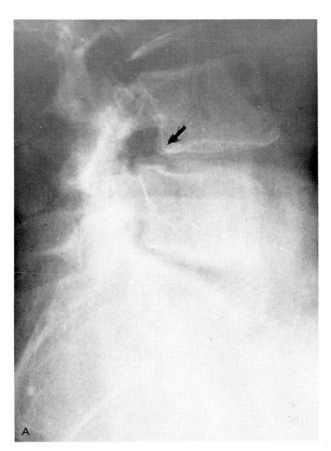 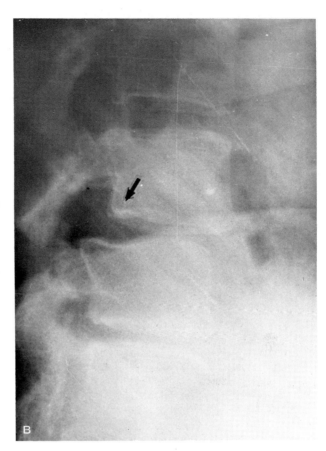

FIG. 20-13. Roentgenograms of a 52-year-old patient with degenerative spondylolisthesis at L4 level: *A,* spine in normal position; *B,* flexion, showing considerable instability, common finding in degenerative spondylolisthesis because of looseness of ligaments at facets and looseness of anulus between bodies. One interesting point to remember is that there is tilting at level of forward slip, but not much anterior-posterior slip.

TABLE 20-2. Paradoxical Occurrence of Degenerative and Isthmic Spondylolisthesis

	Degenerative Spondylolisthesis	Normal Population	Isthmic Spondylolisthesis
Level	L4 9:1		L5 10:1
Sex	Female 4:1		Male 2:1
Age	Over 40		Under 20
Race	Negro 2:1		White 2:1
Spina bifida	Rare (0)	2%	Common (30%)
Sacralization	Common (22%)	6%	Rare (1%)
Trapezoid L5	2 mm.	6 mm.	12 mm.
Lumbosacral angle	145 degrees (Less lordosis)	130 degrees	(More lordosis)

(From Rosenberg N: Degenerative Spondylolisthesis. Paper delivered at the meeting of the American Orthopaedic Association, Hot Springs, Virginia, June 26, 1973.)

slip. This goes along with the belief that L5 stability is increased, which accounts for the development of degenerative spondylolisthesis at L4.

The condition occurs three times as frequently in the Negro female as in the Caucasian, probably because there is increased stability at the lumbosacral angle in the Negro. For example, there is a greater incidence of sacralization of L5 in the Negro, and the body of L5 is more block-shaped.

Hormonal factors might possibly explain why degenerative spondylolisthesis is four times more common in women than in men. For example, it is well known that some ligamentous laxity occurs during pregnancy. Also, some slight change in ligamentous tension occurs with each of the several hundred menstrual periods a woman experiences in her lifetime.

Osteoporosis frequently has been indicted as a cause of degenerative spondylolisthesis, but definite proof is lacking.

Type IV. Peduncular Spondylolisthesis (Fig. 20-14)

This type is caused by fracture or elongation of the pedicles. It is a rare type in the lumbar area and is of little importance. When fractures of the pedicles do occur, they attempt to heal and may do so in a normal or slightly elongated position. Occasionally bone disease, such as osteogenesis imperfecta, may permit stretching of the pedicles, and thus fulfill the criteria for spondylolisthesis. Newman reported such a case.[30]

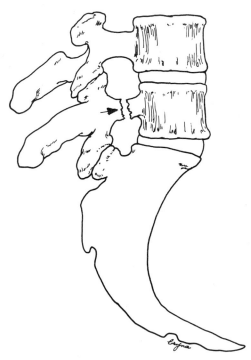

FIG. 20-14. Defect is in pedicle.

Stewart observed fractures of the pedicles in some of his Eskimo skeletons.[44]

Wright and Aase have shown that in Kuskokwim disease the pedicles are elongated (Fig. 20-15).[33,56] Kuskokwim disease is found in Eskimos concentrated in a small area. It is a hereditary recessive condition having some features of arthrogryposis multiplex congenita, yet is quite different.

Osteomalacia occasionally permits elongation of the pedicles, as does achondroplasia.[30]

Reverse Spondylolisthesis

Although reverse or retrograde spondylolisthesis was not mentioned in the classification, it is mentioned here because it bears the name, even though it hardly meets the requirements of spondylolisthesis (by definition, olisthesis means to slip or slide *down* an incline). It would probably be better to call this condition simply "retro displacement."

The appearance of posterior slip of one vertebral body on the one below is seen in the following situations:

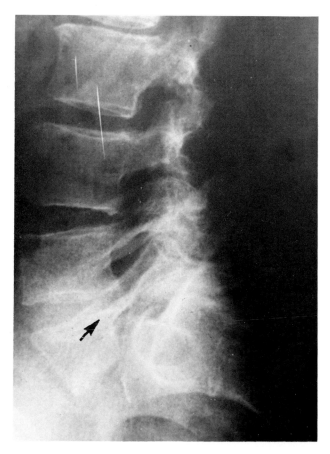

FIG. 20-15. Roentgenogram in Kuskokwim disease. Note elongated pedicle of lower three lumbar vertebrae. (Case courtesy Dr. Gilbert Wright, Sacramento, Calif., 1970.)

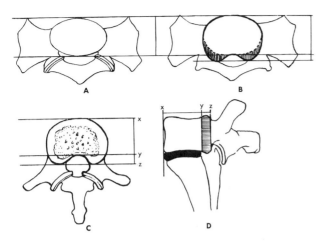

FIG. 20-16. *A,* Note that body of S1 is oval; *B,* body of L5 is kidney-shaped; *C and D,* anteroposterior diameter of L5 is same as that of S1 only in the "hilum" or central portion. Poles of kidney-shaped L5 may lie behind posterior margin of sacrum in lateral roentgenograms, thereby giving illusion of retrodisplacement unless both anterior and posterior margins of vertebrae are viewed and compared. If anterior-posterior diameters of two vertebrae are measured and that of L5 is found to be greater, there may be an illusion of retrodisplacement without true retrodisplacement, that is, pseudo-retrospondylolisthesis. (From Willis TA: Lumbosacral retrodisplacement. J Bone Jt Surg *17:*347, 1935.)

1. When there is an extra thick body of L5 in an anterior-posterior direction with a thinner body of S1 in an anterior-posterior direction, or when the body of L5 is kidney-shaped, thus giving the roentgenographic appearance of being slipped back when actually it is not (Fig. 20-16).[49]

At first glance Figure 20-17 A seems to illustrate a posterior slip of L5 on S1, but if one measures the bodies of these two vertebrae, it will be seen that the anterior-posterior measurement of L5 is greater than that of S1. This could be due either to an actual increase in the anterior-posterior thickness of the body of L5 or to a kidney-shaped body of L5, which causes the corners of the body of L5 to cast a shadow on the roentgenogram posterior to that of the posterior point of the body of S1. This condition is not true retrospondylolisthesis, but might be called "pseudo-retrospondylolisthesis." Figure 17 B represents a case of true retrospondylolisthesis because the anterior-posterior diameters of the bodies of L5 and of S1 are the same, yet L5 is slipped back on S1.

2. When there is a narrowing and degeneration of the disc, but the facets are holding and acting as a fulcrum (Fig. 20-18). This represents a true posterior slip and is a pathologic process. It is true retrospondylolisthesis. The facets remain relatively normal, but the inferior facets of the vertebra above do slide downward on the superior facets of the one below. The

ligaments of the facets stretch, but the cartilage at the facets remains relatively normal.

3. When there is posterior slip only during hyperextension. This is seen in early degeneration of a disc and is the so-called "primary instability."[24] Occasionally this instability is seen as the first visible roent-

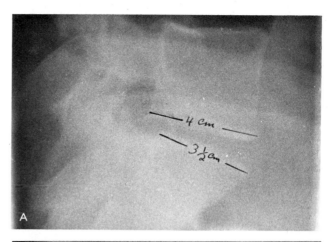

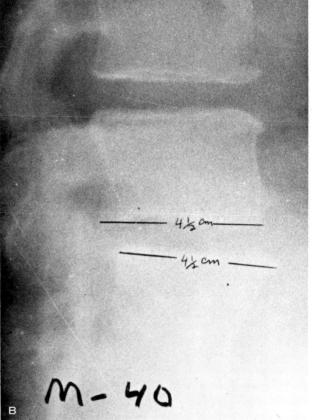

FIG. 20-17. *A,* False retrospondylolisthesis in 45-year-old Caucasian woman. The body of L5 has greater anterior-posterior diameter than does S1 (see Figure 20-17). *B,* True retrospondylolisthesis in 40-year-old Caucasion man. Posterior slip of L5 on S1.

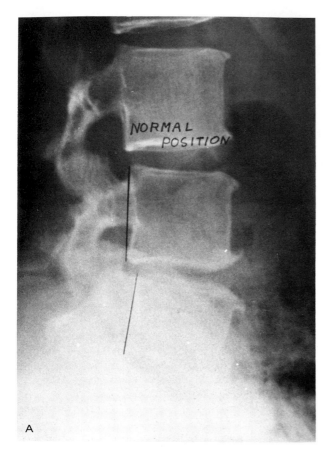
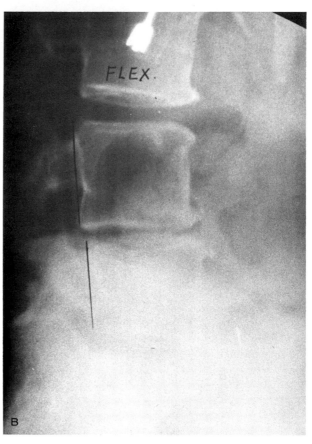

FIG. 20-18. *A,* True retrospondylolisthesis; *B,* note how posterior slip is present in normal position but disappears in flexion.

genographic sign of disc degeneration. It is likely that all cases of true retro- or reverse spondylolisthesis showed this sign initially.

Spondylolisthesis in Other Areas of the Spine

In the cervical vertebrae we often see cases of degenerative spondylolisthesis and we occasionally see the peduncular type due to fracture or non-union of the pedicles.[4] True isthmic spondylolysis or spondylolisthesis in the upper five cervical segments is extremely rare. In the cervical spine the part between the articular facets is extremely short except in C6 and C7, where there is a reasonably well-developed pars interarticularis. I have one case in which I think I can definitely state that there was a fracture of the pars at C6. Azouz et al. reported two cases of spondylolysis at C6.[4] When fractures do occur in this short pars, they probably heal rapidly, and this is why we do not often see them.

Spondylolisthesis in Children

We have found that spondylolisthesis in children behaves somewhat differently from that in adults. At least two different types exist in children: (1) a defect in the pars with a mild to moderate degree of slip and backache predominating, often without leg pain; (2) a high grade of slip and a typical spondylolisthesis build —that is, "short torso and heart-shaped buttocks." This particular shape to the buttocks arises from the fact that the sacrum is vertical rather than at the normal 42 or 43 degrees from horizontal. These children walk with a peculiar "spastic" gait, owing to irritation of the nerves of the cauda equina as they pass over the top of the sacrum. Also, the L5 nerve root may be compressed between the proximal stump of the pars of L5 and the body of S1.

This second type is not common in the general population, but orthopaedists see it relatively often because it is so striking that the pediatrician or family physician immediately refers these children to a specialist. These also are the children who are most often symptomatic.

I have observed cases in which the L5 nerve roots were compressed to thin ribbons between the distal ends of the proximal stumps of the pars and the body of the sacrum. Compression can happen to the other components of the cauda equina—that is, the S1, S2, and S3 nerve roots which also innervate the hamstrings—but these nerves are compressed as they pass over the top of the sacrum. A nerve can function quite normally and still be reduced by compression to 25% of its normal size but, beyond this, some reflex and sensory change is likely to occur.[10] The hamstrings function well and usually show no electromyographic changes, yet are in enough spasm to contribute to the peculiar gait.

Another reason for this peculiar gait is that the pelvis is held in such an extremely flexed position that the hips have reached the limit of their normal extension and still are not in a straight line with the trunk (see Fig. 20-1 B). Notice in the figure that the sacrum is in a vertical position. A line drawn across the top of S1 would be nearly horizontal, instead of 42 or 43 degrees from the horizontal, as is normal for an adult. That means that the pelvis is flexed 42 or 43 degrees. Most people are unable to extend their hips to that extent.

These children often develop a functional scoliosis secondary to compression of the cauda equina as it passes over the top of the sacrum.[35] The so-called "sciatic scoliosis" seen so often in these children may be secondary to the muscle spasm produced by irritation of the nerve elements due to pressure and/or traction. It may also be due to the fact that the L5 vertebra slips forward asymmetrically, causing curvature in the lower lumbar spine. This soon becomes structural scoliosis.

In our series there were just about twice as many girls with this high grade of slip as there were boys, an interesting statistic inasmuch as the overall incidence of the defect is just about twice as high in boys as in girls. In most instances, the parents have not been aware of the child's unusual appearance, and it has been called to their attention by the school nurse or the gymnasium teacher.

We seldom detect the slipping of these vertebrae while it is in progress, a fact that suggests that the slip occurs fairly rapidly once it starts. Therefore, close observation is indicated for children with spondylolisthesis, especially if some slip is already present.

Pain in Spondylolisthesis

It is easy to understand the reason for pain in a child with a high-grade slip, especially with an intact but elongated pars. It is a little more difficult to comprehend the cause of pain in the presence of the ordinary defect in which slip is only 25% or less. In these children the pain is generally coming from the degenerating disc, or at the defect in the pars which may be a fairly acute fracture. It is believed that some, but by no means all, discs are painful during the process of degeneration. Obviously it is not so in every case because we see too many people with spondylolisthesis who have never had any pain and whose L5 disc has degenerated. And, of course, we see many patients without spondylolisthesis who have narrowed discs (which indicates a degenerated disc), but deny ever having had any back pain.

In the adult, the cause of pain has also been studied extensively.[26] It is not known why so many patients develop a lesion in the pars at about age six and then have no problems with it until age 35 or so, when a sudden unusual twisting motion or lifting episode can cause back and/or leg pain. In our series almost 50% of the patients could not associate injury with the onset of symptoms. In an industrial practice, however, probably all patients will report an associated injury. When pre-injury roentgenograms are available, there is rarely any difference between pre- and post-injury findings. A degenerating disc at the level of the defect is more likely to be the cause of pain in the adult than in the child.

There is often a build-up of fibrocartilaginous mass at the defect,[12] which is irritating to the L5 nerve root as it exits at this point. Bony impingement does occur, but not too commonly because, as the vertebra slides forward, the foramen gets larger. In the occasional case, as we have mentioned, true bony impingement is noted between the distal end of the proximal stump of the pars and the body of S1 when the slip approaches 50%.

Macnab has described a corporotransverse ligament which he believes impinges the nerve root of L5 and produces pain.[26] Kinking of the nerve root by the pedicles as the vertebra slides forward also has been incriminated.

As for a bulging or extruded disc at the level of the defect where slipping has already occurred, this is relatively uncommon, probably because the posterior longitudinal ligament gets more taut as slip progresses. In 50 operations during which we took special note,[54] we found a genuinely extruded disc at the level of the defect in only two cases. This is not to say, of course, that this disc space is not causing pain because of degeneration or perhaps pull on the anulus fibrosis.

A ruptured disc at the space above the level of defect can and does occur and may well be the cause of trouble, although involvement of the fourth disc is less likely to be troublesome in spondylolisthesis than in the ordinary case of degenerative disc disease, since spondylolisthesis occurs in a different type of person than does disc disease. Even in the face of a degenerating disc at L4, I am more inclined to perform a one-level fusion in spondylolisthesis than in disc disease. The fact that the fifth disc is unstable may help to preserve the fourth disc, in that a greater-than-normal percentage of the motion occurs at the defective L5 level, thus protecting L4.

When a disc herniation or extrusion occurs at the segment above the slipping vertebra, one has to accept the fact that the patient's symptoms may be stemming solely from the prolapsed disc and the spondylolisthesis is only incidental. If we could be sure of this, discectomy at the offending L4 space would be all that is necessary.

A higher-than-average number of patients, especially men with defective pars, also have Scheuermann's disease in the thoracolumbar area. Although this disease does not usually produce pain at the thoracolumbar level, it is theoretically possible that there might be increased pain in the low back due to increased lordosis at the lumbosacral level, secondary to the kyphosis at the thoracolumbar area due to the Scheuermann's disease.

Patients with spondylolisthesis alone do not have hyperlordosis at the lumbosacral level. In a series of 1009 normal spines which we studied and compared with 125 spines with pars defects, we found that there was no increased lordosis among the cases with spondylolisthesis,[50] but as mentioned above, in patients with high grade slip, the sacrum often becomes nearly vertical. The forward curve of the lumbar spine in spondylolisthesis has been called lordosis, but it is not true lordosis.

Most of the pain experienced by patients past the age of twenty years, especially those with less than 33% slip, is caused by the following: (1) degeneration of the disc at the level of defect; (2) impingement of the nerve roots by the build-up of the fibrocartilaginous mass at the point of defect; or (3) drag on the ligaments, both the anulus and other ligaments around the posterior elements, due to the fact that the bony support is gone.

In cases with more than 50% slip, the cause may be bony impingement between the distal end of the proximal stump of the pars of L5 and the body of S1. In the case of the child with high-grade slip, pain may result from the aforementioned as well as from: (1) stretching of the nerves of the cauda equina over the posterior superior border of S1, (2) in the case with intact but elongated pars, actual impingement of the cauda equina between the posterior-superior border of S1 and the lamina of L5. On myelography in the latter, we often see just a trickle of Pantopaque passing over the posterior-superior border of S1.

To my knowledge, true spondylolisthesis does not occur in the thoracic spine, except with fracture dislocation from severe trauma. Pars defects do rarely occur in the thoracic spine, however, and Friberg has reported the case of a child who had multiple defects, among which were defects in the pars of five vertebrae, at least one of which was in the thoracic area.[11]

TREATMENT

Type I. Isthmic Type

SUBTYPE A. LYTIC TYPE.[30] CONSERVATIVE TREATMENT IN THE ADULT. The "conservative" treatment of the adult with lytic spondylolisthesis is much like that for backache from other causes, particularly from chronic strain or disc disease. The same exercises are prescribed, although I have found them to be less effective in spondylolisthesis than in disc disease. The same is true of traction. The same type of corset is used and with about the same chance of success.

Surgical treatment in the adult. The principal reason for surgical treatment is relief of pain, not, as is the occasional misconception, to prevent the progression of slip. Slip rarely increases in the adult when there has been no surgical intervention (Fig. 20-19). When it does progress, the increase is small and is not in itself an indication for operation. Usually, but not always, it is due to narrowing of the disc space. Occasionally a high grade of slip which has been present since childhood causes neurologic difficulties in an adult and must be treated surgically.

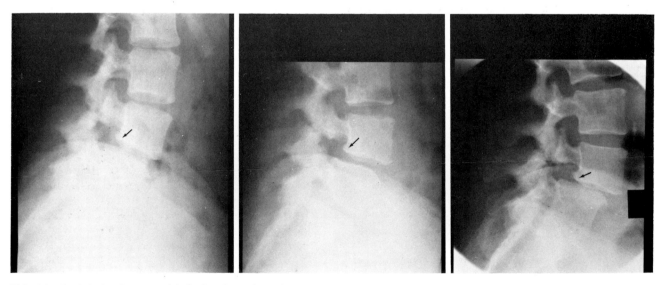

FIG. 20-19. *A,* Isthmic spondylolisthesis at L4, showing a few degrees of slip, in 38-year-old Caucasian. *B,* Same patient at age 44. There have been a few degrees of further slip. *C,* At age 50 there is at least 25% of slip between L4 and L5 with a definite pars defect.

In patients under 25, a one-level fusion is all that is needed in virtually all cases. Whether to extend the fusion to L4 depends on the status of the L4 disc. Although rupture of L4 does occur in younger people, fusion of the L4 disc space is not usually necessary, and we have even performed several one-level fusions on 45-year-old patients. It behooves us to find out, if possible, the status of the L4 disc. The EMG gives valuable information and often confirms the impression gained by the physical examination. The fifth nerve root may be involved, owing either to a bulging disc at the L4 space or to entrapment of the L5 nerve root in the fibrocartilaginous mass at the L5 pars defect. If myelography shows a definitely bulging disc at the L4 space, the L4 disc should be removed and the fusion extended to include L4. If myelographic findings are normal at L4, further study by discography is indicated. If only moderate degeneration is noted on discogram, the fusion can be limited to the L5, S1 space. Serious degeneration and posterior bulging noted on discography, especially if associated with a positive saline acceptance test, requires surgical removal of the disc and inclusion of L4 in the fusion. Often L3 is also severely degenerated, and perhaps L2. Where then does one stop? Under these circumstances, we would perform only a one-level fusion to include only the L5, S1 level. We are well aware of the failings of the discogram as a diagnostic tool. It does give some valuable information in the specific situation mentioned above.

The incidence of successful fusion in our hands is about 94% in the adult if limited to one level. This incidence drops to 84% for two levels. Thus there is a distinct advantage in performing a one-level fusion, even at the risk of having to treat the L4 disc later.

Recently, when we have felt that the L4 disc was the problem, we have done a one-level L5 to S1 fusion and a chemonucleolysis at L4 at the time of operation. These seem to be working out well, but more experience is necessary for us to draw any firm conclusions. When we do this, we use the paraspinal approach (see Chap. 16) and decompress the L5 nerve root on the painful side. Chemonucleolysis does not interfere with the supporting structures as much as do laminotomy and discectomy.

Surgical treatment in the child. In the child, if conservative therapy consisting of time, routine back care, gentle abdominal strengthening exercises, and perhaps a corset does not bring about cessation of pain, spinal fusion is indicated.

Persistent symptoms in a child require operation in a much higher percentage of cases than in the adult, and I also believe that the child should undergo a fusion procedure if slipping is occurring.

Following are the basic differences between the child with spondylolisthesis and the adult, and hence the reasons operation is more imperative in the child: (1) further slipping may occur in the child but almost never in the adult; (2) fusion is effected more readily in the child than in the adult; (3) the child has a great many years ahead of him; (4) if symptoms persist for more than six months in a child, they are likely to persist indefinitely; (5) the child should not be expected to cut down his activities and this is unnecessary with a solid one-level fusion; and (6) the adult can and often is quite willing to cut down on his activities and live within his pain tolerance to avoid a fusion operation.

In the child who has principally back pain, a one-level fusion through the paraspinal approach (see Chap. 16) without decompression is indicated. If he has had much one-sided leg pain with neurologic change, unilateral decompression is recommended, leaving as much of the lamina as possible and always fusing the loose element to the sacrum, but leaving the spinous processes in place and the interspinous and supraspinous ligaments intact. It has not been necessary to keep the child flat postoperatively.

Even in the child with high-grade slip who has tight hamstrings, we would still use the paraspinal approach and leave the loose element in place.

In the same child with bladder or bowel symptoms, we would decompress by removing the loose element, removing the posterior superior corner of the sacrum, and doing a transverse process fusion. In the adult with a high-grade slip, it can be difficult to get a transverse process fusion to "take" if the loose element has been removed and only the transverse processes remain as an area for fusion to the sacral ala. However, this has not been a problem in children.

In the child, the L4 disc is not ordinarily a matter for concern. Thus a one-level fusion is performed. In the presence of very high-grade slip, however, it is often difficult to avoid extension of the fusion to L4 or even to L3. Such an extension does not appreciably lower the incidence of success, since fusion takes place so readily in children.

In the child with nonstructural sciatic scoliosis, a one-level fusion suffices unless there is definite lateral slip of L4 on L5, in which case the fusion should be extended to include L4. If there is definite scoliosis, the scoliosis should be reduced with a Milwaukee brace and a fusion to L4 performed.

If a severe block is suspected, a myelogram is mandatory. Often only a trickle of Pantopaque runs through at the level of defect. Unless there is substantial neurologic change, however, we still simply fuse in situ. We contend that the nerves accommodate themselves to the cramped quarters, and the tightness of the hamstrings disappears over a period of several months.

Reduction of spondylolisthesis. Harrington is convinced that the child with high-grade slip should have the slip reduced.[15]

Reduction of the slip in spondylolisthesis has been attempted by several surgeons over the past 75 years. Reports of these attempts have been sporadic and pessimistic. Reduction by traction methods was usually only partially successful and the slip virtually always returned. Achievement of solid fusion under these circumstances was difficult. It is probably the failure of fusion that permits the slip to return. Fusion across the defect by the posterolateral method without reduction has been so successful in obtaining solid fusion and in relieving pain and hamstring spasm that we do not consider reduction sufficiently beneficial to compensate for the rather enormous difficulties associated with it. However, reduction is in order if it can significantly improve the cosmetically undesirable "spondylolisthesis build"—the short waist with the flat heart-shaped buttocks.

Our own studies indicate that with a slip of 25% this particular build is barely noticeable in most people, but at 50% it is unmistakable.[52] Beyond this, there may be a real cosmetic problem.

With the adaptation of Harrington rods or some modification of this problem, reduction becomes a real possibility.[16] The question then becomes: is it safe and is it worth the effort? If tight hamstrings are the major concern, we can be assured that they will disappear over a period of months after simple "in situ" fusion without decompression or reduction. The child then has a better appearance because he is standing straight and walking normally. However, his torso remains short compared with his other body measurements.

Harrington is of the opinion that the appearance is greatly improved, over and above what can be obtained without reduction. He is in the process of carefully photographing and measuring the children upon whom he has performed a reduction to be sure that such is the case. Recently he reviewed ten cases in which he had reduced a high-grade slip. He had taken standing anterior-posterior roentgenograms from T1 to S1 in all patients. In these he found that the average preoperative measurement was 39.3 cm. Postoperatively the average measurement was 44.1 cm. This is an average gain in height of 4.8 cm., with a range of 2.2 to 7.2. This gain, he believed, was not due to normal growth but secondary to the reduction of the spondylolisthesis.[15]

This is not a procedure to be undertaken by the casual operator, but rather by those skilled in the use of Harrington rods who have studied the whole problem extensively.

To accomplish surgical reduction and fusion, a wide exposure is necessary, with the skin incision beginning over the spinous process of L2 and extending downward onto the sacrum. A subperiosteal dissection is then carried out upon the spinous processes, laminae, facets, and transverse processes. Exposure of the upper sacral segments out to and including the ala is necessary. Caution should be exercised to avoid injuring the unprotected cauda equina at the L5 level in the upper sacral segments because a wide-open sacrum and spina bifida are often present.

Using an osteotome, a window is made in the ala of the sacrum to the sacroiliac joint. A sacral bar is directed through the flair of the ilium and into the ala

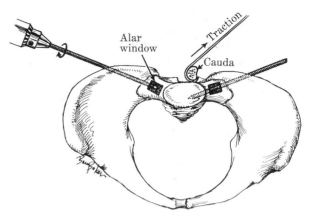

FIG. 20-20. Demonstration of placement of sacral bar into the body of S1. (From Harrington P and Tullos HS: Spondylolisthesis in children. Clin Orth & Rel Research 79:80, 1971.)

of the sacrum. The tip of the sacral bar is introduced into the ala (Fig. 20-20) via the previously prepared window. The dural sac is mobilized in the upper sacral segments. This is not difficult because of the spina bifida which is present in most cases. The sac is retracted medially. With the dural sac under direct vision, the sacral bar is passed under the sac and into the body of S1. A second bar is passed in similar fashion through the opposite side.

A localized distraction is now accomplished, utilizing modified spine instruments. Two blunt hooks, No. 1253, are inserted into the laminae of L1. Two Moe hooks are reversed and inserted through the alar windows into the sacral bars. A ⅛-inch threaded rod with the two hex nuts in place is inserted on each side from the sacral bar below to the hooks in L1. Appropriate distraction force is applied (Fig. 20-21). With this distraction, reduction of the lumbosacral dislocation spontaneously occurs (Fig. 20-22 A, B). Resection of the hypoplastic neural arch of L5 may now be done. This can be done prior to instrumentation if the instruments interfere with visualization.

A posterior interbody fusion is incorporated (Fig. 20-23). A lateral gutter fusion is also performed from L3 to the sacrum. The incision is then closed.

Postoperatively the patient is kept recumbent and "log-rolled" for variation of position. At ten days the sutures are removed and a well-molded body jacket is applied from the trochanters to the xyphoid. Bed rest with position change is required for a few days, followed by a gradual increase in activity. At six months the body jacket is removed and the fusion mass is evaluated.

Significant complications have occurred, the most serious of which was a cauda equina syndrome. In this patient a single sacral bar had been passed posterior to the dural sac with resultant cauda equina pressure. Neurologic deficit occurred in the immediate postoperative period, but subsequently lessened, leaving an S1 nerve root deficit in one leg.

Hall has reported that he has seen two cases reduced by Harrington rods in which the flexion of the pelvis actually increased, causing increased flexion at the hip joints and thus more difficulty in walking.

Ascani has used a technique employing hyperextension of the lumbar spine, putting a localizer over the sacrum and casting from the knees to the sternum.[3] In cases of partial paralysis he has been able to reduce or partially reduce the slip, and in some cases existing bladder and bowel disturbances have disappeared. Through a window in the cast, a posterior fusion is done. Immobilization is continued until fusion is judged to be secure. The patient is then allowed up in a body cast.

It is hoped that the need for reducing spondylolisthesis will be eliminated as people become more aware of the condition and bring it to the attention of the orthopaedic surgeon sooner. This may be a forlorn hope, because for some reason we seldom catch the condition during the slipping phase. It is only after a school nurse or a gymnasium teacher notices that the child's general bodily contour seems to be abnormal that the child is brought to the doctor.

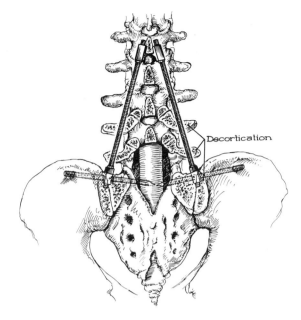

FIG. 20-21. Distraction bars in place. Note inferior hooks seated through alar window onto sacral bar. (From Harrington P and Tullos HS: Spondylolisthesis in children. Clin Orth & Rel Research 79:80, 1971.)

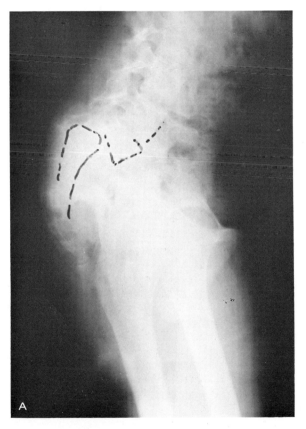 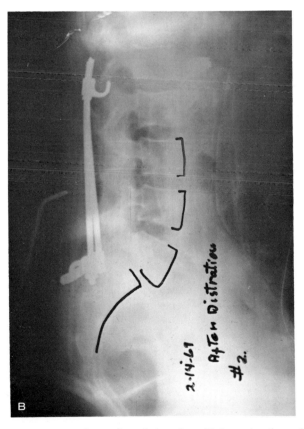

FIG. 20-22. A, White female, age 14, before operation. B, Roentgenogram taken after distraction. Note reduction of L5 on S1.

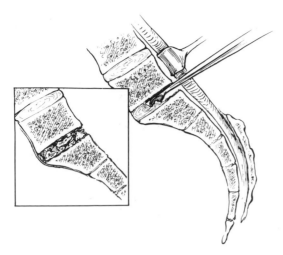

FIG. 20-23. Posterior interbody fusion. (From Harrington P and Tullos HS: Spondylolisthesis in children. Clin Orth & Rel Research 79:80, 1971.)

There is no need to reduce slipping of 25% and probably no need in slipping up to 50% since, with a slip of this magnitude, the body contour is still quite good.[52] The potential candidate for reduction is the one in which abnormal body build results from slippage of L5 clear around anteriorly. One must then weigh the possibility of restoring body appearance to more normal proportions against the magnitude of the operation to decide whether it should be attempted.

Removal of the loose element only. In 1950 Gill described the operation in which the loose element,[12] along with any fibrocartilaginous mass or other material that might be impinging upon the nerve roots, is removed.[1,55] (For a detailed description of the Gill operation, see Chap. 21.) More recently Davis and Baily reviewed their experience with the Gill operation done on 39 patients between 1952 and 1967.[9] Results in 83% were rated as satisfactory from a clinical standpoint. Among their patients those with moderate to severe arthritic changes in the lumbosacral area had the poorest results. Younger adults who had little or no arthritic changes had the best results. This seems like an inconsistency but it is not; the patient who has a lot of arthritic change around the level of defect will get relief from sciatica from simple removal of the loose element, but the degenerated disc and the severe arthritic changes may still give pain.

Unilateral pars separation. The most accurate statistics on the incidence of unilateral pars separations come from the studies of skeletized material.[37] Roche and Rowe found that 18.3% of the pars defects in Caucasian males were unilateral, and 7.2% of the pars defects in Caucasian females were unilateral. The unilateral defect was on the right side twice as often as on the left.

Every vertebra with a unilateral defect showed at least some twisting and deformity of the pars on the opposite side.

As regards treatment of the patient with a unilateral pars defect, I have considered that this level of defect is more susceptible to disc degeneration than are other levels, but the exact degree is not known. Because there is some torsional motion possible, the defect may develop some build-up of fibrocartilaginous mass and, if the disc must be removed, the pathway of the nerve as it exits through the fibrocartilaginous mass should be completely cleared. A spinal fusion is not indicated in the treatment of a unilateral defect in and of itself, except as it might be used following laminotomy for the treatment of disc disease.

Chemonucleolysis in the treatment of spondylolisthesis. We have been able to study 10 patients who have had chymopapain injected into the disc space at the level of the pars defect only. Obviously, if two spaces are injected, no conclusions can be drawn. In these 10 cases, satisfactory relief of pain was obtained in five. At least three in my personal experience were dramatically relieved. None of these had more than 25% slip and all were adults, suggesting that in the adult the pain of spondylolisthesis is probably discogenic. It also suggests possibilities for treatment of patients with spondylolisthesis: (1) in adults, chymopapain injection first and then fusion if necessary: (2) do a one-level fusion and treat the disc above with injection. Injection is not as traumatic as laminotomy and perhaps the rule of always extending the fusion to include the level of laminotomy does not apply to the level where chemonucleolysis is used. Further experience is needed.

Anterior interbody fusion. We have not used anterior interbody fusion as a primary operation for spondylolisthesis but rather as a salvage procedure in patients in whom instability persisted after failure of posterior fusion. In these cases we usually use a Freebody operation at L5 and blocks of ilium at L4 (Chap. 16).

We have found the Freebody technique for interbody fusion to be the most successful of any method in the presence of a high grade of slip. Even so the incidence of failure of fusion is high.

SUBTYPE B. ELONGATION OF THE PARS WITHOUT SEPARATION (FIG. 20-2). Among the patients so affected, a higher degree of slip is noted and most have spina bifida, many with a wide open sacrum. Fusion is the operation of choice and should be done early if slip is progressing. Careful observation is necessary. A single spot lateral roentgenogram, with the child standing, should be taken every four months for a year, then semi-annually until he reaches the age of 15 to be sure slip does not progress. Efforts are made to shield the gonads; this is no problem in boys, but may present some difficulty in girls. Since only a spot lateral need be taken, the total exposure to radiation is actually rather small.

The period of most rapid slip is between ages 9 and 14 in girls and 10 and 15 in boys. Parents should be alerted to signs of increasing slip, which is a clear indication for fusion. The penalty, from the standpoint of function and appearance, for allowing slip to increase is so severe that we prefer to perform a few unnecessary fusions rather than to overlook one (see p. 154 for paraspinal approach). This rule applies whether the child has intact elongated pars or typical pars defects.

In children posterior decompression is not necessary unless significant neurologic changes have taken place. Stopping the slip and stopping all motion relieves the pain, and the tight hamstrings disappear in a few months. Postoperatively no corset or brace is necessary when the paraspinal approach is used. The patient is allowed out of bed immediately. In our experience, early ambulation did not cause any increase in slip, probably because few of the ligaments are sacrificed in the paraspinal approach.

Subtype B is the type most likely to require laminectomy because it carries the greatest danger of impingement of the cauda equina between the lamina of L5 and the posterior superior border of S1. In the occasional case where it is necessary to remove the entire loose element, we use a midline approach rather than the paraspinal, and require bed rest postoperatively until the fusion mass becomes solid.[8]

SUBTYPE C. SPONDYLOLISTHESIS ACQUISITA. Because lateral fusions are now being done instead of posterior fusions, spondylolisthesis acquisita is rare. Its treatment in children consists of immobilization in a knee-to-nipple cast.[45] In the adult, however, this probably would not suffice and, if the symptoms are severe enough, fusion should be extended up one segment. There is no need for treatment in the adult unless symptoms warrant it, since the disease is basically spondylolysis.

SUBTYPE D. PATHOLOGIC SPONDYLOLISTHESIS. When a fracture occurs in a child with generalized bone disease, such as osteogenesis imperfecta or Albers-Schoenberg disease, we believe that treatment is the same as for the normal child who develops the same lesion.

If the surgeon has reason to believe that the fracture is recent, immobilization is in order. If not, symptomatic treatment is the rule. We have never fused one of these spines nor does it seem likely that we will.

SUBTYPE E. ACUTE PARS FRACTURE. For an acute crack in the pars, immobilization promotes healing in most cases (Fig. 20-3). Effective immobilization is best assured by application of a cast from knees-to-nipple (Fig. 20-24). We have occasionally compromised by putting the patient in an ordinary body cast and permitting ambulation, but in these cases healing has only occasionally taken place. It is questionable whether a body cast decreases the motion which takes place at the lumbosacral joint.[48] Braces and body casts do prevent the extremes of bending, but they do not decrease lumbosacral motion with walking. Perhaps the best (if not a knees-to-nipple cast) would be an ordinary corset which reminds the patient to be reasonably careful yet actually makes no attempt to immobilize the lumbosacral area. Two of our patients, a young football player

and a female gymnast, developed pars defects which healed without treatment and while they continued vigorous athletic activities.

The acute fracture has medicolegal significance since, if it can be proved that the lesion was caused by a given injury or accident, it may be compensable. To prove this, however, either roentgenograms taken shortly before the accident must be available or the fracture must heal.

Since the vast majority of patients have had their pars lesions since childhood, one has to assume that a given lesion is old unless proved otherwise.

IATROGENIC SPONDYLOLISTHESIS. The so-called "iatrogenic" spondylolisthesis results from massive decompression posteriorly (Fig. 20-9), when all the support from the posterior elements is removed. If a fusion is to be done on these patients at the time of decompression, it should be a one-level intersegmental transverse process fusion at the level of decompression. If a two-level fusion must be done from L4 to the sacrum, an interbody fusion done through the posterior route by the technique of Cloward may be added at the level of complete posterior instability.[7] Owing to the rather marked instability, neither a two-level intertransverse fusion nor a one-space interbody fusion alone will succeed in solid arthrodesis.[51]

When one considers that, if the posterior elements are removed, about all there is left posterolaterally to fuse is one spindly transverse process to another with a space between them as wide as 4.5 cm., one can see why pseudarthrosis usually occurs. There are some remnants of lateral mass but surprisingly little. Obviously such is not the case when a fusion is being done for isthmic spondylolisthesis at L5 where a rather large well-developed transverse process of L5 is present. These fuse readily. Intertransverse fusion of L4 to L5 across just the one space, not including the sacrum, succeeds in a satisfactorily high percentage of cases if most of the lateral masses remain.

Type II. Dysplastic Spondylolisthesis

In the case of dysplastic spondylolisthesis of L5 on S1, the treatment is the same as for spondylolisthesis of L5 on S1 with an elongated but intact pars. These patients are usually young, often only five to eight years old. A one-level fusion from L5 to S1 can be done on these patients with no fear of complication because of their youth. This type was called congenital by Newman.[30]

Type III. Degenerative Spondylolisthesis

The treatment of degenerative spondylolisthesis is basically the management of degenerative disc disease. The former, however, is often complicated by spinal stenosis that is occasioned by the forward slip, the

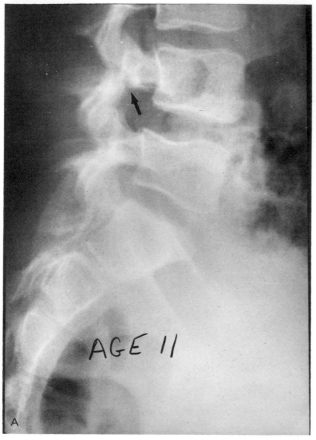

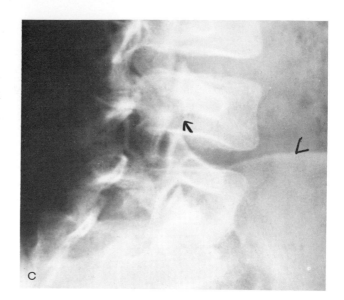

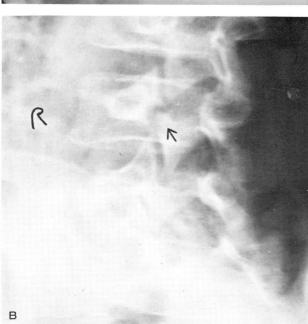

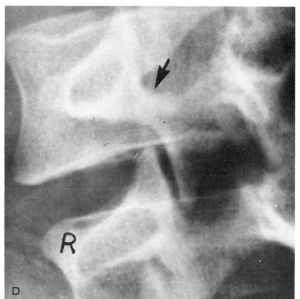

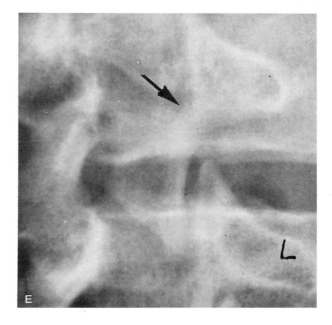

FIG. 20-24. *A*, Lateral view of 11-year-old Caucasian boy who had been playing football. This is believed to represent a fatigue fracture of pars of L4. *B and C,* Right and left lateral oblique views of pars of L4 show definite defects. *D and E,* After immobilization in cast from nipples to knees for four months, pars have healed on both sides.

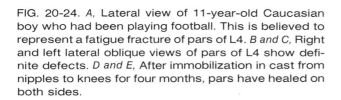

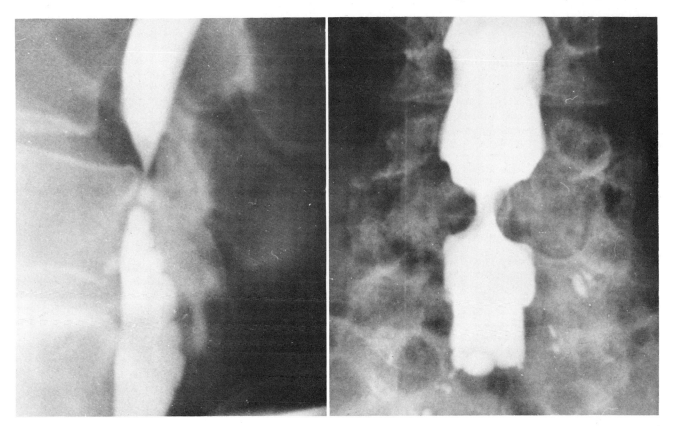

FIG. 20-25. Typical hourglass constriction at level of slip (L4 or L5) in degenerative spondylolisthesis. (Courtesy Norman Rosenberg, Cleveland, Ohio.)

centrally placed facets, and the exuberant bone formation around the facets. There may also be capsular thickening and actual excess fluid in the capsule of the facets, further compromising the lumbar canal (Fig. 20-25).

The initial complaint is back pain or back and leg pain. Often organic findings are surprisingly minimal except for the rather dramatic roentgenographic changes. The patient may even be able to bend forward and touch the floor with knees extended and walk on heels and tiptoes. Many experience pain on walking for any distance or even just on standing, but characteristically find relief by lying down. The symptoms are the classic symptoms of spinal stenosis.

The majority of these patients, as with other degenerative joint diseases, can be treated conservatively by analgesics, physical therapy, training in abdominal exercises, training in back care, corsets, antiarthritic drugs, and reassurance. Spinal stenosis, which is the condition that usually brings the patient to the doctor, is also the condition that makes surgical treatment necessary. Decompression is the procedure of choice.

As the years go by, I find myself performing decompression on more and more of these elderly people. They tolerate the procedure well and are greatly relieved postoperatively. It is my opinion that any person, even

in the late 70s or older, who is genuinely disabled because of spinal stenosis, should have the benefit of surgical treatment.

OPERATIVE TECHNIQUES AND FINDINGS IN DEGENERATIVE SPONDYLOLISTHESIS. A midline incision is made and the laminae denuded of soft tissue. The zygapophyseal joints are large and centrally placed in most cases. Contrary to what one might expect, there is often considerable stability at the level of slip. On removal of the laminae, an absence of epidural fat is noted and the dura may be pale and pulseless, the result of the spinal stenosis that made the operation necessary.

The lateral recesses must be well decompressed so that there is no question that the nerves are completely unroofed. The medial portion of the facet may have to be removed and even foraminectomy may be necessary to ascertain that an adequate decompression has been accomplished. It is best to remove part of the lamina of the vertebra above and below the level of slip. The point of compression where there is a slip of L4 on L5 is on the L5 nerve root as it passes over the body of L5 and out through the nerve root canal. The L5 nerve root should be traced well outward, taking off the corner of the superior articular process of L5 but usually not cutting through the pars of L5. If the pars of L5 must

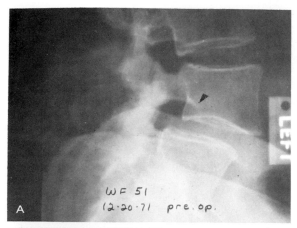

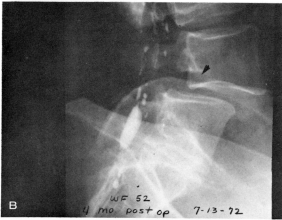

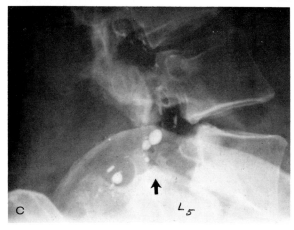

FIG. 20-26. *A,* A 51-year-old female with degenerative spondylolisthesis who had a complete subarachnoid block on myelogram. Decompression was done and posterior stability lost. *B,* Note increased slip 16 months after operation. *C,* Two and one-half years after operation, there is over 50% slip of L4 on L5.

be cut through, then one has two levels of instability, both L4 and L5 and, if a fusion is to be done, it must be from L4 to the sacrum.

When it is necessary to remove all of the stability

supplied by the posterior elements (as with foraminotomy), one is naturally concerned about further slip.

Further slip does usually occur, occasionally to a severe degree (Fig. 20-26 A, B & C). If there was instability on flexion-extension roentgenograms noted preoperatively, one can be virtually certain further slip will take place. Strangely enough, increased olisthesis seems not to make these patients symptomatically worse. Still we now believe that a one-level intertransverse fusion should be done across the level of instability in patients under 65.

We have performed spinal fusion in conjunction with decompression in only a few cases, and so have no statistics regarding the success rate. These have been in younger people (under 65 years of age). We believe it is difficult to obtain a solid fusion when so much bone has been removed, and only the transverse processes and part of the lateral masses remain.

In some cases we have performed an interbody fusion at the L4 interspace through the posterior approach, according to the technique of Cloward,[7] in addition to a transverse process and lateral mass fusion from L4 to sacrum. The outcome has been successful but the procedure is rather formidable.

It is my present belief that, if the patient is below age 65 and arthrodesis is felt to be necessary, only a one-level fusion (L4 to L5 usually) should be done. If the transverse processes are spindly and a lot of the lateral mass has been removed, adding a Cloward interbody fusion by the posterior route, in addition to the intertransverse, will assure solid fusion but unfortunately adds considerably to the operation time.

Type IV. Peduncular Spondylolisthesis

Peduncular spondylolisthesis is so rare that it is little more than a curiosity. Its treatment is usually quite clear albeit rather complex. In the case of fracture of the pedicle, immobilization usually effects healing. If there is an established non-union that is painful, posterior lateral fusion from the vertebra above to the one below is the procedure of choice.

Spondylolisthesis from osteogenesis imperfecta or from Kuskokwim disease (Fig. 20-15), in which the pedicles are actually elongated, usually requires no treatment. In achondroplasia, however, decompression may be necessary.

References

1. Amuso SI, Neff RS, Coulson DB, and Laing PG: The surgical treatment of spondylolisthesis by posterior element resection. J Bone Joint Surg *52-A:*529-536, 1970.
2. Anderson CE: Spondyloschisis following spinal fusion. J Bone Joint Surg *38-A:*1142-1146, 1956.
3. Ascani E: Personal communication.
4. Azouz EM, Chan MD, and Wee R: Spondylolysis in the cervical vertebrae. Radiology *111:*315-318, 1974.
5. Baker DR: Personal communication.

6. Batts M Jr: The etiology of spondylolisthesis. J Bone Joint Surg 21:879-884, 1939.

7. Cloward RB: The treatment of ruptured lumbar intervertebral discs by vertebral body fusion: indications, techniques, after care. J Neurosurg 10:154, 1953.

8. Dandy DJ, and Shannon MJ: Lumbosacral subluxation. J Bone Joint Surg (British Issue) 53-B:578, 1971.

9. Davis IS, and Baily RW: Spondylolisthesis: long term follow-up study of treatment with total laminectomy. Paper presented at the annual meeting of Amer. Acad. Orthop. Surg. San Francisco, Cal. March, 1971.

10. Duncan D: Alterations in the structure of the nerves caused by restricting their growth with ligature. J Neuropath Exper Neurol 7:261-273, 1948.

11. Friberg S: Studies on spondylolisthesis. Acta Chir Scand (Suppl 55) 82:1-140, 1939.

12. Gill GG, Manning JG, and White HL: Surgical treatment of spondylolisthesis without spinal fusion. J Bone Joint Surg 33-A:493-520, 1955.

13. Hall J: Personal communication.

14. Harris RI, and Wiley JJ: Acquired spondylolisthesis as a sequel to spine fusion. J Bone Joint Surg 45-A:1159-1170, 1963.

15. Harrington P: Personal communication, 1973.

16. Harrington P and Tullos HS: Spondylolisthesis in children. CLin Orth & Rel Research 79:75-84, 1971.

17. Hasbe K: Die Wirkelsaule der Japaner. Z Morph Anthrop Stuttgart 15:259-380, 1913.

18. Herbinaux G: Traite sur Divers Accouchemens Laborieux at sur les Polypes de la Matrice. Bruxelles, De Boubers, 1782.

19. Johnson JTH, and Southwick WC: Growth following transepiphyseal bone grafts: an experimental study to explain continued growth following certain fusion operations. J Bone Joint Surg 42-A:1396-1412, 1960.

20. Junghanns H: Spondylolisthesis: 30 pathologisch-anatomisch untersuchte Fälle. Bruns Beitr klin Chir 158:554-573, 1929.

21. Kettelkamp DB, and Wright DG: Spondylolysis in the Alaskan Eskimo. J Bone Joint Surg 53-A:563-566, 1971.

22. Kilian HF: Schilderungen neuer Beckenformen und ihres Verhalten im leben Bassermann und Mathy, Mannheim, 1854 (cit. da Brocher).

23. Klieger B: Personal communication.

24. Knuttson F: The instability associated with disc degeneration in the lumbar spine. Acta Radiol 25:593-609, 1945.

25. Lambl DZ: Zehn Thesen über Spondylolisthesis. Zbl gynak Urol 9:250, 1855.

26. Macnab I: The management of spondylolisthesis. Progr Neurol Surg 4:246-276, Basel, Karger, 1971.

27. Macnab I: Spondylolisthesis with an intact neural arch: the so-called pseudospondylolisthesis. J Bone Joint Surg 32:325, 1965.

28. Morisaki N: The etiology of spondylosis and spondylolisthesis (unpublished). Presented as SICOT Congress, Tel Aviv, October, 1972.

29. Naugebauer F: Die Entschung der Spondylolisthesis, Centralab f Gynäk 5:260-261, 1881.

30. Newman PH: The etiology of spondylolisthesis. J Bone Joint Surg 45-B:36-59, 1963.

31. O Hata H: Spondylolysis: familial occurrence and its genetic implication. J Jap Orthop Assoc 41:931-941, 1967.

32. Penning AL, and Kluft O: Unilateral spondylolisthesis of the sixth cervical vertebra. J Bone Joint Surg 51-A:1379-1382, 1969.

33. Petajan JH, Momberger GL, Aase J, Wright DG: Arthrogryposis syndrome (Kuskokwim disease) in the Eskimo. JAMA 209:1481-1486, 1969.

34. Phalan GS, Dickson JA: Spondylolisthesis and tight hamstrings. J Bone Joint Surg 43-A:505-512, 1961.

35. Risser J, and Norquist D: Sciatic scoliosis in the growing child. Clin Orthop 21:156, 1961.

36. Robert (zu Koblenz): Eine eigentümliche angeborene Lordose, wahrscheinlich bedingt durch eine Verschiebung des Körpers des letzten Lindenwirbels auf die vordere Flache des ersten Kreuzbeinwirbels (Spondylolisthesis Kilian), nebst Bermerlsungen über die Mechanik dieser Beckenformation. Monatsschr Geburtskunde u Frauenkrank 5:81-94, 1855.

37. Roche MB, Rowe GG: Incidence of separate neural arch and coincident bone variations. Anat Rec 109:233-55, 1951.

38. Rosenberg N: Degenerative spondylolisthesis. Paper presented at the meeting of Amer. Orth. Assoc. Hot Springs, Va., June, 1973.

39. Rosenberg N: Personal communication.

40. Rowe GG, and Roche MB: The etiology of separate neural arch. J Bone Joint Surg 35-A:102, 1953.

41. Schultz AH: Personal communication.

42. Steele HH: Personal communication.

43. Stewart TD: The age incidence of neural arch defects in Alaskan natives considered from the standpoint of etiology. J Bone Joint Surg 35-A:937-950, 1953.

44. Stewart TD: Examination of the possibility that certain skeletal characteristics predispose to defects in the lumbar neural arches. Clin Orthop 8:44-60, 1956.

45. Sullivan CR, Bickel WH: The problem of traumatic spondylolysis: a report of three cases. Am J Surg 100:698-708, 1960.

46. Unander-Scharin L: A case of spondylolisthesis lumbalis acquisita. Acta Orthop Scand 19:536-544, 1950.

47. Urist M: Personal communication.

48. Walters RL, Morris JM: Effect of spinal support on the electrical activity of the muscles of the trunk. J Bone Joint Surg 52-A:51-60, 1971.

49. Willis TA: Lumbosacral retrodisplacement. Am J Roentgenol 90:1263, 1963.

50. Wiltse LL: The etiology of spondylolisthesis. J Bone & Joint Surg 44-A:539-569, 1962.

51. Wiltse, LL: Interbody fusion of the lumbar spine. J Western Pac Orthop Assoc 6-No. 1, 1969 (reprint.)

52. Wiltse LL, Bateman JG, Hutchinson RH and Nelson WE: The paraspinal sacrospinalis-splitting approach to the lumbar spine. J Bone Joint Surg 44-A:532-569, 1962.

53. Wiltse, LL: Spondylolisthesis: classification and etiology. Amer Acad Orthop Surg Symposium on the Spine, St. Louis, Mosby, 1969, 143-167.

54. Wiltse, LL: Surgical treatment of spondylolisthesis. Clin Orthop 35:116-135, 1964.

55. Woolsey RD: Simple laminectomy for spondylolisthesis without spinal fusion. J Intern Coll Surg 29:101-105, 1958.

56. Wright DG, Aase J: The Kuskokwim syndrome: an inherited form of arthogryposis in the Alaskan Eskimo. Birth Defects. 5:91-95, 1969.

57. Yano T, Meyagi S, Ikari T: Studies of familial incidence of spondylolisthesis. Singapore Med J 8:203-206, 1967.

21

Spondylolisthesis and Its Treatment: Excision of Loose Lamina and Decompression

GERALD G. GILL

PATIENTS with spondylolisthesis often have marked radicular pain with involvement of the fifth lumbar or of the first sacral roots. On exploration three main causes for the radicular pain have been noted. First, on extension of the spine, the loose lamina of the vertebra caused traction on the first sacral root. Second, upon removal of the loose lamina in patients with evidence of fifth lumbar root compression, it was found that the fifth lumbar root was impinged upon by a mass of fibrocartilaginous tissue and bone at the defect in the pars interarticularis. Third, protrusion or herniation of either the fourth or fifth lumbar disc is found in approximately one-third of the cases. These are handled like any other disc herniation.

Owing to the difficulty in attaining solid posterior fusion in spondylolisthesis and to the presence of bony, dural, and root compression, the decompression should be performed first and the fusion operation later if necessary. We do not recommend the decompression operation for children.

At present our series consists of 65 patients who have been treated by the decompression operation. Over 80% of the patients have had a satisfactory result during a follow-up of over six years. One-half of our patients showed no displacement over an average of five years. The other half showed some displacement occurring over an average period of eight to nine years; males showed an average of 6%, and females an average of 16%. The results in those who showed more forward displacement were as good as in those who did not. We conclude that in adults the displacement is limited, does not necessarily cause symptoms, and is not intrinsically dangerous. The removal of the arch does not cause further forward displacement or influence its degree.

If a fusion is ever considered in these patients, we are firmly convinced that it should be a lateral fusion. Few of our patients, however, have had subsequent fusion operations, and these have not been relieved of residual radicular pain.

INDICATIONS FOR OPERATION

Adults with persistent, recurrent, and incapacitating back and/or leg pain, who do not respond to an active exercise program, should be considered for this procedure. Myelography usually is not necessary, except when the knee jerk is absent, in which cases this study might be required to rule out protrusions of the third lumbar disc.

Our experience with children has been limited. Children who have symptoms and meet Taillard's criteria for the diagnosis of probable forward displacement probably should undergo a lateral fusion and, if they have radicular pain or root compression, subsequent decompression. Taillard's criteria are as follows: (1) a rounded promontory of the sacrum and (2) a decrease in the posterior vertical height of the fifth lumbar vertebra of over one-third of the anterior height. In children who do

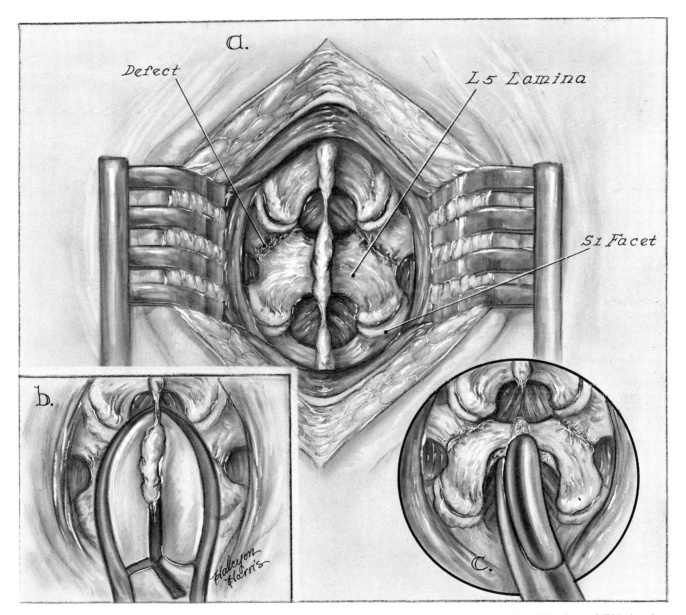

FIG. 21-1. Lumbosacral area in spondylolisthesis as viewed at operation: *A*, exposure of lamina of fifth lumbar vertebra, showing defect in pars interarticularis of fifth lumbar vertebra; *B*, excision of spinous process of fifth lumbar vertebra; *C*, excision of central portion of loose lamina of fifth lumbar vertebra. (From Gill, GG, Manning, JG, White HL: Surgical treatment of spondylolisthesis without spinal fusion. J Bone Joint Surg *37-A*:493–518, 1955.)

not show the criteria of Taillard and have radicular pain, decompression can be performed first, and lateral fusion later if deemed necessary.

SURGICAL TREATMENT

Through a midline incision, the spinous processes of the fourth and fifth lumbar and first sacral vertebrae are exposed subperiosteally (Fig. 21-1 A). The spinous processes of the fourth and fifth lumbar and first sacral vertebrae are then excised (Fig. 21-1 B). With the blunt, double-action rongeur, the entire middle portion of the loose lamina of the fifth lumbar vertebra is then removed (Fig. 21-1 C). The inferior aspect of the lamina of the fourth lumbar vertebra is then bitten away with the blunt-curved, double-action rongeur until the ligamentum flavum is freed from its inferior aspect. By sharp dissection down the midline and upward laterally, the interlaminar portion of the ligamentum flavum between the fourth and fifth lumbar vertebrae is excised. Recently, we have not removed the whole ligamentum flavum below the level of the loose fifth lumbar lamina, merely trimming it to remove a ragged edge, since this may decrease the amount of scar formation over the dura. The lateral portion of the loose arch of

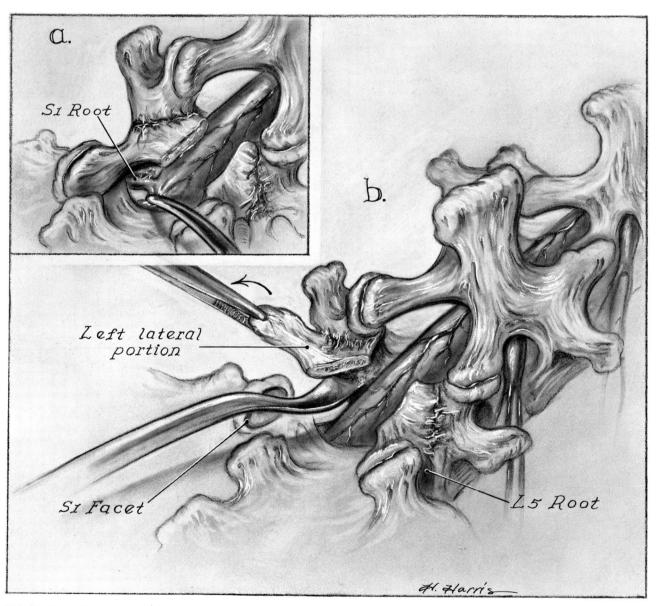

FIG. 21-2. *A*, Relationship of first sacral root to lateral portion of loose arch of fifth lumbar vertebra; *B*, removal of lateral portion of loose lamina of fifth lumbar vertebra. (From Gill GG, Manning JG, White HL: Surgical treatment of spondylolisthesis without spinal fusion. J Bone Joint Surg *37-A*:493–518, 1955.)

the fifth lumbar vertebra is then removed, the attached inferior articular process being freed by sharp dissection from its articulation with the sacrum. This fragment is then elevated and is dissected free from the defect in the pars interarticularis, the dissection being done close to the lamina to avoid injury to the fifth lumbar root (Fig. 21-2 A, B). The fifth lumbar root is exposed somewhat cephalad and is retracted, together with the dura, toward the midline, away from the defect in the pars interarticularis. The defect is almost invariably found to be filled with a mass of fibrocartilaginous tissue compressing the fifth lumbar

root (Fig. 21-3 A). This tissue is removed by means of the Kerrison rongeur.

The fifth lumbar root is identified below the fourth lumbar lamina, and followed out past the foramen to ascertain that the root is free (Fig. 21-3 B). It is important to be sure that this root is not taut across the pedicle of the involved vertebra, and it is mandatory that enough bone be removed with a small osteotome to permit the root to run free and clear. During operation the wound is irrigated with cold Ringer's solution because we believe this reduces the inflammatory response. If bleeding cannot be completely controlled, a

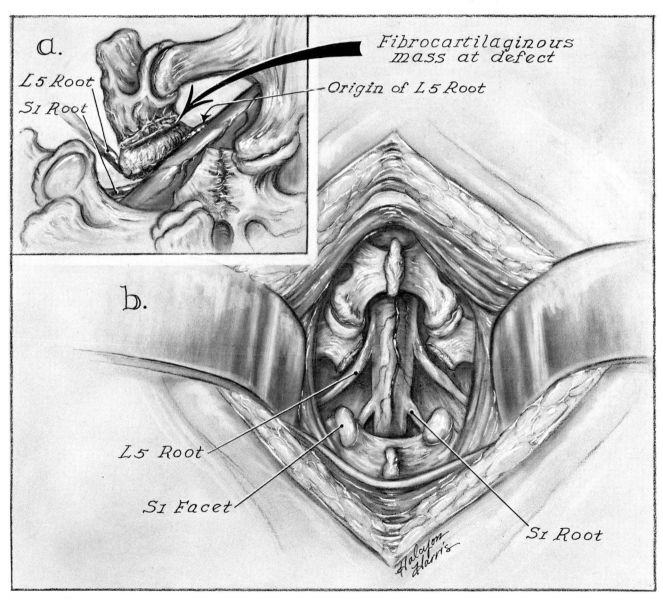

FIG. 21-3. *A*, Fibrocartilaginous mass at defect in pars interarticularis of fifth lumbar vertebra after removal of lateral portion of loose lamina. Fifth lumbar root is compressed from above, posteriorly, and laterally by fibrocartilaginous mass; *B*, completed operative procedure. (From Gill GG, Manning JG, White HL: Surgical treatment of spondylolisthesis without spinal fusion. J Bone Joint Surg *37-A*:493–518, 1955.)

drip and suction tube (Salem sump) is inserted from one side of the wound into the operative area. Suction is applied while Ringer's solution containing a weak antibiotic solution is dripped into the wound. This removes the accumulation of postoperative blood in the wound and thereby decreases postoperative pain. A thin dressing is applied to ensure the patient's comfort.

During operation a polyvinyl sponge is used in place of cottonoid, because it does not fragment; hence the tendency for postoperative scar formation is reduced.

The patients are encouraged to move and turn and move their lower legs and feet. They are allowed to stand and to begin straight leg raising exercises as soon as possible; they are usually discharged from the hospital on the seventh day. Collections of fluid in the wound are aspirated to decrease postoperative discomfort.

After patients have achieved straight leg raising to at least 90 degrees, sitting and toe-touching exercises are begun, to be followed by abdominal exercises. Exercises are performed at least four times a day. Patients are allowed to return to light work at six weeks and heavy work after three months.

References

1. Gill GG, White HL: Surgical treatment of spondylolisthesis without spinal fusion. Acta Orth Scand (Suppl 85) Munksgaard Copenhagen 1965.
2. Gill GG, Manning JC, White HL: Surgical treatment of spondylolisthesis without spine fusion. J Bone Jt. Surg 37A:493–518, 1955.
3. Taillard N: Les Spondylolisthesis. Paris, Masson et cie, 1957.

22

Congenital Anomalies of the Spine

THOMAS K. CRAIGMILE

APPROXIMATELY 60% of all congenital defects involve the central nervous system, alone or in association with defects of other organ systems. A great proportion of these are deformities of the spine, meninges, spinal cord, and nerve roots.[32] Many, particularly those that involve the spinal column but not the neural elements, are asymptomatic and are discovered incidentally at various ages on roentgenograms taken for a variety of other reasons. Most of these defects are of little or no clinical significance and require no treatment or curtailment of activity. Other anomalies, initially asymptomatic, may predispose to spinal or spinal cord injury from relatively trivial, ordinarily harmless forces. In contradistinction are the extensive defects in which the spinal cord is exteriorized. Such defects often are accompanied by craniocerebral abnormalities, which are incompatible with life and for which there is no feasible or desirable treatment.

Between these extremes are a variety of congenital defects that may be classified in one of two categories: (1) defects that are usually successfully treated by a single operation (meningocele, congenital dermal sinus, diastematomyelia, neurenteric cysts, defects in the upper cervical spine that permit subluxation, and congenitally narrowed spinal canal), and (2) defects (mainly myelomeningoceles) that are usually treated surgically in order to prevent meningeal infection or to facilitate care of the child and prevent subsequent occurrence or progression of neurologic defects. Abnormalities of neurologic function are rarely improved by operation.[22,23] In these patients, complications involving impaired cerebrospinal fluid circulation, musculoskeletal deformity, and urinary tract dysfunction are the rule rather than the exception, and the problem is one of never-ending rehabilitation and treatment of recurring complications as they arise.

Embryologic errors resulting in congenital malformations of the spine include failure of fusion of posterior elements of the neural arch, allowing herniation of the meninges and neural tissue; incomplete fusion of the primitive neural tube; defects in notochordal development; and incomplete separation of entodermal derivatives forming the alimentary tract and ectodermal tissue destined to become the spine and its contained neural elements.[3,19,23,26,30] The causative embryologic maldevelopment usually occurs within the first two months of intrauterine life, often between the third and fifth weeks of gestation, when the closure of the neural tube begins in the mid-thoracic region and continues to complete closure at the cranial and lumbar poles.[29]

EPIDEMIOLOGY AND ETIOLOGY

Recent statistical surveys have shown that geography seems to play a significant role in the incidence of congenital anomalies. Defects occur with the greatest frequency in the British Isles, particularly in Ireland and Wales, in Egypt, and in certain smaller geopolitical units.[23,26] In the United States and in most countries south of the equator, the frequency is appreciably lower. No plausible explanation for this geographic variation has been found. Cultural background and environmental factors seemingly have little influence. The incidence of anomalies is higher in infants born during winter months.

Advanced age of the mother and dietary deficiencies are believed to be significant etiologic factors. Hydramnios, abnormal presentations, and toxemias of pregnancy are more common in mothers bearing children with congenital defects, but these complications can hardly be adjudged responsible for embryologic changes occurring in early intrauterine life; indeed, the converse may be true, perhaps the presence of an anomalous fetus causes these difficulties, which occur in the latter stages of pregnancy.

Rubella in the mother during the first trimester of pregnancy, exposure to radiation during the early weeks of gestation, and the use of certain drugs, particularly thalidomide, result in increased incidence of congenital anomalies, but usually affect structures other than the central nervous system. Familial factors, on the other hand, may be considerably more significant. It has been estimated that the likelihood of congenital central nervous system involvement in an infant born to parents who have previously produced a child with such an abnormality is about 150% higher than in the general population.[21]

CLINICAL MANIFESTATIONS

Ordinarily only with such defects as spina bifida cystica, chondro-osteodystrophy, Hurler's syndrome, and achondroplasia does visual inspection disclose the primary defect. In others the first indication may be discovery of a neurologic deficit (motor or sensory change or abnormal sphincter function), musculoskeletal deformity (kyphosis, dislocation of the hip, clubbed feet), cutaneous changes (abnormal pigmentation or hair growth, dimpling of the skin, pathologic accumulations of subcutaneous fat), or a combination of these changes.

Congenital defects of the spine may not become clinically evident until the second or third decade of life. The anomalous state may have been erroneously diagnosed as multiple sclerosis, syringomyelia (in itself congenital in some instances), or neoplasm or vascular malformation of the spinal cord.

PREVENTION

Investigations directed toward alteration of genetic factors have not been effective in eliminating congenital defects. Parents of a congenitally defective child should be counseled regarding the increased risk to subsequent children. Recent refinements in the technique of amniography[11] have made relatively early detection of meningocele and some other defects possible, so that abortion can be performed if the parents desire.

SPINA BIFIDA OCCULTA

In spina bifida occulta there is no visible or palpable external evidence of a defect in the meninges, even though a minimal or major one may be present. In its most insignificant form, this anomaly may consist of incomplete fusion of one or more spinous processes. At the other extreme, there may be complete neural arch deficiencies involving one or more vertebrae. The most common defect is incomplete fusion of a single spinous process extending inward to the ligamentum flavum. Appreciable defects in the adjoining lamina are uncommon.

Etiologic factors include failure of complete development of ossification centers in the neural arch, incomplete fusion of the neural tube, and abnormal notochordal maturation.[26]

INCIDENCE AND SITES OF INVOLVEMENT. The incidence of occult defects of the spine is difficult to assess because many defects remain undiscovered and some, although visualized incidentally on spinal roentgenograms made for some other purpose, are not reported statistically. Meacham estimates that persisting occult spina bifida occurs in 20% of all births,[25] whereas Matson has suggested a figure approaching 25%, but emphasizes that a significant number of the defects discovered early in life disappear during the early years of skeletal maturation.[23]

In those instances of incidental discovery of the defect, the vertebrae most often involved are L5 and S1,

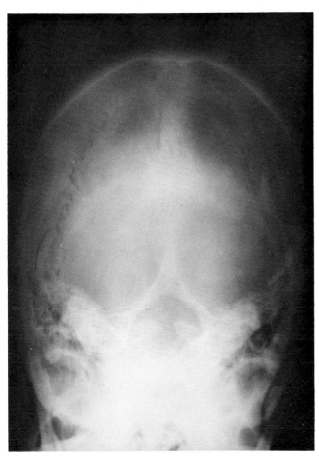

FIG. 22-1. Failure of fusion, C1 arch (spina bifida). Discovered incidentally on routine x-ray examination of skull.

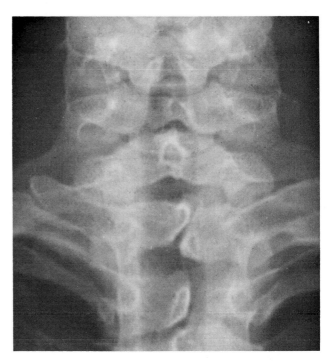

FIG. 22-2. Spina bifida, T1-T2. Such lesions at this level are rare. Patient was free of symptoms or any neurologic deficit.

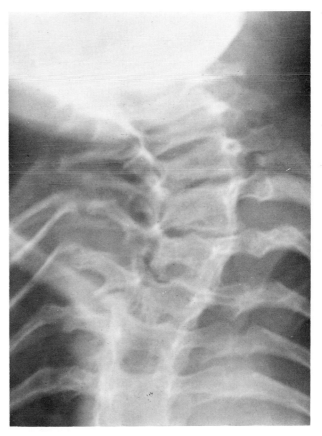

FIG. 22-3. Cervical-thoracic neural arch defect with associated kyphoscoliosis.

with occasional cases occurring in the cervical area (Figs. 22-1 to 22-4). On the other hand, among patients who are examined because clinical manifestations have suggested the presence of a structural spinal defect, the frequency in the caudad portions of the spine increases, since lumbar and sacral spinal defects are more likely to be associated with cutaneous, neural, or musculoskeletal abnormalities than are cervical and thoracic lesions. Matson,[23] in a series of 131 symptomatic patients studied, found that 58% involved the lumbar and lumbosacral portions of the spine, 19% the sacral area alone, and 19% the thoracolumbar spine; the cervical spine was the site of involvement in the remaining 4%. Rarely, and almost solely associated with occult lumbar defects, there may be co-existing diastematomyelia, congenital dermal sinus, or tumor.[1,17,23]

CLINICAL MANIFESTATIONS. In most cases no symptoms or physical findings result from the defect if it is not accompanied by distortion of neural elements. The anomaly is discovered most often on roentgenograms taken after suspected spinal trauma or as a routine measure prior to operation for herniated intervertebral discs. Disclosure of the defect in the latter instance is particularly significant in that dissection can then be

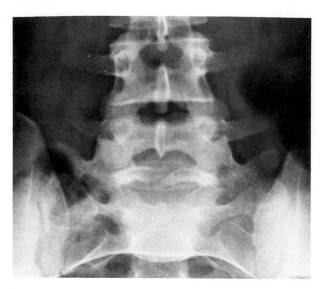

FIG. 22-4. Spina bifida occulta, L5. Asymptomatic defect discovered incidentally. Spina bifida not producing symptoms is most common at this vertebral level.

performed with extraordinary care to prevent injury to the contents of the vertebral canal.

Patients with symptoms display widely varying clinical evidence of spina bifida, particularly cutaneous abnormalities such as localized pathologic pigmentation of the skin and a focal area of abnormal hair growth. Neither in itself is an indication of underlying meningeal or neural defects. On the other hand, when either occurs in the absence of a neurologic or musculoskeletal abnormality, roentgenograms of the entire spine should be made and the child should be examined frequently so that any motor, reflex, sensory, or other deficit may be detected early. Of greater significance is the discovery in the newborn, or older infant, of a cutaneous dimple that may communicate through a dermal sinus to an extradural or intradural cyst, ultimately causing meningitis or cord or cauda equina compression from enlargement of the cyst. Such sinuses, which are discussed later in greater detail, may enter the spinal canal at the site of the spina bifida. The remaining visible midline abnormality of the back represents a subcutaneous collection of fat, usually irregular in contour, nontender, and occupying an area two or more centimeters in diameter. These lipomas may or may not be associated with overlying pigmentation, hair accumulations, or dimpling of the skin. They are more often indicative of occult myelomeningocele formation than are the other cutaneous lesions. Their presence necessitates a thorough clinical and radiologic investigation. Such accumulations of fat should not be excised en bloc because they may contain elements of the cauda equina.

Neurologic abnormalities resulting from occult spinal defects include impairment of motor function (usually symmetrical and flaccid), diminished perception of pain (the only reaction that can be tested with any degree of reliability in the very young), and disturbances of sphincter function. The latter, usually discovered at the time of toilet training, include overflow dribbling of urine, regression to incontinence or urinary retention after seemingly having been trained, and hypotonicity of the anal sphincter.

Musculoskeletal changes associated with spina bifida occulta include kyphosis, congenital dislocation of the hips, and a variety of clubbed foot deformities. Often these defects are present early in life, but remain undetected until the child attempts to walk. When a musculoskeletal deformity, particularly kyphosis, is accompanied by a cutaneous lesion of the lower back, the existence of a congenital deformity of the spine becomes more likely.[26]

Low back pain, which may or may not be associated with lower extremity radiation, may occur in children with spina bifida, but is more common in adults. In the absence of objective neurologic changes it is not an indication for myelography. Any operation on the lumbar spine in such patients rarely relieves the discomfort and may be hazardous if there is an unsuspected occult myelomeningocele.

RADIOGRAPHIC EXAMINATION. X-ray examination of the spine may demonstrate, in addition to the spina bifida, widening of the spinal canal, thinning of the pedicles, a bony spicule arising from the posterior aspect of a vertebral body, or other congenital defects. Occasionally tomograms provide useful additional information. One must keep in mind that a defect in a neural arch in an infant, studied radiographically because of a cutaneous or musculoskeletal abnormality, may close during early childhood.

Positive contrast myelography should be performed in all patients with spina bifida occulta who have a progressive neurologic defect indicating the need for operation. Myelography discloses the size and configuration of the theca and may reveal the presence of unsuspected bony or fibrous spicules, neoplasms, cysts, and occult meningoceles. It may be necessary to introduce the contrast material by way of the cisterna magna if puncture of the lumbar subarachnoid space is contraindicated.

TREATMENT. Asymptomatic occult spina bifida requires no treatment; similarly spina bifida associated with a musculoskeletal deformity or cutaneous abnormality (except in the case of the dimple leading to a dermal sinus) should not undergo myelography and operation unless there is clinical evidence of a progressive neurologic defect. Musculoskeletal defects may be corrected by appropriate orthopedic measures. Angiomatous pigmentation of the skin and abnormal hair growth rarely should be excised. In the absence of neurologic deficits subcutaneous masses of fat are not operated upon for they may contain neural elements. The management of the patient with a cutaneous dimple and a dermal sinus is discussed on page 235.

Should symptoms and signs of a neurologic abnormality appear in a previously asymptomatic individual, or should a seemingly stable neurologic deficit become progressive, plain roentgenograms of the spine should be repeated so that osseous change can be detected and myelography performed. The surgical procedure varies according to the clinical and radiographic findings, but certain features of these widely dissimilar lesions and principles of their surgical treatment are constant.

In many instances surgical treatment is expected to prevent further progression of the deficit, but not to restore function already lost. In other cases, particularly those of an intraspinal dermoid cyst or well-defined lipoma not surrounding the rootlets of the cauda equina, excision of the mass may result in complete or partial recovery of neurologic function.

The procedure is performed with the patient prone and under general anesthesia. The use of magnification may allow more precise dissection. Extensive attempts to free nerve roots encompassed by fat and fibrous tissue may result in increased neurologic deficit. The use of bipolar faradic stimulation to differentiate between neural and fibrous tissue is helpful. When the absence of an overlying lipomatous mass containing neural tissue allows safe access to the spine and laminectomy is planned for removal of an intraspinal cyst or neoplasm, laminae should be exposed for at least one segment above and below the abnormality. Laminectomy should always be started in a normal area and continued in the direction of the defect.

Epidural dermoid sinuses and cysts can be dissected and excised with little difficulty. Those within the dura are usually easily resectable if there hasn't been prior meningitis or local infection. Should a cyst be densely adherent to the cord or roots of the cauda, it is advisable to leave the adherent portion of the cyst wall rather than risk injury to neural tissue; incomplete excision does not necessarily preclude satisfactory return of neurologic function nor greatly increase the likelihood of recurrence. Little is to be accomplished, and irreversible injury to nerve roots may result, from attempts to resect intradural collections of fat surrounding the cauda. On the other hand, discrete lipomas involving no more than one root may be resected with little or no residual neurologic deficit. Fibrous bands or a tense filum terminale tethering the cord should be sectioned. Posteriorly directed meningoceles should be opened, any contained neural elements gently dissected and returned to the spinal canal, and the neck of the sac ligated. Bony or fibrous spurs protruding into the canal should be resected. Complete dural closure should be made, even though a graft is occasionally necessary; the remainder of the wound closure is carried out in anatomic layers.

SPINA BIFIDA CYSTICA

The term spina bifida cystica is applied to all midline fusion defects of the spine in which there is external evidence of herniation of meninges. Although some lesions are covered by intact skin, usually only the periphery of the mass is protected by skin, while its central portion is covered by a thin, fragile transparent membrane. Less than one-third of all cases of spina bifida cystica are meningoceles, which are formed from meningeal layers alone; the remainder, the myelomeningoceles, contain neural tissues, roots of the cauda equina, or, in higher lesions, the spinal cord.

In his review of a large series of patients from the general population, Lorber found the incidence of spina bifida cystica to be three in every thousand births, and that 6.8% of siblings of patients with spina bifida cystica have similar or other congenital anomalies of the central nervous system.[21]

CLINICAL FINDINGS. Meningocele or myelocele usually is located in the lumbar or lumbosacral segments, but any portion of the spinal axis may be involved (Figs. 22-5 to 22-7). Matson found the lesion in the lumbar area in 42%, lumbosacral in 27.5%, thoracolumbar in 10%, sacral in 8%, thoracic in 6.3%, cervical in 3.7%, and anterior or unspecified in the remaining 2.5%.[23]

Rarely does a patient have more than one meningocele or myelomeningocele. Hydrocephalus is the common associated neurologic abnormality; congenital dermal sinus or diastematomyelia rarely accompanies spina bifida cystica.

Meningeal defects vary widely in size, configuration, and nature and extent of cutaneous or membranous coverings. Lesions are usually readily compressible, often with resulting increased tension of the anterior fontanelle, a test for patency of cerebrospinal fluid pathways of doubtful value and safety.

In myelomeningocele with a membranous covering, a complex of neural elements—the neural plaque comprised of nerve roots or spinal cord or both—may be seen partially or completely fused to the membrane at

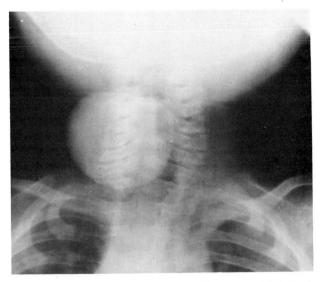

FIG. 22-5. Cervical meningocele. Neural arch defects and soft-tissue shadow of meningocele are apparent. This anomaly is rare.

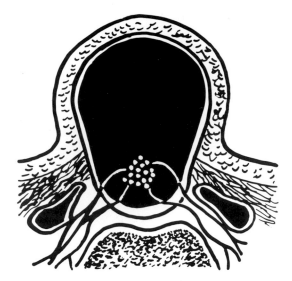

FIG. 22-6. Cross-sectional diagram of lumbar meningocele. Repair can be effected without disturbing neural elements.

the dome of the sac. Rarely does this plaque of nervous tissue lie free in cerebrospinal fluid contained within the meningocele. Membranous myelomeningoceles may be moist, either from escape of cerebrospinal fluid from a defect in the sac or as a result of local transudate (Figs. 22-8 and 22-9).

Most lumbar meningoceles or myeloceles are sessile, at least partially covered with membrane, usually round or ovoid, and varying in diameter from a few centimeters to an area occupying almost the entire width of the back. Narrow-necked defects are most frequently cephalad to the lumbar area, more often protected by intact skin, and less often contain neural elements.

Rachischisis is an extreme defect of the posterior components of the meninges, neural arches, and overlying muscles and integument, with exposure of the spinal cord to the exterior. These lesions are almost always contaminated or grossly infected at birth or shortly thereafter, and are often accompanied by other congenital anomalies of the central nervous system which are not compatible with life.

NEUROLOGIC EXAMINATION. Physical findings in the

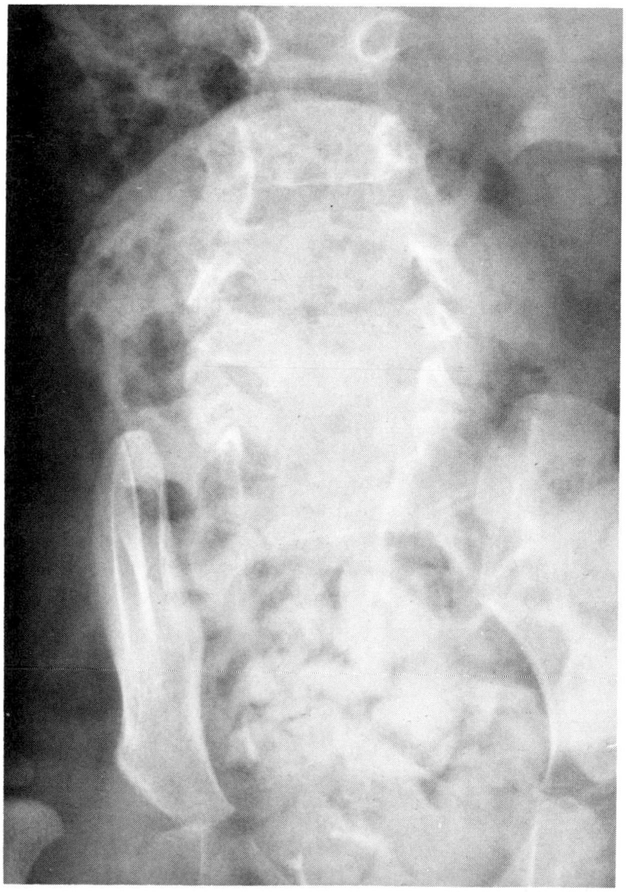

FIG. 22-7. Multiple neural arch defects with soft tissue outline of meningocele.

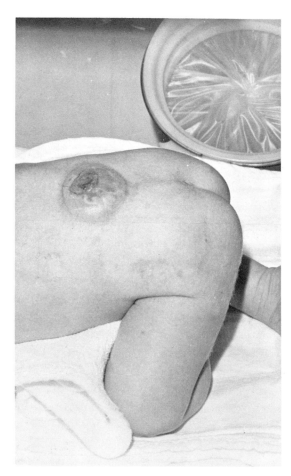

FIG. 22-8. Sessile lumbar myelomeningocele in one-day-old infant with severe lower extremity motor defect.

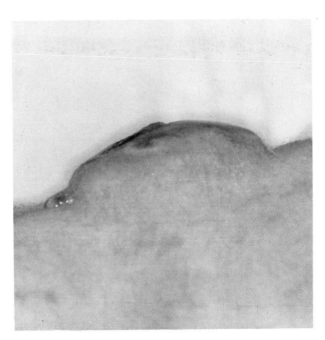

FIG. 22-9. Tangential view of myelomeningocele shown in Figure 22-8. Neural plaque is seen in cephalad portion of lesion, and there is obvious leakage of fluid from defect.

newborn or infant are difficult to assess because of the limitations imposed by the patient's age. Motor evaluation is confined to one's observations of spontaneous movements and responses to painful stimulus. Pain is the only sensory modality that can be tested, the response being a cry or withdrawal of the stimulated extremity. Deep reflexes (quadriceps and Achilles) can be elicited and graded as to degree of activity. The plantar response must be evaluated cautiously, since it may normally be extensor until the age of eighteen months.

In lumbar and sacral lesions the motor deficit may be variable and irregular with little evidence of a lesion at a specific myotomal level, since certain nerve roots may be involved in the cystic deformity while others emerging at a lower level may be spared. Lumbar and sacral defects result in flaccid weakness with diminished or absent deep reflexes, whereas cervical and thoracic myelomeningoceles are associated with hyperactive myotatic reflexes and increased muscular tone. Anal sphincter tone is usually diminished, and in lumbosacral defects, there is no resistance to the examining finger; there may be more or less constant dribbling of urine rather than the periodic emptying of the bladder of the normal newborn.

HYDROCEPHALUS. Many patients with spina bifida have hydrocephalus that is obvious at the time of birth, but often signs of its appearance are delayed. Any infant with a midline fusion defect should be examined at regular intervals for evidence of developing hydro-

cephalus. Head circumference should be measured, and the findings compared with standard head size tables. Rate of growth is more significant than absolute head circumference on any occasion. The examination also includes evaluation of degree of tension of the anterior fontanelle and observation for dilatation of scalp veins, obvious stretching of the scalp, seeming downward displacement of the line of gaze, the presence of a hollow percussion note, and occasionally a cranial bruit. Transillumination of the skull helps in the differentiation between hydrocephalus, subdural hematoma, and anencephaly. Plain skull roentgenograms may demonstrate suture separation, and echoencephalography may distinguish enlarging lateral ventricles from an extracerebral hematoma or hygroma.

ASSOCIATED CONGENITAL DEFECTS. Infants with congenital defects of the nervous system have a significantly higher incidence of other anomalies.[21] Cleft lip and palate and musculoskeletal deformities, for example, are apparent, whereas others are found only after careful examination, and still others (anomalies of the gastrointestinal and urinary tracts) may require special radiographic studies.

ANCILLARY DIAGNOSTIC STUDIES. X-ray examination of the entire spine is essential in all patients with meningocele or myelomeningocele, not only to determine the configuration and extent of the bone defect of the evident anomaly, but to discover any other occult abnormalities. Skull films also are necessary for the detection of suture separation. As opposed to its use in spina bifida occulta, in which case the findings may be an indication for operation, Pantopaque myelography is rarely necessary in spina bifida cystica. Air myelography occasionally may be helpful in defining irregular lesions or those in which transillumination suggests loculation.

INDICATIONS FOR SURGICAL TREATMENT. The decision regarding operation is made after the infant's condition has been evaluated and various factors influencing the ultimate functional result of the operation have been considered. Matson believes the following to be of particular importance: (1) the age and general condition of the patient; (2) the location (spinal level), size, and shape of the sac and width of its base; (3) the nature of the coverings of the sac; (4) the presence or imminence of surface ulceration or leakage of cerebrospinal fluid; (5) the condition of the skin adjacent to the lesion; (6) the presence of arrested or progressive hydrocephalus; (7) the neurologic status of the lower extremities and sphincters; (8) the presence of other congenital anomalies; (9) the family medical history; and (10) the economic and domestic status of the family.[23] Perhaps one should add another factor, i.e., the presence of meningitis at the time the infant is first examined.

Philosophic concepts regarding which patients should be selected for surgical treatment have undergone considerable modification from those generally accepted a decade or two ago.[7,8,16,23] Until recently, most neurosurgeons believed that the majority of newborn infants with large, membrane-covered myelomeningoceles, complete or virtually complete paralysis of the lower extremities, little or no sphincter function, and almost certainly developing hydrocephalus should not be treated actively and should be left to die as "mercifully" as possible. According to follow-up studies, a considerable number of these patients did succumb to meningitis early in life, but many survived with handicaps that could have been partially corrected early in life. Increasing survival rates can be attributed to: (1) improved techniques in the treatment of hydrocephalus; (2) more effective antibiotics in the prevention and treatment of meningitis; and (3) the development of ileal loop diversion of urine to prevent urinary tract infection and ultimate renal failure. With prevention of meningitis through proper treatment of the membrane-covered myelomeningoceles in combination with prophylactic antibiotic use, once-fragile membranes often ultimately become epithelialized with formation of a protective barrier against contamination. An occasional undesirable sequel to secondary epithelialization of the membrane is adhesion formation and incorporation of the neural plaque into overlying scar, with increase in any already existing neurologic deficit.

Considering the fact that many infants with defects that at one time would have been considered incompatible with life are now surviving, more significance is attached to what is termed "quality of life" in those survivors.[7] This includes control or absence of hydrocephalus, freedom from urinary tract infection, correction of musculoskeletal deformities and use of braces or crutches to facilitate ambulation, education, and finally, the capability to be self-supporting. Therefore, the trend is toward earlier and more vigorous surgical treatment, of both the myelomeningocele and the hydrocephalus. It is the opinion of some that almost all patients with myelomeningocele, no matter how overwhelming the deficit from the spinal lesion or other anomalies may be, should be treated surgically as early and as extensively as necessary to forestall immediate and delayed complications and facilitate care.[7,8,36] Shillito, however, believes there are straightforward contraindications to operation; these include spinal defects of such size that closure is not feasible technically, hydrocephalus so marked that significant mental development is not possible, and the presence of other congenital defects incompatible with survival.[34] Meningitis or significant systemic infection are at least temporary contraindications to operation.

If the decision is made to operate on a membrane-covered defect, the procedure should be performed within the first day of life to prevent the almost inevitable infection that occurs if it is delayed. Prophylactic antibiotic therapy is started prior to operation and is continued until wound healing is well established; gentamycin and oxacillin are recommended agents.[34] If hydrocephalus is present at birth, ventriculostomy or ventriculoatrial or ventriculoperitoneal shunting should precede myelomeningocele repair. In cases in which a small myelomeningocele is mainly covered with intact skin, surgical treatment of the hydrocephalus may allow the spinal defect to collapse and the then-undistended membranous portion to heal without further operation.

The management of myelomeningoceles covered by intact skin is appreciably different from that for membrane-covered defects, inasmuch as imminent meningeal infection is not a problem in the former. Postponement of the operation reduces the hazard of a major procedure under general anesthetic because the older infant has greater total blood volume, and his lesion becomes relatively smaller compared to body size as he grows older. Certainly there is no indication that early operation in these patients enhances the outcome from the standpoint of residual neurologic defect. Small skin-covered sessile lesions that do not interfere with care of the infant may never require operation, unless there is evidence of progressive malfunction of the lower extremities or sphincters. In such a patient, hydrocephalus should be treated as soon as it becomes apparent.

OPERATION. General anesthesia is preferred, although local infiltration with lidocaine may be satisfactory in small or premature infants. A well-situated intravenous catheter is inserted prior to operation, and blood is made available for transfusion. The infant is positioned with well-padded supports beneath the shoulders, iliac crests, and ankles to minimize pressure and interference with venous return. The extremities are wrapped to avoid excessive heat loss, and that portion of the back harboring the lesion is elevated slightly to minimize loss of cerebrospinal fluid.

Magnification is recommended to facilitate dissection, and a bipolar faradic stimulator aids in differentiating between neural and fibrous elements.

The skin should be prepared with a povidone-iodine scrub followed by application of a similar solution. The membranous portion of the lesion will not tolerate abrasive scrubbing, but should be painted with the povidone-iodine preparation. A Steridrape with an aperture in its mid-portion, surrounded by lightweight pediatric surgical sheets, provides an adequate drape.

Surgical treatment is directed toward proper placement of the skin incision, meticulous dissection of the neck of the lesion and neural elements, replacement of neural tissues within the spinal canal when feasible, and water-tight closure to prevent cerebrospinal fluid leakage (Fig. 22-10). Initially an elliptical incision is made about the base of the deformity, usually parallel to its long axis. Healing is often facilitated if the general course of the incision is transverse, particularly in the lumbosacral area where the wound is more susceptible to contamination from urine or feces. The operative area should be widely draped, since incisions must often be extended and the surrounding skin and

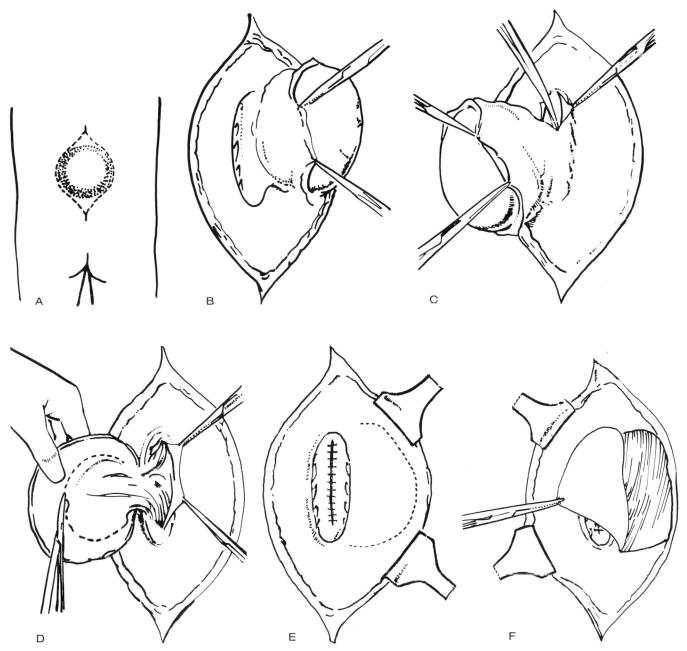

FIG. 22-10. Myelomeningocele repair. *A*, Basic skin incisions used when base of lesion is not excessively broad. *B*, Dissection of base and neck of sac. *C*, Excision of sac. *D*, Lysis of adhesions at base of sac. *E*, Dural closure. *F*, Attached graft of lumbodorsal fascia is dissected, reflected medially, and sutured to fascia on opposite side to form protective layer over exposed dura. (Figs. 22-10*A* to *F* modified from Lassman, LP, in Operative Surgery (Neurosurgery), V Logue, Ed., London, Butterworth, 1971.)

subcutaneous tissues undermined for a considerable distance from the base of the lesion to facilitate ultimate closure. It is occasionally necessary to create skin flaps, which are later rotated to effect closure, but relaxing incisions are to be avoided. The skin and subcutaneous tissue are dissected down to the lumbodorsal or paraspinous muscle fascia at a point cephalad to the sac. At this level the dissection is continued circumferentially about the lesion until the neck of the sac is completely exposed and the surrounding areolar tissue and fat carefully removed. The neck of the sac often is found to be narrower than indicated by preoperative findings. Early in the course of the procedure, the dome of the sac should be opened, preferably in its cephalad portion to avoid the often unpredictable course of nerve root at the caudad pole of the lesion. If there is a true meningocele that contains no neural elements, or certainly none adherent to the wall of the sac, the sac may be ligated at its base after any floating rootlets have been gently replaced within the layer apposed, if it can be done without undue tension or compression of the contents of the spinal canal. The deep fascial layer, subcutaneous tissue, and skin should all be apposed with nonabsorbable sutures, and with little or no tension on the suture lines.

Myelomeningoceles, which are covered in the central portion by a fragile membrane, must be approached differently. Once the cuff of cutaneous and subcutaneous tissue is dissected from about the neck, all viable skin is preserved and separated from the membranous sac. That portion of the skin immediately adjacent to the sac, usually poorly supplied with blood vessels, is discarded. The sac, as in the meningocele, is opened at its superior pole, and the dissection carried toward the neural plaque, which can usually be seen through the transparent or translucent membrane in its usual position near the dome or apex of the lesion. One should not attempt to thoroughly dissect free the various components of the neural plaque because of the hazard of injury to the roots and spinal cord. One may, however, using the stimulator and magnification, safely remove a significant amount of membranous tissue without neural injury, so that the mass that is ultimately replaced within the spinal canal is reduced in size, thereby lessening the likelihood of injury to compressed neural tissue from a tense closure and swelling in the early postoperative period. When the vertebral canal is unusually small or shallow, all of the freed neural tissue cannot be safely returned to the canal and must be left in the space created by the incompletely

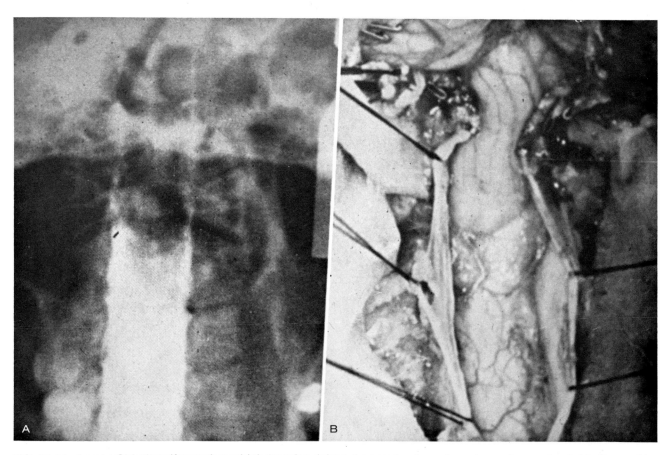

FIG. 22-11. Arnold-Chiari malformation which may be delayed complication of myelomeningocele. A, Myelographic defect; B, appearance at operation.

apposed paraspinal muscles. In such cases an artificial posterior layer of dura may be created from lumbodorsal fascia or any other available fascial layer to prevent escape of cerebrospinal fluid. When the paraspinal muscles are deficient, the defect may be covered by flaps created from lumbodorsal fascia, which may be reflected over the midline. The subcutaneous tissue and skin are closed as for the correction of simple meningocele, except when the rotation of flaps is necessary. Care must be taken to avoid burying cutaneous elements in the wound or dermoid tumor may result.

POSTOPERATIVE CARE AND COMPLICATIONS. Following operation the patient is positioned prone on a Bradford frame or pediatric bed, with an abdominal sling in place to keep the operative site at a level slightly above the foramen magnum, thereby reducing cerebrospinal fluid pressure on the surgical defect until healing is well under way. Lumbosacral wounds are sealed by tightly adherent surgical dressings to prevent contamination. At least daily examinations are performed to determine if there is excessive tension upon the wound, accumulation of cerebrospinal fluid beneath the skin and subcutaneous tissue, or evidence of secondary hydrocephalus. Subcutaneous fluid should be removed by gentle aspiration after the puncture site has been aseptically prepared. Sutures are removed as early as feasible, but usually are kept in place somewhat longer than those in other neurosurgical wounds because of the tension under which these incisions occasionally must be closed.

Complications include leakage of cerebrospinal fluid, wound dehiscence, meningitis and other central nervous system infections, and local superficial wound infections.

Postoperative hydrocephalus, often associated with the Arnold-Chiari malformation, occurs in about 65% of patients with myelomeningoceles and 9% of those with simple meningoceles (Fig. 22-11).[26] When the routine postoperative diagnostic studies indicate progressive hydrocephalus, ventriculography should be performed to evaluate ventricular size and depth of cerebral mantle and, when possible, to locate the site of obstruction. Temporary ventriculostomy, with a plastic pediatric feeding tube inserted through a widened suture or a twist drill hole, may be employed for a few days until it can be determined whether the hydrocephalus will become arrested spontaneously. Drainage should pass into a closed sterile system, with the height of the reservoir adjusted according to cerebrospinal fluid pressure. Prophylactic ampicillin is administered while the ventriculostomy tube is in place and for several days thereafter. Ventriculostomy should be abandoned for a permanent shunt after a few days if it is apparent that hydrocephalus is progressive.

Other complications, which tend to appear later, are the musculoskeletal deformities resulting from paraplegia, urinary infection and renal failure from abnormal sphincter function, pressure sores, infected or ob-

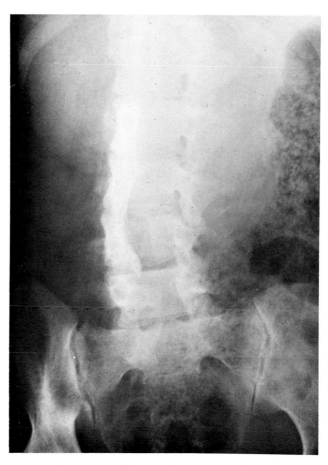

FIG. 22-12. Multiple lumbar neural arch defects. Patient had undergone myelomeningocele repair during childhood and had been paraplegic with sphincter disturbances since.

structed shunts, and delayed progression of a seemingly static motor or sphincter deficit due to scarring at the operative site (Fig. 22-12).

Postoperative care becomes a team effort of neurosurgeon, pediatrician, urologist, orthopedist, psychiatrist, plastic surgeon, social worker, and special education teacher to varying extents. Usually primary neurologic care is supervised by the neurosurgeon or pediatrician, with consultation or treatment provided by the others as indications arise.

INTRATHORACIC MENINGOCELE

Thoracic meningoceles, although rarely producing clinical neurosurgical defect, may display certain features that distinguish them from lumbar and sacral lesions. They are commonly associated with neurofibromatosis. The only clinical manifestations may be those associated with pulmonary dysfunction—dyspnea, chest pain, and cough.

The diagnosis is ordinarily a radiographic one, there being a paravertebral mediastinal mass. Erosion of adjacent vertebral bodies may be seen, and the intervertebral foramen at the level of the deformity is usually enlarged. The diagnosis may be confirmed by myelography or, occasionally, by percutaneous puncture and aspiration of the contents of the sac. Only those meningoceles resulting in pulmonary symptoms and the extraordinary case resulting in neurologic dysfunction require surgical excision.

ANTERIOR SACRAL MENINGOCELE

Anterior sacral meningoceles are rare and result from ventral sacral fusion defects (Fig. 22-13). They may become exceedingly large and may result in increased intracranial tension when intra-abdominal pressure is elevated for any reason. Symptoms include vague or well-defined pelvic pain, disturbances of bowel, bladder, and menstrual function, and, less commonly, alterations in motor and sensory modalities in the lower extremities. The diagnosis can usually be made by the recognition of the large sacral defect on plain roentgenograms. Its full extent and configuration may be established by myelography. When disability is of such extent to warrant surgical treatment, direct excision or a shunting procedure may be performed.

CONGENITAL DERMAL SINUS

Congenital dermal sinuses involving the spine originate during the third to fifth week of embryonic life, when the neural tube is formed by differentiation of neural ectoderm from epithelial ectoderm.[16] Should epithelial closure at that time be incomplete, an externally communicating sinus forms and may extend to any depth toward the central nervous system. Since midline epithelial closure begins in the midportion of the embryo and proceeds in both directions, such defects are most common at the caudal and cranial ends of the spinal axis, with those at the caudal extreme being far more common. Those occurring in the suboccipital region often terminate within the posterior fossa and will not be considered here.

The most frequently encountered congenital dermal sinus, by far, is that occurring in the sacral and coccygeal areas, the pilonidal sinus. It contains hair and keratinous material, often becomes infected, rarely extends to a depth involving the meninges, and is usually excised by a general surgeon when it produces symptoms.

Dermal sinuses involving the spine and its contents are rare in the lumbar and lumbosacral regions and affect the thoracic spine even less frequently. Only a few cases involving the cervical spine have been recorded. They may extend from a point only a few millimeters beneath the skin to inside the dura and, indeed, within the spinal cord. At any point in the course of the sinus, and particularly at its deepest extent, a cystic mass may develop. Those containing only stratified squamous epithelium and epithelial debris are called epidermoid cysts. More common are those surrounding elements of the deepest layers of skin, the dermoid cyst. Occasionally a sinus tract may be the site of more than one cystic dilatation in a "collar-button" configuration.

SYMPTOMS AND PHYSICAL FINDINGS. Examination of the newborn infant may disclose the external communication of the sinus. Being only one or two millimeters in diameter, it can easily be overlooked. The presence of abnormal hair growth or pigmentation in the midline of the back heightens one's suspicion that such a sinus may exist, and inspection of these areas should be particularly thorough. Occasionally the cutaneous opening is discovered only after it has become infected and attention directed to it because of the child's discomfort and the appearance of signs of local inflammation. In an extraordinary patient seen by me, a 23-year-old woman, the outer terminus of the sinus was found during the course of investigation for the cause of low back pain not associated with neurologic symptoms (Fig. 22-14).

Too often the first indication of the presence of a dermal sinus is otherwise unexplained meningitis or symptoms and signs of an intraspinal mass lesion—back pain, paraparesis, disturbances of sphincter function, and reflex and sensory changes below a segmental level. Failure of the cord to migrate in a cephalad direction because of a tethering effect of the sinus and its associated intraspinal cystic mass may produce the first clinical manifestations.

The existence of a dermal sinus should be suspected when meningitis occurs in the absence of systemic infection, cranial or spinal surgery or compound injury, or paranasal sinusitis, otitis, or mastoiditis. The re-

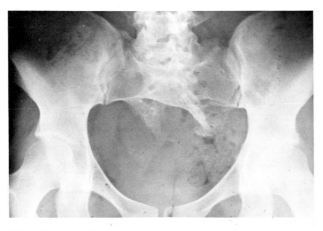

FIG. 22-13. Anterior sacral meningocele. Large bone defect involves primarily right side of sacrum.

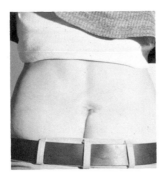

FIG. 22-14. Congenital dermal sinus in adult. Only symptom was nonradiating lumbar pain. There was no history of meningitis and only abnormal physical finding was cutaneous opening surrounded by hair.

sponsible organisms are usually Staph. aureus, E. coli, or H. influenzae.[23] Occasionally aseptic meningitis may follow spontaneous rupture of an intradural cyst.

Signs of an intraspinal tumor with cauda equina or cord compression may be caused by the dermoid or epidermoid cyst or by actual intraspinal abscess formation secondary to contamination from contents of the sinus tract. The mass may be epidural, intradural, or, rarely, intramedullary.

SPECIAL EXAMINATIONS. Radiographs of the lumbar spine may reveal a spina bifida or other neural arch defect at the site of entrance of the sinus into the spinal canal; the dermoid cyst may actually be a segment or two higher within the canal. At the level of the cyst the vertebral canal may be widened and the pedicles flattened. Myelography usually is not necessary because the presence of the sinus, associated with signs of an intraspinal mass or single or recurring attacks of meningitis, makes mandatory the resection of the sinus tract to its innermost extent. Injection of the sinus tract with any dye or radiopaque contrast material should not be performed because of the hazard of introducing infected contents into the epidural or subarachnoid spaces.

OPERATION. It should be emphasized that operation with complete excision of the sinus tract and dermoid or epidermoid cysts with all of their ramifications should be carried out as soon as the diagnosis is made to prevent further episodes of meningitis or enlargement of the cyst. One postpones the operation if there is active meningitis. Surgical excision is deferred until the infection has been successfully treated with antibiotics and sufficient time has elapsed for local inflammation to subside. However, when there are signs of rapidly advancing cord or cauda equina compression, operation becomes imperative even though infection persists.

Preparation of the skin and draping should be carried out as for any laminectomy. Surgical exposure, and the proposed outline of the incision in lumbosacral lesions, should extend for one or two segments below the cutaneous opening and to the level of T12 above, since the sinus tract is virtually always directed diagonally cephalad through the interspinous ligament, with the intraspinal terminal cyst being several segments cephalad to

the external opening (Fig. 22-15). The common site of termination is at the level of the conus.

Prophylactic antibiotic therapy should be instituted at least 24 hours prior to operation. The use of magnification is helpful throughout the operation. It is important to avoid incision through the wall of the sinus as the dissection is carried through the subcutaneous tissues and the lumbodorsal fascia, and as the

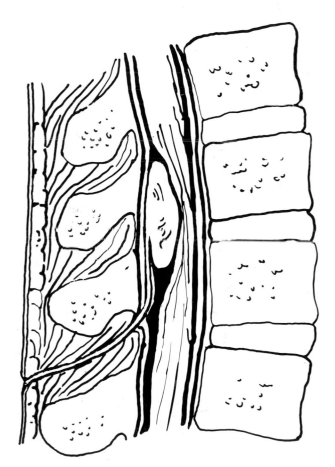

FIG. 22-15. Diagram of sagittal view, congenital lumbar dermal sinus. In lumbar defects intradural termination of sinus may be several segments above cutaneous opening. (Modified from Matson.)

paraspinal muscles are being separated from the spinous processes and laminae. It should be kept in mind that the tract may terminate in a dermoid or epidermoid mass at any point, but it may also continue through a more superficial mass to end in a second cyst outside or within the dura. Therefore one should not be misled into excising a superficial cyst while failing to recognize that the sinus continues, obviously to terminate in a cyst within the spinal canal. Laminectomy should be carried one segment caudad to the point at which the sinus perforates the interspinous ligament, and as far cephalad as is necessary to expose the epidural and intradural portions of the lesion. At any site the tract may terminate as an attenuated sinus or as an epidermoid or dermoid mass. Sinuses penetrating the dura usually do so in or near the midline and extend to any point within the meninges, cauda, or conus. Those rare lesions found in the cervical or upper thoracic spine may actually reach their termination caudad to the external opening.

When infection has not occurred, dissection is usually not difficult because of the absence of adhesions about the sinus and its terminal cyst. After one or more episodes of active inflammation, the existence of adhesions may make complete resection of the cyst so hazardous that a portion of its wall must be left behind. In all other cases removal should be complete to avoid the possibility of recurrent meningitis or secondary cyst formation. The dura should be tightly closed as should the more superficial anatomic layers to prevent escape of cerebrospinal fluid. Antibiotics should be administered for several days following operation.

DIASTEMATOMYELIA

Division of the spinal cord or cauda equina by a midline spicule of bone protruding from the posterior aspects of one or, rarely, more vertebral bodies is termed diastematomyelia. Usually both elements of the divided portion of the cord are completely surrounded by the usual meningeal layers, and the projecting spur, which may be primarily cartilaginous or fibrous rather than osseous, is encased in a layer of dura. Diastematomyelia is not to be confused with diplomyelia, anatomic reduplication of the cord in which there is not vertebral spicule formation, although there may or may not be duplication of the meningeal elements surrounding the divided portion of the cord.[2]

The spicule of osseous or other connective tissue is usually ovoid in configuration and may protrude for varying depths into the lumen of the vertebral canal. It may be attached dorsally to the posterior neural arch. Often one or more posterior elements overlying the diastematomyelia will be bifid with a deficient central element or will display abnormal forms of fusion.[28] The vertebral canal is usually widened for several segments at the level of the spina bifida. Although the inter-

pedicular distances are increased, there is usually no erosion of the pedicles or vertebral bodies as may be seen with intraspinal tumors.[23]

The etiology of diastematomyelia is obscure. Bremer postulated that during the organization of the neural tube from the primitive neuroectoderm in the third to fourth week of embryonal life, aberrant mesodermal cells protrude into ventral neural tissue instead of becoming arranged in a tubular fashion about its periphery.[3] In this central position they persist as a septum of bone or fibrous tissue which may extend for one or more vertebral segments. Other congenital spinal defects are common accompaniments of diastematomyelia. These include kyphosis, hemivertebra, various neural arch defects at unrelated levels, and meningocele and myelomeningocele. Congenital dermal sinus occasionally occurs coincidentally. The condition occurs in females about twice as often as in males.

CLINICAL FEATURES. Symptoms and objective neurologic findings may appear primarily during the course of growth and development or may appear secondarily in a child who seemingly was developing normally. In most cases manifestations are first noted between the ages of 2 and 10.[12] Appearance of symptoms may coincide with onset of exertion of traction upon a tethered cord as the growth of the spine exceeds that of the spinal cord. These include cutaneous abnormalities, spinal deformity, abnormalities of gait and other lower extremity motor changes, and disturbances of the bladder and rectal sphincters. Visible changes in the thoracic or lumbar area include abnormal hair growth, dimpling of the skin, and cutaneous blood vessel malformations; palpable subcutaneous fatty tumors may be present.

Spinal deformity is usually kyphoscoliosis. Often the first evidence of motor change to appear is a disturbance of gait, which may involve one extremity before the other; associated deformities of the feet are common. Hyperactive deep reflexes with extensor plantar responses may occur with thoracic lesions, whereas diminished reflex activity is the result of lesions involving the cauda equina. Sensory changes are less common than are abnormalities of motor function, but may occur in a variety of forms and are often asymmetrical. Urinary incontinence is the most frequently encountered sphincter disturbance and, in many instances, appears in children who were evidently developing normal bladder control.

ROENTGENOGRAPHIC INVESTIGATION. In most instances when the spicule is osseous it may be visualized as an ovoid or, less often, circular density in or near the center of the spinal canal (Figs. 22-16 and 22-17). Tomography may be helpful in identifying the site and configuration of the spur when it is not visualized on routine roentgenograms. When the spicule is primarily fibrous it is not seen on the plain films, and only rarely may a bony spur be seen on films made in the lateral

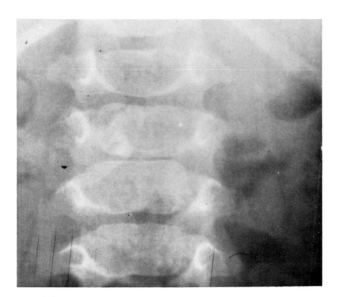

FIG. 22-16. Diastematomyelia at L2 level. Spicule arises lateral to midline.

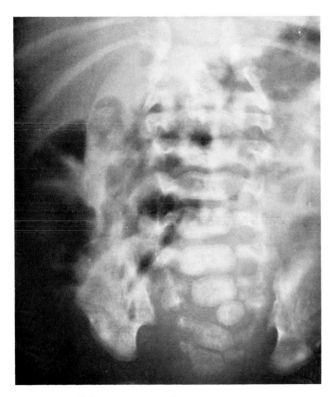

FIG. 22-17. Diastematomyelia at first lumbar level associated with sacral hemivertebrae.

FIG. 22-18. Myelogram in diastematomyelia. Pantopaque column is seen dividing about bony spicule.

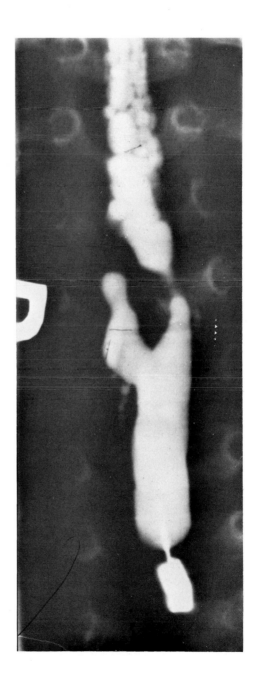

projection. The canal is often widened for some segments above and below the bony abnormality.

Pantopaque myelography is usually necessary to outline the exact size and contour of the lesion and in planning the operation. Ordinarily the contrast material assumes a divided column as it flows past the protruding spicule (Fig. 22-18).

TREATMENT. Treatment consists in removal of the offending spicule of bone and any associated fibrous or cartilaginous tissue contributing to the deformity. Such removal, at least theoretically, prevents further distortion of the upward migrating cord in the growing child. The primary aim of operation is to prevent advancement of the neurologic deficit; reversal of signs probably will not occur. Improvement in sphincter function is more likely to occur than is the return of motor power to the extremities. The only exception to the rule for treating the spicule by laminectomy and surgical excision is the case in which the diagnosis is made incidentally in late childhood or adolescence through roentgenograms made because of suspected injury or other unrelated cause. As long as patients remain free of symptoms or neurologic deficit, they may be re-examined at regular intervals and operation deferred.

Operation is performed with the patient in the prone position and his thighs moderately flexed on the trunk, care being taken to avoid pressure on the thorax or abdomen that would interfere with respiratory exchange or venous return. Endotracheal intubation with assisted respiration is carried out routinely. Transfusion is rarely necessary except in smaller infants.

The proposed midline incision should be of such length to include at least one normal neural arch cephalad and caudad to those anomalous ones at the level of the abnormality. It is not uncommon for two or more arches immediately dorsal to the bony spur to be fused on one side or both. Removal of these laminae, which may have fibrous communications to the underlying dura or even a bony attachment to the spicule, is facilitated and made less hazardous if normal laminae above and below the defect are excised first. As removal of the laminae progresses, adhesions between the dura and the overlying bone must be cautiously separated before the rongeur is applied, to prevent injury. Particular care must be exercised if gentle palpation with a dural separator between the neural arches and the dura indicates there is osseous union between the spicule and the laminae.

Once the adequate dural exposure has been attained, with separation of all fibrous and osseous elements between dura and laminae, the dura above and below the spicule should be incised in the midline. Hendrick believes it is advisable to leave a small cuff of dura immediately surrounding the spur to avoid injury to the underlying neural elements by dissection of the dura and any fibrous adhesions attached to the spur before they are adequately visualized.[12] This method permits thorough inspection of the contents of the dura before lysis of fibrous or vascular communications between bony spicule and cord or cauda equina so that dissection is not begun prematurely. Coagulation of any vessels within the dura should be with the bipolar instrument. The use of magnification and microsurgical instruments is particularly helpful in this phase of the operation. Once the spicule of bone has been isolated it may be removed flush with the underlying vertebral body with a fine-nosed rongeur; any remaining fibrous tissue septum should be carefully excised. The defect in the ventral dural surface requires no special attention; that in the dorsal dural exposure is closed with interrupted fine silk sutures.

Failures of surgical treatment, with subsequent progression of neural defects, have been attributed to incomplete removal of the bony spur or an associated fibrous septum.[12] Postoperative appearance of hydrocephalus or the Arnold-Chiari malformation is rare except in patients with coincidental myelomeningocele.[23]

NEURENTERIC CYSTS

Neurenteric, or enterogenous, cysts may occur when the mesodermal elements forming the supportive structures about the spinal cord fail to develop normally and allow persistent juxtaposition of entodermal and neural ectodermal derivatives.[23] If this connection persists, entodermal tissue may be carried dorsally into the spinal canal to involve neural structures. These neurenteric communications, and the resulting cysts, while exceedingly rare, are most often found in the lower cervical and upper thoracic areas, the level at which the primitive lung bud arises from the foregut.[15]

The entire neurenteric fistula may persist as a partially patent tract or as a fibrous connecting stalk, or only a portion may remain as a solitary cyst lined with a layer of cuboidal or columnar epithelium. The tract or cyst may produce in the vertebral body a defect that persists and is evident on spinal roentgenograms, or there may be widening of the vertebral body secondary to bony proliferation in an effort to obliterate the vertebral defect once occupied by the tract.[23]

Intraspinal neurenteric cysts may be epidural, intradural and extramedullary, or intramedullary; they are generally situated anteriorly in the spinal canal, and produce symptoms and neurologic signs appropriate to the segmental level involved and degree of cord compression. Cysts anterior to the spine may cause difficulty in swallowing or tracheal obstruction.

DIAGNOSIS. The possibility of an intraspinal neurenteric cyst should be entertained when there are clinical manifestations of cervical or thoracic spinal cord compression, particularly if there has been chronic meningismus or episodes of aseptic meningitis. Routine spinal roentgenograms may disclose a persistent vertebral body defect, an unusually broad vertebra, or, rarely, a bony spicule projecting from the body of the vertebra. With myelography, the lesion can usually be outlined and its relationship to the cord and meninges established.[27] When there is a persistent tract anterior to the spinal canal, it may be outlined by the contrast material.

TREATMENT. An attempt should be made to surgically excise the cyst and its contents, preferably using microsurgical techniques. Because of its anterior relationship to the spinal cord, particularly when extensive adhesions are present, complete removal may not be possible. In such instances the contents of the cyst should be evacuated, and the portion of the capsule that

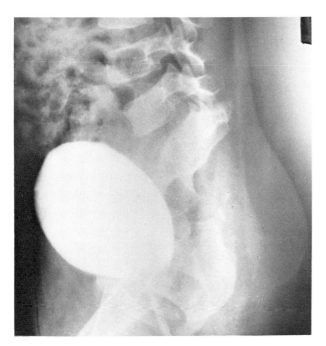

FIG. 22-19. Sacral agenesis. Contrast material is within urinary bladder.

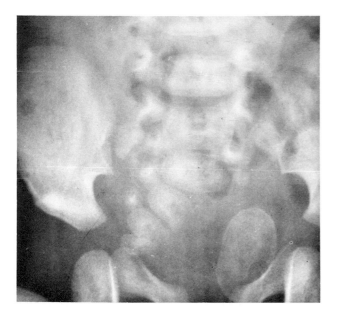

FIG. 22-20. Sacral dysgenesis. Abnormal segments take form of hemivertebrae.

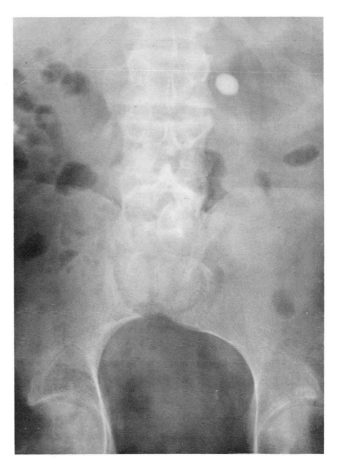

FIG. 22-21. Sacral dysgenesis. Only cephalad sacral segments are formed.

SACRAL AGENESIS

One or more vertebrae may be partially or completely absent. Except in anencephalic monsters, in which the vertebrae most often missing are cervical, those usually absent are lumbar or sacral. Congenital absence of the sacrum rarely occurs as a solitary defect, but usually accompanies other congenital abnormalities of the spine (Figs. 22-19 to 22-21). The iliac wings may be fused posteriorly or may simply be connected by a bridge of connective tissue.[31] The rami of the pubis are ordinarily separated, allowing the ischial bones to evert and the acetabula to face posteriorly rather than laterally.[31] There is no specific treatment.

ANOMALIES OF THE CRANIOVERTEBRAL JUNCTION AND UPPER CERVICAL SPINE

Various congenital deformities occur at the junction of the skull with the spine and in the upper cervical spine which, because of their location, may produce

can be removed without injury to the cord or its vascular supply should be excised. The dura should be closed when feasible. If there is a second cyst in the neck, mediastinum, or thoracic or peritoneal cavities, it may be excised at a separate operation.

symptoms quite unlike those seen in other portions of the spinal axis. Certain anomalies in this region rarely or never are symptomatic and are discovered incidentally on radiographic examinations.

Occipital Vertebra

The occipital bone in man is formed from parachordal cartilage which unites as a single basal plate. In this mass three ossification centers develop which surround the posterior portion of the foramen magnum. Assimilation of the most posterior hypoglossal sclerotome results in the formation of an anomalous occipital vertebra, a bony structure surrounding the foramen magnum.[37] The anterior portion of this ring may be fused to the anterior rim of the foramen magnum, and there may be transverse processes that are fused to the skull and do not contain a foramen for the vertebral artery. The occipital vertebra may be of sufficient mass to encroach on the foramen magnum, particularly in its anterior portion, and compress the lower medulla and upper spinal cord. Symptomatic manifestations of this anomaly, along with others in the craniovertebral area, may not become evident until adult life.

Atlanto-occipital Fusion

Atlanto-occipital fusion differs from occipital vertebra in that some of the normal joints are present and there are foramina for the vertebral arteries within the transverse processes (Fig. 22-22).[37] There may be associated basilar invagination with encroachment on the foramen magnum and its contents. A degree of assimilation and fusion in a combination of forms may occur with the anterior and posterior arches and lateral masses being involved. The Arnold-Chiari malformation is present in about 25% of cases,[24] and cerebellar and cranial nerve dysfunction may be observed.[20] Syringomyelia or hydromyelia also may be present. Long fiber tract involvement occurs in a significant number of cases.

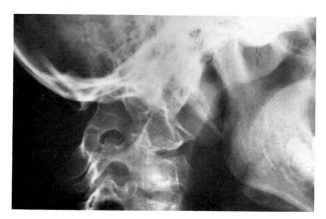

FIG. 22-22. Congenital fusion of occiput and atlas.

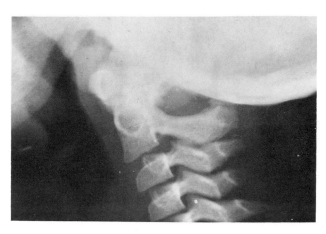

FIG. 22-23. Absent neural arch, C1, with posterior osseous tubercle.

A craniovertebral congenital defect should be considered, along with other diagnostic possibilities, in patients with symptoms and findings referable to the cerebellum, lower cranial nerves, or upper spinal cord, and radiologic diagnostic studies should proceed in a logical and orderly manner. Initially routine films and tomograms of the area should be made and especially inspected for abnormal bony masses, pathologic cranial or vertebral fusion, or failure of normal fusion (Fig. 22-23). Increased dimensions of the cervical spinal canal suggest the presence of syringomyelia or hydromyelia. Pantopaque myelography is usually sufficient to confirm the diagnosis of the displaced tonsils of the Arnold-Chiari malformation or syringo- or hydromyelia with its widened spinal cord, but examination with the patient in both prone and supine positions may be necessary.

Although the cervical cord of the patient with hydromyelia appears distended during Pantopaque myelography, with air myelography performed with the patient in the sitting position the cord is narrower than usual—the "collapsing cord" of hydromyelia or syringomyelia.[6,9,35] Finally, vertebral angiography with demonstration of the posterior inferior cerebellar arteries may be useful in confirming the presence and extent of Arnold-Chiari malformation when other methods have been unsatisfactory.

Treatment of those anomalies of the craniovertebral region characterized by bony encroachment on the foramen magnum or spinal canal or intramedullary distention of the spinal cord usually consists in appropriate surgical decompression. Dissection always should be considered with extreme care because of the likelihood that neural and vascular structures occupy aberrant positions.

Atlantoaxial Fusion

Pathologic postnatal fusion of the first and second vertebrae may be due to undersegmentation of the ossification centers, usually one in each lateral mass of the atlas and one or two in the arch, with one ossification center in the body of the axis and two in its arch. Fusion is complete or incomplete, with varying adjacent positions of the vertebrae being involved. The condition is ordinarily asymptomatic, discovered incidentally, and does not require treatment.

Anomalies of the Dens

The dens, which arises from two ossification centers, may display several congenital malformations. It may never form or may be hypoplastic. Its tip may form but remain separated from the major portion of the dens —the ossiculum terminale. Finally, the dens may form completely but remain ununited with the body of the axis, the os odontoideum. Each of these anomalies permits subluxation of the atlas upon the axis with resulting compression of the spinal cord. Diagnosis can usually be made by examination of the routine roentgenograms and tomograms. The most satisfactory and safest treatment is posterior fusion of the occiput to C1 and C2. Greenberg and his associates advocate transoral decompression followed by posterior fusion.[10] Anterior decompression combined with fusion from this approach has attained less favor. Decompressive cervical laminectomy, which may or may not be combined with suboccipital laminectomy, is strongly contraindicated because it increases the degree of instability and, consequently, the degree of the neurologic deficit.

TIGHT FILUM TERMINALE

Jones and Love[18] and, later, Hendrick[13] have described a syndrome that is due to congenital or acquired tension of the filum terminale. Symptoms include motor and sensory defects, sphincter dysfunction, and kyphoscoliosis, and they occur in the absence of any cutaneous lesion. Diagnosis is made by myelographic demonstration that the conus is situated at an unusually caudad level (it should have advanced to at least L3 level by the age of six months) when no other abnormality is shown. Treatment consists of surgical section of the filum. Hendrick reports that motor and sensory defects may improve significantly after operation, but significant return of sphincter function cannot be expected.[13] It is the opinion of James and Lassman that the syndrome of the tight filum terminale does not exist as a primary entity, but always accompanies some other abnormality.[17]

KLIPPEL-FEIL SYNDROME

The Klippel-Feil syndrome comprises such a variety of primary anomalies of the cervical and thoracic spine, along with other secondary anomalies, that a classic description of the condition no longer is realistic.

Basically there is a reduction in the number of cervical vertebrae with rarely complete absence of the cervical spine. There is fusion of three or more cervical vertebrae (or what may appear to be cervical vertebrae) with partial or complete obliteration of the intervertebral spaces (Fig. 22-24). There may be multiple ribs in the shortened neck, along with reduction in the number of thoracic vertebrae, indicating that seeming cervical vertebrae are actually anomalous thoracic vertebrae.[14] The cervical spinal canal may be widened and the spinous processes and, in exceptional cases, the vertebral bodies bifid or otherwise malformed. Other skeletal abnormalities that sometimes occur are basilar impression, atlanto-occipital assimilation, and atlantoaxial subluxation.

The clinical appearance is that of an absent neck, or of a shortened neck that is unusually broad or webbed. The hairline is abnormally low and there is decreased range of motion of the neck. There may be kyphosis or torticollis and abnormally elevated scapulae (Sprengel's deformity).

The most significant symptoms ascribed to the syndrome are dysphagia and interference with breathing,

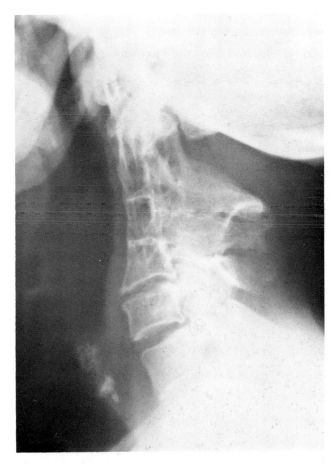

FIG. 22-24. Congenital fusion, C1–C2–C3–C4. Absent neural arch of C1 (Klippel-Feil deformity with atlanto-occipital fusion).

either of which may be life-threatening. Rarely does spinal cord or nerve root compression necessitate decompressive laminectomy or foramenotomy. Patients with the Klippel-Feil syndrome are particularly susceptible to spinal cord injury, often from seemingly trivial forces.

BLOCK VERTEBRAE

Congenital vertebral synostosis, or block vertebrae, results from faulty embryologic vertebral segmentation. There is abnormal intervertebral disc formation and two or more adjacent segments may be involved; it is more common in the cervical area (Fig. 22-25).

In contradistinction to the Klippel-Feil syndrome, this condition usually has no clinical manifestations, but is discovered coincidentally on radiographs made because of trauma or for other clinical reasons. An exception is the rare case in which the abnormal segmentation is not symmetrical with involvement of more than two segments; in such instances scoliosis or kyphosis may result.

The vestige of the intervertebral disc may be partially evident or entirely absent. In the latter situation the trabeculation of the contiguous vertebrae may appear continuous. There may or may not be fusion of the laminae or spinous processes, and the intervertebral foramina between the involved vertebrae are reduced in diameter.

Individuals with block vertebrae formation may be unusually susceptible to fracture-dislocation of the spine at the sites of articulation between normal and fused segments.

CORONAL CLEFT VERTEBRAE

Coronal cleft vertebral bodies result when there is delayed fusion of the dorsal and ventral ossification centers (Fig. 22-26). In some cases the cleft may represent persistence of notochord.[5] One or multiple vertebral bodies may be involved, usually in the lumbar region. The abnormality is observed predominantly in males and usually disappears during the first few weeks of life. The coronal cleft vertebral body is of no clinical significance, but is often seen in association with other congenital defects, particularly chondrodystrophica calcificans congenita.[5]

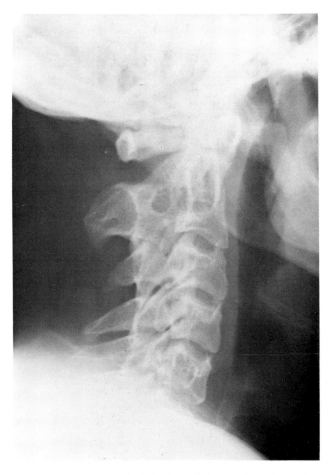

FIG. 22-25. Congenital fusion, C2–C3. (Block vertebrae.)

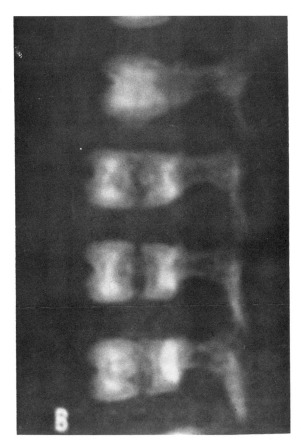

FIG. 22-26. Coronal cleft vertebrae.

SAGITTAL CLEFT VERTEBRAE

Various defects in the configuration of the vertebral bodies may result from persistence of remnants of the notochord. When such remnants extend the length of the vertebral body and are centrally disposed, the sagittally cleft vertebral body with its characteristic butterfly deformity, best visualized in the frontal projection, results (Fig. 22-27). It is rarely associated with clinical manifestations.

HEMIVERTEBRA

Fetal chondrification centers in the vertebral body developing unilaterally or asymmetrically result in hemivertebra (Fig. 22-28). When the abnormality occurs in the thoracic area, abnormalities in rib segmentation are usually associated and congenital hypoplasia of one lung may be observed (Fig. 22-29). Hemivertebra involving only one or two vertebral bodies usually does not produce any clinically evident skeletal deformity or neurologic deficit, but involvement at multiple levels may result in shortening of the trunk, grossly apparent deformity of the spine, and clinical manifestations of spinal cord compression or distortion. Surgical treatment is of little avail, but orthopaedic treatment of scoliosis in certain cases may be helpful.

CHONDRO-OSTEODYSTROPHY (MORQUIO'S DISEASE)

Failure of normal development of epiphyseal cartilage and of cartilaginous bone results in dwarfism due mainly to reduced spinal growth and kyphosis.[33] The principal spinal deformity is usually at the thoracolumbar junction, although in some cases obvious shortening of the cervical portion of the spine may be present. The characteristic radiograph discloses vertebral bodies of diminished height and an anteriorly projecting beak-like deformity. Symptoms often aren't evident until the child begins to walk. Rarely is decompressive laminectomy or a procedure directed toward correcting the scoliosis indicated or of benefit.

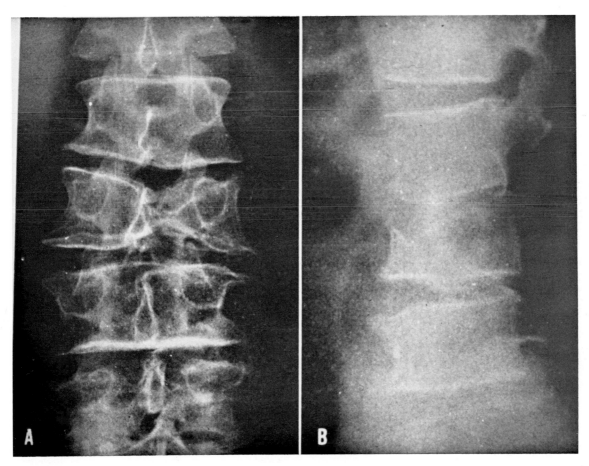

FIG. 22-27. Sagittal cleft vertebrae.

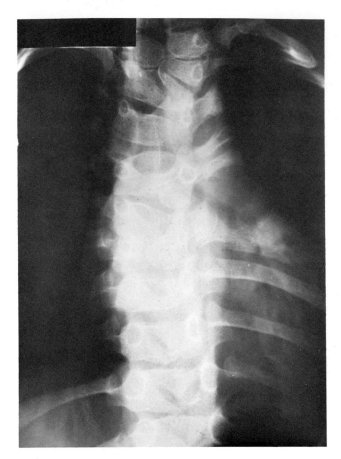

FIG. 22-28. Thoracic hemivertebra with neural arch defect.

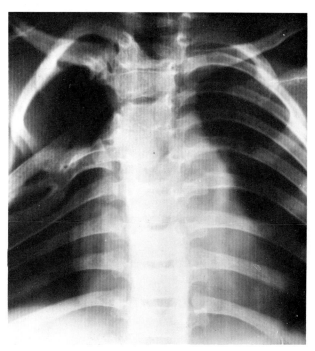

FIG. 22-29. Thoracic hemivertebra with rib fusion.

HURLER'S SYNDROME (MUCOPOLYSACCHARIDOSIS I)

Severe thoracolumbar kyphosis and gibbus formation may accompany Hurler's syndrome owing to wedging deformities of the anterior portions of the vertebral bodies. Rarely does the deformity produce signs of spinal cord compression or distortion, and the short natural history of the disease, along with the fact that other features of the syndrome usually demand prior attention, makes surgical treatment of spinal deformities ineffectual and unwarranted.

ACHONDROPLASIA

Abnormalities of ossification, particularly within long bones and beginning in fetal life, may result in dwarfism that is primarily due to reduced length of the extremities, although the spine is shortened to a varying degree. Strong hereditary factors exist. The lumbar area is most involved, there being an increase in the size of the intervertebral cartilages with reduction in mass of the vertebral bodies. The pedicles are shortened and the spinal canal is narrowed in all planes.[4] Stenosis of the canal, which may or may not be accompanied by kyphoscoliosis, may result in spinal cord compression requiring decompressive laminectomy.[33] Communicating hydrocephalus is a rare complication and may be treated by a valve-regulated shunting device.[23]

OSTEOGENESIS IMPERFECTA

The characteristic radiographic change in osteogenesis imperfecta is osteoporosis; both cortices and spongiosa are defective. In extreme instances there may be compression of the central portions of vertebral bodies with relative increase in the depth of the central segments of adjacent intervertebral discs. The resulting deformity may produce an hourglass configuration of the involved vertebral bodies whose deepest dimensions are usually at the anterior and posterior margins. It has been postulated that small fractures, not radiographically detectable, may contribute to the vertebral deformities, since not all vertebrae are involved and those that are involved are not uniformly distributed.[5] Various abnormal curvatures of the spine may accompany osteogenesis imperfecta, but only those that result in neurologic deficit require surgical treatment.

References

1. Anderson FM: Occult spinal dysraphism. J Pediatr *73*:163–177, 1968.
2. Benstead JG: A case of diastematomyelia. J Path Bact *66*:553–557, 1953.

3. Bremer JL: Dorsal intestinal fistula; accessory neurenteric canal; diastematomyelia. Arch Path 54:132-138, 1952.

4. Caffey J: Pediatric X-ray Diagnosis. Vol 2, 6th ed, Chicago, Year Book Medical Publishers, 1972.

5. Caffey J: Achondroplasia of pelvis and lumbosacral spine. Some roentgenographic features. Am J Roentgenol 84:49-51, 1958.

6. Conway LW: Radiographic studies of syringomyelia. The hydrodynamics of the syrinx in relation to therapy. Trans Amer Neurol Assoc 86:205-206, 1961.

7. Foltz EL, Kronmal R, Shurtleff DB: To treat or not to treat: a neurosurgeon's perspective of myelomeningocele. *In* Clinical Neurosurgery. Vol 20. Edited by RH Wilkins. Baltimore, Williams and Wilkins, 1973.

8. Freeman JM: To treat or not to treat: ethical dilemmas of treating the infant with a myelomeningocele. *In* Clinical Neurosurgery. Vol 20. Edited by RH Wilkins. Baltimore, Williams and Wilkins, 1973.

9. Gardner WJ: Hydrodynamic mechanism of syringomyelia: its relation to myelocele. J Neurol Neurosurg Psychiat 28:247-259, 1965.

10. Greenberg AD, Scoville WB, and Davey LM: Transoral decompression of atlanto-axial dislocation due to odontoid hypoplasia. Report of two cases. J Neurosurg 28:266-269, 1968.

11. Griscom NT, Harris GBC, Umansky I, et al: Internal radiographic anatomy of the intra-uterine fetus. Progr Pediatr Radiol 3:344-371, 1970.

12. Hendrick EB: On diastematomyelia. *In* Progress in Neurological Surgery. Vol 4. Basel, Karger, 1971.

13. Hendrick EB, Hoffman HJ, Humphreys R: Tethered conus medullaris in children. Presented at the 34th annual meeting of the American Academy of Neurological Surgery, Oxford, England, Sept. 6, 1972.

14. Hinck VC: Congenital Abnormalities. *In* The Spinal Cord, 2nd Ed. Edited by G Austin. Springfield, Illinois, Charles C Thomas, 1972.

15. Holcomb GW Jr, Matson DD: Thoracic neurenteric cyst. Surgery, 35:115-121, 1954.

16. Ingraham FC, and Matson DD: Neurosurgery of Infancy and Childhood. Springfield, Illinois, Charles C Thomas, 1954.

17. James CCM, Lassman LP: Spinal Dysraphism: Spina Bifida Occulta. London, Butterworths, 1972.

18. Jones PH, Love JG: Tight filum terminale. Arch Surg 73:556-566, 1956.

19. Lichtenstein BW: Spinal dysraphism. Spina bifida and myelodysplasia. Arch Neurol Psychiat 44:792-810, 1940.

20. Logue V: Syringomyelia: a radiodiagnostic and radiotherapeutic saga. Clin Radiol 22:2-16, 1971.

21. Lorber J: Family history of spina bifida cystica. Pediatrics 35:589-595, 1965.

22. Lorber J: Results of treatment of myelomeningocele. An analysis of 524 unselected cases, with special reference to possible selection for treatment. Develop Med Child Neurol 13:209-303, 1971.

23. Matson DD: Neurosurgery of Infancy and Childhood. Springfield, Illinois, Charles C Thomas, 1969.

24. McRae DL, Standen J: Roentgenologic findings in syringomyelia and hydromyelia. Amer J Roentgen 89:695-703, 1966.

25. Meacham WF: Congenital malformations. *In* Pediatric Neurosurgery. Edited by IJ Jackson and RK Thompson. Springfield, Illinois, Charles C Thomas, 1959.

26. Meacham WF, Dickens RD Jr: Midline fusion defects and defects of formation. *In* Neurological Surgery. Edited by JR Youmans. Philadelphia, WB Saunders, 1973.

27. Neuhauser EBD, Harris GB, Berrett A: Roentgenographic features of neurenteric cysts. Amer J Roentgen 79:235-240, 1958.

28. Neuhauser EBD, Wittenborg MH, Dehlinger K: Diastematomyelia: transfixation of cord or cauda equina with congenital anomalies of spine. Radiology 54:659-664, 1950.

29. Patten BM: Human Embryology. 1st ed., Philadelphia, Blakiston, 1946.

30. Patten BM: Overgrowth of the neural tube in young human embryos. Anat Rec 113:381-393, 1952.

31. Potter EL: Pathology of the Fetus and the Infant. 2nd ed, Chicago, Year Book Medical Publishers, 1961.

32. Record RG, McKeown T: Congenital malformations in the central nervous system. I. A survey of 930 cases. Brit J Sociol 3:183-219, 1949.

33. Rubin A, Friedenberg ZB: Musculoskeletal system. *In* Handbook of Congenital Malformations. Edited by A Rubin. Philadelphia, WB Saunders, 1967.

34. Shillito J Jr: Surgical approaches to spina bifida and myelomeningocele. *In* Clinical Neurosurgery. Vol 20. Edited by J Shillito, Jr. Baltimore, Williams and Wilkins, 1973.

35. Wickbom I, Hanafee W: Soft tissue masses immediately below the foramen magnum. Acta Radiol (Diagn) 1:647-658, 1963.

36. Zachary RB: An appraisal of the surgery for meningocele. *In* Clinical Neurosurgery. Vol 13. Edited by J Shillito, Jr. Baltimore, Williams and Wilkins, 1966.

37. Zingesser LH: Radiological aspects of anomalies of the upper cervical spine and craniovertebral junction. *In* Clinical Neurosurgery. Vol 20, Edited by RH Wilkins. Baltimore, Williams and Wilkins, 1973.

Section VI

Tumors

23

Compressive Lesions at the Foramen Magnum

VALENTINE LOGUE

THE FORAMEN magnum is best regarded as a short tunnel with walls of varying length, forming the uppermost extension of the vertebral canal, rather than as a simple hole in the skull. It is roughly oval in shape, narrower in front than behind, and in vertical extent ranges from about 4 mm. anteriorly, where it is formed by the margin of the basiocciput, to roughly 1 cm. laterally opposite the articular masses, and narrowing posteriorly to 4 to 6 mm. as the rolled margin of the occipital squama.

The structures passing through the foramen are shown diagramatically in Figure 23-1.

SITES OF COMPRESSION. Because of the capacious subarachnoid space, a tumor originating in the foramen magnum may have extended upward into the posterior fossa or downward into the canal or, indeed, in both directions before it has reached a size capable of compromising the neuraxis. Similarly a tumor that originates in the posterior fossa adjacent to the foramen magnum may extend downward to compress the neural structures in the canal (craniospinal), and in the same way a primarily spinal lesion may extend upward through the foramen magnum (spinocranial). We will discuss here not only tumors originating directly at the foramen magnum, but also craniospinal and spinocranial tumors that have extended to compress nervous structures within the foramen.

TYPES OF COMPRESSIVE LESION

Conditions encountered within the foramen magnum are numerous and

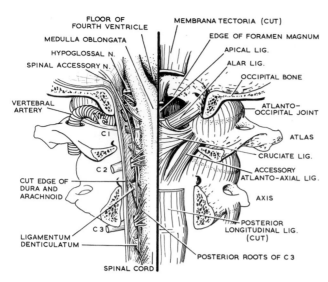

FIG. 23-1. Structures passing through foramen magnum.

varied, but the number found with any frequency in clinical practice is relatively small.

About one-third of all primary tumors of the foramen magnum are intradural and extramedullary, mainly meningiomas and neurofibromas, so that complete surgical extirpation is often feasible. Following is a partial list of tumors that occur in the foramen magnum.

Intradural tumors
  Intramedullary
    Glioma of medulla oblongata and spinal cord
      Astrocytoma
      Ependymoma
      Glioblastoma
      Medulloblastoma
      Hemangioblastoma
  Fourth ventricular tumors
    Craniospinal, consisting of a protruding mass that herniates through the foramen magnum to compress medulla and spinal cord
      Astrocytoma (often cystic)
      Ependymoma
      Papilloma
      Hemangioblastoma
  Extramedullary
    Meningioma
    Neurofibroma
    Schwannoma
    Cysts
      Ependymal
      Enterogenous
      Teratomatous
      Cholesteatoma
      Dermoid
      Aneurysm of vertebral body
Extradural tumors
  Meningioma
  Neurofibroma
  Neurofibrosarcoma
Bony anomalies
  Assimilation of the atlas (with or without dislocation of the atlas; with or without dens separation)
    Basilar invagination
    Hyperplasia of occipital bone and/or articulations
Tumors from bony wall
  Basiocciput
  Jugular process
  Occipital squama
  Atlas
  Dens
    Chordoma
    Chondroma
    Chondrosarcoma
    Metastasis
    Sarcoma
Chiari malformation
  Syringomyelia

DIAGNOSIS

Tumors in the foramen magnum are so uncommon (forming about 2.5% of all spinal tumors) that a surgeon sees only a handful of cases in an active lifetime. This unfamiliarity, combined with the curious presentation of some of the lesions, has given the diagnosis of foramen magnum tumors a sinister reputation.

Symptomatology

Intramedullary Neoplasms

Intrinsic tumors of the medullary-spinal cord junction produce a wide and patchy involvement of cranial nerve and long tracts without raised pressure and their symptomatology is exemplified in the history of Case 1, page 253.

Craniospinal Tumors

The craniospinal group of tumors, usually downward herniating fourth ventricular neoplasms, do not present particular problems in diagnosis. In 90% of cases, intracranial tension rises, demanding investigation on its own account, and the spinal cord signs are mild or absent. Contrast studies demonstrate a lesion low in the posterior fossa, and this finding, coupled with the presence of severe neck pain and/or spinal cord signs, suggests extension of the tumor to the foramen magnum.

Extramedullary Tumors

FORAMEN MAGNUM AND SPINOCRANIAL TUMORS. These tumors are characteristically asymmetrical because they usually arise to one side of the midline. Meningiomas commonly grow from the dura surrounding the entrance of the vertebral artery into the spinal canal, that is, anterolaterally, whereas neurofibromas growing intradurally or extradurally from nerve roots are again situated to one or other side of the spinal cord. It is this extramedullary group that causes the major difficulties in diagnosis.

Lateral and Anterolateral Tumors. A common pattern of evolution may be discerned in about two-thirds of the patients. Pain, a common symptom, is usually due to stretch of the C2 root (the first cervical root frequently having no posterior ramus), and may be the sole symptom, without any physical signs, for months or even one or two years before objective neurologic disturbance appears. If the tumor does not come into contact with the C2 root and so causes no pain, it may grow quite large before symptoms of cord compression appear, at which time the syndrome may progress quickly, leaving the patient quadriparetic, often with respiratory difficulties, in a relatively short space of time.

Pain is usually referred to the neck or subocciput, and sometimes to the occiput. It is nagging, with paroxysmal exacerbations, often made worse by movements of the head, or by coughing, sneezing, and straining, and usually is worse at night.

The next symptom noted is paresthesia, expressed as tingling, "pins and needles," a sensation of numbness or wetness, or peculiar perversions of heat and cold felt in the ipsilateral upper limb.

After a variable period weakness ensues, usually with spasticity (less often hypotonia) in the same arm, but later spreading to involve first the ipsilateral and then the contralateral leg.

Sometimes the pattern is reversed, with symptoms appearing in the leg and spreading proximally to the ipsilateral arm and then to the opposite leg.

By the time the diagnosis is made, a fairly typical picture often can be recognized, and consists of: (1) painful limitation of neck movement; (2) a tri- or quadriparesis more marked on the side ipsilateral to the tumor, with the arm more involved than the leg; (3) a zone of spinothalamic loss, often suspended with its upper level in the cervical region, usually contralateral, suggesting a Brown-Séquard picture; and (4) joint position sense may be reduced, but only mildly, in the ipsilateral limb.

Anterior Tumors. With tumors growing directly anterior, and this is a rare situation, tract involvement tends to affect the limbs bilaterally, and although some asymmetry may still be discerned, the more frank Brown-Séquard appearance tends to be lost.

Other symptoms and signs of these anterolateral and anterior tumors are: (1) trigeminal pain, sometimes paroxysmal, with hypalgesia from pressure on the descending spinal tract and nucleus of the nerve; (2) involvement of the spinal accessory in about one-third of cases, usually mild, but impaired function of other cranial nerves, including the hypoglossal, is uncommon; (3) in this group of cases, raised intracranial pressure is infrequent, occurring in only about 10% of cases.

Posterior Tumors. In tumors growing posteriorly at the foramen, nuchal pain is again frequent. Paresthesia is a common early symptom, is felt often bilaterally in the arms, and is associated early on with reduction of joint position sense, particularly in the hands but extending proximally. In extreme cases this may lead to a pseudo-athetosis, in addition to the tri- or quadriparetic features seen with the anterior tumors.

Extradural Tumors

Tumors in this situation tend to be either extradural neurofibromas or extensions from adjacent bone, the latter frequently being malignant, chordoma or metastasis. Signs of spinal cord compression are similar to those occurring with intradural extramedullary tumors, except for speed of progression.

Differential Diagnosis

In the absence of the foregoing basic symptom patterns, particularly with extramedullary neoplasm, the diagnosis is more difficult and may also be obscured and confused. For instance, neck pain may be relieved for a time by conservative measures, such as traction or the wearing of a collar, suggesting a mechanical disturbance of the cervical discs and joints and diverting attention away from the intraspinal lesion.

Persistence of cervical pain without any physical signs, and sometimes with free movement of the neck, leads to a suspicion that the symptoms may have a psychologic basis, and many patients are dubbed hysterical until neurologic signs appear.

The physical signs may fluctuate considerably over the short or the long term. For example, there are many records of patients who have been rendered almost quadriparetic, only to recover sufficiently in a few months to resume normal activity before deteriorating again; thus multiple sclerosis is a common initial diagnosis.

The majority of these tumors occur in middle life, when cervical spondylosis is rife and the latter's coincidental association with the foramen magnum tumor is quite likely. Thus a diagnosis of spondylotic myelopathy may well be made if the contrast material is screened only up to the foramen magnum and not through it.

Wasting of the small muscles of the hand unilaterally or, more often, bilaterally occurs in about one-third to one-half of benign intradural extramedullary tumors of the foramen magnum, so as to suggest that the site of cord involvement is in the lower cervical region. If cervical spondylosis is shown, the true site of the lesion may be missed, particularly when Pantopaque is not screened actually through the foramen magnum. This may lead to inappropriate operative measures at a lower level.

Wasting of the small muscles of the hand in these patients has been ascribed to involvement of the anterior spinal artery by Symonds, Meadows, and Taylor,[6] and by subsequent authors, but this does not explain all cases, as it has also been observed in lesions lying directly lateral to the cord, which would be incapable of contact with the artery.

The slightly differing and varied features of the Chiari malformation leading to difficulty in diagnosis are described in detail on page 268.

Radiologic Diagnosis

Plain roentgenograms of the skull and cervical spine (with tomography) may show:

1. Bony anomalies (to be described later) such as assimilation of the atlas; dislocation of the occipitoatlo-axial joints with or without assimilation of the atlas; and fusion of vertebrae.
2. Destruction of bone by tumors in the vicinity.
3. Enlarged intervertebral foramen of the occipito-atloid and possibly atlo-axial joint.

In many cases of benign extramedullary tumors, no abnormal features are noted on plain radiography.

Contrast Studies

Myelography by the lumbar route is the basic initial investigation; the cisternal route, when a foramen magnum lesion is suspected, is best avoided.

In performing myelography, it is essential to examine the foramen magnum with the patient both prone and supine. An anxious desire to prevent entry of contrast material into the head, with possible scattering in the posterior fossa, may prevent the Pantopaque from running sufficiently high and the tumor may be missed. However, several techniques to delineate the foramen magnum but avoiding this dissemination of contrast within the intracranial subarachnoid space have been described, a recent one being by Legré et al.[4] Usually a rounded obstruction is seen when the patient is prone, but in some cases Pantopaque may run around

one or both sides of the tumor, apparently demonstrating no block, and it is only with the patient supine that a filling defect is revealed; in these cases the defect is usually the backward displaced spinal cord.

It is important, however, that the upper level of these lesions be delineated (as will be emphasized in the surgical aspects later), and if the contrast material cannot be encouraged to run up past the lesion and then brought down again to cap it, Pantopaque ventriculography or, perhaps, air myelography may be needed to show its cranial extent.

Air Myelography

Air myelography, along with tomography, complements positive contrast myelography and may demonstrate the total extent of an extramedullary tumor; it is also the best method for delineating intrinsic swelling of the cord produced by an intramedullary neoplasm.

Ventriculography

Particularly in the presence of raised intracranial pressure, ventriculography with air, possibly followed by Pantopaque, is the best method of outlining the fourth ventricle and showing the presence of a craniospinal lesion arising within it and herniating downward through the foramen magnum.

Arteriography

Carotid arteriography is of help in demonstrating hydrocephalus, particularly in the craniospinal lesions, when the outlet of the fourth ventricle may be blocked and intracranial pressure is raised (90%), as well as in the 10% of spinocranial lesions causing increased tension.

External Carotid Selective Arteriography

This study may reveal the attachment of meningiomas in the vicinity of the foramen magnum supplied by the meningeal branches of the ascending pharyngeal and occipital arteries.

Vertebral Arteriography

Conditions confirmed or excluded by this study are aneurysm (rare), spinal cord or medullary hemangioblastoma; displacement of the vertebral trunk (and anterior spinal artery) by an extramedullary lesion in its vicinity and its course in relationship to extradural masses; lesions within the fourth ventricle as demonstrated by arterial and venous displacement; tumor circulation; and meningioma attachments to the dura in the vicinity of the foramen magnum, supplied by its anterior or posterior meningeal arteries.

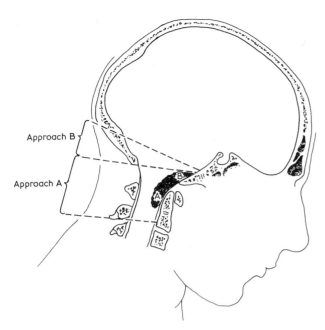

FIG. 23-2. Approach A gives access through laminectomy of C1 and C2, whereas approach B requires a full posterior craniectomy on one or both sides.

It is our practice to employ positive contrast myelography with vertebral arteriography routinely. In most cases the essential information is supplied by these two tests, but if the site and nature of the lesion should remain in doubt, air myelography is next employed, and finally ventriculography using air or positive contrast.

GENERAL MANAGEMENT

In managing a patient with suspected foramen magnum tumor, the observation of certain simple rules may be helpful:

1. Radiographic study of the foramen magnum area, as outlined in the preceding section. The upper level of the tumor should be shown.

2. At operation, when the dura is open, the head should be extended so that the tension on the medulla and spinal cord is relaxed, particularly in the case of anterior masses.

3. If the tumor extends through the foramen magnum into the posterior fossa for a distance greater than 4 or 5 mm., exposure of the posterior fossa is combined with the laminectomy of C1 and C2, for although a tumor reaching just within the posterior fossa may be dealt with safely, and solely, through a laminectomy, if it extends further, possibly involving one or more of the ninth, tenth, eleventh, and twelfth nerves, its precise attachment in relationship to these nerves may not be visualized, so leading to their damage.

The angle between the anterior margin of the spinal canal and the slope of the basiocciput varies between 132 degrees and 164 degrees, a range of over 30 degrees in normal people. In patients with a small angle, the top of the tumor tends to be further forward and becomes less accessible from a laminectomy approach. This feature can usually be assessed preoperatively from contrast studies and is illustrated diagrammatically in Figure 23-2. In the diagram, the angle is in the smaller range, about 140 degrees, and the top of the tumor could probably just be seen through a laminectomy of C1 and C2 (approach A). Nevertheless, to ensure that the attachment of the tumor in its relationship to the jugular foramen, hypoglossal nerve, and possibly small arteries supplying the medulla is clearly visualized, a full posterior craniectomy (approach B) on one or both sides will be required in addition.

SURGICAL TREATMENT

Intramedullary Tumors

GLIOMA OF MEDULLA OBLONGATA AND SPINAL CORD. Ependymomas and hemangioblastomas, situated lower down the spinal cord and in favorable relationship to its posterior surface, often can be removed completely. At the medullary-spinal cord level, unless actually presenting posteriorly, the hazards of attempted tumor removal in this vital zone probably is too great. However, these intramedullary tumors may produce additional symptoms if they block the foramen magnum, often from enlargement by cystic change. These extramechanical factors from external compression may be relieved by decompression, and the surgical exposure of these neoplasms is usually worthwhile.

The method of presentation and the effects of decompression and aspiration of a cyst in an intramedullary glioma are shown in the following case:

Case 1. A 46-year-old woman had, for seven months, experienced diplopia for distant objects—at first intermittent but becoming persistent; for four months, numbness of the right second and third toes, extending to the sole of the foot and then ascending up to the hip; for six weeks, pain and burning around the right eye; for four weeks, loss of sense of taste on the right side; for two weeks, difficulty in swallowing fluids; and for one week, numbness in the right hand. There was no complaint of headache.

Examination demonstrated nystagmus to both sides with a quick component toward the direction of gaze; reduction of light touch and pinprick sensation over all three divisions of the right fifth nerve with reduced corneal reflex; impaired taste over the tongue; reduced pharyngeal sensation; and weakness of the eleventh and twelfth spinal nerves, all on the right side. In the limbs, sensation only was involved: pinprick sensation was reduced over the entire right leg to the groin and over the right hand and forearm, with perversion of touch sensation in the same areas. A clinical diagnosis

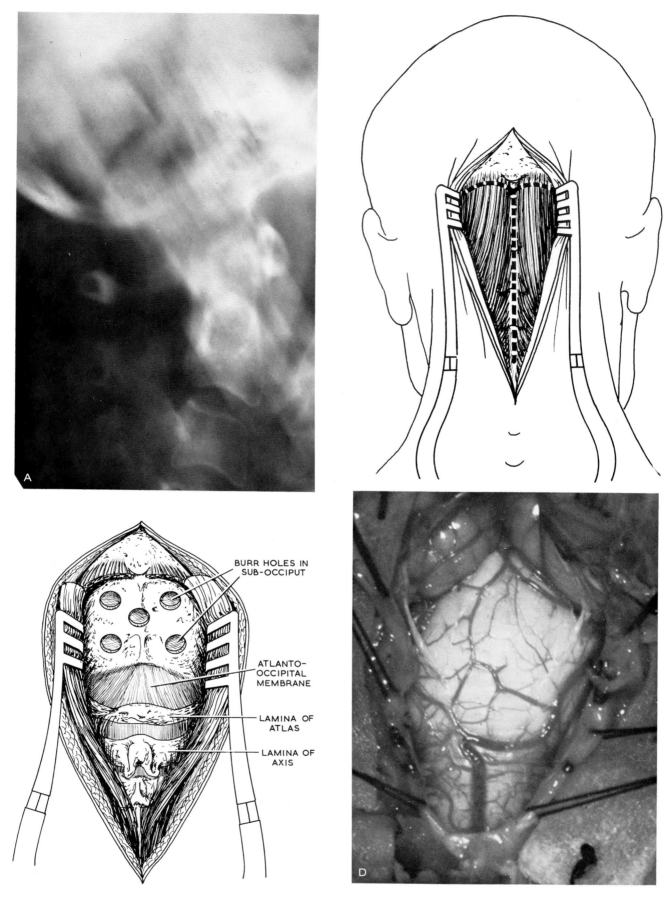

FIG. 23-3. Intramedullary glioma: *A*, air encephalogram; *B*, incision; *C*, craniectomy; *D*, operative photograph of intrinsic glioma showing pale, swollen lower medulla and first cervical cord segment with fine, stretched veins on surface. Tonsils have been displaced upward by mass.

Labels in figure C:

BURR HOLES IN SUB-OCCIPUT

ATLANTO-OCCIPITAL MEMBRANE

LAMINA OF ATLAS

LAMINA OF AXIS

of an intrinsic lesion of the medullary/spinal cord junction was made.

Investigation. Air encephalography (the investigation of choice in this type of case) disclosed a smooth backward expansion of nervous structures extending from the lower margin of the lamina of C1 up to the outlet of the fourth ventricle (Fig. 23-3 *A*).

Operation. With the patient in the sitting position (my preference), and with due precaution taken against air embolus, a bilateral approach to the foramen magnum was undertaken. The incision extended from one inch above the external occipital protuberance to the spine of the fifth cervical vertebra. The skin and subcutaneous tissues in the upper part of the wound were separated from the muscles for 3 cm. on either side of the midline (Fig. 23-3 *B*). Muscles were divided 3 mm. below their attachment to the superior curved line (this subsequently permits a more water-tight closure than if the muscles are completely detached from the bone and reliance is placed on a midline periosteal suture line) and were cleared from the bone with diathermy dissection and from the spines and laminae of C1, C2 and C3 by rugine. Craniectomy of the posterior fossa was made simpler by the sinking of multiple burr-holes with a power drill (Fig. 23-3 *C*). Complete removal of bone to the margins of the exposure was combined with a laminectomy of the first and second cervical vertebrae; care was taken not to insert the blade of the forceps deep to the lamina, but to scale off slivers of bone from the posterior surface. The dura was opened in a Y-shaped fashion starting from below. Thus rupture of the arachnoid was avoided, and massive intracranial CSF replacement by air was prevented at an early stage. The occipital sinuses (which may be as broad as one centimeter) were clipped before incision (or clamped, divided, transfixed, and ligatured). A smooth expansion of the medullary-spinal cord junction measuring 2½ cm. in diameter, displacing the calamus scriptorius and graçile and cuneate nucleii far backward, was exposed, fitting tightly against the dura (Fig. 23-3 *D*). Two milliliters of yellow fluid, from a depth of 4 mm., was aspirated from a grey area in the center. A biopsy was not feasible, but the impression was that of a cystic astrocytoma. The dura was left unsutured and sealed with a layer of gelatin film to prevent ingress of blood in the immediate postoperative phase.

The patient was subsequently given radiotherapy; her symptoms subsided somewhat, particularly that of impaired swallowing, and she remained well five years after treatment.

Craniospinal Tumor

EPENDYMOMA OF FOURTH VENTRICLE ENTERING VERTEBRAL CANAL.

Case 2. This case illustrates the speed at which symptoms may develop with a tumor that has undoubtedly been present a long time. A 33-year-old woman had, for seven weeks, experienced severe transient attacks of neck-ache unrelated to any particular activity and associated with a feeling of paresthesia and numbness over the subocciput, several episodes being associated with vomiting.

Examination revealed tenderness over the left cervical muscles with limitation of neck flexion, but no other abnormality. While she was in hospital, pain increased to become almost continuous, and a final exacerbation was associated with apnea lasting three minutes, during which she developed a flaccid quadriplegia. Following resuscitative measures, respirations returned to normal and there was some improvement in limb weakness.

Ventriculography done as an emergency revealed mild asymmetric enlargement of the ventricles, with an irregular filling defect in the outlet of the fourth ventricle (Fig. 23-4 *A*).

Operation. Bilateral exposure was used, as for Case 1, with craniectomy of subocciput and laminectomy of C1 and C2. When the dura was opened, a tumor mass was seen extending from the fourth ventricle to the lower margin of the C2 laminae covering the back of the cord and overlapping it on each side (Fig. 23-4 *B*). Starting at the lower pole, the tumor was grasped with forceps and steadied, and the portion below was then sucked away (Fig. 23-4 *C*). More and more of the tumor was successively aspirated in this fashion, until its attachment, measuring one centimeter in diameter on the floor of the fourth ventricle, was defined and tumor was gently cut away to leave a plaque about 2 mm. in thickness (Fig. 23-4 *D*). The blood vessels were occluded by bipolar coagulation. Histologic examination showed typical ependymoma with pseudorosettes and blephoroplasts.

The patient remains well 15 years later.

Extramedullary Tumors

Anterolateral Meningioma

Case 3. A 58-year-old man had six-month classic history of an anterolateral foramen magnum tumor as described on page 251.

Investigation. Myelogram in the oblique view with the patient prone shows a tumor located anterolaterally, displacing the cord backward and to the right, with a lobulated margin suggestive of a meningioma (Fig. 23-5 *A*).

Operation. A unilateral exposure was made with the patient in the sitting position. A skin incision was extended from the tip of the mastoid process along the superior curved line to the external occipital protuberance and down to the spine of C5 (Fig. 23-5 *B*). A mechanical advantage was derived from a unilateral exposure in that on insertion of self-retaining retrac-

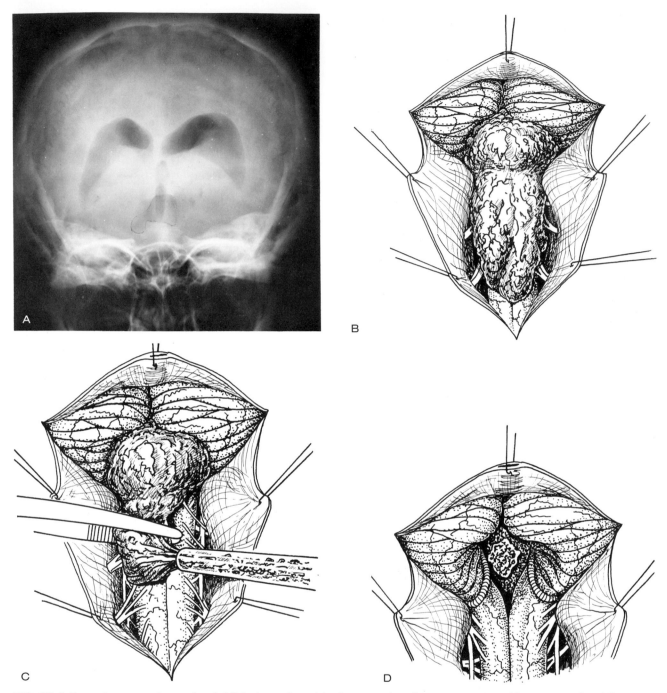

FIG. 23-4. Ependymoma: *A*, semi-axial PA view of ventriculogram showing asymmetry of lower margin of floor and outlet of fourth ventricle (outline of fourth ventricle retouched); *B*, ependymoma of fourth ventricle as viewed on opening of dura; *C*, aspiration of ependymoma of fourth ventricle; *D*, plaque remaining after removal of ependymoma.

tors, the blade resting against the spinous processes rotated the vertebrae so that the anterior wall of the vertebral canal, and tumor, was turned posteriorly to provide better access. Muscles were divided a few millimeters below the superior curved line and cleared from the right half of the posterior fossa and the right hemilaminae of C1 to C4 inclusive. Multiple burr holes

were drilled in the posterior fossa, and a unilateral craniectomy was carried out (reaching sufficiently high to give access to the top of the tumor), combined with a hemilaminectomy of C1 and C2 (Fig. 23-5 *C*). The dura was opened with a curved incision extending laterally across the occipital sinus into the posterior fossa, which permitted reflection of the lateral dural leaf to give

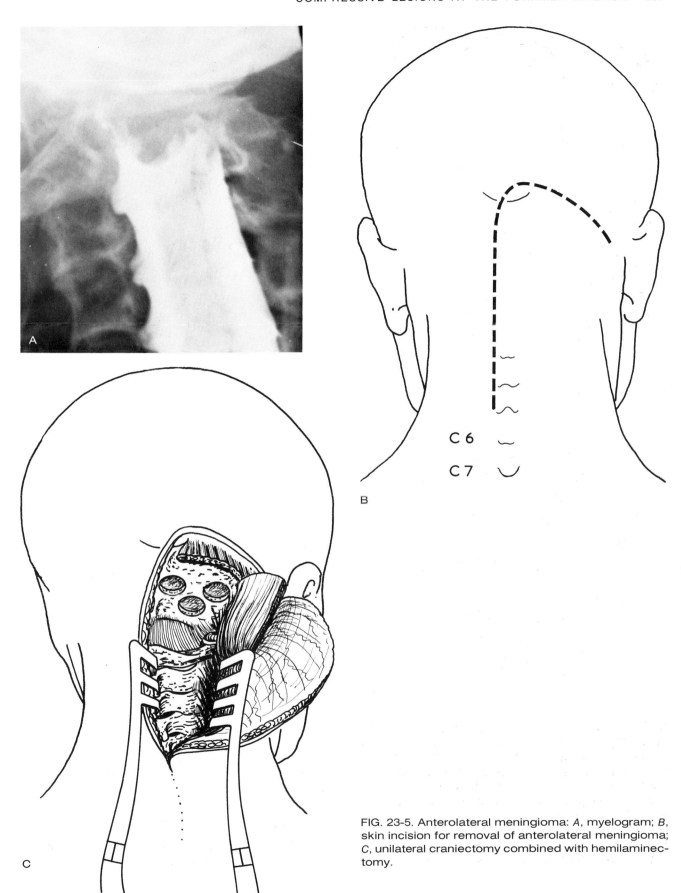

FIG. 23-5. Anterolateral meningioma: *A*, myelogram; *B*, skin incision for removal of anterolateral meningioma; *C*, unilateral craniectomy combined with hemilaminectomy.

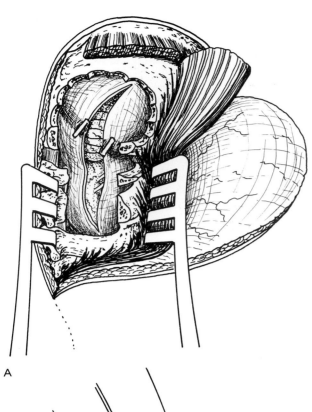

A

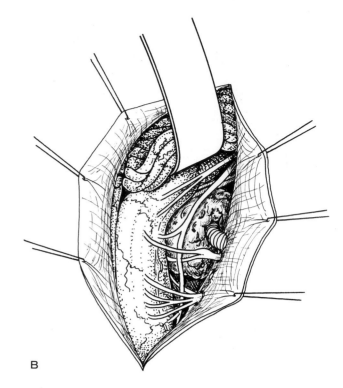

B

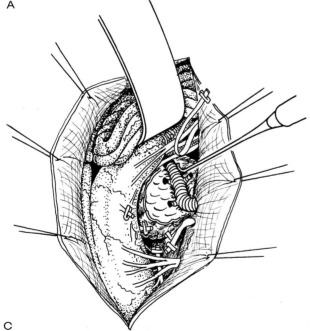

C

FIG. 23-6. Anterolateral meningioma (cont'd): *A*, reflection of lateral dural leaf shows neoplasm overlying entrance to vertebral artery; *B*, blunt hook is inserted between arterial wall and tumor; *C*, spinal accessory and first cervical nerve have been divided to give access to tumor, which is being separated from artery with blunt hook.

better access to the floor of the canal and the top of the tumor (Fig. 23-6 *A*). The neoplasm was found overlying the entrance to the vertebral artery (Fig. 23-6 *B*). A blunt hook was inserted between the arterial wall and the tumor (Fig. 23-6 *C*), and the latter was broken up and removed piecemeal. Several small arteries that entered the tumor after pursuing a short course were coagulated with bipolar forceps or occluded with small hemostatic clips.

With the artery dissected free, it was possible to remove the remaining tumor with rongeurs and to coagulate its base. Retraction and rotation of the spinal cord were kept to a minimum. The use of the operating microscope renders the arterial dissection easier and safer.

Anterolateral Neurofibroma

Most neurofibromas in this situation grow from the C1 nerve roots, either posterior or anterior, but occa-

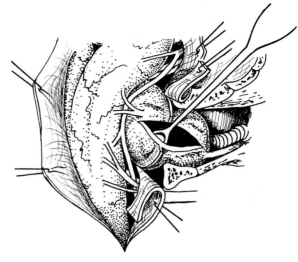

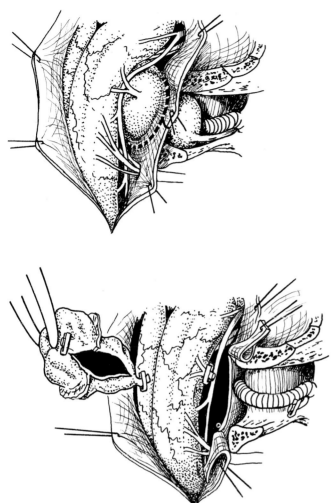

FIG. 23-7. Anterolateral neurofibroma: *A,* dural incision, just short of anterolateral fibroma, is indicated by dotted lines; relationship of vertebral artery in this case is directly anterior to tumor; *B,* incision is made in tumor and contents are evacuated; *C,* course of vertebral artery is indicated, but at operation is usually obscured by adherent plexus of large veins.

sionally a tumor on the C2 root achieves sufficient size to extend upward and cause compression at foramen magnum level. The majority tend to be dumbbell-shaped, partly intradural, partly extradural, the latter part often forming the larger mass. Rarely a neurofibroma on the spinal accessory nerve forms an intradural bilobed tumor, partly spinal, partly cranial.

Case 4. A 45-year-old man had an 18-month history characteristic of an anterolateral lesion, which was confirmed by myelography (see p. 260).

Operation. Unilateral exposure was made, as in Case 3. As soon as the dura was exposed, an extradural extension of the lesion was seen, so that a more radical lateral removal of the margin of the foramen magnum and the arch of the atlas was carried out. Inspection of the extradural portion indicated that it entered the dura, so the latter was opened with a curved flap to give access to the side and front of the cord and exposed the intrathecal extension projecting about one centimeter medially, indenting the cord anterolaterally, and arising from the first posterior cervical root.

The dura was incised vertically to just short of the neoplasm and then extended in circumferential fashion upward and downward to the limit of visibility (Fig. 23-7 *A*). It was now necessary to reduce the bulk of the tumor to avoid unduly disturbing the spinal cord with subsequent manipulations. An axial incision was made in the tumor, and its soft vascular grey translucent contents were evacuated quickly (Fig. 23-7 *B*). Bleeding was arrested with the bipolar coagulator. With the reduction in tension, it was now possible to continue the circumferential incisions until they met anteriorly. The posterior and anterior rootlets, which had no major vessels running on them were now divided between clips, and the mobilized capsule was followed out into the expanded intervertebral foramen and dissected free from the usual adherent plexus of large veins. It was followed laterally until the emergence of the distal end of the root was seen, and this was clipped and divided. The vertebral artery tends to be displaced upward and laterally (Fig. 23-7 *C*), but occasionally it may be posterior to the tumor, and this proximity had to be borne in mind in defining the outer extremity of the neoplasm.

It was often helpful to perform vertebral arteriography, so that the precise relationship of the artery was known preoperatively.

In order to prevent oozing from the muscles into the subarachnoid space, it is advisable to attempt to reconstitute the dura by sewing a patch of either dural substitute or lyophilized dura into the gap.

Anterior Meningioma

Case 5. A 50-year-old man gave a history typical of the progressive pattern of anterior tumors, with patchy involvement, both sensory and motor, of all four limbs developing over a period of two years. Plain roentgenograms revealed no abnormality. Myelography with the patient supine disclosed an anterior lesion with its lower pole at the C1 lamina displacing the spinal cord backward (Fig. 23-8 *A*).

Operation. A bilateral approach was taken, as described for Case 1, the only variation being a wider laminectomy of the C1 laminae to give easier access to the front of the vertebral canal. The tumor was seen directly in front of the first cervical cord segment,

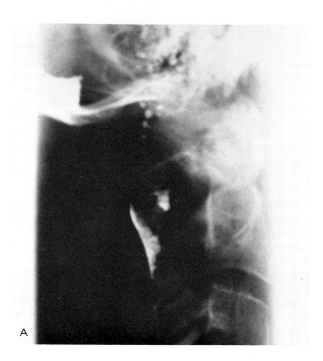

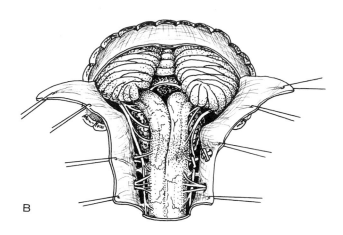

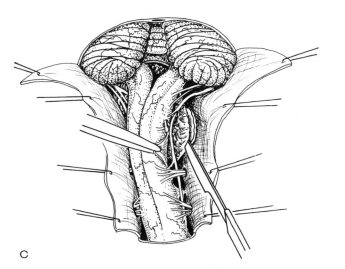

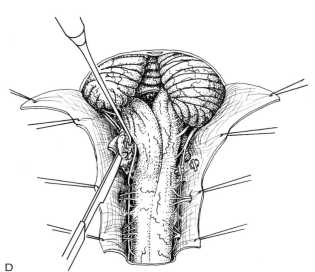

FIG. 23-8. Anterior meningioma: *A*, myelogram; *B*, anterior meningioma bulging first cervical cord segment backward; *C*, tumor is cut away in thin slices (note angle of blade); *D*, blunt hook facilitates removal of tumor pedicle.

bulging the latter backward and extending outward on either side to the lateral margins of the dura (Fig. 23-8 *B*). The head was now extended to relax the tension of the cord over the tumor, and the entry of the vertebral artery was identified. Starting on the right side, the first and second attachments of the ligamentum denticulatum were divided, the cord gently rotated to the left, the relationship of the vertebral artery noted, and, with a thin knife, successive slices of the tumor cut away, with the blade angled medially (Fig. 23-8 *C*). When all the tumor was excised as far as the lateral margin of the cord, a similar procedure was carried out on the left side until eventually the only portion of tumor that remained was that directly in contact with the anterior aspect of the cord and attached to the dura anteriorly only by a slender vertical pedicle. With a blunt hook, this remaining piece was displaced directly forward from its contact with the cord, and then rotated out from under it to its left side (Fig. 23-8 *D*). Further slices were cut away until all that remained was the linear attachment to the dura anteriorly, which could now be gently coagulated.

Excision of the dural attachment of the meningioma in such cases is not as a rule necessary; coagulation of the base usually prevents recurrence.

Ependymal Cyst

Case 6. This case, as does Case 2, illustrates the rapidity with which a benign lesion can produce dangerous complications. A 12-year-old girl had a 17-day history of left-sided neck-ache, subsequently associated with occasional mild headache and paresthesia in the palms of both hands. For seven days, based on the diagnosis of disc disease, cervical traction was applied, followed by a collar, at which time weakness of the legs was noted. Headache became increasingly severe and was associated with vomiting. On examination, there was marked restriction of flexion and extension of the neck, but with free lateral rotation; fine, ill-sustained nystagmus; minimal ataxia of both hands in the finger-nose test; incoordination of the heel-knee-shin test bilaterally; and brisk leg reflexes with a right extensor response. Despite subjective sensory symptoms in the hand, there was no objective loss.

Investigation. Myelogram, with the patient prone and her head fully extended, confirmed a circular obstruction with its lower margin just below the level of the foramen magnum (Fig. 23-9 *A*). In lateral views, this was shown to lie anterior to the cord.

Operation. Bilateral exposure, as in Case 1, showed a blue cyst in front of the cord, displacing the latter backward. The head was extended, clear fluid was aspirated through a sharp needle introduced on the right side (Fig. 23-9 *B*), which collapsed the cyst, allowing it to be drawn out and over to the left side. The cyst's single point of attachment to the front of the

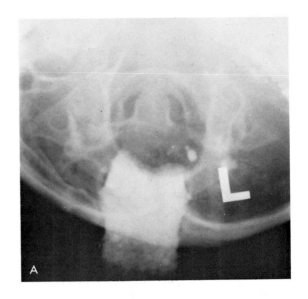

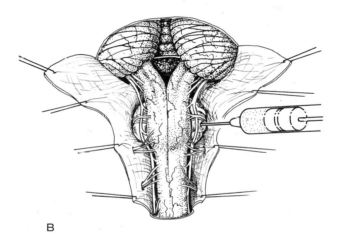

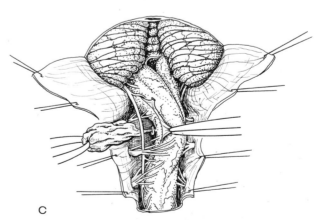

FIG. 23-9. Ependymal cyst: *A*, myelogram; *B*, aspiration of cyst; *C*, complete removal.

cord was divided, and it was removed completely (Fig. 23-9 C).

Histologic examination showed an ependymal cyst with a lining of cubical epithelium.

Posterior tumors

These lesions do not present any particular problems in removal and do not need separate description.

BONY ANOMALIES

Assimilation of the Atlas

The many varieties of this deformity range from virtually complete integration with the base of the skull to various focal fusions involving the anterior arch, the articulation(s), or the lamina, often linked with deformities of the transverse processes. Fusion of the second and third cervical vertebrae is commonly found in association.

The deformity is symptomless and a chance radiologic finding, except in the following conditions:

1. The Chiari malformation, present in some 20% of cases
2. Basilar invagination
3. Displacement of the skull, which, bearing the remnants of the atlas, dislocates forward on the axis, with or without separation of a normal or malformed dens

Treatment of Chiari malformation and basilar invagination will be described later.

In group 3, with cervical cord compression, fixation of the skull to the remaining upper cervical vertebrae is required. Fusion in these circumstances is often more difficult than in the treatment of dislocations resulting from fractures because of the large skeletal gap that may result between the arch of the axis and the occiput if the posterior arch of the atlas is assimilated.

One reliable method of doing this is to utilize bone grafts from the alar of the ilium to fuse the second, third, and preferably the fourth cervical vertebrae to the squama of the occiput. It is carried out in the following stages:

1. Crutchfield skull tongs are inserted and traction applied in an attempt to reduce any deformity, but improvement in position in longstanding cases is often minimal.

2. The usual bilateral exposure of the posterior fossa and upper cervical spine is carried out as described in Case 1 (p. 255). Muscles are cleared from the posterior fossa and from the laminae and spines down to and including the fifth cervical vertebrae (Fig. 23-10 A).

3. The iliac crest is cleared and two slightly curved grafts about 8 cm. in length, 2.5 cm. in width, and to the full thickness of the alar are cut, preserving the iliac crest. Additional bone is taken to pack around the main graft as chips.

4. The grafts have a natural double curve, which permits them to fit into similar curves of the vertebral arches. Each graft is placed in position on the laminae, and where the upper ends come in contact with the subocciput this area is marked out and two slots, one on each side of the midline, are made with the air drill, traversing the bone to expose the dura (Fig. 23-10 B).

5. Drill holes are made on either side of each aperture to take stainless steel wires. The spinous processes are trimmed, and the cortex of the laminae of C2, C3 and C4 is roughened.

6. The grafts, after trimming, are then inserted and their upper ends are held loosely in position in the slots by passing malleable steel wires through a hole drilled in them (Fig. 23-10 C).

7. Each graft is then fixed to the related spinous processes of C2, C3, and C4 by wires passed through drill holes. All wires are now tightened and bone chips are packed in the gaps between the graft and the laminae (Fig. 23-10 D).

8. Traction is continued for six weeks, followed by a Minerva plaster for three months and then a polythene collar.

In some cases, the congenitally fused remnants of the arch of the atlas posteriorly may form a knob that acts as an important compressing agent against the spinal cord, in which case the central centimeter of it may be removed prior to the grafting to provide adequate local decompression of the cord itself.

Basilar Invagination

Basilar invagination may produce disturbance of neurologic function in three circumstances:

1. In association with the Chiari malformation (to be described later) which is present in more than half the cases, possibly on a congenital basis, possibly mechanical from reduction of capacity of the posterior fossa.

2. When the margins of the foramen magnum are so inverted as to constrict the opening and there is direct compression of the cord by bone, particularly posteriorly.

3. By the upward and often backward displaced dens which, with the elevated lower margin of the clivus, indents and angulates the medullary/spinal cord junction from in front. In these cases, there is little chance of posterior removal of bone relieving the compression. This variety may be recognized from the myelogram (Fig. 23-11 A), which will show that there is (a) no Chiari malformation and (b) no encroachment by the inverted bone margins, but (c) a marked angulation of the neuraxis (Fig. 23-11 B).

In this situation probably the only procedure that might help would be a transoral approach to the clivus, and removal of the lower margin of this structure

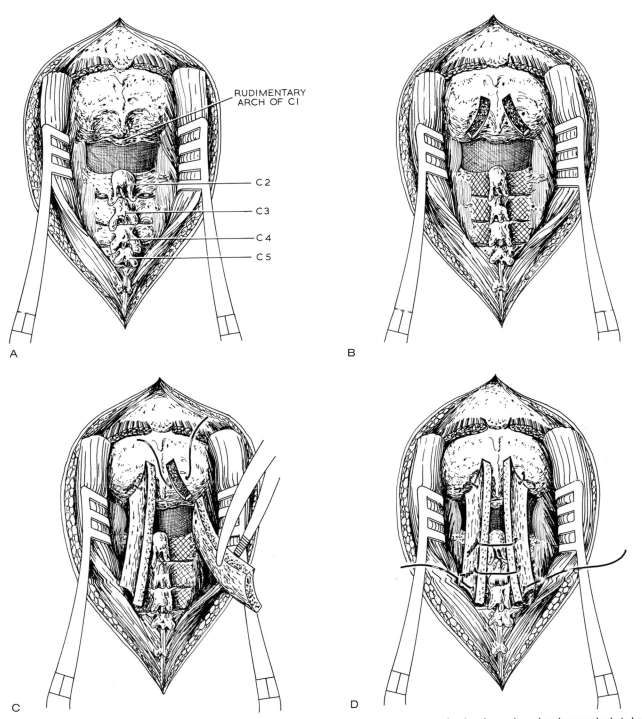

FIG. 23-10. Assimilation of atlas: *A*, exposure of posterior fossa and upper cervical spine, showing large skeletal gap between arch of axis and occiput bearing remnant of atlas; *B*, two slots, one on each side of midline, have been made in subocciput with air drill; *C*, insertion of grafts, held loosely in position with steel wires; *D*, wires are tightened, and bone chips are packed in gaps between graft and laminae.

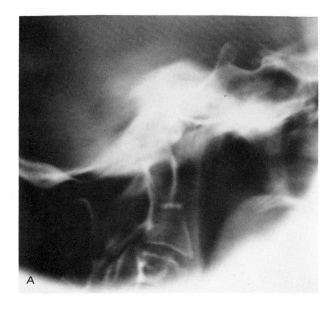

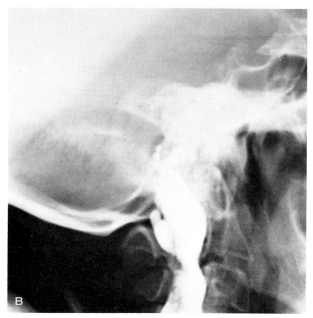

FIG. 23-11. Basilar invagination: *A*, myelogram; *B*, prone myelogram showing sharp angulation at junction of upper spinal canal with lower margin of clivus.

combined with the anterior arch of the atlas and of the dens, a formidable procedure in these abnormal anatomic circumstances.

Operation—Posterior Decompression for Basilar Invagination

The usual bilateral exposure is carried out as in Case 1 (p. 255), but owing to the high elevation of the inverted bony margin, often with the arch of the atlas in close apposition to the skull base, the approach is re-stricted and necessitates removal of the entire sub-occipital bone to give access to the inverted bony margin. Once a wide decompression of the foramen magnum has been achieved, the dura is opened in a Y-shaped fashion, with particular attention to the dividing of a ledge or ridge of dura frequently present directly at the foramen magnum level. Opening of the arachnoid is avoided as far as possible.

In more than half the cases, a Chiari I malformation will be found, and it is essential that the dural opening should extend down the spinal canal for 5 mm. beyond the tips of the tonsils.

Hyperplasia or Hypertrophy of Occipital Bone and/or the Occipito-Atloid Articulation

Case 7. A 67-year-old man had a 24-month history of symptoms and signs of an anterolateral compression of the cord, as described in the introduction under symptomatology.

Investigation. Plain films with tomography demonstrated fusion of the posterior arch of the atlas to the occiput; of the dens to the anterior arch; and of the right occipital articulation, with bone locally showing irregular areas of sclerosis and translucency. *Myelogram.* In the lateral (Fig. 23-12 *A*) and oblique (Fig. 23-12 *B*) views the spinal cord was shown to be displaced backward and to the left at foramen magnum level.

Operation. A bilateral exposure was performed (a unilateral one, as for Case 3, would probably have made the operation slightly easier). The dura was displaced backward and to the left, partly by a greatly enlarged right atlo-occipital articulation projecting medially and posteriorly, and partly by hypertrophied occipital bone lying above the level of the vertebral artery. The hypertrophied bone and posterior margin of the articulation were removed with an air drill with complete relief of pressure on the theca (Fig. 23-12 *C*).

TUMORS ARISING FROM THE BONY WALL

The tumors most difficult to treat are those situated in the dens, in the anterior arch of the atlas, and in the lower anterior margin of the basiocciput, and are frequently chordomas. The management of this type of tumor, with the usual unhappy outcome, is exemplified by the following:

Case 8. A 23-year-old woman, three years previously, had had a swelling removed from the posterior wall of the nasopharynx and diagnosed histologically as a chordoma. Two months prior to admission, following a minor injury, she suddenly developed pain in the neck, which increased and was particularly bad at night,

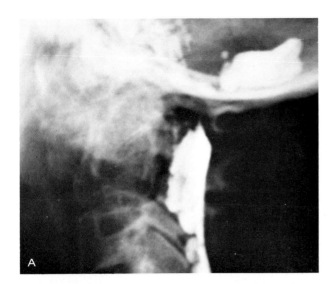

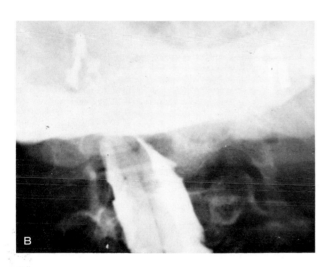

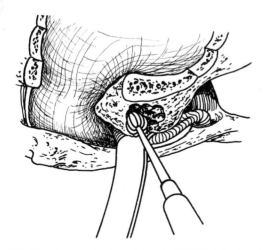

FIG. 23-12. Hyperplasia of occipital bone: *A*, myelogram, lateral view; *B*, myelogram, oblique view; *C*, hypertrophied bone is removed by air drill.

extended up the back of the head, and was exacerbated by coughing, sneezing, and straining. This was followed quickly by weakness in both arms, and for six weeks there had been tingling sensations in both thighs anteriorly, with weakness of both legs and some unsteadiness of gait; for two weeks, difficulty in swallowing; for three days, inability to walk; and for two days, retention of urine.

Examination. Noted were left twelfth cranial nerve palsy; weakness of all four limbs with increased tone; brisk reflexes and extensor plantar responses; a sensory level at C6 dermatome on both sides, below which pinprick, cotton-wool, and temperature sense were all reduced. Joint position sense was impaired in the fingers and wrist on the right side.

Investigations. Tomography revealed destruction of the lower lip of the clivus, and a large, soft-tissue mass in the nasopharynx (Fig. 23-13 *A*). Myelography revealed a complete block at the C2 vertebral level, with backward displacement of the theca (Fig. 23-13 *B*).

First Operation. A unilateral approach was carried out, as detailed for Case 3, with bone removal limited to a right hemilaminectomy of C1 and C2 in order to avoid weakening the occipito-atlo-axial articulation. Typical translucent pinkish-gray friable chordomatous material was present extradurally on the right side and was evacuated from within a tenuous capsule, and followed forward to the anterior wall of the spinal canal and to an eroded hole in the tip of the basiocciput. Despite extension of the head, respirations ceased during the operation and returned to normal on completion of the tumor removal.

Second Operation. An anterior transcervical approach was proposed a fortnight after the first intervention, but during that time roentgenograms showed subluxation of the atlas on the dens (Fig. 23-14 *A*), presumed to be due to detachment of the cruciate ligaments. Crutchfield tongs were applied, and the dislocation reduced. Operation was then carried out through the original posterior fossa incision. The left hemilaminae of C2 and C1 were cleared, and the latter was then encircled with thick stainless steel wire, which was twisted and brought down to run over the bifid spine of C2. The ends of the wires were now separated and taken round each side of the base of the spinous process, and then over its upper surface and twisted together. By bringing the wires as far back as possible onto the spine of C2 (Fig. 23-14 *B*), a better mechanical advantage is obtained in preventing direct displacement forward of C1, which may occur if the arch of the atlas is wired directly down onto that of C2.

Third Operation. Immediately after the fixation procedure, a third operation was performed by means of a transcervical approach similar to that described by Stevenson et al (1966). With the head rotated to the left and extended, a long incision was made from the base of the mastoid process down the anterior border of the sternomastoid, curving medially across the midline at

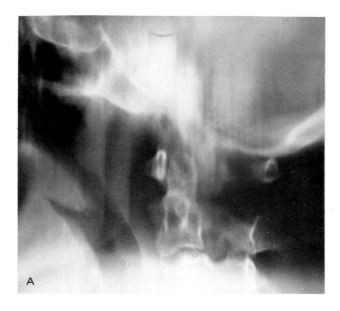

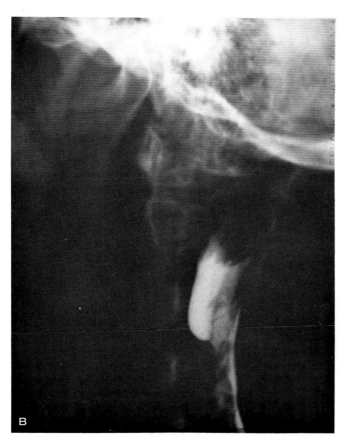

FIG. 23-13. Tumor arising from bony wall: *A*, tomogram showing mass in nasopharynx; *B*, myelogram showing complete block at C2 vertebral level.

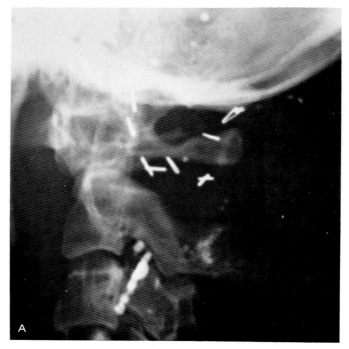

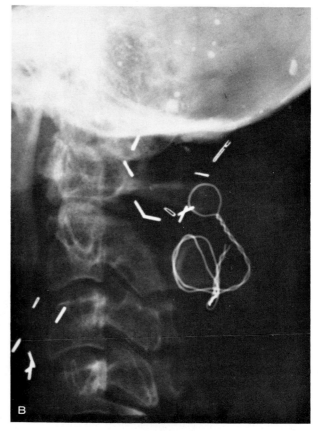

FIG. 23-14. Tumor arising from bony wall: *A*, roentgenogram showing subluxation of atlas on the dens prior to second operation; *B*, postoperative roentgenograms showing stainless steel wire applied to prevent displacement.

the level of the cricoid cartilage (Fig. 23-15 A). The carotid sheath was exposed and the common facial vein ligated and divided. Dissection medially opened the retropharyngeal space and the pharynx was now retracted to the left (Fig. 23-15 B). This maneuver put the hypoglossal nerve on the stretch; the nerve was mobilized throughout its length, while the superior thyroid, lingual, and occipital arteries were divided. To expose the front of the vertebral bodies the prevertebral fascia was divided and finger dissection used to separate the pharyngeal muscles upward until the base of the skull was palpated and the pharyngeal tubercle identified —with some difficulty because of tumor in the vicinity. Blunt dissection was continued laterally to expose the styloid process with its related muscles and the emer-

gence of glossopharyngeal, vagus, and accessory nerves, and the internal carotid artery and jugular vein. The exposure was now adequate for tumor to be seen replacing the rectus capitis anticus and longus colli muscles and sprouting from the anterior arch of the atlas and the bony margin of the clivus. The tumor, including absorbing bone, was removed piecemeal with a rongeur until apparently normal bone was seen in the clivus and lateral masses of the atlas. The dens was not obviously involved. However, tumor tissue was seen extending into the soft tissues on either side of the atlas, but was not accessible. The operation was completed with a temporary tracheostomy and gastrostomy.

The patient made an uneventful recovery and was given a course of radiotherapy, but the tumor recurred and she died three months later.

CHIARI TYPE I MALFORMATION

This condition, which is the most common of the lesions causing compression in the foramen magnum, was first described by Chiari in his paper of 1891, and in

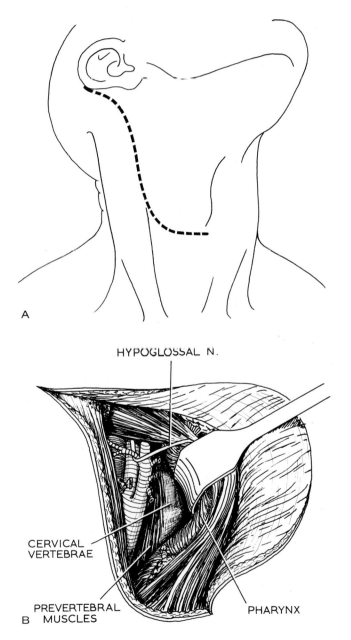

FIG. 23-15. Tumor arising from bony wall: A, incision for third operation; B, retraction of pharynx; C, in drawing, three muscles attached to styloid process have been divided in order to expose tumor; at operation described in text, it did not prove necessary to interfere with muscles or styloid process.

A

HYPOGLOSSAL N.

CERVICAL VERTEBRAE

PREVERTEBRAL B MUSCLES

PHARYNX

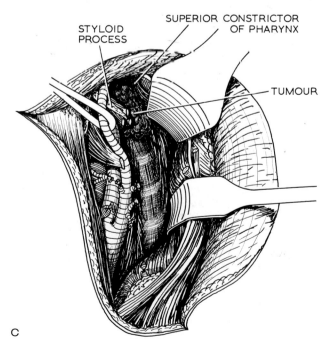

STYLOID PROCESS

SUPERIOR CONSTRICTOR OF PHARYNX

TUMOUR

C

more detail in 1895, when he analyzed 4276 random autopsy reports and found 24 cases of malformation of the hindbrain, which he grouped into four categories: (1) herniation of the cerebellar tonsils, sometimes with the medial surface of the cerebellar hemispheres, through the foramen magnum; (2) herniation of the vermis cerebelli in association with spina bifida and meningocele; (3) cervical meningocele with herniation of the cerebellum into it; (4) agenesis of the cerebellum. The latter two categories have no relevance to this chapter.

The Chiari II malformation is the more common Chiari malformation and manifests itself in infants in association with spina bifida. In contrast, the Chiari I anomaly has been shown to occur usually in the adult, the main incidence being between the ages of 45 and 50. It is characterized by herniation of the tonsils, not the vermis, and is virtually never associated with a meningocele. These two varieties of malformation, Type I and II, are quite distinct therefore in their anatomy and their clinical presentation and run fairly true to form. It is the Chiari I deformity with which this chapter is concerned. Arnold in 1894 added further descriptive details to the anomalies.

It would seem preferable to use the term "Chiari I malformation" rather than "Arnold-Chiari," which covers both types.

Symptomatology

In many of the 80 patients in our series (Table 23-1), the syndromes were not rigidly defined, but they could be categorized without much difficulty according to their major symptomatology.

Headache, which was the sole complaint in nine of our patients, was also present in 12 patients who had other symptoms. Headache was of several varieties: (1) a cough headache precipitated by coughing, sneezing, or straining; (2) persistent dull suboccipital pain; (3) paroxysmal, severe, bursting, generalized headache, although unrelated to high intracranial pressure. *Hydrocephalus* was an uncommon complication, but it could be severe. Although intracranial pressure was high in occasional cases, it was usually low or normal. *Bulbar and cranial nerve symptoms* brought some patients initially to consult the otolaryngologist. *Ataxia of gait,* as an almost isolated symptom, occurred in four elderly women. *Long tract involvement,* seen in nearly one-third of the cases, comprised permutation and combination of disturbance of pyramidal tracts, spinothalamic tracts, and posterior columns, often asymmetric, and usually mild. *Radiculopathy* consisted of wasting and weakness, particularly of the C5 and C8 innervated upper limb muscles, with a surprising lack of involvement of the legs. Symptoms usually progressed slowly, and often fluctuated, but sometimes they were static for long periods. The degree of neurologic damage was usually mild to moderate.

The course does not resemble the steady, fairly rapid progress made by tumor compression at the foramen magnum. Differentiation from posterior fossa tumors with herniation of cerebellar tonsils is not difficult, because raised intracranial pressure is extremely rare with the Chiari anomaly, and cerebellar involvement is unusual. The more important differential diagnoses concern disseminated sclerosis (many cases having been so diagnosed initially), motor neuron disease, and cervical spondylosis; they are resolved eventually by the radiologic studies.

Radiologic Diagnosis

PLAIN ROENTGENOGRAPHIC CHANGES. Assimilation of the atlas is the most significant feature and is noted in 20% of cases; basilar impression is noted in 11%, fused vertebrae in 3%. In nearly two-thirds of cases, however, no changes are demonstrated on the plain roentgenogram. The diagnosis derives therefore from a positive decision, taken on the history and clinical findings in the face of normal roentgenograms, to outline the craniospinal junction by myelography.

CONTRAST INVESTIGATION. The most reliable method of confirming tonsillar herniation is by myelography, using Pantopaque by the lumbar route, with the patient supine. With the patient in the prone position, the tonsils often may not produce any significant obstruction. The defects produced by the tonsils are usually rounded, are best seen in the oblique views, and are often asymmetric, sometimes with a little notch be-

TABLE 23-1. Chiari Type I Anomaly—
Clinical Features

Features	Cases
Headache	9
Hydrocephalus	3
Bulbar involvement with cranial nerve nucleii 5–12 and their connections: difficulty in swallowing and speaking; vertigo; oscillopsia	11
Cerebellar disturbance: ataxia of gait	4
Long tract involvement: pyramidal, spinothalamic, posterior column	14
Upper limb radiculopathy	2
Syringomyelia	37
Total	80

It will be noted that in 37 cases, nearly half, the condition is associated with syringomyelia. Conversely, of all patients with syringomyelia, about 85% have Chiari I malformation.

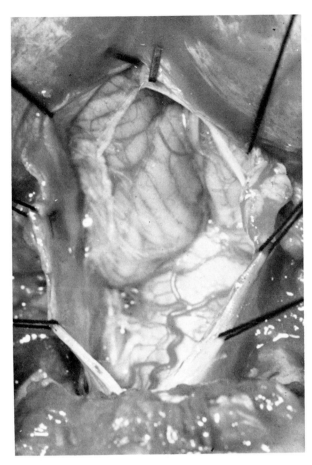

FIG. 23-16. Operative photograph of Chiari I malformation. Posterior fossa decompression has been done and vertical portion of dural incision carried out which will be extended in form of Y. Asymmetric enlargement and herniation of tonsils is seen with expansion of first cervical cord segment. In this patient arachnoid is opened widely.

tween them (see Fig. 23-17 A). Their lower limit may extend just through the foramen magnum or down to the arch of the axis, or even as far as C3.

AIR ENCEPHALOGRAPHY. This confirmatory method of diagnosis is not so reliable as Pantopaque myelography, for in some cases air passes upward between the tonsils or around them, and an obstruction may not be demonstrated.

VERTEBRAL ARTERIOGRAPHY. Often this study shows the caudal loops of the posterior inferior cerebellar arteries to descend below the foramen magnum, but this may occur in normal people and is by no means a conclusive diagnostic feature. Its main value is in excluding the presence of a posterior fossa tumor.

If a tumor is strongly suspected, air or Myodil *ventriculography* is necessary, as is *scintiscan*. The normal tonsils are usually symmetric and their lower borders are no nearer than 3.8 mm. to a line joining the lower

border of the foramen magnum with the lower margin of the clivus, so that any actual herniation of the tonsils through the foramen magnum is significant. However, as a Chiari I malformation is a congenital condition and presumably exists from early fetal life, remaining for many years symptomless, it may occur as a coincidental finding with some other disease of the central nervous system, and the significance of any herniation of the tonsils must be assessed in the light of the symptomatology.

Operation

The essential feature is the wide decompression of the posterior fossa and particularly of the foramen magnum with the upper two, sometimes three, cervical vertebrae, depending on the degree of herniation of the tonsils. A bilateral exposure is carried out as detailed for Case 1 (p. 255). The dura is opened in the usual Y-shaped fashion, preserving the arachnoid intact, where the tonsils will be seen protruding through the foramen magnum. They may be symmetric or asymmetric, altered in color, and gliotic, often with a fringed lower margin. Typically they are pressed together in the midline, and overlie the exit of the fourth ventricle enveloping the upper cervical cord both posteriorly and round its sides, reaching forward to, and sometimes beyond, the transverse meridian. Inferiorly their tips tend to indent and heap up the gracile and cuneate nuclei into a large white eminence (Fig. 23-16). The dural incision must extend at least 5 mm. beyond the tip of the tonsils.

Previously the arachnoid was opened wide and the tonsils were separated to free the outlet of the fourth ventricle. With the present technique, however, the arachnoid is preserved, if possible, in order to prevent postoperative entry of blood and muscle ooze into the CSF pathways. Such seepage could provoke a brisk inflammatory reaction and ultimately a communicating hydrocephalus.

Results of Decompression Surgery

For the assessment of these results, the patients' disabilities were graded mild, moderate or severe, and change of one grade in either direction was defined as improvement or deterioration. Virtually no patients showed a change of more than one grade.

SYRINGOMYELIA

Although syringomyelia was recognized as a nosologic entity in 1827, its association with the Chiari I malformation has been established only in the last 15 years, owing mainly to WJ Gardner's work from 1950 onward,[3] and it is now generally conceded

TABLE 23-2. Results of Decompression
Surgery in 41 Survivors*

Symptoms	Number of Cases	Results
Headache	9	8 cured
		1 improved
Hydrocephalus	2	2 cured
Bulbar and cranial nerve symtoms	10	7 improved
		2 arrested
		1 deteriorated
Cerebellar disturbance	4	3 improved
		1 arrested
Long tract symptoms: pyramidal, spinothalamic, posterior column	14	7 improved
		6 arrested
		1 deteriorated
Upper limb radiculopathy	2	2 improved
Total	41	

*Of 43 cases; mortality rate, 4.7%. Results are reasonably encouraging, with improvement or prevention of deterioration the rule.

that syringomyelia is associated in something like 95% of cases, with some form of obstruction of the outlet of the fourth ventricle. The Chiari I malformation is present in 85% of cases; adhesive obstruction, tumors, cysts, and the Dandy-Walker syndrome comprise the remaining 10%. The rare syringomyelias resulting from traumatic spinal lesions, arachnoiditis, and the like are not relevant to this chapter.

Symptomatology

The symptoms of syringomyelia derive from three mechanical disturbances: (1) the excavation of the spinal cord by the cyst, which may be central, eccentric, or multilocular; (2) the compression of the medulla oblongata, with its cranial nerve nucleii and their connections, and of the upper cervical cord by the tonsillar prolapse of the Chiari malformation; and (3) stretch of the cranial nerves by the downward displacement of the medulla in a number of cases. The interplay of these three factors produces a permutation and combination of signs resulting in many variations of the "typical" syringomyelic pattern.

Thus there may be involvement of cranial nerves V to XII, simulating "syringobulbia" (but without any cystic excavation of the brain stem): wasting and weakness of the arm, particularly hand muscles with reduced reflexes; a suspended area of dissociated sensory loss over the trunk, or of the cape or halfcape distribution; and spasticity in the legs. Posterior column involvement and sphincter disturbance are less common, and trophic changes of skin or joints usually occur very late.

In some patients with minimal or no physical signs a large cyst in the cord may be demonstrated by radiography; conversely, a gross syringomyelic picture may be present with a spinal cord of normal size, although there is an excavating cyst within it.

Radiologic Diagnosis

The two characteristic radiologic features are widened cervical cord and obstruction to the outlet of the fourth ventricle, usually a Chiari I malformation. Swelling of the cord is best confirmed by positive contrast myelography (Fig. 23-17 A), which demonstrates, with the patient prone particularly, the widened cervical cord, and with the patient supine, a Chiari I anomaly in most instances. Occasionally an irregular obstruction by adhesions is revealed. Though such confirmation is not essential, it is possible to ascertain by air myelography that the expansion of the cord is caused by displaceable fluid and not by a solid or partly cystic tumor. The study requires a large, almost total replacement of spinal fluid by air, while the patient is in the lateral position. Tomographs taken with the patient head-down show the cord to be dilated; those taken with the patient head-up show the cord to be deflated (Fig. 23-17 B).

Surgical Treatment

The principles underlying operative treatment are based on Gardner's partial explanation of the mechanics responsible for excavation of the cord,[3] which can be stated briefly as follows:

With each cardiac systole, cerebrospinal fluid is normally ejected from the fourth ventricle, but if this is obstructed by the Chiari I malformation (or any other lesion), the fluid tends to be diverted down the central canal. The cisterna magna is also blocked by the tonsils, so that no CSF can be displaced from it into the cervical subarachnoid space surrounding the cervical cord. Thus there is a differential pressure gradient between the inside and the outside of the cord, and although the hydrodynamic pressures involved are very small indeed, the pulsation over many years produces a syrinx.

Operation

The operation comprises essentially a bilateral exposure of the posterior fossa as in Case 1 (p. 255), with a large decompression, particularly of the foramen magnum far laterally with the arches of C1, C2, and also C3, if the degree of downward herniation of the tonsils warrants it. This decompression, with a Y-shaped division of the dura, relieves its constricting effect and, indirectly, the obstruction of the outlet of the fourth ventricle by the impacted tonsils.

Some advocate a wide opening into the fourth ventricle by separation of the tonsils, exposure of the

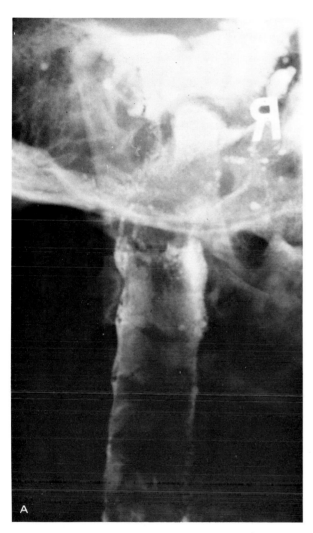
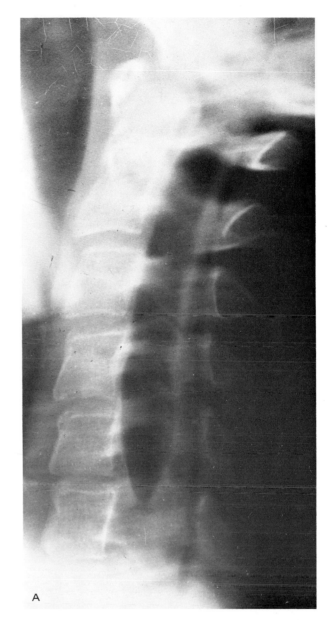

FIG. 23-17. Syringomyelia: *A*, myelogram demonstrating expanded cervical cord with asymmetric curved filling defects below foramen magnum, indicating herniated tonsils; *B*, midline tomogram of air myelogram with patient in lateral position with head uptilt of 15 degrees. Spinal cord has "deflated" to form a band 4 mm. in cross section up to its junction with medulla. At level of C6 vertebra, spinal cord is beginning to expand.

opening of the central canal, and plugging of the opening with a piece of muscle or gauze to prevent the ingress of CSF.

We have found this wide exposure to sometimes result in aggravation of the physical signs and in subsequent development of communicating hydrocephalus and/or meningocele, owing to the entry of blood and muscle ooze into the subarachnoid space. In recent years a change of technique has been adopted whereby the arachnoid is not opened, but all dural compression is completely relieved, if necessary, by the

addition of lateral incisions just below foramen magnum level.

That this procedure is efficacious in causing contraction of the cyst can be seen in Figure 23-18, which depicts the preoperative Pantopaque myelogram, and one done a year postoperatively, following a simple decompression with preservation of the arachnoid. The tracing shows the measurements of the actual reduction in cord size.

In the few patients with widespread adhesions obliterating the outlet of the fourth ventricle, often

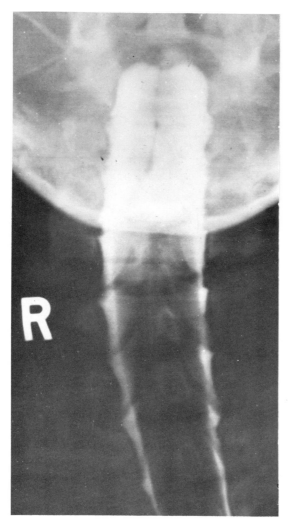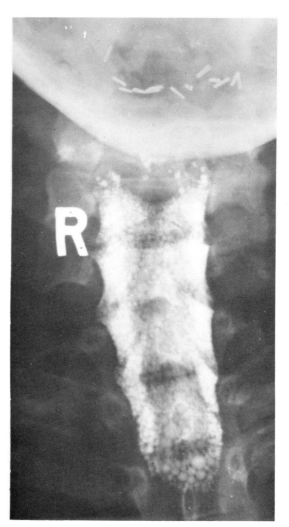

FIG. 23-18. Syringomyelia: *left,* preoperative myelogram; *right,* postoperative myelogram.

binding the tonsils together and also onto the upper cervical cord, an attempt to dissect these adhesions free has led on occasion to an increase in symptoms. Although it is now possible, with the operating microscope, to carry out this dissection with greater accuracy and care, the simple decompression maneuver is capable of producing an amelioration of symptoms without serious risk.

The syrinx, as a rule, does not extend upward to the level of the tonsils, but ends two or three segments below, so that the expanded cord is not usually seen in the cervico-occipital decompression.

Results of Surgical Decompression

In assessing the results of surgical treatment, we must recognize the nature of this condition—a chronic and slowly progressive neurologic disease with multiple neurologic signs, not all of which are susceptible to influence by operation. It is erroneous to draw conclusions concerning the arrest or deterioration in a patient with, say, a ten-year history in a follow-up period of a mere one to two years.

The flouting of this principle, among others, has led to confusion concerning the efficacy of operative treatment for this condition. Figure 23-19 shows the response of individual symptoms and signs in 41 patients (most of whom, of course, had more than a single symptom or sign), in whom the mean follow-up period was 5 years 9 months, with a range of $3\frac{1}{2}$ to $11\frac{1}{2}$ years. As a generalization, it appears that in roughly two-thirds of cases, there was no significant change in the overall symptomatology during the period of follow-up, and one hopes that this represents permanent arrest of progression. In one-third of the cases, there was some recovery, which varied according to the neurologic modality involved.

The greatest improvement occurs with regard to

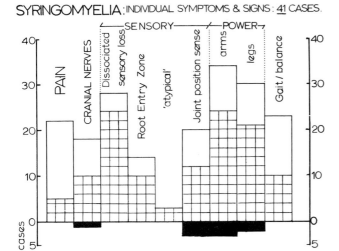

FIG. 23-19. Results of surgery in 41 cases of syringo-myelia. Each symptom or sign was allocated one of three degrees of severity: mild, moderate, or severe. In no patient was there change of more than one degree, whether in the direction of improvement or deterioration. Mean followup period was five years, nine months, with a range of 3½ to 11½ years. Crossed areas represent no change; clear zone, improvement; and dark areas, deterioration in three patients.

pain, whether it was felt locally in the neck, in radicular distribution, or remotely over the trunk or limbs. Less change is noted in gait and balance, and less still in cranial nerve involvement, joint position sense, and root entry zone sensory loss.

Motor power improved in about a third of the patients, but dissociated and atypical sensory change showed minimal response. Three patients, roughly 7% of the total number, had several modalities significantly and permanently worsened by the operation. The follow-up is still short, particularly for those with long histories, and it is probable that relapse will occur in some cases.

Indications for Surgical Treatment

For a long-standing disease process that is usually slowly progressive and sometimes even self-arresting, the major aim of surgical treatment is to arrest deterioration, rather than obtain improvement. The operation is a major procedure and results in considerable discomfort to the patient. Surgical manipulation in an area containing so many important structures must entail a risk to life, and may induce such complications as communicating hydrocephalus, traumatic meningocele, and a worsening of established symptoms.

The following guidelines dictate our choice of investigative measures and our decision to operate:

1. In patients with symptoms of syringomyelia, whatever their duration, provided the condition is still progressive and the patient is not chair- or bed-bound, investigation by myelography with air or Myodil is justified.

2. If distention of the cord is demonstrated with herniated tonsils, operation may be considered on the following grounds:

a. Severe pain, whatever its site, needing treatment on its own account, regardless of the general neurologic picture, when the chances of relieving it are good.

b. Symptoms that are rapidly progressive over a period of weeks to months and would become severely crippling without surgical treatment.

c. When "syringobulbia," unilateral spinothalamic loss, or severe posterior column involvement is a predominant symptom, suggesting that direct pressure on the lower medulla and cervical cord by the herniated tonsils is the paramount mechanical feature.

Difficulties in decision arise when a patient's disease has progressed slowly over a period of many years. In such cases operation should be contemplated at a stage when it is still possible to prevent total upper limb crippling by preserving some intrinsic hand muscle power and retaining sensation, particularly joint position sense, in the fingers.

Patients who, at the time of initial consultation, present a classic progressive picture of the disease, are already chair-bound or require help with a walking frame or tripod, and/or have reduced respiratory capacity are in danger of having their condition worsened by surgical intervention. Such patients are best regarded as being beyond surgical aid, but even so, severe pain or "syringobulbia" might justify operative decompressive relief as a calculated risk.

References

1. Chiari H: Ueber Veranderungen des Kleinhirns in Folge von Hydrocephalie des Grosshirns. Deutsch Med Wschr 17:1172-1175, 1891.
2. Chiari H: Über die Veranderungen der Kleinhirns der Pons und der Medulla oblongata in Folge von Congenitaler Hydrocephalie de Grosshirns. Denkschr Akad Wissensch Wien Math Naterw KL 63:71-116. 1895.
3. Gardner WJ: Hydrodynamic mechanisms of syringomyelia. Its relationship to myelocele. J Neurol Neurosurg Psychiat 28:247-259, 1965.
4. Legré J, Dufour M, Debaene A, Alliez B, Dalmas J: Exploration des tumeurs du trou occipital par myelographie opaque et iodoventiculographie. Neurochirurgie 17:481-492, 1971.
5. Stevenson GS, Stoney RJ, Perkins RK, Adams JE: A transcervical transclival approach to the ventral surface of the brain stem for removal of clivus chordoma. J Neurosurg 24:544-557, 1966.
6. Symonds CP, Meadows SP, Taylor J: Compression of the spinal cord in the neighbourhood of the foramen magnum. Brain, 60:52, 1937.

24

Bone Tumors and Tumor-Like Lesions of Vertebrae

J. VERNON LUCK AND DAVID C. G. MONSEN

PRIMARY bone tumors with a clinically significant incidence of vertebral involvement are uncommon.[10,21,28] Descriptions of the bone tumors and tumor-like lesions which involve vertebrae with extreme rarity have been omitted. Entities excluded: osteogenic sarcoma, chondrosarcoma, fibrosarcoma, reticulum cell sarcoma, desmoplastic fibroma of bone, neurofibromas of von Recklinghausen's neurofibromatosis, solitary osteochondromas, hereditary chondrodysplasia, fibrous dysplasia, and Hodgkin's disease.

Hemangioma is the most frequently encountered benign bone tumor of a vertebral body. Of the primary malignant bone tumors, myelomatosis has by far the highest incidence of vertebral involvement.

BONE TUMORS WITH POTENTIAL VERTEBRAL INVOLVEMENT

I. Benign Bone Tumors
  A. Angiogenic
    1. Hemangioma
  B. Osteogenic
    1. Osteoid osteoma
    2. Benign osteoblastoma
  C. Mesenchymal (specific origin unknown)
    1. Giant cell tumor
II. Primary Malignant Bone Tumors (Unicentric)
  A. Notochordal remnant (probable)
    1. Chordoma
  B. Mesenchymal (origin uncertain)
    1. Ewing's tumor
III. Primary Malignant Bone Tumor Multicentric
  A. Hematopoietic (primitive marrow reticulum —probable)
    1. Myelomatosis
IV. Secondary Malignant Bone Tumors
  A. Carcinoma metastatic to vertebrae
    1. Osteolytic metastases
    2. Osteoplastic metastases

TUMOR-LIKE LESIONS OF VERTEBRAE

Of the many tumor-like lesions of the skeletal system, two, aneurysmal bone cyst and eosinophilic granuloma, are characterized by a clinically important incidence of vertebral involvement. It is not uncommon for their ominous roentgenographic appearance to be interpreted as that of a malignant tumor.

Of these two entities, aneurysmal bone cyst has the higher incidence and is more locally aggressive, possessing the potential of creating a path of osseous destruction spanning two or more vertebrae. In such cases a pathologic fracture and a major neurologic deficit are a constant threat.

An eosinophilic granuloma remains confined to one vertebral body. It usually destroys most of the vertebral body, and a near-total collapse is the rule.

MILESTONES

Since most malignant primary tumors of bone are rare, their diagnosis and treatment remained in a state of disorganized confusion until the 1920s. In 1922 the indomitable surgeon-pathologist, Earnest Codman organized the first Bone Tumor Registry.[21,28] Under the auspices of the American College of Surgeons, a large number of case studies was rapidly collected, enabling the Registry Committee—Doctors Codman, Bloodgood and Ewing—to publish the first practical classification of bone tumors in 1928. This long-needed classification had far-reaching influences. Widespread acceleration of interest in this previously neglected subject steadily advanced the quality of patient care and effectively upgraded teaching. Subsequent revised classifications have reflected the expanding area of knowledge. A proliferation of the research projects centered on one or more facets of skeletal neoplasia further documented the new interest. Oncologic investigations in recent years have increased in a virtually geometric progression. Codman, were he still with us, would be elated—and doubtless, irascible.

In the diagnosis of vertebral body tumors and tumor-like lesions, the development of practical needle biopsy techniques has been helpful. Ottolenghi and Ray are skillful proponents of this method.[36,38,47] Vertebral rods for selected cases of vertebral collapse, such as those in the set developed by Harrington,[16] are likely to be employed more frequently in the years ahead, and when there is osteoporosis, methylmethacrylate cement can offer essential adjunct support.[43]

DIAGNOSIS

Conditions and studies requiring evaluation include:

1. PAIN. Location(s) of localized and radiating pain, severity, variations, type(s), timing, duration, changes since onset, nocturnal pain and influence on sleep, medications taken for relief and their effectiveness.

2. TENDERNESS. Location(s), degree, type (e.g., diffuse, trigger-point).

3. CONDITION OF MUSCLES. Spasm, guarding, atrophy.

4. MOBILITY OF SPINE. Segmental limitation of motion; "poker spine."

5. NEUROLOGIC EXAMINATION. (Presented in Chapter 4.)

6. ROENTGENOGRAPHIC STUDIES. Employ all methods available for the best protrayal of vertebral lesion(s). The constellation of diagnostic methods has progressively and impressively advanced into higher levels of sophistication, and has ushered in higher quality patient care. For skeletal system studies, the "workhorse" of the diagnostic radiologist is still his "regular" x-ray machine, just as the "plain light" microscope continues to serve as the "workhorse" of the surgical pathologist. Eventually, these great old "workhorses" will be displaced by ingenious equipment and methods developed in creative minds of investigators yet unborn.

7. LABORATORY STUDIES. Space permits only the briefest overview of diagnostic methods in regular use or employed in specific oncologic diagnostic problems.

Microscopy. The phase microscope, on occasion, brings out added cellular details. The electron microscope is a magnificent research instrument and no doubt will encompass an expanded role in the future.

Enzymatic studies. Alkaline and acid phosphatase levels are useful.

Tumor tissue transplants and cultures. Seldom have a practical application.

Radioactive scanning. While opinions vary regarding the added diagnostic value of routine radioactive skeletal system scans, the method is widely employed and has many proponents. In cases in which there are carcinoma metastases, the skeletal system is involved in more than 50% (Jaffe contends that 70% + is more accurate).[21] Of all of the sites of skeletal metastases, vertebral bodies are the most common. Metastases are delivered via arteries to the marrow of the cancellous trabecular system within the peripheral cortical walls of the vertebral body. When the metastasis is the osteolytic type, it can become relatively advanced before routine roentgenograms clearly portray it. Proponents of skeletal scintiscans present convincing evidence that scintiscans reveal vertebral and other skeletal osteolytic carcinoma metastases one to several months earlier than do roentgenograms. However, the more aggressive (anaplastic) metastatic foci, as well as the extremely slow-growing (indolent) foci, may not generate a sufficient reactive osteoblastic response to permit a useful scintiscan portrayal. When scintiscans are made, their interpretations, as with other diagnostic studies, are correlated with the clinical and roentgenographic findings.

Immunologic methods. Increasingly employed for diagnostic information and for therapy. Immune surveillance is utilized to determine whether the host's immune response to the tumor is strong, weak, or absent.

When a previous surveillance indicated a strong immune response and a later determination reflected a weak response, the tumor may have either recurred locally or metastasized.

Virus studies. For the most part, they are exciting experimental explorations.

PATHOLOGIC VERTEBRAL FRACTURES CAUSED BY TUMORS

Pain originating from a vertebral tumor can be an ominous symptom. In most cases it is pain in the back or neck that motivates the patient to see a physician. Potential causes of pain directly related to vertebrae include:

MICROFRACTURES. These fractures frequently develop as fatigue fractures that are too small to be visualized roentgenographically. In addition to causing disabling back or neck pain, they are capable of generating reflex-type pain radiations that can simulate referred pain from nerve root lesions. Paravertebral muscle spasm, often severe, may last only a few days. A series of microfractures can cause protracted severe pain and muscle spasm, and later paravertebral muscle

atrophy in the area overlying the involved vertebrae. It is reasonable to presume that a microfracture communicating with an intervertebral foramen could, through creating reactive changes, cause nerve root irritation. This type of fracture also may develop in a vertebral body, e.g., at a site adjacent to a disc. A later enlargement of the fracture may permit the nucleus pulposus to protrude into the vertebral body, producing a Schmorl's node. Most microfractures heal rapidly. When a tumor mass undergoes aggressive growth, a major pathologic fracture generally develops.

GROSS FRACTURES. These are classified according to the degree of vertebral body compression: (minimal, moderate, near-total).

Minimal to moderate compression fractures. Generally these fractures are not associated with a neurologic deficit, but the patient should be meticulously examined and closely observed. When the intact portion of the vertebral body reveals moderate to advanced weakening, caused either by tumor infiltration or osteoporosis, it is mandatory to protect the vertebral body from further collapse, and an associated neurologic deficit.

Methods of management include (1) bed rest, on a turning frame or on a mattress moderately arched at the fracture level (until a better method can be arranged); (2) hyperextension body cast, with or without a chin-occiput extension; and (3) a "halo" incorporated into the body cast for selected cases in which the involved vertebral body is in either the upper dorsal or cervical region.

Near-total pathologic compression of a vertebral body. In fractures of this extreme degree, a neurologic deficit is the rule. Evaluation and clinical management of the neurologic lesion is well described elsewhere in this treatise. Plaster of paris casts, frequently incorporating a "halo" for traction and added stability, can be an important component of the total management.

BENIGN VERTEBRAL TUMORS

Hemangioma

A vertebral hemangioma involves the body.[10,21,24,28,45] Involvement within the cortical walls of a major part of the body is usually present when conventional roentgenograms clearly portray the hemangioma (Fig. 24-1). Small hemangiomas of vertebrae are a common autopsy finding in the elderly. Whether the hemangioma should be classified as a benign tumor or a hamartoma is academic. In many cases the hemangioma is an incidental roentgenographic finding. A lower thoracic or upper lumbar vertebra is the usual location, and involvement of more than one vertebra is decidedly rare. When lesions of two or more adjacent vertebral bodies are predominately osteolytic, and there is protrusion of the

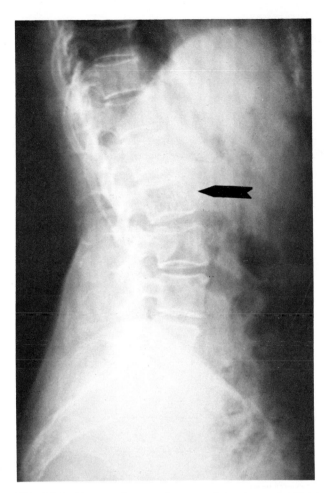

FIG. 24-1. Hemangioma of second lumbar vertebral body (arrow). Pain relieved by irradiation. No recurrence of pain and no change visualized in vertebral body during nine-year follow-up.

peripheral margin of one or more vertebrae, the diagnosis is far more likely to be an aneurysmal bone cyst than a hemangioma. When the hemangioma involves nearly all of a vertebral body, severe pain may develop and may be caused by microfractures. Involvement to an extreme degree, if untreated, can cause vertebral body collapse. The collapse can be sudden and create a major neurologic deficit.

SEX INCIDENCE. More frequent in females.

AGE INCIDENCE. Seldom appear before the middle decades.

ROENTGENOGRAPHIC PORTRAYAL. In the roentgenograms, the classic honeycombed appearance of the vertebral body reflects osteoporosis in combination with a few large bony trabeculae, the larger and more prominent of which extend from the superior aspect of the vertebral body to the inferior.

SYMPTOMS. When there is virtually total involvement of the vertebral body, there is likely to be moderate to severe pain and muscle spasm. This must be interpreted as evidence of a major deficit in the mechanical strength of the vertebral body. If this deficit is untreated, collapse is a serious threat. Moderate to pronounced tenderness over an extensively involved vertebra is the rule.

TREATMENT. Even though an involved vertebral body appears intact, if it is producing pain and muscle spasm, there should be no delay in carrying out radiation therapy; 3,000 or more rads are recommended. The involved vertebra should be appropriately protected during the period of radiation therapy. A body cast may be required to prevent collapse of the vertebral body. Protection of a greatly weakened vertebral body should be continued for many weeks following radiation therapy, since a considerable period of time is required before the re-ossification process establishes sufficient strength for the vertebra to withstand normal mechanical loading. When the lesion is an incidental finding, and there is roentgenographic portrayal of good strength, there may be no need for therapy. Hemangiomas of this type should be followed. The patient should be informed of the presence of the hemangioma and the importance of promptly seeking appropriate therapy, if pain and muscle spasm at the involved spine level should evolve. The hemangioma may remain unchanged and symptom-free indefinitely.

DIFFERENTIAL DIAGNOSIS. Although no other entity is likely to create the classic honeycombed hemangioma appearance, the possibility that the lesion represents a giant cell tumor, an aneurysmal bone cyst, an osteolytic carcinoma metastasis, or a myelomatosis focus is kept in mind. When the roentgenographic diagnosis of hemangioma is viewed as unequivocal, a biopsy is not required. When a biopsy is indicated, a needle biopsy is generally the technique of choice, since most vertebral hemangiomas are located in either one of the lower four thoracic vertebrae or in a lumbar vertebra, all of which are accessible for a safe needle biopsy.

Osteoid-Osteoma

This unique, painful "pea size" solitary benign tumor may develop anywhere in the skeletal system, including a vertebra.[6,10,20,21,24,29,31] It is remarkable that a tumor so small can generate so much pain. In long bones, where the incidence of osteoid-osteoma is far higher than it is in vertebrae, an unexplained peripheral formation of dense periosteal bone is one of the most consistent features, and this reactive bone may be so dense and thick that the nidus (which is the tumor) may be difficult to identify roentgenographically. This tumor has been known to occur in a neural arch adjacent to or in one facet of an intervertebral joint, and in a lumbar transverse process. We do not know of a case in which the tumor was in a vertebral body. Reactive peripheral ossification is absent. Figure 24-2 portrays a "pea size" osteoid-osteoma in the sacral facet of the left lumbosacral facet joint. The typical radiolucent ring directly

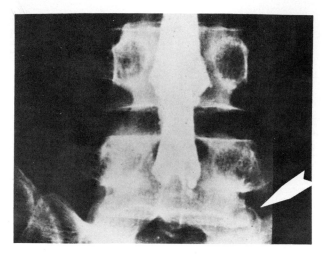

FIG. 24-2. Osteoid osteoma (arrow) on sacral facet of left L5–S1 facet joint. Confirmed histologically.

peripheral to the nidus delineates the tumor (arrow). A reflex type of radiating pain is not an unusual clinical feature.

TREATMENT. Radiation therapy is not useful. The only successful method of treatment is the surgical removal of the tumor. As in osteoid-osteomas of bones of the extremities, the surgical identification of the tumor can be difficult. Therefore, every effort should be made to determine the exact location of the nidus, prior to (and frequently during) the operation. Since there is no surrounding area of dense periosteal ossification, the tumor, when seen at operation, usually appears as a small spherical reddish brown lesion. If the operation fails to remove the "nidus," the deep-boring bone pain returns after operation, and the patient, clearly aware that the tumor was not eliminated, will emphatically inform the surgeon that he "missed." In order to locate exactly this tumor nidus in the bone of an extremity, Kirschner wires are inserted in two planes as guides or, when available, an intensified fluoroscopic screen is employed. In the spine, obviously, Kirschner wires would not be used. Whether or not a vertebral nidus could be visualized by an intensified fluoroscopic screen is not known. This tumor, once completely excised, does not recur. A second osteoid-osteoma develops with such extreme rarity as to have no significance for clinicians.

Benign Osteoblastoma of Bone

This is the term used by Jaffe and Lichtenstein.[20,24] Dahlin and Johnson recommended the term "giant osteoid-osteoma."[11] Benign osteoblastoma of bone is the term now in vogue.[6,21,29] During recent years, several cases of osteogenic sarcoma have been misinterpreted histologically as benign osteoblastomas. Since a benign osteoblastoma is characterized by numerous osteoblasts, tumor bone, and tumor osteoid, selected fields in micro-sections can simulate the histologic features of osteo-

sarcoma. Therefore, those who accept this lesion as a benign bone tumor do so with adherence to strict histologic and roentgenographic criteria. Correlative studies are meticulously performed to avoid errors in diagnosis. Figure 24-3 shows, in a 16-year-old male patient, a benign osteoblastoma involving the left lamina of C7 and the left C7–T1 facet joint. The lesion was excised and a one-level fusion performed. Three weeks after the operation, the site was irradiated (Cobalt—low dose). No recurrence was noted during an 18-year follow-up.

Jaffe has reported a benign osteoblastoma involving the entire spinous process of the third cervical vertebra in a 16-year-old male patient, and another in a 15-year-old male patient in whom a major part of the sacrum was destroyed by the tumor. In both instances, surgical resection of the tumor established a cure. In large osteoblastomas, irradiation is appropriate. Benign osteoblastomas of bone are radiosensitive, whereas osteoid-osteomas are not.

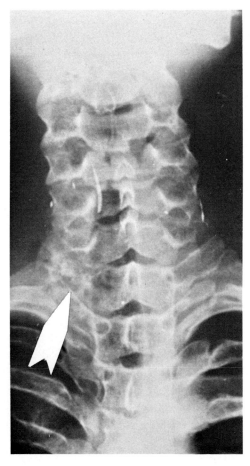

FIG. 24-3. Benign osteoblastoma of bone (arrow). Tumor destroyed major part of left lamina of C7, and left C7–T1 facet joint. No recurrence during 19-year follow-up. Treated by surgical excision and low dose of cobalt radiation.

Giant Cell Tumor

This distinctive tumor has been clearly separated from several lesions, formerly termed giant cell variants, and from malignant giant cell tumor.[5,8,14,19,28,29,34,48] It is designated giant cell tumor, not benign giant cell tumor. It may be appropriate to classify a giant cell tumor as a locally aggressive primary bone tumor. In its nonmalignant form, a giant cell tumor characteristically displays a local aggressiveness, requiring complete eradication of the tumor, to prevent recurrence. Several giant cell tumors have been reported in which a solitary pulmonary metastasis possessed the same nonmalignant histopathologic appearance as the primary tumor. However, these have been extremely exceptional cases, and cures have been reported following resection of the solitary lung lesion. Nearly all giant cell tumors of the extremities develop in the ends of the long bones at the site where epiphyses once existed. Most occur in patients past the age of 20 years, more commonly in females than in males.

Vertebral Giant Cell Tumors

During adult life, it is not rare for a giant cell tumor to develop in a vertebral body. The peak incidence is between ages 30 and 60.[11,21] Since this tumor is osteolytic, the vertebral body becomes extensively involved. Without treatment, the locally aggressive character of the tumor ushers in a pathologic compression fracture. Since the tumor tissue is soft, a needle biopsy of an accessible vertebral body will provide adequate tissue for the histopathologic diagnosis. Aneurysmal bone cysts, more common in the vertebrae than are giant cell tumors, may be erroneously diagnosed as giant cell tumors.

TREATMENT. This tumor is radiosensitive. When it is neither feasible nor appropriate to surgically resect the tumor, radiation therapy is employed. Because the site of skeletal radiation therapy has the potential for ultimately developing a radiation-induced sarcoma, many authorities believe that when a surgical resection is feasible, it is the treatment of choice.[22] The surgical procedure must remove every vestige of tumor cells, to prevent a recurrence. Strut grafts may be mandatory. One or two segments from the middle third of the fibula may serve well. Rib grafts also may be used, but are not so strong as fibular grafts. In replacing a large vertebral body, two fibular struts are likely to be required to achieve adequate bone graft mechanical support and effective osteogenesis. The spine must be supported while the bone grafts become fused to the vertebra above and below the site of the tumor. In rare instances a giant cell tumor has developed in the sacrum. Treatment has been surgical—by cryotherapy, by irradiation, or by a combination of these therapies. If treatment is surgical, bone grafts must fill the need for mechanical support. If the junction of the lumbar spine with the sacrum has been weakened by radical resection of the tumor, iliac and (or) fibular bone grafts are appropriate. If a major part of the sacrum between the sacroiliac joints has been resected, strut grafts from the fibula should be effective. Postoperatively, roentgenograms of the tumor site should be taken every three months for the first one to two years. Because of a relatively high recurrence rate following the treatment of giant cell tumors, meticulous, unbroken follow-up surveys are essential. At the first sign of a recurrence, which is the presence of a small or moderate-sized osteolytic focus at the former tumor site, the area, if accessible, should be re-explored and the recurrent tumor widely excised. If this is not done, an advancing osteolytic process delineates the enlarging tumor. Surgical procedures for the resection of a recurrent giant cell tumor become complex. When the surgical elimination of the tumor is not feasible, the astute employment of nonsurgical therapies is mandatory.

PRIMARY MALIGNANT BONE TUMORS (UNICENTRIC)

Chordoma

When a chordoma is encountered by an orthopaedic surgeon, it is likely to be a sacrococcygeal chordoma.[2,17,35] The diagnosis prior to a biopsy has a relatively low rate of accuracy. Chordomas may appear anywhere in the spinal column, but are more common at the ends of the spine—the occipital cervical junction and the sacrococcygeal region.[12,18,39] This slow-growing malignant tumor is believed to originate from cell rest remnants of the nodal cord. Our experience is limited to chordomas of the sacrococcygeal region. The tumor is osteolytic and grows slowly at its peripheral margin. Although this tumor is rare, it is clinically important to have an awareness of its existence. This point deserves emphasis, because in the majority of chordomas there has been a delay in establishing the correct diagnosis. Histologically this is a distinctive tumor and, with adequate biopsy, material is readily identified by the pathologist.

SEX INCIDENCE. Sacrococcygeal chordomas have occurred more frequently in males.

AGE INCIDENCE. They may appear at any decade of life. However, most sacrococcygeal chordomas develop during middle age.

Sacrococcygeal chordomas cause pain that frequently is identified as coccygeal. The tumor and likewise the osteolytic process of the tumor extends equally to the right and left sides of the tumor-bearing area. Foci of calcification may or may not be present. Metastases occur via the blood. The incidence is low—plus or minus 15% in sacrococcygeal chordomas.

TREATMENT. The treatment is surgical, and resection of the tumor should be as radical as is feasible. When the involvement of the sacrum is extensive, the resection is likely to leave the ilia without sacral support. Fibular struts set securely between the iliac sides of the sacroiliac joints can offer good mechanical support and active osteogenesis. Frequent roentgenographic evaluation should be carried out postoperatively, and the first sign of a recurrent osteolytic focus calls for re-exploration to widely resect recurrent tumor. This is a type of tumor in which a routine second exploration and excision, as indicated, has an important place. The second resection is carried out four to six months following the first resection. Fibular struts placed between the ilia in a first procedure naturally would not be removed at the second exploration. Irradiation of the tumor has been employed, but generally has not been helpful.

PROGNOSIS. In the past, chordomas have been viewed as tumors that will ultimately be fatal to the patient. However, if diagnosed before extensive involvement has developed, and if the surgical excision is repeated, the entire tumor may be eradicated and the prognosis in such cases should be reasonably good. There have been cases in which it was not feasible to totally resect the tumor, but since the tumor was slow-growing, it was partially resected at intervals of one to several years. These resections, though not ablating the entire tumor, have given the patient many years of comfortable life.

Ewing's Tumor

AGE DISTRIBUTION. The incidence of Ewing's tumor during the first decade of life is higher than that of other primary malignant bone tumors.[10,21,45] However, the peak incidence occurs during the second decade and the first half of the third decade. This is the most catastrophic of the solitary primary malignant bone tumors. Fortunately, this tumor is rarer than any of the osteogenic sarcomas.

SEX DISTRIBUTION. Although a bone in an extremity is the usual site, location in a vertebra or in the sacrum is not rare. For the most part, little reactive bone is formed other than the so-called multilayer "onion peel" periosteal ossification seen best when the tumor involves a long bone diaphysis. In rare instances this tumor metastasized to other sites in the skeletal system. Some authorities interpret these foci as multicentric sites of the primary tumor rather than as metastases.

In the larger reported series of Ewing's tumor, a clinically significant number were located in the spinal column. In the series of 210 cases reported by Dahlin (Mayo Clinic),[10] there were 16 in which Ewing's tumor was located in the spine.

Fortunately, this catastrophic tumor is relatively rare. Although it is rarer than osteogenic sarcoma, the incidence of the latter in vertebrae is nil.

TREATMENT. Irradiation therapy is the most widely used treatment of this tumor. Chemotherapy and immunotherapy are being added in multifaceted therapy programs and cure rates substantially higher than the former 5 to 10% are being reported.

PRIMARY MALIGNANT BONE TUMOR (MULTICENTRIC)

Myelomatosis (Multiple Myeloma)

This malignant and fatal disease originating in the bone marrow hematogenous cells ultimately involves a major portion of the skeletal system. In myelomatosis, involvement of vertebrae occurs in approximately two-thirds of all cases. The two cancers that are capable of literally riddling the spinal column with osteolytic foci are myelomatosis and carcinoma with osteolytic metastases.[10,15,21] Myelomatosis is two or three times as common in men as in women, and the period of life when this malignancy becomes manifest is during middle age or later. It is rare to see this process in patients under 30 years of age.

Vertebral body involvement generally appears more or less simultaneously in many vertebrae, more frequently in dorsolumbar vertebrae than in the cervical vertebrae (Fig. 24-4 B). Extensive osteolytic involvement of vertebral bodies causes pathologic compression fractures, some of which are associated with a serious neurologic deficit. Multiple vertebral bodies may become so riddled by myelomas that virtually all normal bone is replaced by tumor tissue, leading to vertebral collapse. Collapse is likely to be the most catastrophic where mechanical stresses reach the highest levels, such as the dorsolumbar junction. An intervertebral disc may expand to develop convex surfaces that project into adjacent vertebral bodies. It is common for a nucleus pulposus to rupture into an adjacent vertebral body.

ROENTGENOLOGIC FEATURES. In addition to the involvement of the vertebrae, the classic circumscribed so-called "punched out" foci frequently may be found in the pelvis, ribs, and skull (Fig. 24-4 A). Ultimately most of the skeleton may show roentgenographic evidence of involvement.

SYMPTOMS. Often it is pain from the spinal involvement that brings the patient to a physician. This pain may be from microfractures or from a compression fracture.

DIAGNOSIS. Ordinarily, myelomatosis is not difficult to diagnose.[7,26,36,46] The roentgenograms taken alone may simulate those of carcinomatosis with osteolytic skeletal metastases. There is generally a secondary anemia, an increase in the blood sedimentation rate, and a characteristic electrophoretic pattern in the serum and urinary proteins. In less than 50% of the cases, Bence Jones proteinuria is present at least intermittently. A sternal puncture will confirm the diagnosis in a high percentage of cases by revealing the presence of plasma cells in levels of 15, 20 or 30%, or higher. Of course the higher the percentage, the more certain the

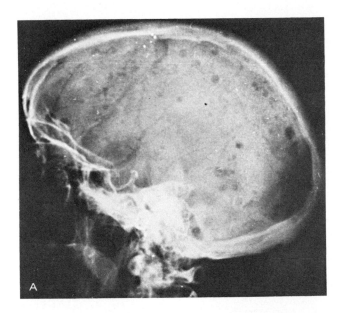

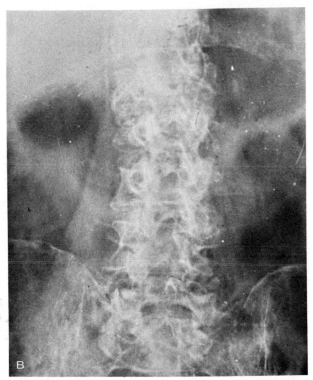

FIG. 24-4. *A*, Myelomatosis. Classic "punched out" osteolytic tumor foci are best seen in lateral view of skull. *B*, Patient became paraplegic from collapse of lower thoracic vertebral bodies.

diagnosis of myelomatosis. Biopsies of a site of skeletal involvement also reveal the diagnosis. Needle biopsies of vertebral bodies can be carried out if this is needed.

TREATMENT. A wide variety of methods of treatment have been utilized. Protection of the vertebrae against pathologic compression fractures and compression of the spinal cord is of the highest importance. Irradiation,

chemotherapy, and possibly immunotherapy, or combinations of these methods, are utilized.

PROGNOSIS. While there have been many cases in which the patient's life appeared to be prolonged and catastrophic complications prevented, this malignancy is 100% fatal.[7] While survival beyond two years from the time of diagnosis was formerly exceptional, the use of combined therapies in a multifacet program is prolonging life beyond three years. It should be pointed out with regard to radiation therapy that when the process reaches the stage of wide skeletal dissemination, irradiation appears to have little benefit. If there is a specific site in the spinal column where the pain is severe, radiation therapy can be beneficial in relieving pain, albeit temporarily.

SECONDARY MALIGNANT BONE TUMORS

Carcinoma Metastases

The tumors affecting the vertebrae most frequently by far are carcinoma metastases. In fact, carcinoma metastases are the most common of all skeletal system tumors, primary or secondary.[1,10,21,24,45]

AGE INCIDENCE. Highest during the middle and later decades.

SEX INCIDENCE. While the overall sex distribution is approximately equal, osteoplastic metastases develop principally in males, since cancer of the prostate is the predominant source of osteoplastic metastases.

DISTRIBUTION. While any part of the skeletal system may become the site of a carcinoma metastasis, relatively few appear below the elbow and knee. The femur, pelvis, vertebrae, humerus, and skull are the skeletal sites of predilection.[40,42,44]

Osteolytic Metastases

Thoracic and lumbar vertebral bodies are the most frequently involved (Fig. 24-5). As previously stated, the osteolysis associated with replacement of bone by soft tumor tissue is responsible for the high incidence of pathologic compression fractures. When an osteolytic metastasis is discovered prior to a compression fracture, every effort should be made to prevent a major fracture and secondary neurologic deficit.[32,16,43] Unfortunately, the symptoms caused by a pathologic fracture frequently represent the initial "catastrophic" evidence that a carcinoma has metastasized. In instances when a primary carcinoma has not been identified or cannot be located, a biopsy may be appropriate to establish the diagnosis. Needle biopsies of accessible vertebral bodies nearly always yield an accurate diagnosis.[36,38,47]

Carcinomas with a propensity for dispatching osteolytic metastases to the spine include carcinomas of the thyroid, kidney, and adrenal. Although most skeletal metastases from carcinoma of the breast are osteolytic,

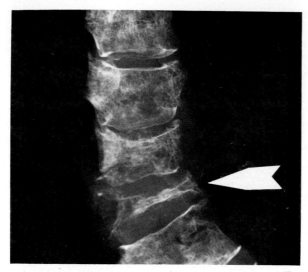

FIG. 24-5. Osteolytic carcinoma metastases. Lateral roentgenogram of postmortem specimen of lower thoracic, upper lumbar vertebral bodies. Patient became paraplegic following near-total collapse of vertebral body behind arrow.

an occasional osteoplastic metastasis is seen. Most vertebral osteolytic metastases become painful at an early stage. The metastatic cells are delivered by the blood via a nutrient artery, inside the vertebral body. Until the osteolytic focus exceeds 1 cm. in diameter, it

will not be visualized by routine roentgenograms. Microfractures can develop early, and produce sharp pain but remain "invisible." By contrast, osteoplastic vertebral metastases tend to remain silent, even for long periods, provided the reactive new bone forms diffusely in the metastatic tissue and is strong enough to give the vertebral body the mechanical support required to maintain integrity of the cortical walls.

Partial to extensive re-ossification at sites of osteolytic metastases may occur if: (1) the vertebral body collapses and destroys a major part of the metastatic tissue through mechanical crushing and by disrupting blood supply; (2) necrosis of the metastatic tissue follows irradiation; (3) involution and resorption of metastatic tissue is caused by immunologic influences; (4) metastatic tissue is resolved through chemotherapy; or (5) metastatic tissue disappears spontaneously without a known cause.

Osteoplastic Carcinoma Metastases

In osteoplastic metastases the reactive new bone formation, so characteristic of these metastatic foci, forms from the influences of the tissue in the metastases.[28,45] This is in striking contrast to osteolytic foci, where host bone is destroyed and replaced by soft carcinomatous tissue. As would be anticipated, relatively small osteoplastic metastasis may be portrayed

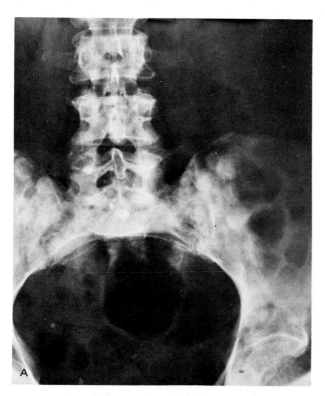

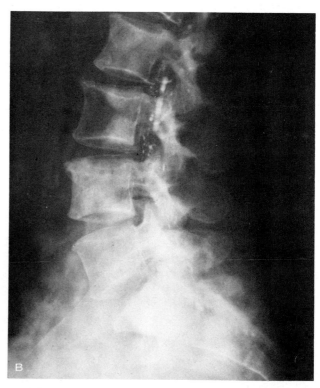

FIG. 24-6. Osteoplastic carcinoma metastases. Primary was in prostate. Pronounced reactive osteoplasia encompassing each metastatic focus prevented pathologic fracture. *A*, Anteroposterior view. *B*, Lateral view.

roentgenographically. Although the degree of reactive osteoplasia within osteoplastic metastases is widely variable, pathologic fractures are uncommon, except when weak osteoplasia combines with osteolysis. The most dense osteoplastic metastases originate from a primary carcinoma of the prostate (Fig. 24-6 *A* and *B*). The tumor cells do not directly participate in forming the bone trabeculae whose network delineates the metastatic focus. A major component of calcium in metastases from a keratinizing epidermoid carcinoma of the lung can cause these metastases to roentgenographically simulate osteoplastic metastases. Histologically there are no bony trabeculae.

Carcinomatosis is likely to produce hypercalcemia. Higher levels of hypercalcemia may be associated with gastrointestinal upsets, malaise, and even disorientation. Both acid and alkaline phosphatase may be elevated, but it is acid phosphatase that frequently reaches high levels when osteoplastic metastases originate from carcinoma of the prostate.

TUMOR-LIKE BONE LESIONS OF VERTEBRAE

Aneurysmal Bone Cyst

This widely variable osteolytic entity is neither an aneurysm nor a cyst.[3,21,24] When it forms in vertebral bodies or the sacrum, it can be progressively destructive. Early diagnosis and effective treatment have prevented many disasters. This little understood skeletal entity, once classified as a giant cell tumor variant, is not believed to be a neoplasm.[3,5] Investigators who view it as vasculogenic admit that the numerous blood-filled channels, so characteristic of this lesion, rarely possess an endothelial lining.

There is no sex predilection. In contrast to giant cell tumor, with a peak incidence in middle-aged women, an aneurysmal bone cyst generally develops during the first or second decade of life. While long bone metaphyses are the principal sites, the lesion does involve vertebrae. The erroneous diagnosis of a vertebral aneurysmal bone cyst as a giant cell tumor continues to occur.[24] An aneurysmal bone cyst develops more frequently in a vertebra than does a giant cell tumor. While the lesion may remain intraosseous, the classic aneurysmal bone cyst is characterized by a prominent soft tissue component bulging from the surface of the host bone, with a thin margin of fibrous bone overlying the "bulge" (Fig. 24-7—arrows). Jaffe uses the term "blowout" to describe the soft tissue bulge and the "tell-tale" thin margin of bone demarcating the bulge.[21] Vertebral sites have occurred more often in spinous and transverse processes than in vertebral bodies. A conspicuous and highly important feature is the capacity of this lesion to advance from one vertebra to adjacent vertebrae.[30,48] Therefore, when a vertebral

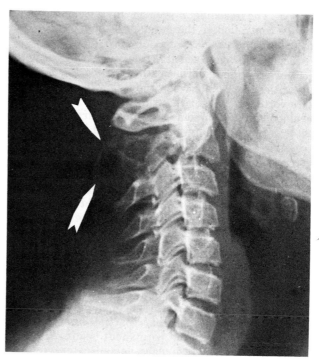

FIG. 24-7. Aneurysmal bone cyst of spinous process C2 (arrows).

body is the initial site, the lesion has the potential of advancing through an intervertebral disc to involve an adjacent vertebra. Likewise, when a spinous process is involved, the lesion may advance to one or more spinous processes in the immediate vicinity of the initial lesion. From a lumbar transverse process, it can advance to an adjacent facet joint, lamina, and pedicle.

The blood channels, usually large, that characterize the inner area of the mass may riddle the mass until it resembles a sponge. These channels, since only rarely do they have a semblance of endothelial lining, are not blood vessels; they are simply channels of blood flowing through clefts in a tissue mass possessing little cohesion. As previously stated, this lesion may acquire a truly ominous appearance, leading the unwary to erroneously diagnose the condition as malignant.

TREATMENT. Even when the tumor is large and aggressive, surgical ablation can be the treatment of choice.[4,37] When feasible, a block resection and not merely curettage is required. The recurrence rate following simple curettage exceeds 20%. If the lesion recurs, and is accessible, resection is repeated. We do not know of a case in which the recurrent tumor was malignant. Resection of a large lesion creates a large skeletal defect. Frequently, the defect can be well bridged by one or more fibular struts, combined when appropriate with iliac grafts. Internal spine fixation may be required (rods).[16] It should be kept in mind that the blood channels that may be numerous within the mass can cause profuse hemorrhage when the mass is

38. Ray RD: Needle biopsy of lumbar vertebral bodies. J Bone Joint Surg *35A:*760, 1953.

39. Robbins SL: Lumbar vertebral chordoma. Arch Path *40:*128, 1945.

40. Rubin P and Ciccio S: Status of bone scanning for bone metastases in breast cancer. Cancer *24:*1338, 1969.

41. Sherman MS: Osteoid-osteoma. Review of the literature and report of 30 cases. J Bone Joint Surg *29:*918, 1947.

42. Sherman RS and Ivker M: The roentgen appearance of thyroid metastases in bone. Am J Roentgenol *63:*196, 1950.

43. Sim FH, Daugherty T and Ivins JC: The adjunctive use of methylmethacrylate in fixation of pathological fractures. J Bone Joint Surg *56A:*40, 1974.

44. Sklaroff DM and Charkes ND: Diagnosis of bone metastasis by photoscanning with strontium 85. JAMA *188:*121, 1964.

45. Spjut HJ, Dorfman HD, Fechner RE and Ackerman LV: Atlas of Tumor Pathology, Second Series, Fascicle 5, Tumors of Bone and Cartilage. Armed Forces Institute of Pathology, Washington, D.C., 1970.

46. Tong EC and Rubenfeld S: The strontium 85 bone scan in myeloma. Amer J Roentgen *103:*84308, 1968.

47. Valls J, Ottolenghi CE and Schajowicz F: Aspiration biopsy in the diagnosis of lesions of vertebral bodies. JAMA *136:*376, 1948.

48. Verbiest H: Giant cell tumors and aneurysmal bone cysts of the spine. With special reference to the problems related to the removal of a vertebral body. J Bone Joint Surg (Brit) *47:*699, 1965.

49. Yabsley RH and Harris WR: Solitary eosinophilic granuloma of a vertebral body causing paraplegia. Report of a case. J Bone Joint Surg *48A:*1570, 1966.

25

Spinal Cord Tumors

DANIEL RUGE

A SPACE-TAKING mass within the vertebral canal may cause a variety of neurologic symptoms ranging from a slight increase or decrease in sensitivity to total paralysis. Owing to the small lumen of the canal and the limited tolerance of neural tissue to abnormal external pressure and ischemia, a seemingly small tumor may cause serious compression of the spinal cord and spinal nerve roots resulting in dramatic clinical neurologic signs.

Although direct surgical removal of the tumor is perhaps the most straightforward and logical approach to the problem, such a procedure is not always feasible, for if the tumor is intimately attached to the spinal cord, removal may result in unwarranted injury. Alternative procedures to the total excision of the tumor include subtotal removal, surgical decompression of the spinal cord, chemotherapy, and radiation therapy. Sir Victor Horsley has been credited with the first successful surgical removal of a spinal cord tumor. William Gowers diagnosed compression of the spinal cord by a thoracic spinal tumor in a certain Captain Gilbey, who had sustained a painful back injury in 1884. After Sir William Jenner gave a concurring diagnosis, Horsley successfully removed the tumor on June 9, 1887. Within one year Captain Gilbey had made a good recovery.

SYMPTOMS AND SIGNS

In 1918, Frazier presented a schematic framework of three cycles in which to interpret the development of symptoms during the life history of a spinal cord tumor.[18] Though undoubtedly no patient's symptoms conform exactly to Frazier's cycles, his scheme provides a useful starting point for our discussion. The first or root cycle is characterized by unilateral symptoms resulting from compression of either the dorsal (sensory) or ventral (motor) nerve roots. The second cycle is the Brown-Sequard syndrome, which is characterized by paralysis and by loss of fine tactile discrimination, position sense, vibratory and proprioceptive sensibility on the side of the body ipsilateral to the tumor, and loss of sensation of pain and temperature on the side contralateral to the tumor. Finally, the third cycle progresses to bilateral motor and sensory deficit, paralysis of the bladder and rectum, hyper-reflexia, and vasomotor and trophic disturbances.

Since an accurate chronology of the onset of symptoms cannot always be obtained from the history, it is not easy to assess the validity of any developmental scheme of symptoms (see also Chapter 4). However, our experience has confirmed the general outline of Frazier's findings. Typically, initial symptoms include hyperesthesia and hyperalgesia at the dermatome related to the level of the tumor, presumably due to compression of the dorsal roots serving the dermatome. This hypersensitivity can be correlated to the patient's complaints of shooting or radiating pain, which may travel down the extremities, and girdling or constricting pains of the abdomen and chest. Frequently patients complain that these symptoms are intensified by sneezing, coughing, or exertion upon defecation.

Since spinal cord tumors rarely hemisect the cord discretely, the term "modified Brown-Sequard syndrome" has been applied to cases of more marked loss of motor function ipsilateral to the lesion and more marked loss of sensory function contralateral to the lesion.

The initial flaccid paralysis ascribed to "spinal shock" (mimicking a lower motor neuron lesion) gives way eventually to the spastic paralysis characteristic of an upper motor neuron lesion. Tumors of the cauda equina always cause lower motor neuron symptoms and signs because the compressed cauda equina is comprised of nerve roots, not descending motor tracts.

Finally, the neurologic evaluation reveals a variety of pathologic reflexes and signs in patients with spinal cord compression due to tumors. Corticospinal tract involvement indicated by the Babinski reflex, Beevor's sign (suggesting paralysis of the rectus abdominis inferior to the umbilicus), and ankle clonus characteristic of spasticity are a few of the important signs.

DIFFERENTIAL DIAGNOSIS OF EXTRADURAL, INTRADURAL EXTRAMEDULLARY, AND INTRADURAL INTRAMEDULLARY TUMORS

Although it is often impossible to ascertain preoperatively the exact position of a spinal cord tumor in relation to the meninges, a few differentiating characteristics are noted. In 1932, Mixter found that in contrast to intradural tumors, extradural tumors exhibit a more rapid clinical course, typified by back and girdle pains, less symmetric cord involvement, and erosion of the vertebral canal.[28]

In diagnosing intradural tumors, Elsberg found, in 1916, that while extramedullary tumors were more common in the thoracic spine and tended to extend transversely, intramedullary tumors were more common in the cervical spine and tended to extend longitudinally.[16] Furthermore he found that the symptoms of extramedullary tumors began with radicular pains that progressed to symptoms of spinal cord involvement, whereas intramedullary tumors were characterized by numbness, tingling, variable root symptoms, dissociation of sensations, and early muscular atrophy. In 1954, Oberhill associated intramedullary tumors with lack of radicular irritation and the presence of long tract involvement.[29]

Whereas extramedullary tumors cause greatest sensory loss in the most caudal dermatomes and least sensory loss in the level near the lesion, the opposite is true for intramedullary tumors. Since the lateral spinothalamic tract and the ventral spinothalamic tract are laminated in such a way that fibers related to more caudal segments of the body lie closer to the periphery of the cord, extramedullary compression more severely involves fibers innervating segments removed from the lesion, whereas intramedullary pressure more severely affects fibers innervating segments near the lesion.

DIAGNOSTIC PROCEDURES

To complement the patient's history and neurologic evaluation, a variety of laboratory tests are available for investigating the vertebral canal. The most easily tolerated examination is the plain radiograph of the vertebral column, which may be helpful in detecting extradural tumors and certain intradural tumors. Extradural tumors may be evidenced by erosion of the pedicles, widening of the vertebral canal, or scalloping of the posterior surface of the vertebral bodies. Confirmation of this degeneration of the vertebrae is sometimes found in abnormal acid phosphatase and alkaline phosphatase levels in the blood. Banna et al. have reported three cases that were initially diagnosed as idiopathic scoliosis from the plain radiograph, but on further investigation the condition proved not to be idiopathic, but due to intramedullary astrocytomas.[4]

A helpful test is the lumbar puncture and examination of cerebrospinal fluid. Since this procedure is often painful and may exacerbate the patient's symptoms, one should attempt to incorporate related tests, such as the Queckenstedt test and myelography, with the initial effort. Normally the cerebrospinal fluid is clear, containing no red cells and only 0 to 10 white blood cells per high-power field and a total protein of 20 to 40 mg. per 100 cc. of fluid. When a tumor partially or totally impedes the flow of cerebrospinal fluid, the fluid below the tumor is not mixed and exchanged for fresh cerebrospinal fluid from the ventricles and may be xanthochromic with an elevated protein content. In the extreme condition, known as Froin's syndrome, the protein is so concentrated that the fluid coagulates on standing. The cellular content of the cerebrospinal fluid is not elevated in Froin's syndrome.

In conjunction with the lumbar spinal tap one may determine whether there is a subarachnoid block to the flow of cerebrospinal fluid by compressing the patient's jugular veins (Queckenstedt test). Under normal conditions this causes a rapid rise in cerebrospinal fluid pressure, which rapidly returns to normal on release of jugular compression. If subarachnoid block is incomplete, it will be reflected in a decrease in the amplitude and rate of pressure changes, whereas complete block results in the absence of all pressure changes.

Ehni and McNeel, who simulated the Queckenstedt test with a physical model, emphasize that dynamic manometry measures the rate of flow of fluid and not its stable pressure.[15] They also stress that impedence to fluid flow is determined by the region of smallest cross-sectional area regardless of whether that region is the spinal needle or the passage around the subarachnoid block. Finally they report that lesions containing fluid which the rising cerebrospinal fluid pressure can displace (e.g., venous blood) may present a block to myelographic examination but not to dynamic manometry. They point out that these conclusions must be accepted with caution because of deviations between their model and physiologic conditions.

Our experience has shown the Queckenstedt test to be of variable reliability, and the danger of dislodging tumors of the subarachnoid space militates against all but judicious use of this test. One should be prepared for emergency surgery should the tumor become dislodged and cause an increase in neurologic deficit.

Myelography is almost always indicated for the localization of spinal cord tumors, since it provides the most accurate determination of the level of the spinal cord compression. In the presence of a complete block, the introduction of 1 cc. of Pantopaque (a radiopaque oil) is adequate to determine the inferior level of the space-taking mass, and one need not subject the patient to the risks and discomfort of removing such a small quantity of contrast medium. Obviously, if there is no block, or if it is incomplete, a larger quantity of contrast medium will be used.

Although proponents of the cisternal approach to radiopaque oil injection argue that it aids in delineating the superior extent of the subarachnoid block and may reveal additional tumors at levels superior to a subarachnoid block determined by lumbar injection, in our judgment only rarely do these advantages outweigh the serious risk of damaging neural tissue via a cisternal puncture, and hence the lumbar approach is preferred.

Almost invariably the level of subarachnoid block found by myelography is superior to that anticipated in the neurologic evaluation of symptoms and signs. This occurs because the spinal nerve roots enter the spinal cord at levels superior to their entrance into the vertebral column and because of the lamination of the long tracts of the white matter.

PATHOLOGIC CLASSIFICATION

Extradural Tumors

Discussion of extradural tumors arising from the vertebrae appears in Chapter 24, but is omitted here.

Chordomas arise from the remnants of the embryonic notochord and are found at either end of the vertebral column, though more commonly in the sacral region. These pink, vascular, jelly-like tumors, though seldom truly metastatic, regionally invade and destroy local osseous tissues and compress neural tissue. In other respects they are essentially benign.

Hematomas containing effused blood, though rare, can be found extradurally, and speculations on their etiology have included trauma, blood dyscrasias such as hemophilia and leukemia, toxic febrile illness, and anticoagulant therapy. Although hematomas have been discovered in conjunction with herniation of the nucleus pulposus, it has also been reported that by themselves they mimic the low back pains and sciatica caused by a protruded intervertebral disc.[8,41]

Blood-borne *metastases of tumors* whose primary locations are outside the central nervous system and its associated connective tissues most frequently reside extradurally. In rare instances metastatic tumors have been found to be intradural extramedullary and even intramedullary.[11,17] Feiring and Hubbard postulated a metastasis of breast carcinoma via the perineural lymphatics of the brachial plexus to a cervicothoracic extramedullary site in two female patients.[17] In the female patient reported by Davis et al.,[11] either metastasis from breast carcinoma or seeding from a solitary cerebral metastasis may have resulted in the intramedullary tumor at T6. Metastatic carcinomas lying in the extradural space may derive from a variety of primary sites, including the breast, thyroid, prostate, lungs, and kidney. According to Davis and Davis, the most common primary sites for metastatic tumors of the extradural space are carcinoma of the breast, prostatic carcinoma, and hypernephroma.

Intradural Extramedullary Tumors

On rare occasions tumors arising from the meninges or the nerve root sheaths are found outside the dura mater, but they are usually found to be intradural extramedullary. In contrast to the extradural tumors, these intradural extramedullary tumors are generally benign.

Meningiomas ostensibly arise from the dura mater to which they are frequently attached, but it is likely that arachnoid villi, which are adherent to the dura, may contribute to their origin. Although they can be found attached to any of the three meninges, most of them are subdural with a broad dural attachment. They are usually laterally or posterolaterally situated and in proximity to the emergence of the nerve roots. Commonly they are bulbous in shape with encapsulated and circumscribed smooth or unevenly nodular surfaces. They are much more common in women than in men, and as Davis and Washburn report,[13] they are particularly prevalent in the thoracic spine of women 50 to 60 years of age. Meningiomas may occur in the cervical spine, but rarely in the lumbar spine.

Neurofibromas, which are called neurinomas, neurilemomas, and schwannomas have an uncertain origin, although Russell and Rubinstein favor the hypothesis that they are derived from Schwann cells, and hence prefer the designation schwannoma.[33] These circumscribed and encapsulated ovoid tumors lie in close association with the nerve roots and seem to have a predilection for the posterior roots of the thoracic and the lumbar segments of the spinal cord. On occasion the neurofibroma will extrude itself through an intervertebral foramen and assume an hourglass or dumbbell shape. In contrast to meningiomas, neurofibromas have more extracellular matrix, such as collagen fibers. Graham and Bond described one neurofibroma in which the center had become completely ossified.[20] Their closer association with the nerve roots brings on early radicular irritation, although the early symptoms are those of direct cord compression. Whereas the meningioma is more common in women, the neurofibroma is more common in men. Multiple neurofibromas occurring in von Recklinghausen's neurofibromatosis are transmitted as a mendelian dominant genetic disease.[42]

Teratomatous, dermoid, and *epidermoid cysts* are not easily distinguished. Theoretically the dermoid cysts contain only dermal elements and not the other embryonic elements found in teratomatous cysts. Epidermoid cysts do not contain the hairs and various skin appendages found in dermoid cysts. All of these cysts may have developed from the abnormal migration of ectodermal cells into the neural groove. Trauma has been implicated in the etiology of dermoid and epidermoid cysts, but there is not always certainty that it is either responsible or contributing. Although these intradural cysts can exist both within and outside the neural tissue of the spinal cord, we shall discuss them collectively here.

Teratomatous cysts are frequently posteriorly or posterolaterally situated in the spinal cord at all levels. Dermoid cysts are ovoid masses containing a thick, yellow, mucus-like substance intermingled with hairs.

Russell and Rubinstein cite the presence of a dermal sinus as diagnostic of an underlying dermoid cyst.[33] Dermoid cysts are especially common in the lumbosacral region and seem to predominate in males.[33] The epidermoid cysts, which are circumscribed and smoothly encapsulated and contain cholesterin, also seem to be more common in males.[24]

A variety of other intradural cysts have been reported. Loculated collections of fluid entrapped in the juxtamedullary subarachnoid space are commonly referred to as *arachnoid cysts,* but they may have ependymal cells lining their walls. This subarachnoid entrapment of cerebrospinal fluid may simulate the symptoms and signs of spinal cord compression, and on occasion may produce myelographic defects suggestive of an intradural neoplasm. Stewart and Red have described intradural cysts of the arachnoid membrane, which communicate via rostral ostia with diverticula visible on myelography.[40] Some of their patients had signs indicating progressive myelopathy. Such lesions will on occasion be encountered when one suspects a neoplasm, and at times may be anticipated from the myelographic study. In any case surgical eradication of the membrane is recommended if neurologic deficit exists.

In addition to extramedullary ependymal lined cysts, there are also those that communicate with the ependyma of the central canal. These cysts are *syringomelia* or *hernial protrusions of the central canal.* Finally *hydatid cysts,* which are most frequently observed in the body and lamina of the vertebra, may occur as extramedullary subarachnoid cysts and have also been observed within the spinal cord itself.[23]

Intradural Intramedullary Tumors

The *ependymoma,* a relatively benign neoplasm of neuroglial origin which comprises the majority of all gliomas of the spinal cord and filum terminale, is derived from the ependymal lining of the central canal. The tumors, though not encapsulated, are demarcated and circumscribed. Appearing as soft, friable, granular brownish red or bluish gray masses, they usually cause a fusiform or cylindric swelling of the spinal cord or filum terminale and may be accompanied by cysts. Somewhat more common in males,[38] they have a predilection for the lumbosacral segments.[33] Sloof et al. found half of all ependymomas to be associated with the filum terminale.[38] Though they are relatively benign, spinal ependymomas have been known to metastasize to the extravertebral soft tissue, and intracranial ependymomas have on rare occasions seeded new tumors via the cerebrospinal fluid. Subependymal gliomas are rare tumors which Russell and Rubinstein classify as a type of ependymoma. Arising from the subependymal layer, they are rich in fibers characteristic of astrocytes, but their nuclei are more characteristic of ependymal cells.

In addition to ependymomas there are wide varieties of intramedullary gliomas which are difficult to classify. At one extreme the Bailey and Cushing classification system accommodates the histogenetic origin of tumors,[3] whereas at the other extreme the Mayo Clinic classification system better accommodates the anaplastic origin of tumor cells.[38] Without attempts at classification, the characteristics of the more commonly identified gliomas are presented below.

Of the 273 intraspinal intramedullary gliomas presented by Sloof et al., 169 were ependymomas (62%), 86 were astrocytomas (32%), 8 were oligodendrogliomas (3%), and the remainder a variety of types. The *astrocytomas* are circumscribed and cause a limited fusiform swelling of the spinal cord. Composed of firm fibrous tissue with granular outer surfaces, their cut surfaces may vary in color from gray or yellow to beefy red. Astrocytomas also may be accompanied by cysts or syringomyelia. Predominating somewhat in males, these tumors are more often encountered in the upper segments of the cord,[33] in contrast to the lumbosacral localization of ependymomas.

Frequently considered as astrocytomas or related to them are the astroblastoma, the polar spongioblastoma, and the glioblastoma multiforme. The *astroblastoma* is a well-defined tumor that appears homogeneous, soft, and pinkish gray when cut. The polar *spongioblastoma*, which is similarly well demarcated, firm, and grayish white, may metastasize in the meninges, forming a thick soft gray sheet of tissue over the spinal cord.[33] Composed of a variety of histologic types, the *glioblastoma multiforme* presents itself as a spherical or elongated growth that may metastasize in the leptomeninges via the cerebrospinal fluid of the subarachnoid space and form nodular growths over the posterior aspect of the spinal cord or cauda equina. Somewhat more common in males, the glioblastoma multiforme has its maximum incidence among those aged 45 to 55 and is rare before the age of 30.

Another group of tumors distinct from the astrocytomas and their relatives are the *oligodendrogliomas*, which are solid, well-demarcated tumors varying in color from grayish pink to purple or brown. Sometimes accompanied by cysts these tumors are often heavily calcified. Spread along the cerebrospinal pathway is possible and may be chronic, leading to meningeal fibrosis, or it may be massive, highly cellular, and rapidly fatal.

Mixed gliomas formed from combinations of astrocytomas and ependymomas with oligodendrogliomas have been observed.

Distinct from gliomas, which arise from the neuroglial cells, are the *tumors of the neuron series*, which arise from nerve tissue proper. One type, the *medulloblastoma*, is believed to arise from the fetal granular layer of Obersteiner, a subpial layer of primitive cells of the cerebellar cortex.[33] These soft, friable tumors, which appear red or purple when exposed at operation, are especially prevalent in the fourth ventricle of children (64% occurring between birth and the age of 14).[33] These highly malignant tumors may subsequently seed the subarachnoid space, forming a discrete or diffuse opalescent infiltration over the posterior surface of the spinal cord.

Another type of tumor of the neuron series is the *ganglioneuroma*, which appears as a small, firm, well-circumscribed tumor, whose gray cut surfaces are finely granular. It may be cystic and contain foci of calcification.

Extradural and Intradural Tumors

Lipomas of the spinal cord are juxtamedullary, subpial masses of firm, lobulated adult fat, which do not present a clear cleavage plane and usually lie posterior to the spinal cord. According to Ehni and Love, these intradural lipomas are most commonly found in the cervicothoracic region, and extradural lipomas are more common in the lower thoracic spine.[14] In patients with congenital anomalies, most frequently spina bifida occulta, intradural lipomas may communicate with extradural lipomas. In a lipomeningocele, a subcutaneous lipoma becomes continuous with a lipoma of the cauda equina via a spina bifida occulta, and additional herniation of neural elements into the meningocele sac forms a lipomyelomeningocele. If these tumors occur near the cervical enlargement, they may cause a lower motor neuron flaccid paralysis of the upper extremities while the lower extremities are exhibiting spastic paralysis. Ehni and Love suggest that this is due to "stretching," by the lipoma, of the nerve roots serving the brachial plexus.

SURGICAL TREATMENT

Extradural Tumors

Extradural tumors are usually metastatic, and osteolytic invasion of the bony elements may have caused collapse of the vertebral bodies. In such cases, spinal fusion, along with decompression and extirpation of the tumor, may be indicated. Dissection and removal of a highly vascular extradural tumor is facilitated by separation of the tumor from the dura mater and control of bleeding by electrocoagulation of blood vessels of the tumor as they are separated from the dura mater. A combination of suction and sharp and blunt dissection utilizing curettes, rongeurs, scalpel, and scissors may be useful, depending on the situation. In general the extirpation of the tumor proceeds more successfully by the removal of large fragments rather than many small ones. Schneider cautions that the dura mater should never be opened in the presence of malignant extradural tumors, for this can only encourage intradural metastases.[35]

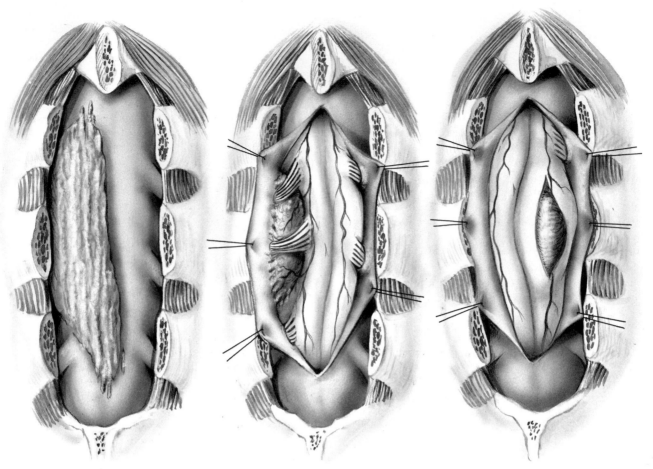

FIG. 25-1. *A*, Extradural neoplasm; *B*, intradural extramedullary neoplasm; *C*, intradural intramedullary neoplasm.

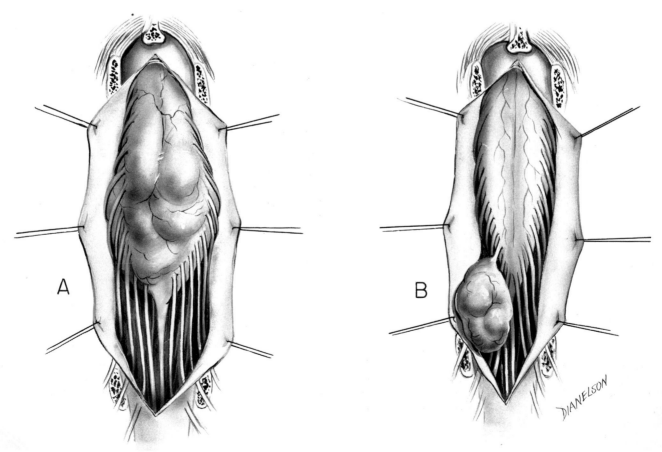

FIG. 25-2. *A*, Tumor of the conus medullaris; *B*, tumor of the cauda equina.

There is some freedom in retraction of the cauda equina at lumbar levels, but caution is essential in the protection of both the emerging nerve roots, and those that still remain within the dura mater.

Intradural Extramedullary Tumors

Paucity of extradural fat and absence of dural pulsation may indicate a tumor. After the extradural fat has been elevated, an incision is made in the dura mater rostral to the lesion to avoid spinal cord damage accompanying the sudden initial release of fluid caudal to the tumor, and to avoid damaging a posteriorly displaced spinal cord through an incision made directly over the site of the lesion.[25] The dura mater is then opened and tied back with sutures.

Posteriorly situated intradural extramedullary meningiomas are most easily removed along with their dural attachments, and this facilitates control of bleeding. While others recommend the closing of the dural defect with a dural graft, Gelfoam, or a gelatin sponge,[9,30] we do not believe a dural substitute is necessary. Instead the dura may be partially sutured or left open to enhance decompression, and attention should be directed toward a watertight muscle and fascia closure. Meningiomas of the anterior or anterolateral aspect are less accessible and require a more generous laminectomy around the tumor. The spinal cord may be gently rotated by one or two divided dentate ligaments, and piecemeal intracapsular evacuation of the meningioma may carefully proceed. Finally the capsule may be removed.

Neurofibromas tend to present themselves more laterally than do meningiomas and are commonly in close association with the nerve roots. Removal of the laminae to the pedicles may be necessary to facilitate the delivery of anterior and anterolateral tumors. Nerve fibers commingling with the tumor are sacrificed, and intracapsular piecemeal removal of the neurofibroma with a curette may be facilitated by rotation of the spinal cord by a divided dentate ligament. A neurofibroma may extrude through the intervertebral foramina and assume an hourglass or dumbbell configuration. Removal of the extraspinal parts of the tumor may proceed through the unroofing of the intervertebral foramen and the removal of the posterior part of a rib.

Intradural Intramedullary Tumors

Since incision of the neural tissue invariably causes an increase in neurologic deficit, it is not indicated in patients with only minor symptoms and signs of neurologic deficit who have intramedullary lesions which are not cystic. Instead decompression of the spinal cord is performed by leaving the dura mater unsutured and dividing the dentate ligaments. Follow-up radiation therapy may be of value. If the patient has major symptoms and signs of neurologic deficit, and if he is aware of his problem, one may choose to search for an attenuated area of the posterior median sulcus of the spinal cord and incise it vertically, being careful to avoid the lateral corticospinal tract. Subsequent enucleation of the tumor may be possible if the tumor is well encapsulated, as is fortunately the case with many ependymomas. When easy separation of the neoplasm from the spinal cord is not possible, attempts at removal may only worsen the neurologic deficit. Occasionally inaccessible intramedullary tumors may extrude themselves through a vertical myelotomy and become operable at a later time. Though we have not employed this technique, we believe that closure of the dura mater is only proper if the tumor has been completely removed. Love advises suturing the dural edges to the laminectomy margins to prevent constriction of the cord from postoperative edema, and to provide for long-term decompression of the spinal cord should the tumor recur.[25]

Poppen advocates postoperative intravenous urea solutions to control spinal cord swelling[30]; more recently mannitol and steroids have been employed.

The surgical removal of intramedullary and juxtamedullary cysts is handled in much the same manner as are intramedullary tumors, with the exception that hemilaminectomy may be sufficient. If possible, decompression of the spinal cord may be achieved by aspiration or drainage of the cyst. While arachnoid cysts, which are juxtamedullary, need merely to be punctured, Stewart et al. report on a cyst of the conus medullaris which was surgically drained by a siliconized tube, 1 to 2 cm. long, inserted into the cyst through a small myelotomy.[39] If possible, the walls of the cyst are excised except for portions directly adherent to the spinal cord. If the cyst must remain intact, a subarachnoid fistula made from silastic tubing may be constructed to allow drainage of an intramedullary cyst into the subarachnoid space.[37] Recurring symptoms of cystic lesions, suggesting that a previously drained cyst has become filled, may be treated by either reoperation or aspiration percutaneously, if one is absolutely certain of its location. Booth and Kendall have used percutaneous aspiration via two concentric needles. The outer needle is inserted in the midline and passed obliquely upward until its tip lies posterior to the dura mater and inferior to the cyst as determined by posteroanterior and lateral radiographs. The inner needle is then advanced until it enters the cyst. They caution, however, that there is considerable risk of spreading infection if the lesion is an intramedullary abscess or granuloma.[7]

References

1. Austin G: Spinal cord tumors. The Spinal Cord. Edited by G Austin. Springfield, Charles C Thomas, 1972, ed 2.
2. Bailey IC: Dermoid tumors of the spinal cord. J Neurosurg 33:676–681, 1970.

3. Bailey P, Cusing H: A Classification of Tumors of the Glioma Group. Philadelphia, Lippincott, 1926.

4. Banna M, Pearce GW, Uldall R: Scoliosis: a rare manifestation of intrinsic tumours of the spinal cord in children. J Neurol Neurosurg Psychiat 34:637-641, 1971.

5. Barone BM, Elvidge AR: Ependymomas. J Neurosurg 33:428-438, 1970.

6. Beatly RA: Cold dysesthesia: a symptom of extramedullary tumors of the spinal cord. J Neurosurg 33:75-78, 1970.

7. Booth AE, Kendall BE: Percutaneous aspiration of cystic lesions of the spinal cord. J Neurosurg 33:140-144, 1970.

8. Boyd HR, Pear BL: Chronic spontaneous spinal epidural hematoma. J Neurosurg 36:239-242, 1972.

9. Connolly RC: Thoracic laminectomy for tumor. *In* Logue V (ed : Neurosurgery, volume 14 of Operative Surgery, edited by C Rob and R Smith. London, Butterworths, 1971, ed 2.

10. Cross GO, White HL, White LP: Acrylic prosthesis of the fifth cervical vertebra in multiple myeloma. J Neurosurg 35:112-114, 1971.

11. Davis RA, Brochner R, Ruge D, Wetzel N: Notes on some unusual causes of spinal cord compression. Q Bull NUMS 32:329-337, 1958.

12. Davis L, Davis RA: Principles of Neurological Surgery. Philadelphia, WB Saunders, 1963.

13. Davis RA, Washburn PL: Spinal cord meningiomas. Surg Gynec Obstet 131:15-21, 1970.

14. Ehni G, Love JG: Intraspinal lipomas. Arch Neurol Psychiat 53:1-28, 1945.

15. Ehni G, McNeel D: The spinal manometric (Queckenstedt's test). The effects of certain factors as seen in a hydraulic model. J Neurosurg 33:654-661, 1970.

16. Elsberg CA: Diagnosis and Treatment of Surgical Diseases of the Spinal Cord and its Membranes. Philadelphia, WB Saunders, 1916.

17. Feiring EH, Hubbard JH: Spinal cord compression resulting from intradural carcinoma. J Neurosurg 23:635-638, 1965.

18. Frazier CH: Surgery of the Spine and Spinal Cord. New York, D Appleton, 1918.

19. Giuffre R: Intradural spinal lipomas. Acta Neurochir 14:65-69, 1966.

20. Graham DI, Bond MR: Intradural spinal ossifying schwannoma. J Neurosurg 36:487-489, 1972.

21. Larson S, Wetzel N, Brochner R, Ruge D: The surgical treatment of metastatic epidural tumors. Q Bull NUMS 35:42-44, 1961.

22. Lassman LP, James CCM: Lumbosacral lipomas: a critical survey of 26 cases submitted to laminectomy. J Neurol Neurosurg Psychiat 30:174-180, 1967.

23. Ley A Jr, Marti A: Intramedullary hydatid cyst. J Neurosurg 33:457-459, 1970.

24. List CF: Intraspinal epidermoids, dermoids and dermal sinuses. Surg Gynec Obstet 73:525-538, 1941.

25. Love JG: Laminectomy for the removal of spinal cord tumors. J Neurosurg 25:116-121, 1966.

26. Lyons JB: The Citizen Surgeon. London, Peter Dawnay, 1966.

27. Merritt HH: A Textbook of Neurology. Philadelphia, Lea and Febiger, 1973, ed 5.

28. Mixter WJ: Spinal column and spinal cord. *In* Practice of Surgery. Edited by D Lewis. Hagerstown, WF Prior, 1932.

29. Oberhill HR: Spinal cord tumors. Surg Clin N Amer 34:1113-1130, 1954.

30. Poppen JL: An Atlas of Neurosurgical Techniques. Philadelphia, WB Saunders, 1960.

31. Rogers HM, Long DM, Chou SN, French LA: Lipomas of the spinal cord and cauda equina. J Neurosurg 34:349-354, 1971.

32. Ruge D: Surgery of the lumbar spine. *In* Logue V (ed): Neurosurgery, volume 14 of Operative Surgery, edited by C Rob and R Smith. London, Butterworths, 1971, ed 2.

33. Russell DS, Rubinstein LJ: Pathology of Tumors of the Nervous System. Baltimore, Williams and Wilkins, 1971, ed 3.

34. Schmidt MB: Ueber die pacchioni'schen granulationem und ihr verhaltniss zu den sarcomen und psammomen der dura mater. Archiv fur Pathologische Anatomie und Physiologie und fur Klinische Medicin 170:429-464, 1902.

35. Schneider RC: Intraspinal tumors. *In* Correlative Neurosurgery. Edited by EA Kahn, EC Crosby, RC Schneider, JA Taren. Springfield, Charles C Thomas, 1969.

36. Scoville WB, Palmer AH, Samra K, Chong G: The use of acrylic plastic for vertebral replacement or fixation in metastatic disease of the spine. J Neurosurg 27:274-279, 1967.

37. Silvernail WI, Brown RB: Intramedullary enterogenous cyst. J Neurosurg 36:235-238, 1972.

38. Sloof JL, Kernohan JW, MacCarty CS: Primary Intramedullary Tumors of the Spinal Cord and Filum Terminale. Philadelphia, WB Saunders, 1964.

39. Stewart DH Jr, King RB, Lourie H: Surgical drainage of cyst of the conus medullaris. J Neurosurg 33:106-110, 1970.

40. Stewart DH Jr, Red DE: Spinal arachnoid diverticula. J Neurosurg 35:65-70, 1971.

41. Svien HJ, Adson AW, Dodge HW Jr: Lumbar extradural hematoma, report of case simulating protruded disc syndrome. J Neurosurg 7:587-588, 1950.

42. Turner OA, Gardner WJ: Familial involvement of the nervous system by multiple tumors of the sheaths and enveloping membranes. Amer J Cancer 32:339-360, 1938.

43. Weber EL: Electrophoretic analysis of fluid proteins in patients with central nervous system mass lesions. J Neurosurg 36:679-686, 1972.

44. Wisoff HS, Ghatak NR: Ependymal cyst of the spinal cord: case report. J Neurol Neurosurg Psychiat 34:546-550, 1971.

26

Operating Microscope in Spinal Cord Surgery

ROSS H. MILLER

In RECENT years, the operating microscope has been used more frequently in neurosurgical procedures. The increasing popularity has been due to improved equipment, and with the greater sophistication of equipment, better illumination of the operative field has resulted. Magnification of the structures of the spinal canal has enabled the surgeon to operate more safely on spinal cord lesions, with increased visibility of the blood vessels of the lesion and, in some cases, the fiber tracts of the spinal cord.

Vascular anomalies of the spinal cord are the most frequent lesions for which the microscope is used. Meningiomas with vascular attachments to the cord, neurofibromas, and intramedullary tumors are also occasionally easier to remove with the aid of the microscope.

Magnification enables one to handle the tissues more gently, thus minimizing postoperative complications resulting from manipulation of the spinal cord. The operating microscope also enables the surgeon to visualize and preserve important normal blood vessels that supply the spinal cord and are involved in a vascular anomaly, as well as those vessels that are being compromised by a spinal cord tumor. The nerve roots are often encased by meningiomas and hemangiopericytomas of the spinal cord. The nerve roots may be preserved by the careful dissection of the tumor. The dissection of the capsule of an intramedullary tumor, such as an ependymoma or astrocytoma, may be easier when the surgeon can define, by magnification, the plane of change between the tumor wall and the spinal cord tissue. The magnification also enables the surgeon to see small bleeding vessels in a tumor bed and to coagulate them with a bipolar current.

go back to work if he can find a somewhat lighter job, his work foreman is telling him he must be absolutely cured so that he can lift and stoop in unlimited amounts before he should even think about returning to work. Behind all this is the insurance company with its millions of dollars and the possibility that, if he really is disabled permanently, a huge monetary settlement is in the offing.

Our studies indicate, as do many others, that the industrial patient is much slower in returning to work than is the private patient.[12] In addition, however, our studies show that the industrial patient actually has a much higher hysteria and hypochondriasis level as measured by psychologic tests than does the private patient.[21] We have theorized that this is due to the milieu in which the industrial patient finds himself.

The back sufferer should be made to recognize that what has gone wrong with his back is not life threatening, and in fact is not likely to get worse. Further, that the natural history of the condition is to get well. Also, generally speaking, the condition is not amenable to being "fixed" by operation, and about all he can expect from operation is to convert an intolerable situation into a tolerable one. True, some are dramatically relieved by operation.

Often the less educated person equates the human body with his automobile. If there is something wrong with it, if he can just get the right mechanic, it can be restored to complete normalcy.

He should be apprised of the fact that, once he has had a disabling back condition, especially if he has undergone operative treatment, he is likely to have episodes of trouble in future years. He should learn how to care for his back, should learn the proper exercises, and probably should immediately start training for a lighter job. We realize that this is difficult for many people, but the alternative is to spend the rest of his life on a dole from the state or from an insurance company. Often the dole is fortified by income from a working spouse or children—a bitter solution for a once proud head of a family.

It is well known that people in the upper echelons of society have as much disc disease as those in the lower.[7] They are also as subject to acute attacks of lumbago and sciatica. However, the havoc such trouble wreaks on them and their families is infinitely less for many obvious reasons, the most important being that the better educated can keep on working, often in a nearly normal fashion, while the person who must do heavy work cannot.

TREATMENT OF THE ACUTE ATTACK

Our usual course of treatment for an acute attack of lumbago, perhaps with the patient bent over or listed to one side, is to give meperidine hydrochloride (Demerol) immediately following the examination, and to send him first to the x-ray department for a spine series and then to the physical therapy department.

As a routine, large anteroposterior and lateral roentgenograms on 7 × 17 inch plates are requested. A spot lateral focusing over the lumbosacral joint is taken, as are 45-degree lateral oblique views of the lumbosacral area and a 20 degree caudocephalad view, sometimes called a Ferguson view. In addition, a standing AP of the pelvis is taken. Differences in leg length can be determined in this way.[5]

Physical therapy provides hot packs and massage. Assuming that the roentgenograms have revealed a basically normal low spine, manipulation is used, and should be gentle. If applied in the early phase of an acute attack, when relaxation has been effected with meperidine hydrochloride, hot packs, and perhaps an injectible muscle relaxant, manipulations may be of great benefit to the patient.[2,9,10,19]

As the patient gets over his acute attack, he is trained in exercises and instructed in routine care of his back. It is essential that a careful physical examination be done along with a careful neurologic examination. A patient in the acute state may be difficult to examine properly, but later this is not a problem.

Every effort should be made to uncover other causes of low back pain, such as Marie-Strumpell arthritis, tumor, disc infection, tuberculosis, metastatic malignancy, and abdominal or pelvic disease. Laboratory studies are essential to rule out active rheumatoid arthritis or gouty arthritis. A routine arthritis study consists of a nonfasting blood uric acid, a sedimentation rate, and a latex fixation test.

A trial with a potent antarthritic such as phenylbutazone or indomethacin is often ordered. Dramatic relief may be obtained, but it is important to instruct the patient in stomach care to avoid producing an ulcer. Potent antarthritic drugs are contraindicated in patients who have or have had gastric ulcer.

Muscle relaxants and analgesics may be ordered as indicated. Physical therapy is used, but the principal function of the physical therapy department has been training in exercises and otherwise instructing the patient in care of his back. Corsets are occasionally ordered, as are heel lifts, to partially level the pelvis.

The injection of trigger points with 1% lidocaine hydrochloride and a corticosteroid is a valuable adjunct in the treatment of acute or chronic low back pain, and one that has been overlooked to some extent in recent years. These injections are simple procedures and virtually harmless. Marked temporary relief is the rule, and even prolonged relief is not uncommon. Some patients obtain permanent relief after several injections of the same area, done at weekly intervals.

Injection of the facets, or even filling the facets, with lidocaine hydrochloride and a corticosteroid sometimes is done, under fluoroscopic control, especially if the source of pain appears to be the facets and not the disc.[12] The facet joints may be filled with sodium iothalamate (Conray-60) before the lidocaine is injected. This gives some information about the condition of the facets and proves that the needle is indeed in the facet joint.

Injection of the posterior primary divisions of the lower three lumbar nerve roots on the painful side can be beneficial, and also requires fluoroscopic control. These divisions are located posteriorly just above the most medial point of the transverse process and, of course, the sacral ala.

The vast majority of patients gradually get over their acute attack in a matter of two or three weeks and have no further trouble. They should all be given detailed instructions in low back care by which they are to live for the rest of their lives. They should be trained in exercises in the hope of avoiding future attacks.

ROUTINE INSTRUCTIONS FOR CARE OF THE LOW BACK

The patient with chronic back and/or leg pain is given a set of routine instructions on a printed sheet and is asked to study them. On his next visit, these are reviewed carefully with him to ensure his complete understanding. These instructions are as follows:

1. Sleep alone or in a king-sized bed.
2. Use a firm, level bed. It need not be hard.
3. Sleep on your side with the knees drawn up. *Do not* sleep on your abdomen. If you must sleep on your back, use a rolled-up blanket or pillow under your knees.
4. In getting out of bed, turn over on your side, draw up your knees, then swing your legs over the edge.
5. Do not sit with the legs out straight on an ottoman or footstool.
6. When you are driving, hitch your car seat forward.
7. When riding in a car, not driving, on a long trip, use a low (2- to 3-inch) footstool if you are a short person.
8. Sit with the buttocks "tucked under" so that the hollow of the back is eradicated.
9. Avoid deep sofas.
10. Avoid stooping or lifting. If you must lift, set your abdominal muscles and bend with your knees.
11. Do not bend forward with the knees straight. Always squat.
12. Do not lift loads in front of you above the waistline.
13. Avoid bending backward.
14. Avoid long standing as much as possible, but if unavoidable, place one foot on a low footstool.
15. Always stand and walk with the buttocks "tucked under."
16. To get relief from back pain when walking, try to form a crease across the abdomen, elevating the front of the pelvis and shortening the abdominal muscles.
17. Women should avoid very high heels.

EXERCISES

It is essential that the doctor and the therapist understand each other. When exercises are ordered, particularly in a large therapy department, one is frequently surprised at what he actually gets when a therapist who is not accustomed to treating his patients administers the training.

The success of exercises, which are said to represent the "white hope" for back pain sufferers, varies directly with how strongly the surgeon and the therapist believe in them. The help of a physical therapist who is thoroughly trained in the use of these exercises is mandatory. Movies are a valuable adjunct to instruction. The vigor with which the exercises are performed should be graduated as his return to normalcy progresses. The exercises we use are basically those of Williams:[18]

1. *Abdominal setting.* The patient lies on his back on a firm surface with his arms folded on his chest and his knees drawn up. First the lumbar spine is flattened so that the spinous processes in the mid lumbar area touch the pad. Then the abdominal muscles are tightened until the thorax is lifted or nearly lifted off the surface (Fig. 27-1). This exercise should be done isometrically at first. It can be done completely isometrically under most circumstances.

2. *Gluteal tightening.* The hands are placed on the abdomen in the region of the umbilicus. The heels are a little closer to the buttocks than in Exercise 1. Again the abdominal muscles are contracted and the lumbar spine is flattened. The gluteal muscles are contracted and the buttocks are raised just off the mattress (Fig. 27-2).

As a general rule, Exercises 1 and 2 should be used by postoperative patients and those experiencing acute episodes. Virtually all patients can do these two exercises without hurting themselves, if they do them by simple muscle setting. The patient is given instructions to do the exercises morning and night, but not to the point of causing pain. Pain, either immediate or delayed, is an indication that the patient is exercising too strenuously; if he quits, he is doing no good. There is a fine balance, just tolerable to the patient, that will eventually strengthen his abdominal muscles.

3. *Knees to chest.* This exercise is used in young people or in people who have a healthy spine but need some limbering of the spine and some stretching of the posterior structures. It is to be avoided in postoperative patients and in those with severe osteoarthritis, degenerative spondylolisthesis, or isthmic spondylolisthesis with high grade slip (Fig. 27-3). This exercise can be done by drawing up both legs or one at a time. When both legs are drawn up, the thighs should be spread apart to avoid contact with the abdomen.

Patients are instructed to do their exercises morning and night. They can be done in bed but the bed should

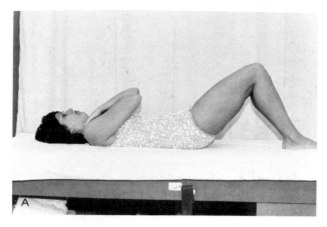 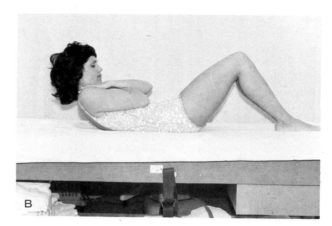

FIG. 27-1. *A*, Model has flattened her back and eliminated her lumbar curve. Eliminating lumbar curve is first step in performing this exercise and is hardest instruction to get across. It is important to keep legs relaxed and not to use legs to tilt pelvis and flatten back. If this maneuver is not done properly, this exercise does more harm than good. This exercise is all that need be done at first because abdominals are set and building abdominals is the most important single goal. Abdominal muscles should be contracted for five seconds, then relaxed slowly. Even patients with acute back condition can perform this one, as can the many who have neck problems. *B*, Model has begun movement into sitting position while holding her back flat (with the lumbar curve eliminated). This is about as high as patient should ever raise upper part of her body. Note that her arms are folded across her chest. An alternate position for arms, to be assumed later as tolerance permits, is to hold ear lobes. We do not have patients clasp their hands behind their head. Raising the chest in this exercise is done only by younger people with relatively normal spines. Older people do only isometric exercises.

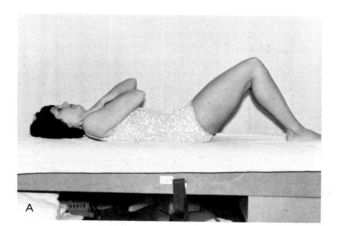 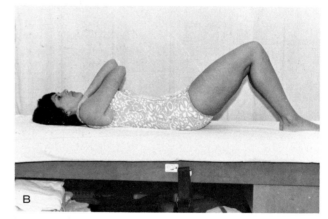

FIG. 27-2. *A*, Hands are normally placed over umbilicus, but were placed higher in this picture to show flattening of back. Prelude to this exercise, that is, flattening of back, is same as shown in Figure 27-1 *A*. *B*, Buttocks are tightened as if to pick up a marble. They need not be lifted more than one inch off table (at first, very little). Buttocks should never be raised so high that lumbar spine is extended.

be firm. It is better if they are not done immediately upon awakening, since there is a tendency to injure the back at that time due to some generalized stiffness early in the morning.

As a routine, the therapist instructs the patient in his exercises on the first visit, then again one week later. The doctor sees the patient one month later. On this second visit, and then periodically thereafter, he is again checked to see if he is doing the exercises correctly. The success of the exercises varies directly with the enthusiasm of the doctor and his physical therapist. As the condition of the back improves the exercise program becomes more advanced.

CORSETS

Considerable controversy exists as of this writing regarding the reasons a corset so often relieves some back pain. Waters and Morris believe it effects a slight

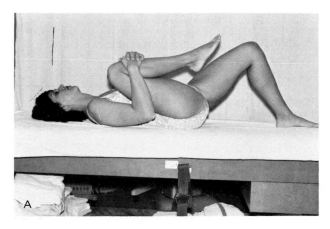
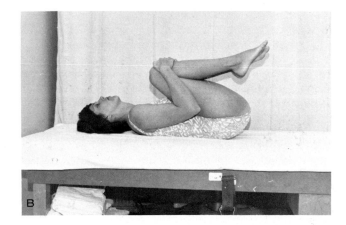

FIG. 27-3. *A*, In instructing patient in this exercise, we often start with one leg at a time. As his tolerance increases, he flexes both hips at a time. *B*, As knees are drawn toward chest, they are separated and pulled toward arm pits. This exercise is done two or three times in each training period. Thighs are held in flexed position to count of five. If there is disease in knee, popliteal area can be grasped and pulled by hand and knee allowed to remain partially extended.

but definite relief of pressure on the disc. This decrease in pressure can actually be demonstrated by means of a pressure gauge inside the tip of a needle. Farfan attributes this relief to the limitation of rotation afforded by the corset. He argues that abdominal pressure of sufficient magnitude to relieve significant pressure on the disc would shut off the return flow of blood in the large veins.[4]

It is our opinion that the relief of pain which the patient so often reports from a corset is most often secondary to the increased intra-abdominal pressure and the resultant decreased load on the disc. This decrease is small but definite. Batson's plexus of veins, being extra-abdominal, is not shut off by increased intra-abdominal pressure and continues to return blood uninterrupted even at moments of extreme increase in intra-abdominal pressure. Results of extensive studies indicate that braces actually increase motion between L5 and S1 in ordinary walking.[17] However, a brace reminds the patient not to bend and rotate his back, and this deterrent is especially advantageous in patients whose disease is situated above L5. The small corset is a compromise, but probably helps more people than does a high rigid brace. As a practical matter, a corset is used if it relieves symptoms, but discontinued if it does not.

SHOE LIFTS

According to results of population studies,[7,8] a discrepancy in leg length, as much as $1\frac{1}{2}$ inches, which the patient has had most of his life, does not predispose to low back trouble. However, many who already have back trouble can be helped by partial leveling of the pelvis. Complete leveling is not recommended immediately, for example, for a $\frac{3}{4}$-inch difference, a $\frac{1}{2}$-inch

correction can be made in the heel height if $\frac{1}{4}$ inch is removed from one shoe and added to the other. Later, perhaps, one might pursue complete correction.

The patient who has a short leg secondary to recent fracture or other injury should have his pelvis leveled completely without delay.

TRACTION

Sciatica severe enough to preclude ambulation requires treatment by traction in the hospital. Pelvic traction, with a weight of 20 pounds, is applied. The head may be elevated 25 degrees and the knees flexed to the limits of the hospital bed. Bathroom privileges are extended for bowel movement only, but at times the weight might be removed and the bed flattened to allow the patient to curl up on his side if he desires. Sedation and muscle relaxants are dispensed generously.

It is debatable whether traction is better than bed rest alone. Traction forces the patient to be more quiet and certainly has some placebo effect, but probably has little other value. Numerous patients who have been ordered to bed at home for two weeks and have made no improvement have improved greatly in the hospital in traction, probably because of the enforced bed rest.

Studies on intra-discal pressure indicate that the least intra-discal pressure is produced when the patient lies flat on his back with hips and knees flexed 90 degrees each.[12] Certainly, this position is well known to relieve acute sciatic pain, but it has not been used extensively, largely because the foot of most beds will not raise that high.

If improvement is noted after two weeks of traction, the patient should be sent home to continue the traction, in a hospital-type bed, for another two weeks. If no further improvement is made after two more weeks, it must be decided whether operative treatment is warranted. A myelogram is seldom performed, when ruptured disc is suspected, until the patient has had an adequate trial of conservative treatment and operation seems inevitable.

Electromyography is a safe means of confirming the presence of nerve root compression or irritation and of establishing which lumbar nerve is involved.

Discogram is of particular diagnostic value in spondylolisthesis in patients aged 30 to 45. In the planning of a spinal fusion, if there is some question whether the fusion should be extended to include the L4 interspace, a negative myelogram at the L4 space and a reasonably normal discogram signify that one can safely do an L5 to S1 fusion, leaving the L4 space open. The words "reasonably normal" are used because few are absolutely normal.

Laminectomy or laminotomy with removal of the nucleus pulposus has been used for 40 years. Chemonucleolysis is very promising. (See Chapter 31 for details of chemonucleolysis.)

Far fewer spinal fusions for disc disease have been done in recent years than previously. For example, it is no longer believed that a narrowed disc space at L5 in the presence of a herniated disc at L4 is an indication for spinal fusion if laminectomy is to be done. Likewise, such congenital anomalies as asymmetric vertebrae are no longer considered indications for fusion. Except in a patient past 60, however, it would not be advisable to perform a laminectomy for spondylolisthesis or spondylolysis without fusing.

Recently chemonucleolysis is being done to a limited extent on patients with spondylolisthesis where no more than a first degree slip is present. A fair percentage have been relieved of their pain and fusion has not been necessary. If the patient is not relieved by the chemonucleolysis, fusion can be done with as good or perhaps better chance of success than if the injection had never been done.

The very elderly should, of course, be treated conservatively (nonoperatively) as long as there seems to be hope of their getting over their pain. Conservative treatment should not be continued indefinitely, however. In recent years an increasing number of elderly people are being given low back operations because of intractable sciatica who in years gone by would have been condemned to spend several years of the remainder of their lives in semi-invalidism. Elderly patients have fewer emotional problems than do younger people, and relief of pain actually occurs in a higher per cent.[20] However, most of the patients who come to surgery at an advanced age have a lot of "washboarding," that is, blocking of the subarachnoid space may result from a buildup at the disc space, with choking off of the spinal canal, giving the symptoms and signs of spinal stenosis. Decompression is very successful in these cases.

HYSTERIA AND MALINGERING

Every doctor who treats pain is confronted with the problem of deciding whether musculoskeletal symptoms in a given patient originate from somatic or psychogenic disease. Learning to make the proper diagnostic decisions on the basis of logical analysis rather than by mere intuition presents a thorny challenge.[6]

Psychometric studies have been used by us to evaluate the degree of hysteria a patient may have and also to predict the subjective end results following operation.[20] This method shows considerable promise, and studies along this line are being pursued vigorously.

It must be recognized at the outset that most patients who come to the doctor with pain as their principal complaint have both a somatic and a psychogenic component to their problem. Likewise deliberate feigning of illness is rather rare as compared with the subconscious conversion of emotional problems to organic symptoms. The following are nine rules of thumb that may help spot the hysterical patient:

1. Dramatic description of pain, often with use of superlatives.

2. Poor localization. "The whole left side hurts."

3. Usually prescribed treatment of no help.

4. Reverse or bizarre action of drugs unaccountable by any known pharmacologic action.

5. Disparity between appearance of health and protestations of pain.

6. Veiled hostility toward previous doctor.

7. History vague, a lot of extraneous matter thrown in.

8. Accompanying neurotic symptoms.

9. History of many operations on other areas of body.

During a routine physical examination of the low back, the following observations should be made.

BACK MOTION. A great deal of diagnostic importance is attached by the insurance companies to lumbar spine motion. Actually there is such a wide range of normalcy as to make recording simple range of motion virtually valueless.

It is true that, if a patient can bend symmetrically in all directions and in an amount that would appear to be adequate for his age, this is strong evidence that his back pain is not due to discogenic disease nor to instability.

If the physician is concerned that the patient may be consciously or subconsciously misleading him as regards his ability to bend, considerable information can be obtained by watching the patient get undressed (if he is a male), while pretending to be reading the chart or otherwise engaged. Especially observe him when he bends over to pick up something from the floor.

MUSCLE SPASM. Unless there is a list, it is difficult to be sure of muscle spasm. If a list remains even while bending forward, this is good evidence of organic disability. Also, if on bending to the right or left, the level at which motion occurs is different on one side than on the other, we have evidence of muscle spasm.

If one has ever examined a patient with an acute disc space infection, he has seen true back muscle spasm and will probably not forget it, but it is wise to consider carefully before labeling a patient as having back muscle spasm.

MUSCLE WEAKNESS. Ask the patient to walk on his tiptoes and then on his heels. Then ask him to stand and balance himself by touching his index fingertips to the top of a high desk or x-ray viewbox. While he is balancing himself with his fingertips, have him stand on his painless leg, flexing the knee on the painful side. Then ask him to rise on tiptoe first and then on the heel while standing on the one leg. Have him repeat the maneuver, standing on his painful leg. He may have said his leg is weak but, if he can rise on the heel and toe while standing on one leg, he does not have much weakness in the lower leg. If the physician wishes to check further for weakness, he can ask the patient to rise several times on heel and toe to see which side tires sooner.

Extensor hallucis longus strength must be tested in addition. Quadriceps weakness should also be checked if it seems appropriate.

ATROPHY. The patient who complains that he has had severe sciatica for several months would be expected to have some loss of girth in the thigh or calf. If he does indeed have loss of size, especially if there is an inch or more at the maximum point of muscle development in the thigh and one-half inch or more in the calf, then it probably is due to the pain. The major leg may normally be slightly larger than the minor.

One must remember that the painful leg, because it is not exercised much, may develop edema that will deceive the examiner into believing the patient is hysterical or a malingerer because he has no loss of size in the leg.

SPECIAL TESTS. In cases where the patient has the prospect of monetary gain, the doctor must always be wary. There is no doubt that the average patient who is being paid while he is ill takes longer to return to work than the one who is not. Most of the time this attitude cannot be considered true malingering.

The following are some of the tests that can be used as a help in revealing the patient whose back condition is strongly affected by psychosomatic factors or the one who is malingering.

BURNS TEST. In this test the patient is asked to kneel on a firm but padded stool (Fig. 27-4). If a chair is used, an ordinary kitchen-type chair is best but should be padded with a blanket or pillow. The back of the chair should be either to the patient's right or to his left. Ask him to bend over and touch the floor. He may rest his buttocks on his heels if he wishes, but he should touch the floor with his fingertips. If he does not have severe hip joint disease or acute lumbago, he will be able to accomplish this. The examiner should stand in front of him so that the patient can fall against him if he

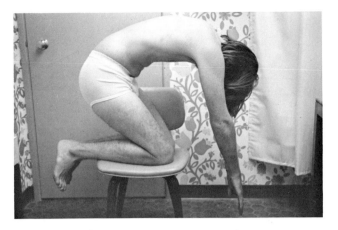

FIG. 27-4. Burns test (described in text).

decides to fall forward to give a very convincing demonstration of how "bad off" he is. If a patient complaining of chronic lumbago cannot be persuaded to touch the floor, his is either partially or completely an emotional problem or he is a malingerer. This is a good test and in my experience very reliable.

FLIP TEST. This test was described by Michele in 1958.[11] The mechanics of the flip sign are as follows (Fig. 27-5 A, B, C).

The patient is instructed to sit squarely on the examining table with his legs dangling off its side and holding his back erect, sitting as tall as possible. The arms hang at the side of the body or may be used by the patient for supplemental fixation on the table. The examiner places the open palm of one hand against the distal thigh (suprapatellar area) of the affected extremity, depressing the thigh against the table with the heel in the other hand. The affected limb is then extended at the knee. The patient's attention should be diverted when this is done.

Even in cases of genuine sciatica, no resistance or complaints may be noted until the 45-degree arc is reached, but continuance of elevation past this point is attended with an acute reversal of the lumbar lordosis and the patient tends to lean backward, frequently needing to hold the table with his hands to prevent a complete backward fall on the table.

In cases of genuine sciatica it is also noted that the individual is unable to sit erect on the table with both knees extended. He must either flex the knee of the affected extremity or lean backward to avoid the pain associated with nerve root tension. The simulator evidences no difficulty in sitting erect on the table with the knee on the side where he claims to have sciatica fully extended.

In the reinforced flip test the patient is asked to sit tall on the table with his legs hanging over the side as before but with the ankle dorsiflexed. If the knee can be extended without sciatic pain when the foot is dorsi-

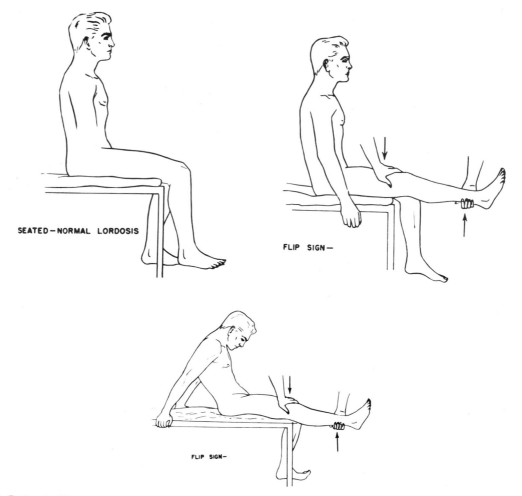

FIG. 27-5. *A,* Patient sitting erect on examining table with legs dangling. He is asked to sit as "tall" as possible and grasp the edge of the table with his fingers (not shown). *B,* Negative flip sign, knees extended and spine erect. *C,* Positive flip sign is present when examiner, pressing distal thigh against table with one hand and with other gradually elevating heel and extending knee, produces reversal of lumbar lordosis with backward flexion of trunk. (From Michele AA: The flip sign in sciatic nerve tension. Surgery *44:*940, 1958)

flexed and without the patient leaning back, then he does not have sciatica.

LIST. If the patient who is showing a list is seated on a stool and asked to bend forward, a genuine list will remain but a simulated one will disappear as he bends forward to touch the floor with his fingertips. The test will be used infrequently, but it is quite accurate.

PLANTAR FLEXION OF FOOT TEST. It is well known that in a case of sciatica, if the leg is brought up in straight leg fashion to the point where pain is produced, then dropped back down just to the point where the pain is disappearing, sciatic pain will be reproduced by dorsiflexing the ankle on the extended knee. If the sciatic pain is also made worse by plantar flexing the ankle under the same circumstances, then we have presumptive evidence that at least to this extent there is an emotional overlay or deliberate malingering.

FLEXED THIGH TEST. We know that the straight leg test may cause pain in the patient with lumbago or sciatica. After performing the straight leg test, the knee is flexed as it is brought up toward the abdomen. It is not pushed so hard as to cause movement of the lumbar spine. If the patient complains of severe pain on this maneuver it may, except in the very acute case, be considered an indication of exaggeration, either conscious or unconscious. This conclusion does not hold true if there is hip joint disease on the side being tested.

FORWARD BENDING IN A SITTING POSITION. This test can be used for the person who is simulating inability to bend forward. In a sitting position, with hips and knees normally flexed, even a person with a totally stiff back will be able to bend forward to where his chin is nearly level with his knees, unless he had hip joint disease or an acute spinal condition. If he will not bend forward when in a sitting position, his problem is probably not organic.

ELY TEST. This test is performed with the patient on his abdomen. The knee is flexed while gentle pressure is put on the area of the sacrum.

The patient with true sciatica often complains of pain down the course of his leg to the area where it has been radiating. This is due to the pull of the rectus femoris and quadriceps mechanism on the pelvis, which causes hyperextension at the lumbosacral joint. If pain is felt only in the front of the thigh and the sciatica is not reproduced, we cannot say his sciatica is not genuine, but we can say it is probably not too severe.

Pain in the front of the thigh on execution of the Ely test is normal. If he reports pain at the lumbosacral level on bending backwards, but does not when his attention is diverted as the Ely maneuver is performed, then we have an inconsistency in his pain pattern and presumptive evidence that it is hysterical.

ANTERIOR TIBIAL TEST FOR FOOT DROP. Calliet has described the anterior tibial test, which is performed as follows: The patient is asked to stand with weight distributed equally on both feet. The examiner then pushes backward on the patient's sternal area. If the foot drop is not genuine, his tibialis anterior muscle will automatically contract and the tibialis anterior tendon will bowstring across the front of the ankle and dorsum of the foot. He is not able to prevent this.

SUMMARY

Whatever our approach to the treatment of low back pain, it is clear that disc degeneration represents a more or less normal physiological process which in the majority of cases has a favorable prognosis. There is even some question if disc degeneration per se ever produces back pain. Therapeutic management should be tailored to the severity of the clinical manifestations. If the patient can curtail some of his more vigorous activities, follow a set of rules for care of the low back, persistently carry out exercises that will keep his pelvic flexors and abdominal muscles strong, keep his weight down and use harmless, non-addicting drugs as necessary, the vast majority of those who suffer from the syndrome can live comfortable lives.

Operations such as interlaminar disc removal (laminotomy), chemonucleolysis, and spinal fusion, should be done sparingly and only as a last resort after an adequate trial of conservative therapy. What constitutes *adequate* conservative therapy varies considerably between treating physicians.

It is likely that, on the average, more back operations than necessary are performed. Patients virtually force the surgeon to "do something" when they have not found relief after weeks or months of nonoperative treatment.

The younger surgeon especially suffers loss of self esteem when one of his patients consults another surgeon who will take a more aggressive approach. We must be constantly on guard against such pressures; better to lose a patient to another physician than to suffer loss of reputation by doing unnecessary back surgery.

In a recent report, it was estimated that one hundred thousand laminectomies are performed each year in the United States alone.[16] Of these about 70% obtain a really satisfactory result. This leaves 30,000 poor results annually in the United States alone. This grim statistic should make us treat our back patients nonoperatively if possible. Second operations are notoriously unsatisfactory.

As regards hysteria and malingering, it can be said that subconscious exaggeration of symptoms is extremely common in low back disease. True malingering, while much less common, does exist.

How to apprise the patient of the fact that his pain may have an origin other than organic without his taking offense, and still better, to persuade him to sincerely work to do something about his emotional problems would tax the wisdom of Solomon.

References

1. Calliet, R: Personal communication. February, 1974.
2. Chrisman OD, Nittnacht A, Snook, GA: A study of the results following rotatory manipulation in the lumbar intervertebral disc syndrome. J Bone Joint Surg *46-A*:517–524, 1964.
3. Fisher T: Manipulative Surgery Principles and Practice. HK Lewis, London, 1937.
4. Farfan HF: Mechanical Disorders of the Low Back. Philadelphia, Lea & Febiger, 1973.
5. Ford L, Goodman FG: X-ray studies of the lumbosacral spine. Southern Med J *10*:1123, 1966.
6. Frost HM: Diagnosing musculoskeletal disability of psychogenic origin in orthopaedic practice. Clin Ortho & Rel Res *82*:108–122, 1972.
7. Hult L: The Munk Fors investigation. Acta Orthop Scand Supp. 16, 1954.
8. Hult L: Cervical, dorsal and lumbar spine syndromes. Acta Orthop Scand Supp. 17, 1954.
9. Mennell J: Back Pain. Boston, Little, Brown, & Co., 1960.
10. Mensor MC: Nonoperative treatment, including manipulation, for lumbar intervertebral disc syndrome. J Bone Joint Surg *37-A*:925, 1955.
11. Michele AA: The flip sign in sciatic nerve tension. Surgery, *44*:940, 1958.
12. Mooney V: Personal communication, 1973.
13. Nachemson A, Morris JM: In vivo measurements of intradiscal pressure; discometry, a method for the determination of pressure in the lower discs. J Bone Joint Surg *46-A*:1077, 1964.
14. Nordby EJ, Lucas GL: A comparative analysis of lumbar disk disease treated by laminectomy or chemonucleolysis. Clin Ortho Rel Res *90*:119–129, 1973.

15. Norton PL, Brown T: The immobilizing efficiency of back braces. J Bone Joint Surg *39-A:*111, 1957.
16. Rothman R: Report given at American Academy Orthopaedic Surgeons Instructional Course, October, 1973, Philadelphia, Pa.
17. Waters RL, Morris JM: The effect of spinal supports on the electrical activity of the muscles of the trunk. J Bone Joint Surg *52-A:*51-60, 1970.
18. Williams PC: The Lumbosacral Spine. New York, McGraw Hill Book Co., 1965.
19. Wilson DG: Manipulative treatment in general practice. The Lancet *1:*1013-14, May, 1962.
20. Wiltse LL: Lumbosacral strain and instability. American Academy Orthopaedic Surgeons Symposium on the Spine, CV Mosby Co., 1969, pp. 54-82.
21. Wiltse LL, Rocchio P: Predicting success of low back surgery by psychological tests and physician's rating of functional component. Paper presented at the annual meeting of the American Orthopaedic Assoc., Hot Springs, Va., June, 1973.

28

Low Back Pain of Sacroiliac Joint Origin

HOMER C. PHEASANT

In the early part of the century, an appreciable percentage of low back pain problems were attributed to sacroiliac disease. Fusion of the sacroiliac joint as a form of specific treatment was popularized by Smith-Peterson.[3,4]

Identification of sacroiliac disease was dependent on the patient's subjective identification of a pain pattern in the posterior thigh, leg, and groin, and the early writers believed that the most important single diagnostic finding was the localization of tenderness about the inferior sacroiliac ligaments and in the sacrosciatic notch, together with intrarectal tenderness about the front of the sacroiliac joint.[2-4]

More recently, Coventry has reported instances of sacroiliac laxity and pain, together with symphyseal symptoms which followed the removal of bone grafts from the posterior iliac crest.[1] He uses stress roentgenograms to demonstrate pelvic instability.

One should strongly suspect sacroiliac disease when the pain is localized to the region of the posterior superior iliac spine and radiates to the groin or anterior medial thigh. To further incriminate the sacroiliac joint as the source of chronic low back pain, an injection procedure can be carried out either under image intensifier control in a hospital, or with standard x-ray equipment in a physician's office. When it has been confirmed that the needle has been directed into the sacroiliac joint, a small amount of 1% Xylocaine, with or without intra-articular corticosteroid, is injected and its clinical effect observed. Under some circumstances, Renografin has been injected in an effort to confirm the needle position, but this rarely has been successful, since the sacroiliac joint has no actual joint space and no capsular laxity. Conversely, in a few controlled cases, normal saline has been injected to test patient response.

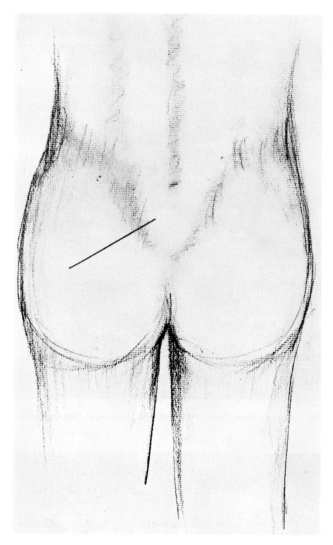

FIG. 28-5. Position of skin incision.

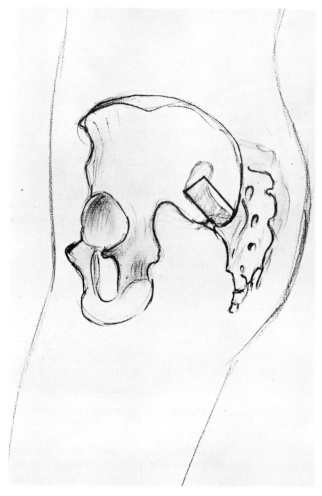

FIG. 28-6. Rectangle of bone removed is about 1 inch in width by 1½ to 1¾ inches in length and, as shown, extends into horizontal arm of sacroiliac joint and includes posterior superior iliac spine.

the sacrosciatic notch is carefully identified. This area is then exposed with a Cobra retractor. A Taylor retractor is used with the tip of the retractor imbedded in the external table of the ilium to identify the lateral extent of the iliac exposure, which should be about 2½ to 3 inches lateral to the posterior superior iliac spine. Figure 28-5 illustrates the placement of the skin incision. Figure 28-6 shows the rectangular block of bone that is removed and later reversed and countersunk into a ⅜ to ½-inch defect, which is surgically created through the sacroiliac joint into the sacrum. The articular cartilage of the sacroiliac joint is curretted with an epiphysiodesis fine currette and cancellous bone packed into the created defect before the graft is tamped into place. The margins of the iliac defect are then rongeured, so that the fragments infold over the countersunk graft. Closure is largely a reapproximation of the gluteal fascia laterally and medially.

Postoperatively the patient is allowed out of bed with crutches on the third to fourth day, but is advised not to bear weight on the side of the fusion until there is roentgenographic evidence of beginning consolidation, which takes three to four months.

References

1. Coventry MV, Tapper EN: Pelvic instability. J Bone Joint Surg 54-A:Td3-101, 1972.
2. Gaenslen FG: Sacro-iliac arthrodesis. JAMA 89:2031-2035, 1927.
3. Smith-Peterson MN, Rogers WA: Arthrodesis for tuberculosis of the sacroiliac joint. JAMA 86:26-30, 1926.
4. Smith-Peterson MN, Rogers WA: End-result study of arthrodesis of the sacroiliac joint for arthritis; traumatic and non-traumatic. J Bone Joint Surg 8:118-36, 1926.

29

Spondylosis

DANIEL RUGE

PATHOLOGIC changes in an intervertebral disc vary from an acute herniation of the nucleus pulposus without associated degenerative changes in the surrounding anatomy to chronic alterations in the disc and all adjacent structures (Fig. 29-1).

In acute herniation the nucleus pulposus passes through a weakened or torn part of the anulus fibrosis. Owing to the thinness of the posterior anulus, the rupture is usually in a backward direction, and the restraint of the posterior longitudinal ligament tends to direct the herniation laterally. The protrusion enters the vertebral canal or intervertebral foramen as a single sessile mass, or as several masses, with some fragments remaining between the vertebral bodies. Frequently, the fibers of the anulus fibrosus are only partially torn, causing a bulge into the vertebral canal or intervertebral foramen.

Occasionally a nucleus pulposus may rupture either up or down through the cartilaginous plate into the vertebral body (Schmorl's node); rarely, a herniation will pass anteriorly, avoiding both the vertebral canal and vertebrae.

Chronic degenerative changes in intervertebral discs probably result from desiccation of the nucleus pulposus. Decrease in the height of the intervertebral space produces a bulge of the anulus fibrosus, and its fibers become hyalinized and coarsened. The anulus bears much of the stress of normal movement, and an osteophytic reaction occurs at the attachment of its fibers to the bone. Spurs appear on the adjacent vertebral lips to form bony ridges with a thin central portion of fibrocartilage between them. Osteophytes may be situated on any portion of the vertebral body, but neurologic sequelae result when either the spinal cord or nerve root is impinged.

315

A   B   C   D

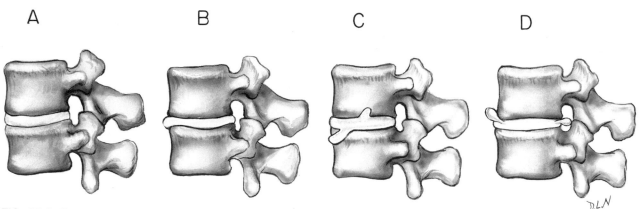

FIG. 29-1. Spondylotic degeneration: *A*, normal intervertebral relationships; *B*, weakening of anulus fibrosis with bulging of disc and narrowing of disc space; *C*, herniation of disc into vertebral body (Schmorl's nodes); *D*, herniation of nucleus pulposus.

CERVICAL SPONDYLOSIS

Acute nuclear prolapse is infrequent in the cervical spine, occurring much less often than chronic degenerative change. Symptoms and signs depend on the location of the protrusion. Central posterior protrusions cause myelopathy, lateral protrusions cause radiculopathy, and intermediate protrusions may cause both. Rarely, lateral protrusions occur and compress the vertebral artery and veins. Presumably ventral protrusions also occur, and then symptoms may result from secondary degenerative changes in the spinal column.

Acute herniations are more frequent at the C5-C6 and C6-C7 interspaces. These are the areas of the smaller lumen, the thicker cord, and the largest nerve roots; the signs of myelopathy plus C6 and C7 radiculopathy are noted.

Bull estimated that the nucleus pulposus constituted approximately 15% of the disc's volume, and that in cervical discs the maximum volume, if spherical, would have a diameter of 7 millimeters. This could cause either cord or root symptoms if the herniation occurred into a narrow area of the vertebral canal or intervertebral foramen. The signs and symptoms would be even more profound in an older patient who has osteophytes and fibrosis of tissue surrounding the cord and roots.

Below the level of the axis, the inferior facet of the vertebra above is in contact with the superior facet of the vertebra below. The point of contact of the facets forms the interpedicular (zygapophyseal) joint, and becomes the posterolateral wall of the intervertebral foramen. During youth, the facets form a synovial joint, which, with age, succumbs to arthritic change. At times degenerative changes are present in the joints even though the disc has not degenerated. If osteophytes are present on the margins of the articulating facets, there may be encroachment on the vertebral canal and on the intervertebral foramina.

Disappearance of the intervertebral spaces produces a degree of telescoping of the laminae; the upper edge of a lamina may come to lie inside the lower edge of the lamina above it. As a rule, the settling is greater posteriorly than anteriorly, a condition that increases the lordosis. Although there is doubt that the ligamentum flavum undergoes hypertrophy, it does buckle and encroach on the dorsal aspect of the spinal cord. At the same time, bars at the intervertebral space compress the ventral surface of the cord, resulting in further narrowing of the sagittal diameter of the canal. This not only compresses the cord, but also compromises the flow of blood, particularly in the anterior spinal artery.

Marginal lipping of vertebrae and narrowing of the intervertebral space result in the formation of osteophytes of the articular processes, causing narrowing of the foramina. Probably as a consequence of the external constriction, the dural root sleeve thickens and the arachnoid becomes fibrotic. All these factors combine to compress the nerve root producing radiculopathy.

SYMPTOMS. Pain is the primary complaint. Its onset may be dramatic or insidious, but in either case, it is ultimately intermittent and the exacerbations are not always related to activity. There is a wide variation in the segmental distribution of nerve roots, but a point of some value in localization is that the brachialgia arising from cervical spondylosis generally affects the radial aspect of the hand—the thumb, index finger, and middle finger. Irritation of the C6 nerve root affects the thumb and index finger, whereas irritation of the C7 nerve root also affects the middle finger. Irritation of any of the lower cervical roots produces generalized aching in the proximal muscles about the scapula and pectoral area, as well as in the brachium.

PHYSICAL FINDINGS. The patient frequently tilts his head forward and to the opposite side and resists most movements, particularly extension.

The motor signs in the upper extremities are usually

those of lower motor neuron variety: atrophy, decreased reflexes, and weakness. Rarely, one finds increased reflexes in the arm, and this strongly suggests compression of the cord as well. In fact, one may see signs of both lower motor neuron and upper motor neuron lesions in the same extremity. Should the pyramidal tract be affected, spasticity, as evidenced by homolateral ankle clonus and the Babinski sign, may be seen.

RADIOLOGIC STUDIES. The nature of the disease may be deduced from the history and radiographs. Sudden onset of symptoms and the absence of osteophytes on lateral and oblique films tend to suggest acute herniations, whereas a long history and films showing posterior lipping and encroachment of the intervertebral foramina are more likely to signify chronic spondylosis. Positive myelographic defect in the presence of normal films also supports the probability of acute herniation, but certainly does not guarantee that such is the situation. It is generally agreed that, in the cervical spine, chronic disease is far more frequent than acute herniation.

Myelography is useful in supplementing the information gained from lateral and oblique radiographs of the cervical spine. A disc showing a good deal of osteophytosis on plain roentgenograms may produce little indentation of the Pantopaque column if the osteophytes are placed far laterally. On the other hand, a disc only slightly involved by spondylosis may show a large indentation of the Pantopaque column if some of the cartilage has protruded. The typical appearance is a filling defect corresponding to the interspace, with lack of definition of the root pouches. If there is a large protrusion or osteophyte, the Pantopaque may be hung up, resulting in a long, vertical filling defect. There is great value in obtaining lateral films to determine both backward protrusion of disc material or forward protrusion of ligamentum flavum.

INITIAL TREATMENT. The key to initial treatment is immobilization. Bed rest, traction devices, and braces are most commonly employed. One or all should be utilized unless the patient is manifesting signs of paresis of the upper extremities or long tract spinal cord signs. Neck exercises and neck manipulation are contraindicated.

SURGICAL TREATMENT. Surgery will be considered only if conservative measures are ineffective. Physical findings and results of the myelogram influence the decision to operate. Signs of spinal cord compression, with or without root symptoms, are indications for laminectomy.

The upright, sitting position is favored, and if laminectomy is to be done, the neck should be in a neutral (not flexed) position. Removal of two laminae may be sufficient, but should the cord be displaced dorsally, further removal is indicated. A clue to the degree of spondylosis within the vertebral canal may be the extent of degenerative changes in the muscles, tendons, and laminae. In the extreme, one may encounter palpable fibrotic and calcified masses in the muscles and tendons quite superficial to the laminae. It is noteworthy that similar changes may be present adjacent to the spinal cord. Vertical incision of the dura mater and division of the dentate ligaments permit gentle but adequate retraction of the spinal cord, so that one might assess the nature of the mass. If a soft mass is palpated, there is justification for incising the ventral dura to effect removal. If there is a bony projection, as is usually the case, it is probably not wise to attempt removal, because in the majority of cases the operation, which has made proper inspection possible, has also given adequate decompression. It is advantageous to preserve the arachnoid, particularly if one finds that it is not possible to suture the dura mater. Crandall and Batzdorf, in reviewing their patients, reported better results when the dural incision was not closed, and they have recommended insertion of a dural graft.[5]

For the intraforaminal protrusions and the arthritic hypertrophy of the zygapophyseal joints, which produce root signs, laminectomy does not extend sufficiently laterally to expose either a herniation or a spur, and removal of bone is directed to the posterior wall of the foramen (Fig. 29-2). This consists of removing the medial half of the joint with a small portion of the adjacent lamina. The surgery is facilitated if the neck is flexed, and this may permit access through an adequate interlaminar space laterally. One is usually obliged, however, to utilize a burr and small curettes to expose the intraforaminal course of the nerve and any protrusion lying deep to it. If one removes adequate bone in performing the medial facetectomy, one can see the dural sleeve of the nerve root project laterally and perpendicularly from the dura mater of the spinal cord. Inferior to the dural sleeve of the nerve root, there is an area corresponding to an axilla, and in this region one may encounter either a soft fragment of protruded nucleus pulposus or a spur. Gentle upward retraction of the dural sleeve of the nerve root is safe, but medial retraction of the dura mater of the cord is to be avoided. Protruded nucleus may be removed easily. If there is a compressing spur, it may be meticulously curetted, with all movements of the curette being directed toward the surgeon and away from the neural structures. Regardless of the finding at surgery, there is great need for restraint, because too much vigor exercised in searching for a nucleus pulposus or in removing spurs may have hazardous consequences. Certainty that operation will disclose a soft herniated nucleus pulposus may frustrate the surgeon, and his insistence that the operation must produce such a specimen may be harmful to his patient.

The patient with severe spondylosis, consisting of subluxations and multiple angulations of the vertebral column, may require a more extensive surgical procedure. If quadriparesis exists, extensive laminectomy of three, four, or more vertebrae may be required. Simultaneous fusion lateral to the laminectomy, utilizing a

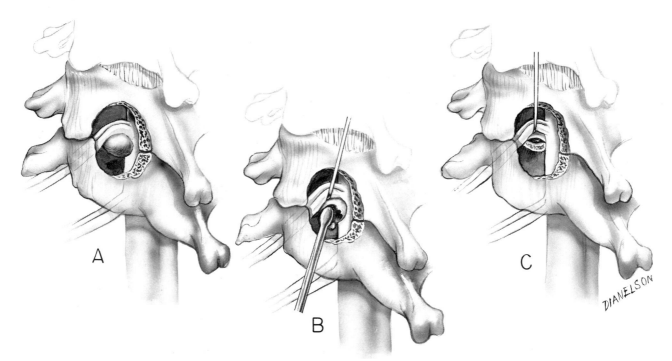

FIG. 29-2. Surgical treatment of herniated cervical disc: *A*, hemilaminectomy revealing disc protrusion; *B*, gentle retraction of nerve roots allowing piecemeal removal of disc; *C*, completed removal of herniated cervical disc.

bone graft extending from C2 to T1, is advised. Not only will this support the spine, but hopefully, stability and immobility of the spine result in the disappearance of spurs.

LUMBAR SPONDYLOSIS

The lumbar spine has some similarities to the cervical spine in that there are normally a lordosis and considerable mobility. The supporting structures are subject to similar morphologic deterioration, and so the pathologic states described for the cervical spine are equally applicable to the lumbar spine. The lumbar vertebrae and intervertebral discs are larger, and the lumbar vertebral canal contains primarily nerve roots because the conus rarely extends lower than the L1-L2 interspace.

We encounter acute herniations of the nucleus pulposus more commonly in the lumbar spine than in the cervical, but the frequency of low back syndromes in the absence of disc extrusions also attests to a high incidence of chronic degenerative states.

SYMPTOMS. The patient's story is characteristic, with pain being the prominent feature. The pain may be in both the low back and leg, with emphasis on the latter. Physical activities such as lifting, jumping, and falling may be contributing factors and, in the patient's view, are usually associated with the onset, particularly if the backache precedes the sciatica.

The leg pain may be bilateral, but is usually uni-lateral, and Nashold and Hrubec, in a recent survey of over 1,000 patients, noted a more frequent occurrence on the left.[11] Coughing, sneezing, straining, and walking often aggravate the pain in both back and leg. When specifically questioned, the patient may admit to numbness or bladder disturbance, but it is the pain that makes him seek assistance.

The study reported by Nashold and Hrubec revealed that among the group with lumbar disc disease, 4.4% also had cervical disc rupture and 1% had thoracic disc rupture.

PHYSICAL FINDINGS. *Posture.* Paravertebral muscle spasm, spinal tilt, loss of lumbar lordosis, and immobility are characteristic posture changes. The tilt is generally to the side opposite the sciatica, but exceptions have been noted. Attempts at extension are considerably more limited than flexion. There is frequently a limp, and on standing the affected limb is gently flexed at both hip and knee.

Motor Signs. Atrophy, weakness, and decreased deep tendon reflexes are anticipated lower motor neuron sequelae of nerve root compression.

One can observe the loss of bulk and tone to the gluteus and muscles of the leg. The anterior tibial muscle, when atrophied, causes the anterior crest of the tibia to be prominent. Comparative measurements at the greatest circumference about the calves will give an approximate estimate of the atrophy.

Weakness is a consequence of the atrophy, but may occur in its absence. It is easily tested in the extensor hallucis longus muscle by asking the patient to dorsiflex the great toe against resistance. A paretic anterior tibial muscle will not permit heel walking nor strong dorsiflexion of the foot.

The ankle reflex is usually decreased in the patient with an L5-S1 lesion, but may also be altered with a lesion at L4-L5. Depression of the patellar tendon reflex suggests a lesion at L4-L5 or higher.

Sensory Signs. Pain on straight leg raising is regarded as very significant and suggests nerve root compression. It is a very consistent finding, and its absence suggests that the protrusion is probably above the nerve root. Restriction of straight leg raising is probably more a sensory phenomenon than motor because the patient stops raising the leg when pain appears and resists passive elevation of the limb because this aggravates the pain.

Other sensory findings consist of hypesthesia and hypalgesia. Numbness on the dorsum of the foot and anterolateral aspect of the leg are common findings, but localization of the level by sensory findings is not precisely reliable. Davis, Martin, and Goldstein concluded, on the basis of their study of 500 patients that sensory findings are unreliable,[7] and Wilson reached the same conclusion in analyzing the results of examinations on 1,000 patients.[18]

RADIOLOGIC STUDIES. A patient with symptoms suggestive of a lumbar herniated disc requires radiologic survey of the lumbar spine, sacrum, and pelvis, not only to assess the architecture of the spine, but also to exclude the presence of other osseous disease. It is particularly helpful to note the presence or absence of spondylolisthesis or other congenital anomalies.

Positive contrast myelography is not required to make the diagnosis, but is valuable in localizing the herniation or herniations that have occurred. As a rule, the results of myelography aid the decision for surgery and may assist in planning the surgical approach.

INITIAL TREATMENT. Bed rest is the ideal initial treatment. It is more comfortable on a firm bed, which permits one to lie with flexion at the hips and knees. It should be total—with or without traction—and its duration, unfortunately, is influenced by many factors including economic. It is frequently not possible for the patient to have an appropriate trial of rest outside a hospital, and a stay of many weeks in a hospital for this purpose constitutes questionable utilization of both space and funds. Whenever possible, a month of greatly reduced activity should precede consideration of surgical interference.

SURGICAL TREATMENT. The generally accepted indications for surgery are the following:

1. Failure of adequate rest to greatly diminish pain.
2. Massive central protrusion causing severe and sudden motor deficit of extremities and bladder.
3. Progressive and severe weakness of a muscle group.
4. Recurrent sciatica which affects the patient's productivity.

Most herniations of nucleus pulposus occur at the two inferior interspaces (Fig. 29-3), and for these we prefer to limit the elevation of the muscles to the affected side. The sacrum offers an ideal landmark, and exposure of the sacrum and lowermost interlaminar space permits accurate localization.

To explore the L5-S1 interspace, one removes the inferior portion of the L5 lamina to uncover approximately 2 cm. of ligamentum flavum (Fig. 29-4). The superior portion of the sacrum at this interspace is then removed until one encounters the termination of ligamentum flavum and the appearance of extradural fat or dura mater. The ligamentum flavum is generously excised, while an attempt is made to preserve the fatty tissue. Exposure at superior levels is accomplished in a similar manner after appropriate portions of superior and inferior laminae are removed with rongeur.

The nerve root is retracted medially to expose the herniated mass in most instances. Rarely, when a fragment of disc has presented medial to the root, a portion of the disc is removed before one completes the retraction. The irritability of the root is worthy of note. Frequently, even though the herniation is not extensive, mere handling of the root will result in strong muscle contraction. It is also occasionally observed that a root that has been compressed for a long time is not irritable. The higher the level, the more roots are retracted, and so great care is required to obtain exposure. Retraction of a root is facilitated if the surgeon refrains from excessive packing of sponges within the vertebral canal.

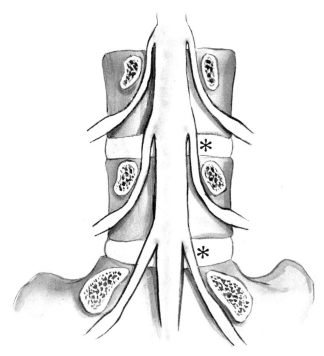

FIG. 29-3. Asterisks mark where disc protrusions compress nerve roots. Hence L5–S1 herniated disc would compress S1 not L5 nerve root.

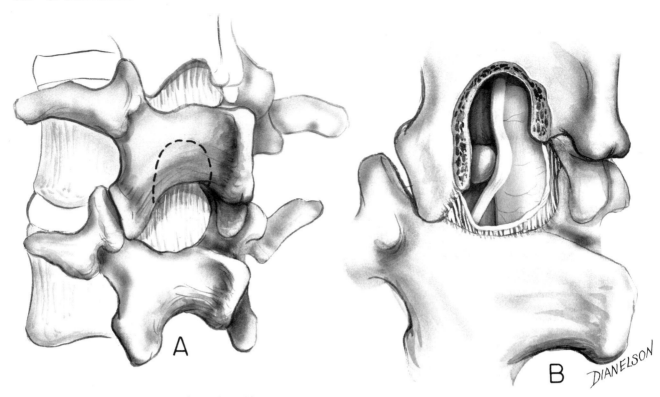

FIG. 29-4. Surgical treatment of herniated lumbar disc: *A*, dotted line indicates bone to be resected; *B*, resection of inferior portion of lamina and removal of underlying ligamentum flavum reveals protruding disc compressing nerve root.

If the nucleus has extruded, it is often easier to remove a large fragment, but search should be made for additional fragments outside and inside the interspace. In the passing of instruments into the interspace, care must be exercised to avoid injury to vessels anterior to the vertebral body. It is prudent to forego attempts to reach the area of the anterior longitudinal ligament, particularly with instruments requiring opening and closing of the jaws.

The proximity of the great abdominal vessels should be a deterrent to the reckless removal of "the last" fragment of disc material. However, the surgeon should not let his pride deter him from realizing that he may have inadvertently entered a major artery or vein. Palpation of a strong femoral pulse after completion of the surgical procedure will assure that vessels have not been injured. The wise surgeon will have a plan of procedure for such an eventuality.

Complete laminectomy is seldom required, but it may be appropriate for the infrequently occurring midline or large herniation in the superior interspaces of the lumbar spine. The technique is then similar to that utilized for removal of a cauda equina tumor. If much retraction is required to extricate the herniated nucleus pulposus anterior and lateral to the dura mater, one would be well advised to incise the dorsal dura mater, retract the nerves of the cauda equina, and then incise the ventral dura to remove the disc material.

Occasionally, it is expedient to utilize less than total laminectomy. One may remove the inferior portion of the spinous process above and the superior portion of the spinous process below to gain access to the ligamentum flavum (Fig. 29-5). By cutting further cephalad and caudad with a rongeur, one can decompress the dorsal aspect of the cauda and gradually expose more of the dura mater. This will permit bilateral access to the interspace and is useful for removing disc material while minimizing retraction.

If one is not satisfied with the removal of a herniated nucleus pulposus and if one is interested in searching for further cause of root symptoms, passing a nerve hook underneath the root and into the foramen may disclose the cause of root compression. Spurs may be removed with a gouge or curette.

NARROW LUMBAR CANAL

A variety of conditions that affect the lumbar spine defy precise classification. They have in common a narrow vertebral canal, which is presumed to be congenital, but since symptoms appear in adulthood, one may conclude that changes in the morphology of supporting structures have etiologic importance. Variations in the size of the lumen, plus variations in the acquired alterations, may account for multiple symptom complexes ranging from minor sensory complaints to severe sensory and motor impairment.

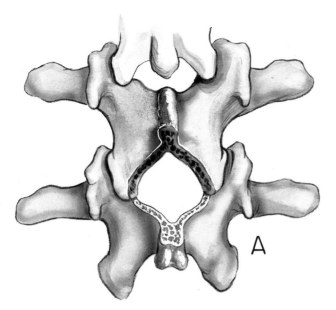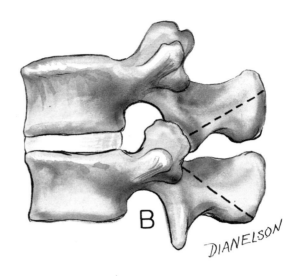

FIG. 29-5. Wedge removal: *A*, Inferior portion of spinous process above and superior portion of spinous process below are removed; *B*, dotted lines indicate bone to be resected.

Verbiest published the histories of seven male patients who were found at operation to have a generalized narrowing of the vertebral canal, probably of developmental origin.[16] Symptoms appeared in adult life and always implicated the cauda equina. Walking or standing produced radicular pains, with disturbance of sensation and paresis of the legs. On lying down, there would be remission of symptoms and only minimal physical findings. He observed that the normal lumbar vertebral canal has the form of a pentagon, with its greatest diameter between the pedicles. His patients were found to have preservation of the interpedicular space, but had sagittal constriction, primarily at L3–L4, with the encroachment being primarily from the articular processes.

Payne and Haung consider a contrast column of 20 mm. transversely and 15 mm. sagittally to be a proper minimal size, and that any reduction indicates spinal stenosis.[12] Blau and Logue suggested that ischemia of the nerve roots produced the symptoms,[1] and Wilson believes that in addition to an ischemic etiology, there might be postural effects.[17] In the ischemic variety, pain results from muscular contraction and is relieved by rest, including standing still; in the postural type, pain results from lordosis and is relieved by changing the posture, but not by standing still. Yamada et al. implicate the ligamentum flavum, and point out that if there is a narrow canal, increasing the lumbar lordosis will thicken the ligamentum with the result that the cauda equina is compressed posteriorly and laterally.[19] It should be remembered that this posture may also cause a bulge of an intervertebral disc toward the cauda equina.

Lateral lumbar myelograms made with the patient erect and extended show the greatest narrowing to be at L3–L4 and L4–L5. Surgical decompression should include extensive removal of the ligamentum flavum, and Verbiest has found it necessary to remove the medial part of the articular processes in most instances.

We have, on occasion, noted that the facets are unusually large and that the entire lamina sinks forward, the superior portion encroaching on the dura and its contents from behind. Frequently, the large facets crowd the dura and nerve roots from the side, and if the distortion of the vertebral column causes a bulge of the intervertebral disc or ligaments, the constriction is further increased from in front. It is difficult to conceive of adequate decompression without removal of the medial facets in those instances when they are chiefly responsible for compression.

Epstein et al. have reported on a group of patients whose sciatica resulted from nerve root entrapment in the lateral recesses.[8] Except for very positive straight leg raising, the neurologic findings were not striking, and myelography on the whole was normal or nearly normal. Surgical exploration revealed the nerve root (or roots) to be locked into the lateral recess by the superior (which is also the medial) facet, and adequate facetectomy decompressed the affected roots and brought about relief of symptoms.

COMPRESSION BY REDUNDANT NERVE ROOTS

Cressman and Pawl reported on a patient whose myelogram revealed a serpentine configuration and block at L3–L4, which operation showed to result from a redundant nerve root and median bar.[6] Schut and Groff reported on a patient whose myelogram appeared to be quite similar but in whom surgery revealed three redundant nerve roots.[15] Both patients were relieved by decompression, which included vertical dural incision.

References

1. Blau JN, Logue V: Intermittent claudication of the cauda equina. An unusual syndrome resulting from a central protrusion of a lumbar intervertebral disc. Lancet 1:1081–1086, 1961.
2. Brain L, Wilkinson M: Cervical Spondylosis. Philadelphia, WB Saunders, 1967.
3. Brish A, Lerner MA, Braham J: Intermittent claudication from compression of cauda equina by a narrowed spinal canal. J Neurosurg 21:207–211, 1964.
4. Bull JWD: Cervical spondylosis. Proc Roy Soc Med 41:513, 1948.
5. Crandall PH, Batzdorf U: Cervical spondylotic myelopathy. J Neurosurg 25:57, 1966.
6. Cressman MR, Pawl RP: Serpentine myelographic defect caused by a redundant nerve root. J Neurosurg 28:391–393, 1968.
7. Davis L, Martin J, Goldstein SL: Sensory changes with herniated nucleus pulposus. J Neurosurg 9:133–138, 1952.
8. Epstein JA, Epstein BS, Rosenthal AD, et al: Sciatica caused by nerve root entrapment in the lateral recess: the superior facet syndrome. J Neurosurg 36:584–589, 1972.
9. Friedman H: Intraspinal rheumatoid nodule causing nerve root compression. J Neurosurg 32:689–691, 1970.
10. Logue V: Cervical spondylosis. In Neurology. Edited by D Williams. New York, Paul B Hoeber, 1957.
11. Nashold BS, Hrubec Z: Lumbar Disc Disease. St. Louis, CV Mosley, 1971.
12. Payne KWE, Haung PWH: Lumbar disc syndrome. J Neurosurg 37:75–82, 1972.
13. Raaf J: Removal of protruded lumbar intervertebral discs. J Neurosurg 32:604–611, 1970.
14. Ruge D: Surgery of the lumbar spine. In Logue V (ed): Neurosurgery, volume 14 of Operational Surgery, edited by C. Rob and R. Smith. London, Butterworths, 1971, ed 2.
15. Schut L, Groff RA: Redundant nerve roots as a cause of complete myelographic block. J Neurosurg 28:394–395, 1968.
16. Verbiest H: A radicular syndrome from developmental narrowing of the lumbar vertebral canal. J Bone Jt Surg 26B:230–237, 1954.
17. Wilson CB: Significance of the small lumbar spinal canal: cauda equina compression syndrome due to spondylosis. J Neurosurg 31:499–506, 1969.
18. Wilson CB: Clinical signs by physical examination, in Lumbar Disc Disease. Edited by BS Nashold and Z Hrubec. St. Louis, CV Mosby, 1971.
19. Yamada H, Ohya M, Okada T, Shiozawa Z: Intermittent cauda equina compression due to a narrow spinal canal. J Neurosurg 37:83–88, 1972.

30

Degenerative Diseases of the Thoracic Spine

DONALD R. GUNN

THIS CHAPTER deals with aspects of thoracic pain of spinal or paraspinal origin not related to fracture, infection, or neoplasm. The term thoracic disc derangement embraces intervertebral disc protrusion, herniation, narrowing, calcification, and degeneration. Thoracic radicular pain is the term used to describe pain that radiates from the spine around or through one or both sides of the chest. Pain in the chest is a common complaint with a wide variety of causes, and it is not generally appreciated that it frequently arises from the spine or paraspinous regions. In 1937, Ollie reviewed 600 consecutive cases of chest pain and concluded that in about one-third of the patients, the pain was of spinal origin.[4] Thoracic pain of spinal or paraspinal origin may be attributed to thoracic disc derangement, posterior primary ramus entrapment syndrome, costovertebral joint syndrome, or other causes.

In his book, *Radicular Syndromes with Emphasis on Chest Pain Simulating Coronary Disease*, Davis emphasized that pain may result from stimulation of either a ventral or dorsal root and gave details of segmental patterns, symptomatology, and diagnostic signs. The literature on thoracic disc disorders as a cause of thoracic radicular pain is not large, but gives adequate coverage of the signs and symptoms produced. Older references to surgical treatment are very depressing, but more recent papers are quite encouraging.[3,6] The outstanding impression, however, is the relative paucity of literature devoted to thoracic pain of other than visceral origin.

ANATOMY AND PATHOGENESIS

In 1822, Magendie stated that, in animals, stimulation of the peripheral

323

cut end of a ventral motor root gave rise to a pain response as long as the dorsal sensory root was intact. The role of the ventral nerve roots in the production of radicular pain was studied in man by Frykholm who made the following observations:[2]

1. Stimulation of a normal ventral nerve root apparently produces no pain, but stimulation of a compressed and chronically irritated ventral nerve root produces typical ventral root pain.

2. Whereas stimulation of the dorsal root produces a typically dermatomal distribution of pain, ventral root pain is referred to the muscles innervated by that root (myotomal distribution).

3. Blocking the dorsal nerve root with local anesthetic abolishes all pain, whether of dorsal or ventral root origin.

If a painful stimulus is severe and is maintained for a long period, its input into the spinal cord will spread through interconnecting neurons so that appreciation of pain will spread both proximally and distally as well as across the midline. Thus the area in which pain is described may be much greater than one would anticipate with a purely radicular distribution.

COSTOVERTEBRAL JOINT. A rib head has two articular facets separated by a ridge. Each facet is part of a synovial joint, which articulates with a facet on the appropriate vertebral body, and the ridge between the facets is in contact with the anulus. The head of the rib is held in position by the triradiate ligament, which consists of a superior fasciculus to the vertebral body above, an inferior fasciculus to the vertebral body below, and a middle fasciculus, which blends anteriorly with the anulus deep to the anterior longitudinal ligament.

COSTOTRANSVERSE JOINT. A typical rib tubercle also has two facets. The medial facet, covered with articular cartilage, articulates with a reciprocal facet on the tip of the corresponding transverse process. The lateral facet gives attachment to the lateral costotransverse ligament (lateral facet of the rib to the tip of the transverse process). The middle costotransverse ligament occupies the space between the neck of the rib and the anterior aspect of the corresponding transverse process. The superior costotransverse ligament runs from the crest of the neck of the rib to the inferior surface of the transverse process above.

DISTRIBUTION AND COURSE OF ANTERIOR AND POSTERIOR PRIMARY RAMI. The anterior primary rami supply the skin forward of the posterior axillary line, and the posterior primary rami supply the skin from the posterior axillary line to the middle of the back. Each posterior ramus runs backward immediately after leaving the intervertebral foramen and traverses a narrow gap between the lateral margin of the inferior articular facet and the medial border of the superior costotransverse ligament. It is here that entrapment may occur.

SYMPTOMS AND SIGNS

SYMPTOMS. Pain is the outstanding complaint and varies widely in severity and distribution. The patient often implicates a specific incident, automobile injuries being the most commonly mentioned cause of disc derangement. Some patients describe an acute onset of pain but no specific injury; others describe a slow onset of pain, also with no distinct origin. The most common site of pain is the mid or low thoracic region, and it is described as either encircling the chest wall to the axilla and pectoral region or as piercing directly from back to sternum. Occasionally it extends over a wide area. The pain is usually aggravated by activity, particularly that which requires maintaining the arms at or above the shoulder level. Heels striking on hard surfaces, or the driving of vehicles with poor or absent suspension, such as forklift trucks, often exacerbates the pain. Some patients learn that coughing or sneezing must be avoided. Most patients find rest to be salutary, but about half of them also learn that lying supine aggravates the pain. The pain is variously described; occasionally it is said to be crushing or constricting, reminiscent of pain of cardiac origin. Others describe a boring or stabbing pain, beginning posteriorly and coming through to the sternum or epigastrium. Paresthesia in the lower limbs is not uncommon, and a feeling of numbness, heaviness, or "pins and needles" of the anterior thigh region is the commonest of these. According to Davis, tingling, numbness, and stiffness of the fingers often accompanies chest pain, though this is difficult to explain on an anatomical basis.

LOCAL SIGNS IN THE THORACIC REGION. Spasm is not as noticeable a feature as it is in the lumbar spine, but may be detectable particularly in the lower thoracic paravertebral muscles. Deformity is rare, but occasionally one sees an increase in kyphosis. Tenderness is commonly present, and its distribution must be accurately defined. It may occur under the following circumstances:

1. If there is a lesion of an intervertebral disc, it is common to find that the two adjacent spinous processes are tender, but occasionally the tenderness is confined to only one of them.

2. Tenderness of an interspinous ligament rather than of the adjacent spinous processes suggests irritation of the segmental nerve supplying that ligament.

3. Although paraspinal tenderness in the thoracic region is often said to indicate changes in the costovertebral joints, it more probably indicates tenderness of the paraspinal muscle. The costovertebral joints are, of course, not available for palpation. Tenderness of the paraspinal muscles may be an expression of nerve root irritation.

4. The presence of pain and tenderness of the muscles at the anterior end of an intercostal space (parasternal tenderness) is interesting and not

uncommon. It is believed that pressure over the anterior end of a rib may produce pain, and therefore the costovertebral joints are blamed. This is a rare phenomenon, and careful palpation usually reveals that the tenderness is muscular and not bony.

Some sensory change is usually present. The best method of testing appears to be the drawing of the end of an opened paper clip across the skin (this instrument has proved to be more satisfactory than either a pin or pinwheel). The most common finding is a well-defined proximal level of hyperesthesia accompanied by another, often less well defined, band of hyperesthesia distally. The distance between these two levels of hyperesthesia may be narrow, apparently representing the boundaries of one dermatome, but more often the hyperesthesia levels are many centimeters apart. Between the upper and lower bands of hyperesthesia, the sensation is often surprisingly normal, although some hypoesthesia may be present. The sensory changes are bilateral in 50% of cases and often occupy the distribution of both posterior and anterior primary rami. If only the posterior primary ramus is involved, the sensory change extends from the midline of the back to the posterior axillary line, whereas with only anterior primary ramus involvement it extends from the flank to the front. The importance of posterior or posterior and anterior rami involvement will be discussed later.

LONG TRACT SIGNS. In every case of thoracic pain of spinal origin, assessment of the function of the spinal cord distal to the level of pain is essential. The abdomen and the lower extremities will be examined for diminished superficial reflexes, spasticity, hyperactive deep tendon reflexes, clonus, and the Babinski sign. In addition, it is not uncommon to find some degree of sensory change, such as hypesthesia of the anterior aspect of the thigh, which may indicate involvement of a root of the genitofemoral nerve.

ROENTGENOGRAMS AND SPECIAL TESTS

ROENTGENOGRAMS. A normal thoracic spine roentgenogram does not exclude disc derangement. One should look for narrowing of an interspace and/or calcification of the disc space. Degenerative changes at one or two interspaces are particularly important, and unilateral changes may produce root signs on that side only. Myelography of the thoracic region is difficult and exacting, but is worth attempting. The myelograms should be taken in both left and right oblique views. Occasionally it helps to remove the needle and observe the flow of contrast agent with the patient supine. In lesions of T11 to T12, the use of a large volume (40 cc.) of material may be helpful in differentiating between a flow defect and a small, but significant, disc protrusion. Tomography has been employed in the diagnosis of

spinal lesions since 1940.[7] Lateral tomographic cuts may show evidence of posterior osteophyte or ridge formation that cannot be visualized on regular films.

SPECIAL TESTS. Electromyographic testing of intercostal muscles may be helpful. Intercostal blocks under fluoroscopic control may provide significant diagnostic information and suggest methods of treatment. The Minnesota Multiphasic Personality Index is an essential part of the examination of all cases of long-standing thoracic spinal pain. Graduated spinal anesthesia is of great help in assessing the degree of pain relief one may anticipate if an organic lesion can be removed.

DIFFERENTIAL DIAGNOSIS

THORACIC DISC DERANGEMENT. Derangements of thoracic intervertebral discs are characterized by a definite history of injury; pain and sensory changes, usually bilateral, involving anterior as well as posterior primary rami distributions; tenderness over one or two spinous processes and at the anterior end of the corresponding intercostal space; evidence of spinal cord involvement; disc space changes on radiologic examination; and a filling defect on myelography.

POSTERIOR PRIMARY RAMUS ENTRAPMENT SYNDROME. Entrapment of a posterior primary ramus may occur where it passes between the medial border of the superior costotransverse ligament and the lateral margin of the inferior articular facet. Characteristically, the onset is usually acute and unrelated to trauma; pain is unilateral and local; sensory change is limited to the distribution of the posterior primary ramus (i.e., it does not extend beyond the posterior axillary line); and tenderness over the spinous processes is absent.

COSTOVERTEBRAL SYNDROME. Although a severely deformed costovertebral joint undoubtedly can cause pain, it rarely does because the intercostal nerve is not intimately related to the costovertebral joint.

TREATMENT OF THORACIC DISC DERANGEMENT

NONSURGICAL TREATMENT. There is little place for physical therapy in the treatment of thoracic back pain. Heat in one form or another may be soothing, but may also exacerbate the symptoms. Manipulation of the thoracic spine is not recommended.

Cervical traction has been used extensively both diagnostically and therapeutically. It may produce relief of pain and also diminish both spinous and parasternal tenderness.[1] The traction should be relatively heavy and should reach 20 to 30 pounds for 15 to 20 minutes, two to three times a day. Braces such as the

Thomas or Taylor posterior spinal supports may provide some relief.

Infiltration of interspinous ligaments with local anesthetics may give temporary relief. Even if pain relief is complete, the sensory changes remain unaltered and the pain returns within several hours. Since the innervation of the interspinous ligaments is segmental, the relief of pain by infiltration of one ligament may be helpful in determining the level of radicular irritation. Infiltration of a costotransverse joint often also blocks the intercostal nerve at that level, while infiltration of a costovertebral joint frequently blocks one or both of the adjacent intercostal nerves. Intercostal blocks should be carried out under fluoroscopic control. A marker is used to identify the level of the space and then a spinal needle is inserted at the predetermined level 4 cm. from the midline. The needle should pass just below the transverse process and the neck of the rib, and lie with its tip just lateral to the upper part of the intervertebral foramen. This position is confirmed in two planes. If the needle puncture is made not more than 4 cm. from the midline and is inclined medially, it is unlikely that it will enter the pleura and it is almost impossible for it to enter the vertebral canal. After the tip of the needle is confirmed as being lateral to the upper part of the selected intervertebral foramen, 1 to 2 ml. of a 1% solution of local anesthetic is injected. If the correct level has been selected, sensory testing shows disappearance of the upper and lower bands of hyperesthesia and their replacement by a narrow band of hypesthesia along the appropriate intercostal space, accompanied by relief of pain. A small amount of steroid may be added, and a film is taken to provide confirmation of the level of the needle before it is withdrawn. Some patients get considerable relief from a course of four to six blocks done at weekly intervals.

A change of occupation is often an important aspect of treatment. For example, the change from the constant trauma of driving an unsprung forklift truck to a sedentary job may reduce pain to more acceptable levels.

SURGICAL TREATMENT: THORACIC DISCECTOMY. Normally the patient is placed in the lateral position with the left side up, but the approach may be through the right side if indicated. The level of the thoracotomy is dictated by the findings on an anteroposterior film. The rib selected for removal is the one that is seen to cross the midaxillary line at the level of the involved disc (e.g., the seventh rib would probably be removed in order to reach the disc space between the ninth and tenth thoracic vertebrae). After the pleura has been incised, the lung is retracted and the involved disc is identified by a count downward from the first rib and also upward from the twelfth or thirteenth rib. Preoperative radiologic studies are essential to this kind of localization. When the spine is being palpated, the ridges that are felt are the intervertebral discs, and the concavities between the ridges are the vertebral bodies. After identification of the correct disc, a longitudinal incision is made in the parietal pleura. The incision lies just anterior to the heads of the ribs, which are easily palpated, and extends at least to the discs above and below the one to be removed. The pleura is lifted and undermined both anteriorly and posteriorly until the anterior longitudinal ligament and the head of the rib are visualized. The intercostal arteries and veins above and below the intervertebral disc are then identified. These vessels, which cross transversely in the concavity of each vertebral body, are isolated, ligated, and divided. Division of only two intercostal vessels does not appear to jeopardize the blood supply to the spinal cord. It is possible to raise the anterior flap of pleura to allow blunt dissection to continue across the anterior longitudinal ligament until the opposite side of the intervertebral disc can be palpated.

The head of the rib is first removed, and an incision is then made into the anulus and continued through the anterior longitudinal ligament. At this stage it helps to locate the appropriate intercostal nerve in the intercostal space and to trace it back to the intervertebral foramen. The dissection of the nerve in the region of the foramen is not easy, but when it has been done the posterolateral corner of the disc is identified and excision can be continued. One of the great advantages of this exposure is that work on the disc space can always be in a postero-anterior direction (i.e., away from the spinal cord). Excision is continued usually with fine curet until the posterior longitudinal ligament is visualized. With the nerve root used as a guide, a fine dissector is then carefully inserted between the posterior longitudinal ligament and the dura. The posterior ligament can then be removed to whatever extent appears necessary. The end plates of the bodies are then removed by curet or chisel until bleeding cancellous bone is visualized, and portions of the removed rib are then inserted as bone grafts. One may cut two shallow transverse grooves in each body with a curet and insert a segment of rib into each and then pack the intervening space with finely cut bone chips.

The longitudinal incision in the parietal pleura is sutured over the grafted area. A chest tube is inserted and the chest wound closed.

Thoracotomy is a very painful operation, and a careful balance must be struck between control of pain and depression of respiration. Postoperatively deep breathing and coughing are encouraged, and blow bottles are used to stimulate pulmonary function. As soon as good breath sounds are present and a roentgenogram shows re-expansion of the lung—usually 24 to 36 hours after operation—the chest tube is removed. The patient is rolled from back to side every two hours until turning can be achieved actively. The sutures are removed at about ten days, and anterior and posterior plaster shells are then made. The shells are applied when the patient is helped out of bed, but as soon as he can stand easily, a complete body cast is applied. This is worn for eight to twelve weeks.

Our only postoperative complication has been a single instance of bilateral clonus of two days duration. The incidence of post-thoracotomy pain of a radicular distribution seems to have been higher in this series than in the thoracotomies done for other reasons, probably owing to isolation of the intercostal nerves at the intervertebral foramen. Intercostal blocks may relieve the pain, but it subsides in time.

SURGICAL TREATMENT: EXCISION OF SPINOUS PROCESSES AND INTERSPINOUS LIGAMENTS. As noted above, pain is sometimes relieved by infiltration of an interspinous ligament. Unfortunately, excision of spinous processes and interspinous ligaments does not remove the cause of pain and will, at best, achieve only temporary relief.

TREATMENT OF THE POSTERIOR PRIMARY RAMUS ENTRAPMENT SYNDROME

An attempt is made to infiltrate the posterior primary ramus as it passes backward through the narrow gap bounded medially by the lateral margin of the inferior articular facet, superiorly by the inferior aspect of the transverse process, and laterally by the medial border of the superior costotransverse ligament. To do this, a needle is inserted about 2 cm. from the midline and is "walked" laterally off the edge of the inferior facet. A 1% solution of local anesthetic is used, and is followed by a small amount of steroid. If the diagnosis is correct, pain relief should be complete.

TREATMENT OF THE COSTOVERTEBRAL SYNDROME

Costotransversectomy in the treatment of thoracic radicular pain is rarely indicated, and this when there is gross and obvious deformity of the head and neck of a rib or a severely deformed single level costovertebral joint. Through a wide exposure, the costotransverse ligaments are divided and the transverse process removed with rongeurs. The rib is then divided at about the angle and after the stripping of soft tissue, the costovertebral joint is opened. The rib head is forced from its attachments to the anulus and adjacent vertebrae.

References

1. Davis D: Radicular Syndromes With Emphasis on Chest Pain Simulating Coronary Disease. Chicago, Year Book Publishers, 1957.
2. Frykolm R: Deformities of dural pouches and strictures of dural sheaths in the cervical region producing nerve root compression. A contribution to the etiology and operative treatment of brachial neuralgia. J Neurosurg 4:403-413, 1947.
3. Logue V: Thoracic intervertebral disc prolapse with spinal cord compression. J Neurol Neurosurg Psychiat 15:227-241, 1952.
4. Ollie JA: Differential diagnosis of pain in the chest. Canad Med Assoc J 37:209-216, 1937.
5. Raney FL: Costovertebral-costotransverse joint complex as the source of local or referred pain. J Bone Jt Surg 48A:1451-1452, 1966.
6. Ransohoff J et al: Transthoracic removal of thoracic discs. J Neurosurg 31:459-461, 1969.
7. Weinbren M: A Manual of Tomography. London, HK Lewis and Company, 1946.

31

An Approach to Failure of Lumbar Spine Operations

RICHARD N. STAUFFER

FAILURE to gain symptomatic relief after an operation on the lumbar spine is a cause of suffering and disability to the patient, and a source of great consternation to the treating physician. Many patients undergo multiple spinal operations only to have problems increase with each operation. A typical history includes laminectomy for disc excision followed by re-exploration and, finally, one or more spinal fusions. Statistics are not available to determine how many people are disabled because of unsuccessful operations, but if one accepts a mean failure rate of 20% (a rough average of many clinical reports), the number may total many thousands.

INDICATIONS FOR SURGICAL TREATMENT

Although it can be agreed that meticulous handling of delicate structures (dura mater, spinal roots, and facet joints) during operation contributes to good results, it is probable that proper indications for operation are a greater determinant of the outcome than is the method of operation. There can be little argument about the *absolute* indications for lumbar disc operation, which are: (1) massive midline disc herniation, and (2) increasing neurologic deficit. These generally require immediate operation. Unfortunately, the vast majority of cases are not so clear-cut and fall into the large "grey zone" of *relative* indications, which are: (1) failure of adequate conservative management to relieve symptoms, and (2) recurrent episodes that respond to conservative measures but are frequent enough to effectively incapacitate the patient. Surgeons probably have not agreed on what constitutes "adequate conservative management," but to us it implies an effort to obtain considerable relief of pain and remission of signs by means of strictly enforced bed rest (with local heat, anti-inflammatory agents, and muscle relaxants) for a period of three weeks. It is from within this large, ill-defined area of relative indications that most of the failures arise. However, there is statistical information available which, if heeded, will help to refine indications within this relative category and help to decrease the number of failures.

It is often stated that the success of a disc excision depends on whether nerve root pressure is relieved or whether a nuclear prolapse actually did exist. Hirsch found that when definite evidence of disc herniation and nerve root compression was found at operation, 96% of the patients had a satisfactory result.[6] The clinical results after excision of the so-called "bulging disc" or a negative exploration were much less satisfactory. Sprangfort reported an almost linear relationship between the degree of disc herniation found at operation and the clinical end result.[11] Ninety-five percent of the patients in his series who had a so-called "complete herniation" obtained complete relief of pain, whereas only 40% of those with a "negative exploration" had any pain relief. Those with bulging discs and equivocal findings ranged somewhere between these two figures. These papers have pointed out that there are elements of the patient's history and physical examination and ancillary diagnostic measures that have statistically predictive value in determining the presence of definite disc herniation and hence predictive value as to the success of the surgical procedure.

There are also important nonstructural factors that bear on the success or failure of surgical treatment. Social and psychologic factors play a significant role in the production of disability, particularly with regard to low back problems. Wiltse has done a prospective clinical study of the predictive value of various preoperative factors in patients having chemonucleolysis.[15] He found that elements of the preoperative Minnesota Multiphasic Personality Inventory correlated highly with the clinical results achieved by this method of treatment. Specifically, when the Hs (hysteria) or the Hy (hypochondriasis) parameters were elevated above the eighty-fifth percentile, the patient had less than a 10% chance of obtaining a good result from treatment. The percentage of satisfactory results rose to 16% between the seventy-fifth and eighty-fourth percentiles.

Wiltse also found that patients with compensation claims had a high statistical correlation with failure. This has been documented in a number of retrospective studies of the results of laminectomy and disc excision[1,4,6] and lumbar fusion.[9] In our follow-up of patients having anterior interbody disc excision and fusion,[12] and posterolateral fusion,[13] a total of 32 patients were receiving, or suing for, compensation. Only 12 of them had achieved a satisfactory result from treatment and returned to work. This represents a percentage far

below the satisfactory results of the overall series. The most significant factor predisposing to a poor clinical result was the presence of compensation claims, and the presence of a preoperatively diagnosed personality disorder or psychoneurosis ranked second. Beals and Hickman have documented the prevalence of emotional abnormality and the prolonged disability associated with the industrially injured low back.[2] This is probably a symptom of a social ill, and there is little the physician can do about it, except to realize that compensation elements have a highly significant predictive value in the surgical treatment of patients with low back problems.

To reduce the number of failures, patients must be selected judiciously for treatment with lumbar fusion techniques. In recent years there has been a definite tendency toward conservatism and constriction of indications for fusion. Lumbar fusion is rarely, if ever, absolutely indicated as a primary treatment of degenerative disease. The implicit indication for lumbar spinal fusion is localized segmental instability (whether caused by degenerative disease or spondylolisthesis), when conservative measures have failed. However, our present inability to define spine stability in precise biomechanical terms makes this an intuitive diagnosis in most cases. The vast majority of patients suffering low back pain of mechanical origin can be restored to a productive, comfortable existence by conservative measures, including isometric muscle-strengthening exercises, treatment of emotional disorders, and alteration of recreational and vocational activities.

There is more disparity of opinion regarding the role of lumbar fusion combined with disc excision. We believe this combined procedure to be necessary when (1) there is a history of severe, incapacitating mechanical low back pain prior to acute disc syndrome, and (2) when there has been excessive bone removal, predisposing to an unstable vertebral unit. DePalma and Rothman found a high degree of correlation between relief of back pain and relief of sciatica following disc excision.[4] Overall, 48% of their patients had persistent low back pain postoperatively. However, by combining fusion with disc excision they lowered the incidence by only 5% (a figure of no statistical significance). The addition of bone grafting, regardless of technique, adds greatly to the length and blood loss of the surgical procedure, the incidence of postoperative complication and morbidity, and the length of postoperative convalescence. Therefore, combining fusion with disc excision in order to reduce the number of failures does not seem justified, except in patients with localized degenerative disease and a history of incapacitating mechanical low back pain predating the acute disc syndrome, and in patients in whom an extensive laminectomy is required, predisposing him to segmental instability and postoperative back pain. Figure 31-1 illustrates a case in which disability resulted from extensive laminectomy and partial facetectomy. A subsequent posterolateral fusion was successful.

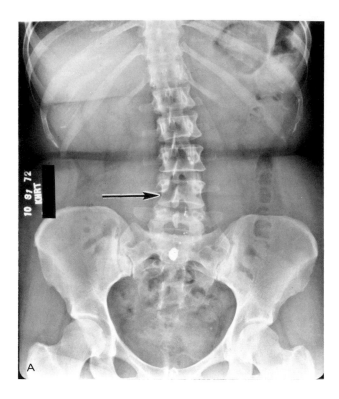

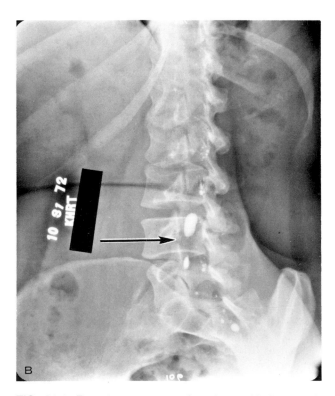

FIG. 31-1. Roentgenograms of patient with incapacitating mechanical low back pain subsequent to large laminectomy. Note complete absence of inferior facet of fourth lumbar vertebra on right (arrow): *A*, anteroposterior roentgenogram; *B*, right oblique roentgenogram.

EVALUATION AND TREATMENT

Obviously the first step in the management of failure of a lumbar spine operation is a thorough evaluation of the patient. Treatment without diagnosis is futile and inevitably leads to yet another failure, and serves to perpetuate the patient's suffering. Because of the complexity of the problem, this evaluation is best accomplished by a multidisciplinary approach involving concerned, interested, open-minded individuals in several fields who will seek out the causes of the failure and try to establish the important elements in the patient's disability. Some of the potential causes for failure, in rough order of decreasing occurrence, are:

1. Poor indications for initial procedure[4,6]
2. Psychoneurosis and compensation elements[2,15]
3. Arachnoiditis and perineural scarring
4. Unrelieved bony compression of neural elements[5,7,14]
5. Recurrent extrusion of disc material at the same or another level[1]
6. Segmental vertebral instability
7. Postoperative discitis (infection)
8. Extradural pseudocysts[3]
9. Retention of foreign body (sponges)

With Combined Bone Grafting:

10. Pseudarthrosis
11. Residual motion of successfully fused segments[8]
12. Spinal stenosis due to exuberant new bone formation[10]
13. Instability above fused segments
14. Scarring and denervation of paravertebral musculature
15. Bone graft donor site pain

Figure 31-2 represents the organizational schema of the structured approach we are currently using. We believe that the most logical initial step is a thorough medical examination conducted by an internist who is quite aware of the extraspinal causes of back and leg pain. This evaluation gives us an outline or medical silhouette of the patient. The details of the portrait are then painted in with evaluation by the orthopedist, neurologist, neurosurgeon, psychologist, psychiatrist, and physiatrist. All of these people bring to bear a point of view and knowledge that may contribute to unraveling the patient's problem. Ancillary diagnostic aids, such as roentgenograms of the spine, myelography, electromyography, discography, straight leg raising test under Pentothal anesthesia, the Minnesota Multiphasic Personality Inventory (MMPI), and graphic self-image portrayal, are used when appropriate and helpful.

Once the individual evaluations are done, a period of communication is vital. It is obvious that all of the specialists must be able to speak to one another rationally and effectively. At this point it should be possible to identify, at least in general terms, the most important elements of the patient's disability. A major

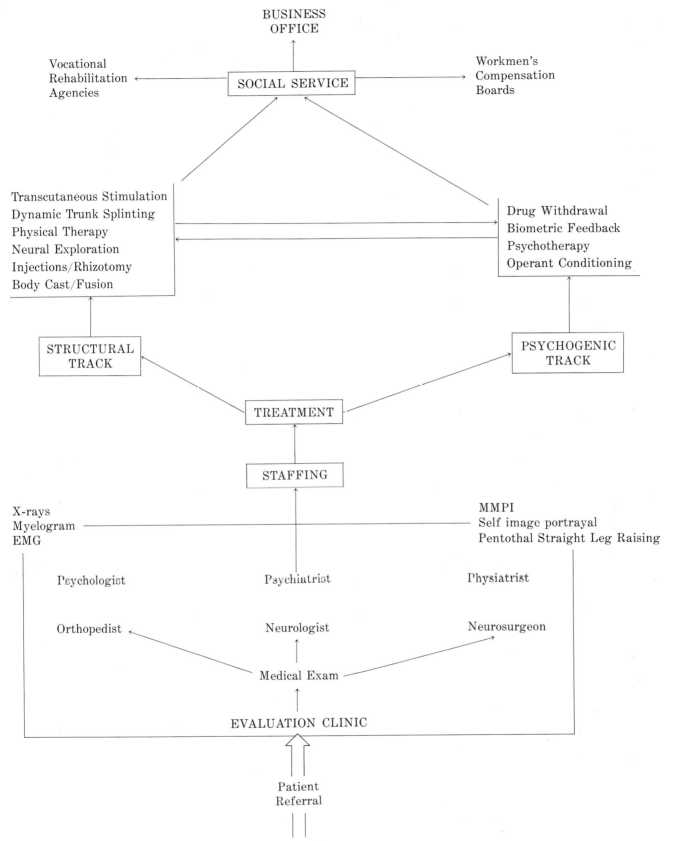

FIG. 31-2. Schematic representation of evaluation and treatment program.

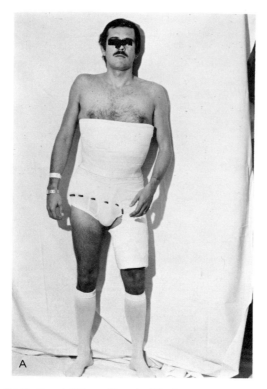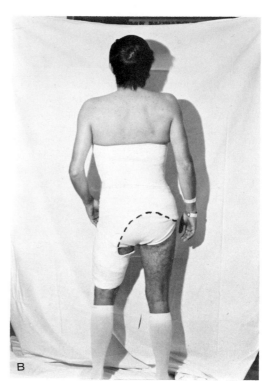

FIG. 31-3. Front (A) and back (B) views of body cast incorporating least symptomatic thigh. Note careful molding about iliac crests.

contribution to solving the problem can be the decision whether the problem is chiefly structural or chiefly psychogenic. Of course, most patients who have undergone several operations on the back will have some elements of both, but it is important to determine which is more significant.

If the patient enters, then, the "psychogenic track," his period of treatment begins, generally in an in-hospital, controlled environment under the direction of the psychiatrist and psychologist. Such techniques as operant conditioning, controlled drug withdrawal, and intensive psychotherapy may be employed to break the cycle of depression and chronic pain and invalidism.

If organic elements are believed to be of primary importance, the patient enters the "structural track" and a number of treatment techniques are employed. It should be noted that the patients are not irrevocably tracked in one direction or the other. In fact, most are crossed back and forth between treatment programs before their therapy is completed. Some of the structural treatment modalities available include transcutaneous stimulation (which we prefer to dorsal column electrode implantation), physical therapy rehabilitation programs, dynamic trunk splintage, facet joint injections under image intensifier control, and facet rhizotomy, neural exploration, and lumbar fusion.

We attach considerable importance to a trial of six weeks' immobilization in a body cast with thigh ex-tension prior to considering lumbar spinal fusion. Careful questioning of the patient just prior to and after removal of the cast may yield useful information. If the patient's symptoms of back and/or leg pain are relieved or improved by a period of fairly firm immobilization of the lumbar vertebral segments, a spinal fusion has a reasonable chance of affording relief. If a fusion procedure is to be done, a posterolateral type is preferred. Our follow-up studies[12,13] indicate that the chance of a satisfactory result in patients who have been previously operated upon is 81% with the postero-lateral, and only 53% with anterior interbody fusion.

References

1. Armstrong JR: The causes of unsatisfactory results from the operative treatment of lumbar disc lesions. J Bone Joint Surg 33B:31, 1951.
2. Beals RK, Hickman NW: Industrial injuries of the back and extremities. J Bone Joint Surg 54A:1593, 1972.
3. Borgeson SE, Vang PS: Extradural pseudocysts: a cause of pain after lumbar-disc operation. Acta Orthop Scand 44:12, 1973.
4. DePalma AF, Rothman RH: Surgery of the lumbar spine. Clin Orthop 63:162, 1969.
5. Harris RI, MacNab I: Structural changes in degeneration of the lumbar intervertebral disc: their relationship to low back pain and sciatica. J Bone Joint Surg 36B:304, 1954.

6. Hirsch C: Efficiency of surgery in low-back disorders. J Bone Joint Surg *47A*:991, 1965.

7. Paine KWE, Haung PWH: Lumbar disc syndrome. J Neurosurg *37*:75, 1972.

8. Rolander SD: Motion of the lumbar spine with special reference of the stabilizing effect of posterior fusion: An experimental study on autopsy specimens. Acta Orthop Scand Suppl *90*:1-144, 1966.

9. Sacks S: Anterior interbody fusion of the lumbar spine. J Bone Joint Surg *47B*:211, 1965.

10. Singh SH, Kirkaldy-Willis WH: Experimental anterior spinal fusion in guinea pigs: a histologic study of the changes in the anterior and posterior elements. Canad J Surg *15*:1, 1972.

11. Sprangfort EV: The lumbar disc herniation: A computer-aided analysis of 2,504 operations. Acta Scand Orthop Suppl *142*:1-95, 1972.

12. Stauffer RN, Coventry MB: Anterior interbody lumbar spine fusion: Analysis of Mayo Clinic series. J Bone Joint Surg *54A*:756, 1972.

13. Stauffer RN, Coventry MB: Posterolateral lumbar spine fusion: Analysis of Mayo Clinic series. J Bone Joint Surg *54A*:1195, 1972.

14. Verbiest H: A radicular syndrome from developmental narrowing of the lumbar vertebral canal. J Bone Joint Surg *26B*:230, 1954.

15. Wiltse LL, Rocchio PD: Predicting success of low back surgery by preoperative tests. Paper read at AOA meeting,

Section VIII

Roentgen Survey

32

Roentgen Survey

Radiographic anatomy and methods of study are found in Chapter 5, and the applicability of radiographs to the evaluation of spinal disorders is discussed in many of the chapters dealing with specific diseases. This chapter is intended to further illustrate roentgenographic characteristics of some of the disorders discussed in these earlier chapters.

METABOLIC DISORDERS

Radiographs of metabolic disorders such as osteoporosis and osteomalacia display the composition of bone, or perhaps more accurately, the paucity of bone.

OSTEOPOROSIS. According to Jaffe, osteoporosis is characterized by a reduction of osseous tissue per unit of bone volume, sparsity of the spongy trabeculae, and thinning and porosity of the cortices.[8] Figure 32-1A illustrates parallel vertical striations and mild compressive changes in thoracic vertebrae.

In advanced osteoporosis, the trabeculae are unable to resist the weight of the body and the internal pressure of the intervertebral discs. As a result, the central portion of the vertebral body collapses, producing a biconcave vertebra and biconvex expansion of the nucleus pulposus and disc.[6] Figure 32-1B illustrates paucity of osseous tissue, compressed vertebrae, and widened disc spaces in the lumbar spine. Even in the presence of the osteoporotic skeletal state, a medical consultation may be necessary to rule out or ascertain osteoporosis the disease (see p. 88).

OSTEOMALACIA. Any condition that depletes the body's calcium can cause

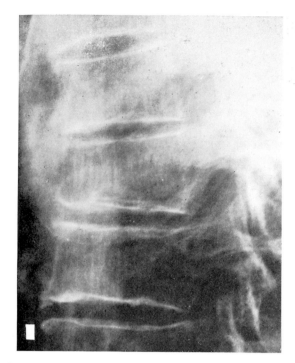

FIG. 32-1. Osteoporosis. Lower thoracic vertebrae in 64-year-old woman with osteoporosis. Roentgenogram shows parallel vertical striations and mild compressive changes. (From Epstein BS: The Spine. A Radiological Text and Atlas. 4th ed. Philadelphia, Lea & Febiger, 1976.)

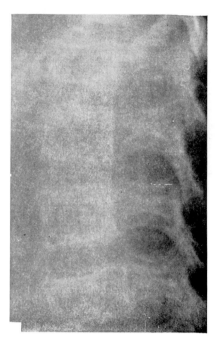

FIG. 32-2. Osteomalacia in lumbar vertebrae of 8-year-old boy. There is demineralization with maintenance of borders. (From Epstein BS: The Spine. A Radiological Text and Atlas. 4th ed. Philadelphia, Lea & Febiger, 1976.)

osteomalacia. The demineralization is shown in Figure 32-2, in which the lumbar discs are moderately bulging in appearance, and vertebral peripheries are slightly denser than their central portions.

INFECTIONS

In nontubercular infections of the spine (discussed in Chapter 8), the radiologic appearance depends on the time sequence of the disease, and one or two months may elapse before there is any radiologic evidence. Initially, small foci of rarefaction appear adjacent to the cartilaginous plates. The destructive progression and/or interbody fusion depends on the response to treatment or the individual's ability to cope with the infection.

In discitis, there is progressive loss of the intervertebral disc space. The adjacent vertebral margins of the infected disc become eroded, the degree of erosion depending on the amount of destruction resulting from the infection. As healing occurs, the areas of erosion become recalcified, and ultimately an interbody fusion denotes the successful resolution of the disease (Fig. 32-3).[6]

In tuberculous infections of the spine (discussed in Chapter 9), the initial site of involvement is at the cartilaginous plates, but the infection may spread throughout and beyond the vertebral bodies into the ligamentous and soft tissues, permitting severe scoliotic and kyphotic deformities. Because of the many radiographic appearances that this disease may produce, we are reproducing here some roentgenograms additional to those appearing in Chapter 9 (Figs. 32-4 to 32-7).

SCOLIOSIS

Most scolioses are noninfectious and result from congenital vertebral malformations or from muscular imbalances secondary to myopathies and neuropathies, or the condition may be idiopathic. As shown in Chapter 19, entitled Scoliosis, the curvatures are primarily lateral.

In cases of scoliosis, radiologic examinations of the spine should extend from the iliac crests up to the cervical region, with the patient in the supine, sitting, and erect positions (Fig. 32-8). For pre- and postoperative roentgenograms of this condition the reader is referred to Chapter 19.

SPONDYLOLISTHESIS AND CONGENITAL ANOMALIES

Radiographs of spondylolisthesis, revealing slippage of vertebrae, are shown in Chapter 20. A large group of

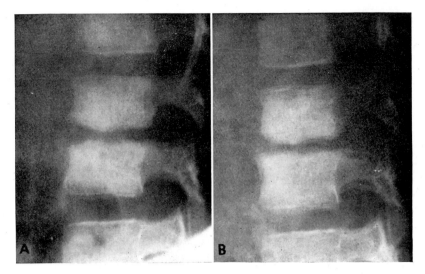

FIG. 32-3. Discitis of L3 interspace in 9-year-old boy with severe back pain, muscle spasm, and mild fever. Onset of symptoms mild, about four weeks prior to first examination. *A,* Discal narrowing and early sclerotic changes at end plates. He was treated with immobilization and antibiotics, and ten weeks later was greatly relieved. *B,* Reexamination shows irregular discal narrowing and sclerosis extending deep into centra of L3 and L4. (From Epstein BS: The Spine. A Radiological Text and Atlas. 4th ed. Philadelphia, Lea & Febiger, 1976.)

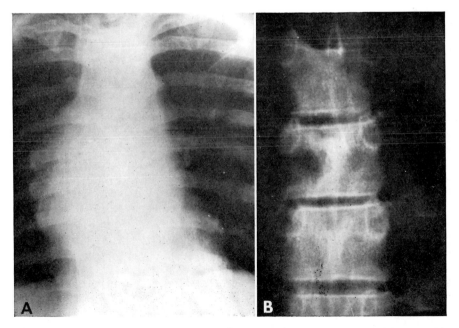

FIG. 32-4. Tuberculous paravertebral abscess in thorax of 25-year-old man with back pain and radicular symptoms referable to T6. *A,* Posteroanterior chest film reveals spindle-shaped mass extending from upper to lower thorax. On lateral film (not shown), trachea is displaced anteriorly. *B,* Excavating lesion is present on lateral margin of T6. (From Epstein BS: The Spine. A Radiological Text and Atlas. 4th ed. Philadelphia, Lea & Febiger, 1976.)

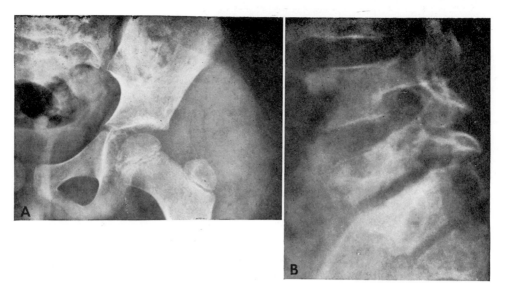

FIG. 32-5. Lumbosacral tuberculosis in 6-year-old girl. *A,* Large soft tissue swelling is present over left hip, with pain and limitation of motion. *B,* Tuberculosis at lumbosacral vertebrae is manifested by bone destruction with some effort at repair. Fifth lumbar vertebra is partly collapsed, lumbosacral interspace is narrowed, and anterior aspect of vertebra is partly destroyed. Slight sclerotic changes are seen posteriorly and inferiorly. On anteroposterior film (not shown) the transverse process is partly destroyed as well. (From Epstein BS: The Spine. A Radiological Text and Atlas. 4th ed. Philadelphia, Lea & Febiger, 1976.)

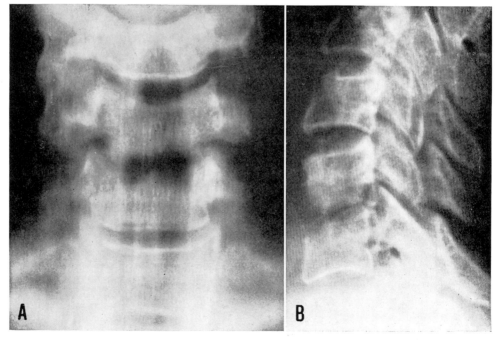

FIG. 32-6. *A,* AP laminagram and, *B,* lateral view of lower cervical spine of patient with tuberculous spondylitis. Disc between C6 and 7 is affected, and bony margins of adjacent vertebrae are destroyed. Soft tissue swelling is present in front of involved joint. (From Epstein BS: The Spine. A Radiological Text and Atlas. 4th ed. Philadelphia, Lea & Febiger, 1976.)

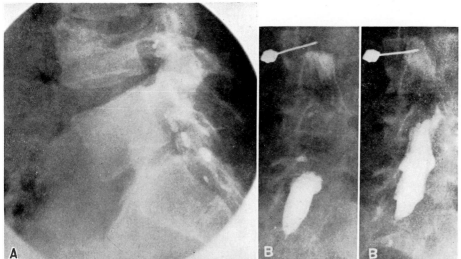

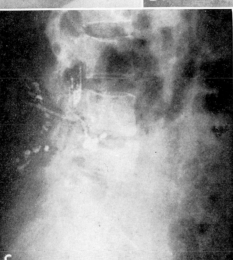

FIG. 32-7. *A,* Tuberculosis of fourth lumbar vertebra in 35-year-old man with symptoms of cauda equina compression. *B,* First myelogram in erect posture shows Pantopaque held up at third lumbar interspace. Note dentate pattern of inferior margin of upper Pantopaque. Next myelogram was made in head-down position. Inferior margin of intraspinal protrusion is delineated as corresponding with lower aspect of destructive process in fourth lumbar vertebra. *C,* Draining sinus persisted five months after operation. This was injected with Lipiodol, and led to posterosuperior aspect of body of L4. (From Epstein BS: The Spine. A Radiological Text and Atlas. 4th ed. Philadelphia, Lea & Febiger, 1976.)

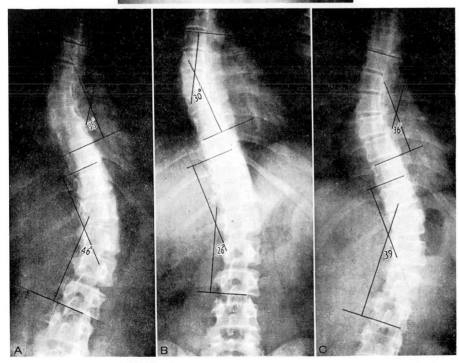

FIG. 32-8. Scoliosis study. *A,* Erect posture; *B,* supine position; *C,* sitting position. (From Epstein BS: The Spine. A Radiological Text and Atlas. 4th ed. Philadelphia, Lea & Febiger, 1976.)

339

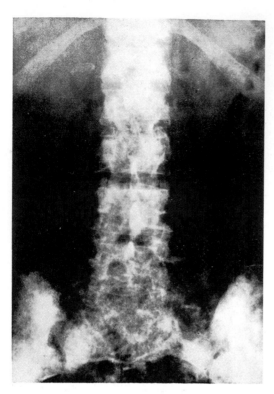

FIG. 32-9. Anteroposterior roentgenogram of lumbosacral spine showing lytic and osteoblastic metastases from carcinoma of breast. (From Epstein BS: The Spine. A Radiological Text and Atlas. 3rd ed. Philadelphia, Lea & Febiger, 1969.)

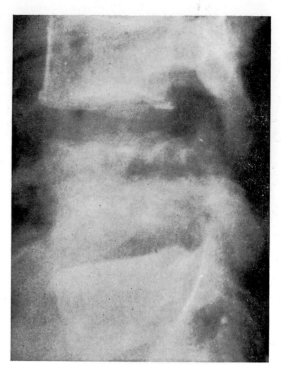

FIG. 32-10. Osteogenic sarcoma of L4 with considerable destruction of bone in dorsal aspect of body of vertebra and pedicles. (From Epstein BS: The Spine. A Radiological Text and Atlas. 3rd ed. Philadelphia, Lea & Febiger, 1969.)

congenital anomalies involving osseous and/or neural structures, many of which produce great deformity, are adequately illustrated in Chapter 22. The primary pathology is in the bone or neural tissue itself—not a secondary change resulting from extraneous influences.

BONE TUMORS

Bone tumors and tumor-like lesions of vertebrae lend themselves to radiographic diagnosis. Metastatic neoplasms account for most tumors of the spine. Figure 32-9 demonstrates extensive lytic and osteoblastic metastases from carcinoma of the breast. The diagnosis was not difficult, given a history of malignant disease. In contrast, primary osteogenic sarcoma, as shown in Figure 32-10, which shows destruction of the body and pedicle of L4, was not anticipated in an otherwise healthy individual who complained of backache and sciatica following trauma.

SPINAL CORD TUMORS

Tumors of the meninges or its contents may escape radiographic recognition without the aid of contrast studies. Large tumors may enlarge foramina or destroy pedicles (Fig. 32-11), but early diagnosis may require

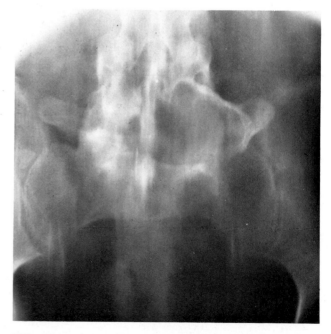

FIG. 32-11. Lumbosacral erosion in 63-year-old man with neurofibromatosis. (Courtesy of Dr. Richard Davis, Philadelphia, Pa.)

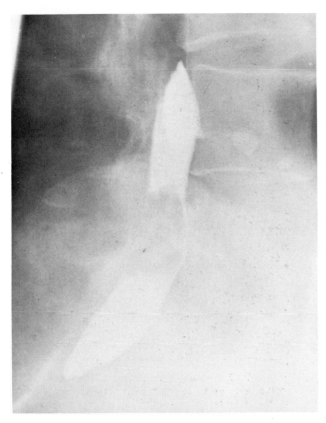

contrast studies (Fig. 32-12), which reveal encroach-ment of the mass upon the spinal fluid compartment.

ARTHRITIS

The structures making up the spine, as do other tis-sues of the body, undergo constant change in varying manner and degree. An important variation is found in the ability to replace new for old cells, and the failure to renew is part of the ageing process. The subtle and progressive changes occurring in the spine with ad-vancing years, or from uncertain etiology, are fre-quently diagnosed as arthritis. *Itis* implies inflamma-tion; strictly applied, therefore, the term *arthritis* should be reserved for inflammation of joints, but gen-eral usage has extended the term to also include degen-eration of the joints.

Degenerative Disorders

A description of the pathologic progression of spon-dylosis appears in Chapter 29. Two distinct entities are recognized radiologically: osteoarthritis and osteophy-tosis (spondylosis deformans).

OSTEOARTHRITIS. A morbid condition of synovial joints, osteoarthritis in the spine limits strict usage of

FIG. 32-12. Pantopaque myelogram reveals incomplete block in 58-year-old man with intradural neurofibroma. (Courtesy of Dr. Richard Davis, Philadelphia, Pa.)

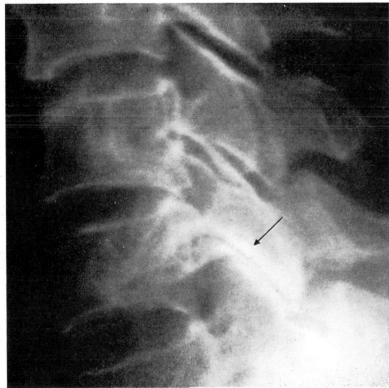

FIG. 32-13. Sclerotic osteoarthritis involv-ing facets of lower cervical spine. (From Brain, Lord and Wilkinson M: Cervical Spondylosis. Philadelphia, W. B. Saunders Company, 1967.)

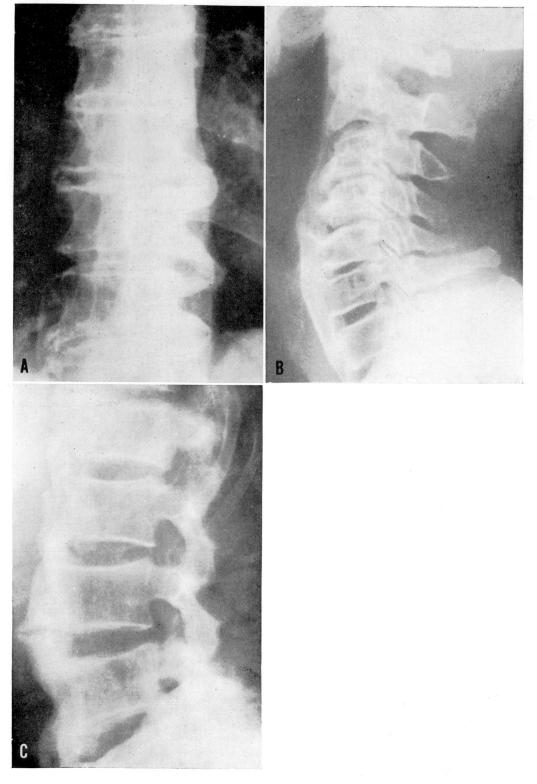

FIG. 32-14. *A*, Left lateral marginal osteophytosis of thoracic spine. In this instance, usual rule of absence of these changes in proximity of thoracic aorta is not observed. *B*, Cervical spine presents advanced calcification and ossification of anterior spinal ligament. *C*, Similar and even heavier changes are present in lumbar region. (From Epstein BS: The Spine. A Radiological Text and Atlas. 4th ed. Philadelphia, Lea & Febiger, 1976.)

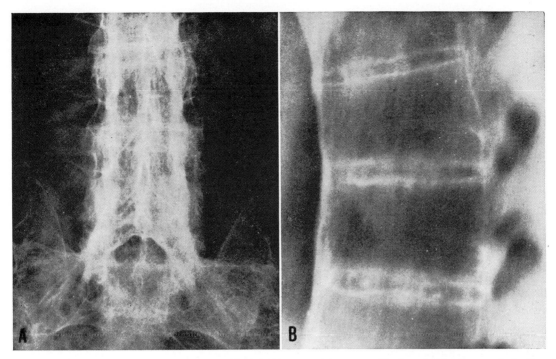

FIG. 32-15. *A,* AP view of lumbar spine of 58-year-old man with long-standing ankylosing spondylitis. Track formation is prominent and sacroiliac joints are fused. Diffuse demineralization of bone is evident. *B,* Lateral laminagram of upper lumbar vertebrae reveals narrowing of discs, calcification of anterior and posterior spinal ligaments, and intradiscal calcifications. (From Epstein BS: The Spine. A Radiological Text and Atlas. 4th ed. Philadelphia, Lea & Febiger, 1976.)

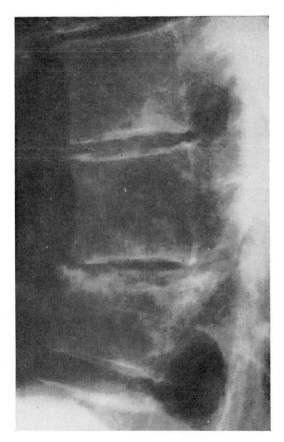

FIG. 32-16. Superior surface of vertebral body is depressed because of granulomatous involvement of bone with rheumatoid arthritis. Some sclerotic reaction is present as well. (From Epstein BS: The Spine. A Radiological Text and Atlas. 3rd ed. Philadelphia, Lea & Febiger).

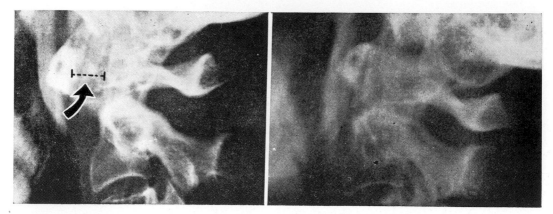

Fig. 32-17. Bilateral subluxation of atlanto-axial joints in rheumatoid arthritis. *Left,* Flexion. *Right,* Neutral. Atlanto-odontoid interval (arrow) is increased in flexion and exceeds 2.5 mm. This is common in this disease and is due to ligamentous laxity. (From Hollander JL and McCarty DJ Jr.: Arthritis and Allied Conditions. 8th ed. Philadelphia, Lea & Febiger, 1972.)

the term to the degeneration of the diarthrodial posterior apophyseal joints (the facets). Joint cartilage is destroyed by friction acting in conjunction with an intrinsic process of cartilage degeneration as shown in Figure 32-13.

OSTEOPHYTOSIS. In this condition the initial change is degeneration and flattening of the intervertebral disc. As the disc flattens, the anulus expands and carries periosteum with it, which when calcified forms osteophytes. Disc tissue actually extends outward to lie between the osteophytic lips. The larger rounded excrescences lie in front of the vertebral column, but on occasion small osteophytic spurs grow around a posterior herniation. Finally, the spurs and surrounding ligaments become calcified and more apparent radiologically (Fig. 32-14).

Inflammatory Disorders

Ankylosing spondylitis and rheumatoid arthritis are the most common types of inflammatory diseases and the etiology is frequently uncertain. Epstein has stated that "the question whether ankylosing spondylitis and rheumatoid arthritis are the same basic disease is still unresolved."

ANKYLOSING SPONDYLITIS. This condition appears in early childhood and is more common in males than in females. The inflammation of joints begins in the sacroiliacs and slowly progresses upward, occasionally sparing the cervical spine. The interbody and facet joints are primarily affected, and the small joints that hinge the ribs to the spine may also become involved. The disease progresses very slowly, and in two or three years the joints become obliterated. In approximately ten years the active disease subsides, but the osseous changes are permanent. When the paraspinal ligaments become calcified, the anteroposterior roentgeno-

grams of the spine have a "trolley-track" appearance (Fig. 32-15), which aids in differentiating the condition from rheumatoid arthritis, for in the latter calcification is not the rule.

RHEUMATOID ARTHRITIS. Also known as polyarthritis, rheumatoid arthritis is the most disabling type of arthritis. Although it affects primarily the extremities, it also has an affinity for the joints of the spine. It is more prevalent in females than in males, and may appear in childhood, but usually appears in the third to fifth decades. Figure 32-16 illustrates that the inflammation extends to destroy the articular cartilage, and ultimately the joints become affected, with trabecular dissolution extending to the end plates, bringing about collapse and compression of the body.

The cervical spine is particularly prone to attack, and there is a proclivity toward softening of the ligaments that hold the vertebrae together, permitting vertebral displacement and luxation (Figs. 32-17 and 32-18).

TRAUMA

Management of traumatic afflictions of the spine requires roentgen studies as a guide to treatment, but demands great care to minimize manipulation, which could lead to progression of neural insult. The lateral film illustrates an obvious compression fracture of C6 with retrodisplacement (Fig. 32-19A). Oblique films reveal fractures in the left and right pedicles (Fig. 32-19 B and C)

In the event that the symptoms and physical findings are profound and the plain films show no evidence of fracture-dislocation, contrast studies frequently aid in establishing a diagnosis (Fig. 32-20 A). Figure 13-20 B is an air study of the same patient, taken after operation, and shows the column of air lying between the vertebral bodies and the spinal cord.

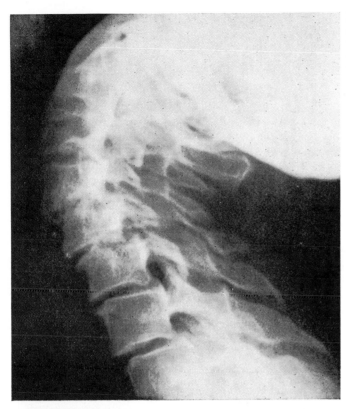

FIG. 32-18. Advanced rheumatoid arthritis. Cervical spine, lateral view. There are multiple, "stepladder" subluxations with reduction in height of intervertebral discs and erosions of vertebral endplates, apophyseal joints, and posterior arches. Note tapering of lower spinous processes. Dens (not clearly depicted) was almost totally destroyed. (From Hollander JL and McCarty DF Jr.: Arthritis and Allied Conditions. 8th ed. Philadelphia, Lea & Febiger, 1972.)

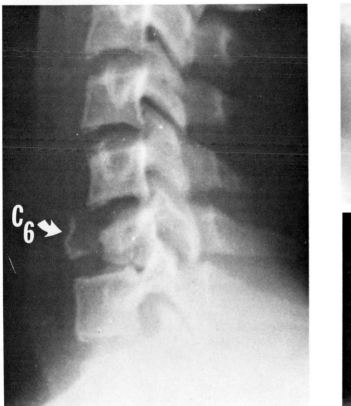

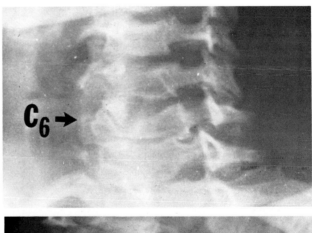

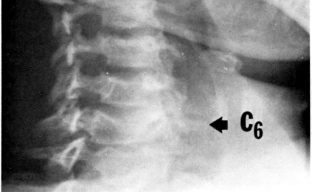

FIG. 32-19. A, Lateral roentgenogram reveals compression fracture of C6 with retrodisplacement of body. B and C, Oblique films of same patient reveal fractures of left and right pedicles. (From Hardy AG and Rossier AB: Spinal Cord Injuries: Orthopaedic and Neurological Aspects. Stuttgart, George Thieme Publishers, 1975.)

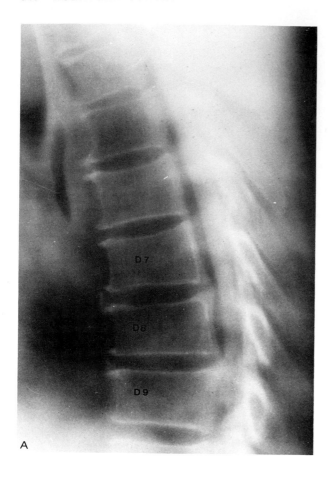
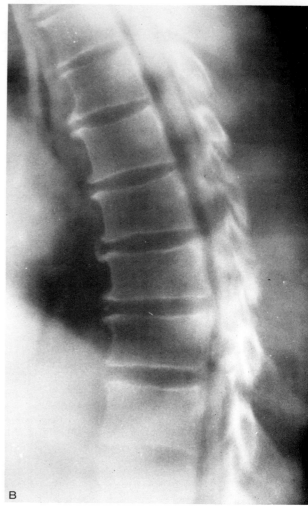

FIG. 32-20. Air myelogram of 39-year-old patient with sensory and motor paraplegia reveals block caused by herniated nucleus pulposus at T8-T9. *B,* Air myelogram made after removal of herniated nucleus pulposus reveals that there is no longer a block. (From Hardy AG and Rossier AB: Spinal Cord Injuries: Orthopaedic and Neurological Aspects. Stuttgart, George Thieme Publishers, 1975.)

References

1. Adams JC: Arthritis and Back Pain. Baltimore, University Park Press, 1972.
2. Bailey RW: The Cervical Spine. Philadelphia, Lea & Febiger, 1974.
3. Brain, Lord, and Wilkinson M: Cervical Spondylosis. Philadelphia, W. B. Saunders Company, 1967.
4. Collins DH: The Pathology of Articular and Spinal Diseases. Baltimore, Williams & Wilkins, 1950.
5. Cook HA: Fluoride studies in a patient with arthritis. Lancet 2:817–819, 1971.
6. Epstein BS: The Spine. 4th ed. Philadelphia, Lea & Febiger, 1976.
7. Hollander JL and McCarty DJ: Arthritis and Allied Conditions. 8th ed. Philadelphia, Lea & Febiger, 1972.
8. Jaffe HL: Metabolic, Degenerative and Inflammatory Diseases of Bones and Joints. Philadelphia, Lea & Febiger, 1972.

Section IX

Trauma

33

Head and Neck Injuries from Acceleration-Deceleration Forces

JACK WICKSTROM AND HENRY LaROCCA

The term "whiplash," a colloquialism coined in 1928 by Crowe,[4] and "reactivated" in 1945 by Davis,[5] reporting a series of patients who sustained neck injuries in rear-end collisions, became a part of our language, and the controversy over the term "whiplash" was kindled.

Macnab succinctly summarized the controversy by saying "the emotional overtones associated with the lesion converted it into a cause rather than a clinical syndrome."[13] The controversy has continued primarily on a philosophic basis rather than on a scientific one.

Patients who have been involved in rear-end collisions that have exposed them to sudden acceleration-deceleration forces frequently complain of headaches and neck pain, which may not begin at the time of the accident but may occur as long as 48 hours afterward. These symptoms are frequently associated with pain in the shoulders and paresthesias or numbness in the arms and hands, particularly with pain in the back of the head and in front of the neck. Some patients also complain of hoarseness, dysphasia, blurring of vision, and vertigo.

The physical findings in such patients frequently vary in significance immediately following the injury; however, examination at the end of 24 hours usually reveals some swelling in the sternocleidomastoid muscles, and limited motion of the neck, particularly in rotation and extension.

This frequent disparity between the patient's claims and physical signs and the negative roentgen findings has fostered differences of opinion regarding the extent of injury and the significance of the symptomatology as well as the need for a rationale of treatment.

The physician seeing a patient who complains of neck pain, vertigo, blurred vision, headache, and dysphasia frequently considers the symptoms bizarre and attributes them to a desire for secondary gain. The physician who explains to the patient "nothing was seen on the x-rays," and therefore decides that nothing could be wrong, further adds to the confusion. The feeling of insecurity engendered in the patient by such confusion seems to magnify his symptoms and convinces him that there must be collusion between the treating physician and the insurance carrier.

Extensive research on this subject has been stimulated by Gotten,[7] Braaf and Rosner,[3] Macnab,[13] Hohl,[8] Liu,[12] Martinez,[14,15] Ommaya,[16,18] Selecki,[20] and Severy.[21-25]

The electroencephalographic work reported from our laboratory indicated that the abnormal electroencephalogram is a poor indicator of subclinical brain injury.[12] It is significant that 24% of the 29 animals with "normal" electroencephalograms had identifiable neurologic lesions not indicated in the electroencephalograms recorded from brain surface electrodes.

Tsuchiya's work with subcortical electrodes in the mid-brain of rabbits,[27] which revealed abnormal brain wave patterns beginning seven to 45 days after acceleration, has stimulated us to study a group of primates using flexible electrodes inserted stereotaxically into their mid-brain along with scalp electrodes. These animals have been subjected to acceleration before and after electrode insertion. We have found spike discharges in the subcortical leads without abnormality of the scalp leads in those animals with electrode insertion after acceleration. We anticipate that by using signal averaging techniques developed by Saltzberg,[19] and digital matched filters, we may one day be able to detect subcortical spike activity on scalp leads and increase the sensitivity of electroencephalogram evaluation to detect abnormal activities.

MANAGEMENT OF THE PATIENT

Although it is unwise to extrapolate experimental findings directly into clinical situations, our studies over the past ten years have shown that significant damage can be produced in the cervical spine and brain in animals subjected to acceleration forces similar to those experienced by occupants of vehicles struck from the rear.

The majority of injuries from acceleration forces are relatively minor and consist of muscle strains, tears of muscle fibers, and some injuries to ligaments. In our extensive clinical experience, however, we have seen a sufficient number of patients who have had enough residual damage to convince us that all such patients need repeated evaluations and careful management. We cannot agree with those who say that treating such patients only prolongs the symptoms and causes the condition to be more difficult to overcome as it becomes more firmly fixed in the patient's mind.[4] However, we do agree that *overtreatment* with prolonged bracing,

protracted application of heat and other forms of physical therapy, or excessive sedation given as "muscle relaxants" is dangerous and contributes to the patient's disability.[5]

Successful management of these cases requires the same careful evaluation that the rational therapy of any pathologic condition requires. This evaluation begins with an assessment of damage to the car, which should give some indication of the force of impact. The greater the force or energies involved at the time of impact the greater the damage produced. It is also important to determine, if possible, the position of the patient and of his head at the time of impact, since rotation to one side or another at this time restricts extension and thus subjects anterior soft tissues to greater tensile forces, increasing the danger of tearing.

As part of the initial assessment, careful examination of the head, neck, and upper extremities, as well as of the low back, may reveal evidence of soft tissue damage in the anterior aspect of the neck, particularly pain and tenderness in the sternocleidomastoid muscles. Localization of tender areas in the posterior mus-

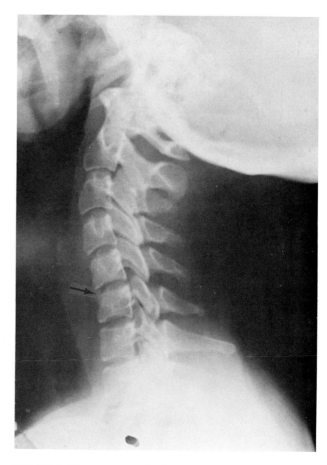

FIG. 33-1. Sharp reversal of cervical curve seen here is significant and was associated with delayed degenerative changes in 60% of patients studied by Hohl.

culature and osseous structures in the neck and shoulder girdles should be defined. Brachialgia and paresthesias in the upper extremities are usually the result of soft tissue injuries and muscle spasm in the scalene group, and probably do not represent direct injury to nerve roots. The work of Inman on segmental telalgia produced by injection of hypertonic saline into the ligamentous structures of the spine is important to remember.[10] Assessment of motion and systematic search for localized tenderness over the skeletal elements must be recorded. This initial evaluation allows the physician to establish some baseline for comparison as further swelling occurs or restriction of mobility becomes apparent. Patients who complain of dizziness, particularly dizziness with any change of head position, should have the benefit of electronystagmograms and complete evaluation by an otolaryngologist.

Initial x-ray examination should consist of routine anteroposterior, open-mouth anteroposterior, lateral, and oblique views. If no widening of the intervertebral space or bone damage is visualized, additional flexion and extension laterals should be taken. Loss of lordotic curve on the lateral view is a frequent finding. Some discredit its significance;[3,4] others believe it is significant.[1,6] Hohl believes "deeply lordotic, shallow lordotic, and flat cervical curves are normal variations," but that sharp reversal of the curve is significant (Fig. 33-1); the latter was associated with delayed objective degenerative changes in 60% of the series of patients he studied.[8]

Instability or true subluxation may be noted, and widening of an intervertebral space is indicative of disc disruption (Fig. 33-2). Avulsion of a portion of the anterior edge of a vertebral body must not be confused with calcification in the anterior longitudinal ligament associated with degenerative disease (Fig. 33-3). Roentgenologic findings indicating significant trauma are invariably associated with positive physical findings, such as localized skeletal tenderness, restriction of mobility, and protective palpable spasm, whereas those of degenerative disease may not be associated with such signs.

Re-evaluation by x-ray examination is indicated if symptomatology persists and should definitely be repeated in those patients who demonstrate sharp rever-

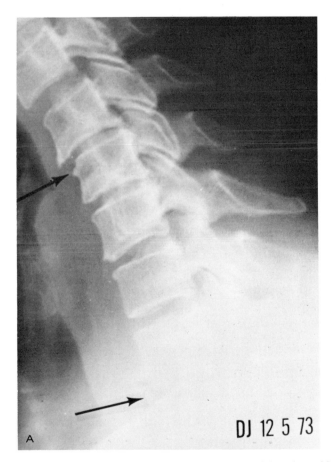
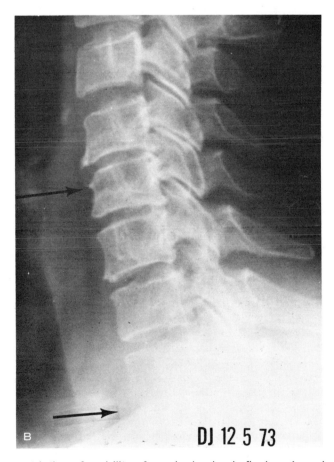

FIG. 33-2. Roentgenogram of D.J., 55-year-old patient. Note restriction of mobility of cervical spine in flexion, *A*, and extension, *B*. Also note subluxation of C4 on 5 (upper arrow in *A*). The subluxation and changes seen in superior surface of C5 were not present in films made in November 1972 after injury.

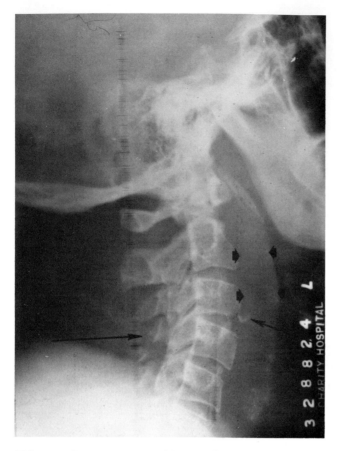

FIG. 33-3. Radiographic evidence of severe damage of cervical spine resulting from hyperextension forces. Note widening of retropharyngeal space indicating massive hemorrhage plus avulsion of anterior inferior edge of body of C3 and widening of intervertebral space between C2–3 and C3–4. Also note laminar and spinous process C4 fractures, the result of impact of neck against millwork protruding above back of seat from truck body.

sal of the normal lordotic curve on their initial films. The rapidity with which deterioration can occur is shown in Figure 33-4. However, acceleration of degenerative changes usually appears more slowly, as shown in Figures 33-5 and 33-6.

Once evaluation has been accomplished, and the extent of soft tissue, intervertebral disc, or osseous injury has been defined, a mode of therapy is selected to match the patient's requirements. In cases with minimal symptoms and findings, simple explanation of the nature of the injury and its expected course toward spontaneous resolution is all that may be required. When symptoms of pain are more substantial, and are associated with positive physical findings, drug therapy with appropriate sedatives, analgesics, and anti-inflammatory medication is prescribed. In either case, the patient should be advised of the possibility of an increase in symptomatology within 48 hours following the incident,

and instructed therefore to return for repeat examination at the end of 24 to 48 hours. The findings in the second examination, and all subsequent examinations, are compared with those of the initial one. Should symptoms become moderate to severe, management should also include rest in bed at home, or even hospitalization if indicated. The acute phase generally subsides within the first two weeks following injury, but low-grade discomfort and motion restrictions may persist for as long as 8 to 12 weeks. Treatment in the majority of cases in this subacute phase is dictated by the intensity of symptoms and by the patient's reaction to these symptoms. The use of a cervical collar is indicated when motion of the neck repeatedly stimulates pain or when the application of gentle manual traction to the chin and occiput by the examiner is associated with an increase in comfort. In patients with neurologic deficits in the upper extremities associated with neck pain and brachialgia, more intense treatment is mandatory and should include hospitalization for traction and for regular examination of the status of the neurologic function. Persisting neurologic deficit that is refractory to this form of management may indicate the need for further assessment with electromyography and myelography. Operative treatment may be required, depending on the results of the special assessment.

The majority of patients who have no neurologic deficit respond favorably to the approach described. Some develop local areas of irritation within muscular and ligamentous structures, and if these are not satisfactorily controlled with anti-inflammatory drugs given systemically, local injections of steroid may provide the desired relief. Such localized areas are commonly seen at the occiput, vertebra prominens, upper inner pole of the scapula, and anterior aspect of the shoulder joint at the intertubercular groove. Recurring occipital headache may be caused by the presence of a hyperirritable area at the insertion of the capital extensors into the skull, and may be reduced with local steroid injection. If occipital neuritis develops, diphenylhydantoin may provide relief. In the presence of more generalized headache, not specifically associated with an area of hyperirritability at the occiput, electroencephalography and neurologic consultation are in order.

The use of isometric exercises for neck and shoulder muscles, described by Ilfeld, have proved most beneficial, particularly in overcoming spasm and pain in the trapezius and paraspinous muscles.[9]

If symptoms abate, but mobility of the neck does not increase or return to normal after three weeks, intermittent cervical traction with preliminary heat, followed by rotary manipulation, usually effects restoration of mobility; with increased mobility a decrease in symptoms occurs. Although application of traction by a therapist is preferred, it can be used at home once its application has been demonstrated. The patient must understand that traction is used solely to increase his

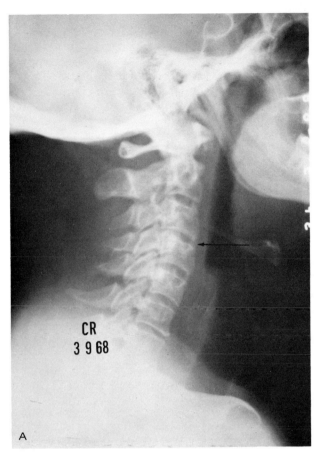
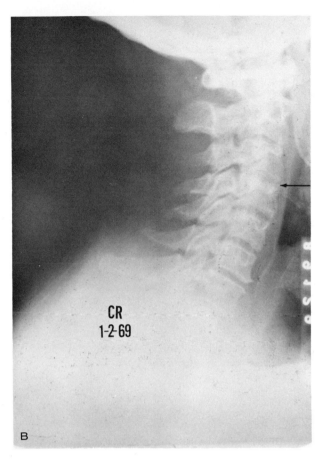

FIG. 33-4. Roentgenograms of patient who had restriction of motion and disabling pain after acceleration injury. *A*, immediately after injury; *B*, changes between C2–3 and C3–4 occurring in less than 9 months.

comfort, and, to make it worthwhile, relief of pain should continue after the traction has been completed. Traction should be applied with the neck in approximately 10 to 15 degrees of flexion. Intermittent, rather than continuous, traction is more comfortable for the patient and seems to be more efficient. Traction applied to increase mobility requires that muscles actually be stretched so that at least 20 to 35 pounds of intermittent traction force should be prescribed for 20 minutes. It must be emphasized that if traction irritates the occipital nerve or increases headaches, it should be discontinued immediately. We would again caution that a protracted period of traction or other unnecessary physical therapy increases the expense unduly, and may convince the patient that his condition is extremely serious.

In spite of adequate early management, a small percentage of patients continue to suffer disabling symptoms, and to demonstrate consistently restricted motion, persisting muscle spasm, and muscular irritability. Such problems can continue even in the absence of discrete neurologic deficits. The total clinical problem interferes with their work capacity and disrupts their pleasure and activities of daily living. The few in whom

the disorder is intractable should be further evaluated by myelography and discography, in preparation for operation, if necessary. When operation is contemplated, adequate psychologic assessment is advised to determine whether an element of psychic disorder is contributing to the overall trauma. However, the psychologic problem may be the result of intractable pain rather than the cause of it. Admittedly, distinguishing one situation from the other is difficult, and the surgeon is required to rely on his own intuition regarding the patient as a whole.

Operative treatment should be considered only after attempts at conservative management have failed to relieve symptoms and when disability has been present for six to twelve months. A time factor is inserted into the decision-making simply because in many cases pain is sufficiently reduced by the end of six months to make operation unjustifiable. On the other hand, sometimes disability is so great in the early phase that surgical treatment may be necessary before the sixth month. Once surgical management is indicated, assessment with contrast roentgenography is mandatory. This not only validates the clinical impression of organic disease, but localizes the levels of disease and rules out some

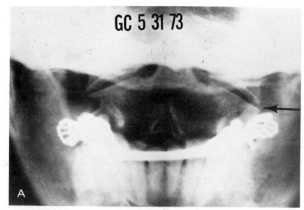

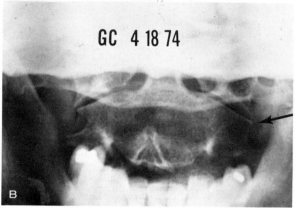

FIG. 33-5. Roentgenograms of G.C., 52-year-old woman who complained of and demonstrated progressive loss of ability to rotate her head: *A,* A-P views of atlanto-axial joint; *B,* comparable view, made almost 11 months later, showing increased loss of joint space between C1–C2 zygoapophyseal joint on left. This also corresponded to point of tenderness and reproducible pain on forced rotation.

unusual and unsuspected lesion, such as a tumor. In individuals under the age of 30, myelography is more often than not negative in the type of patient under discussion, but does remove the concern about unsuspected tumor. In individuals over 30 who may have degenerative disease before their traumatic episode, myelography may demonstrate bar defects in the anteroposterior view or compression defects anteriorly on the lateral views. The commonest level for such defects is at C5-C6, the joint at which the lower neck motion is concentrated and disease is most frequently found.

If results of myelography are positive, the study is highly accurate in pinpointing the level of defect. The surgeon may proceed with confidence under these circumstances. Negative results, on the other hand, are an indication for further study, since negative findings on myelogram in no way imply that the patient's symptoms are not organic. In our hands, discography has proved to be of substantial value in spite of the prevailing controversy regarding this test. Discography should

be performed with the patient awake, so that information regarding the reproduction of symptoms can be obtained. This reproduction is perhaps the most important of the results of the test, although abnormal volumes of fluid accepted are also indicative of disc disease. Likewise, abnormal roentgenographic patterns of dispersal of the contrast material are also indicative of disc disease. However, the patient's response to intradiscal injection is the only parameter that indicates which disc is probably the source of pain if several discs are degenerative. Discography should begin at the C5-C6 level, the most common level of this disorder; if findings are normal, then C4-C5 and C6-C7 levels are studied.

Once full assessment has been completed and the levels of cervical disc disease have been defined, an operation is planned to attend to these specific levels. The operative procedure that has provided the greatest degree of satisfactory outcome is anterior intervertebral disc excision with interbody fusion, in which a rectangular mortised graft, obtained from the iliac crest, is used. The technique allows for full exploration of the uncovertebral joint regions and the posterior longitudinal ligament. It also provides for immediate stability of the fused segments and for early bone union, since cancellous bone surfaces are opposed to one another under compression. Recovery from such an operation is rapid, although elimination of preoperative symptoms is somewhat slower. Experience indicates that only some of the patients enjoy a complete cure, but the majority do enjoy conversion of their problem from a daily and constant one to an episodic one at a reduced level of intensity. Some patients fail to achieve any alteration in their symptoms in spite of obtaining a solid fusion; they remain as a challenging enigma. The simplest expression of this enigma is that such patients have exactly the same identifiable disease as those who enjoy an excellent result, and are given the same treatment, which fails to produce a satisfactory outcome for reasons completely unexplained.

In reviewing a group of 362 patients of the original group of 488 patients who had experienced acceleration injuries to the cervical spine, we found twelve who required disc excision and anterior fusion. Of the original group of 488 patients, 126 were lost to follow-up. Of the 12 who had disc excisions and anterior interbody fusions, 41.6% had solid fusions and some improvement of symptoms, but only three (25%) had complete relief of all symptoms.

The third group of seven patients undergoing operation following acceleration injury to the cervical spine failed to obtain relief, even in the presence of solid fusion. The ultimate agent responsible for the pain must in some way be different from that in the previous two categories; otherwise the operation should be equally as effective. Unfortunately, there is no way to determine preoperatively what this factor is or whether it is present.

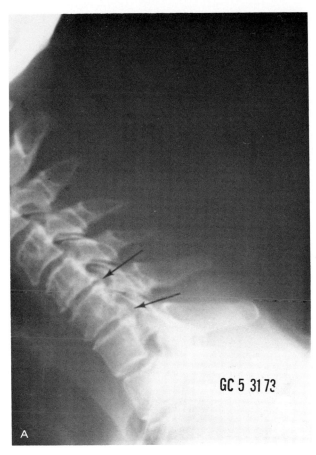
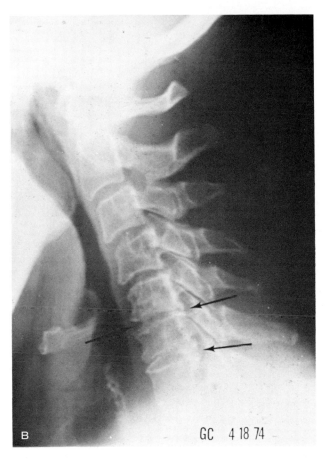

FIG. 33-6. Roentgenograms of G.C., 52-year-old woman whose films are shown in Figure 33-5. Lateral views of cervical spine show increase in size of posterior osteophytes between C5–6: *A*, at the time of injury, and *B*, made less than 11 months after injury.

In reviewing the characteristics of those patients who experienced satisfactory results as compared with those who experienced unsatisfactory results, no clear-cut difference emerges which would have distinguished one group from another before operation. What these few cases seem to indicate is that success follows the first procedure in a number of cases, but if not, repeated operations at the same level do not alter appreciably the patient's clinical problem. Analysis of the features of these patients and other groups like them indicates the necessity for a great deal more research. It has been suggested that in those who respond satisfactorily to conservative management, or to one operative procedure, injury to the soft tissues and intervertebral discs in the neck has been responsible for the patient's pain syndrome. However, failure to respond probably indicates involvement of structures more complex than the musculoligamentous and intervertebral disc tissues in the neck, and the question of more subtle injury to other structures in the neck, or even to intracranial contents, is raised, especially in the light of the experimental data being gathered.

References

1. Abel MS: Moderately severe whiplash injuries of the cervical spine and their roentgenologic diagnosis. Clin. Orthop. *12*:189-208, 1958.
2. Barnett JR: Whiplash injuries of the spine. J. Fla. Med. Assn. *43*(11):1099, 1957.
3. Braaf MM, Rosner S: Symptomatology and treatment of injuries of the neck. New York State J. Med. *55*:237-242, 1955.
4. Crowe HE: The conservative management of neck injuries. Monograph, The Defense Research Institute, Inc. Feb., 1964, pp. 25-27.
5. Crowe HE: A new diagnostic sign in neck injuries. Monograph. The Defense Research Institute, Inc. Feb., 1964, pp. 21-23.
6. Gay JR, Abbott KH: Common whiplash injuries of the neck. JAMA *152*:1698, 1953.
7. Gotten NM: Whiplash injuries—a survey of 100 cases subsequent to settlement of litigation. JAMA *162*:865-867, 1956.
8. Hohl M: Soft tissue neck injuries in automobile accidents—factors influencing prognosis. Presented at Annual Meeting of the American Academy of Orthopaedic Surgeons, Las Vegas, Nevada, 1972.

9. Ilfeld, Frederic, Beverly Hills, California. Personal communication, 1974.

10. Inman VT, Saunders JB: Referred pain from skeletal structures. J. Nerv. Ment. Dis. *99*:660-667, May, 1944.

11. Kornhauser M, Gold A: Application of the impact sensitivity method to animate structures, an impact acceleration stress. Publication 977, National Academy of Science, 1962, pp. 333-344.

12. Liu YK, Wickstrom JK, Saltzberg B, Heath RG: Subcortical EEG changes in rhesus monkeys following experimental whiplash. 26th ACEMB, 404, 1973.

13. Macnab I: The whiplash syndrome. Orthop. Clin. N. Amer. *2*:389-403, July, 1971.

14. Martinez JL: Acceleration produced head and neck injuries. Proc. Am. Soc. Engng. Education, Ann Arbor, Michigan, June, 1967.

15. Martinez JL: Study of whiplash injuries in animals. Monograph (paper No. 63-WA-21), ASME, September, 1963.

16. Ommaya A, Corrao P: Pathologic biomechanics of central nervous system injury in head impact and whiplash trauma. Accident Pathology, U.S. Government Printing Office, Washington, D.C., June, 1968, pp. 160-179.

17. Ommaya AK, Faas F, Yarnell P: Whiplash and brain damage. JAMA *204*:285-289, April, 1968.

18. Ommaya AK, Hirsch AE, Martinez JL: The role of 'whiplash' in cerebral concussion. Proc. 10th Stapp Car Crash Conf., Paper No. 660804, November, 1966, pp. 197-203.

19. Saltzberg B, Lustick LS, Heath RG: Detection of focal depth spiking in the scalp EEG of monkeys. EEG Clin. Neurophys. *31*:329-333, 1971.

20. Selecki BR, Williams HBL: Injuries to the Cervical Spine and Cord in Man. Australiasia Medical Publishing Co., Ltd., New South Wales, 1970.

21. Severy DM, Bunk HM, Baird JD: Backrest and head restraint design rear end collision protection. Presented at Automotive Engineering Congress, January, 1968.

22. Severy DM, Mathewson JH: Automotive and barrier rear end collision performance. SAE, Reprint 62C, 485, Lexington, N.Y.

23. Severy DM, Mathewson JH: Automotive barrier impacts. Highway Research Board Bulletin *91*:39, 1954.

24. Severy DM: Automobile crash effects. Presented to Engineering Section, California Traffic Safety Conf., Sacramento, California, October 7, 1954.

25. Severy DM, Mathewson JH, Bechtol CO: Controlled automobile rear-end collisions, an investigation of related engineering and medical phenomena. Can. Serv. Med. J. *XI*:727, 1955.

26. Torres F, Shapiro S: Electroencephalograms in whiplash injuries. Arch. Neurol. *5*:40-47, 1961.

27. Tsuchiya K, Hiyama K, Kawahara M, Tsuchiya T, Sekimoto A: A study of the deep EEG pattern from the brain stem of rabbits with experimental whiplash injury. J. Jap. Orthop. Assn. *42*:1057-1065, 1968. (In Japanese with English abstract.)

28. Wickstrom J, Martinez JL, Johnston D, Tappen NC: Acceleration deceleration of the cervical spine in animals. Proc. 17th Stapp Car Crash Conf., Springfield, Charles C Thomas, 1965, pp. 182-187.

29. Wickstrom J, Martinez JL, Rodriguez R Jr.: Cervical sprain syndrome: Experimental acceleration injuries of the head and neck. Proc. Symp. Prevention of Highway Injury, University of Michigan, 1967, pp. 182-187.

30. Wickstrom J, Rodriquez R, Martinez J: Experimental production of acceleration injuries of the head and neck. Accident Pathology, U.S. Government Printing Office, Washington, D.C., 185-189, June, 1968.

31. Wickstrom J, Martinez JL, Rodriguez R Jr., Haines DM: Hyperextension and hyperflexion injuries to the head and neck of primates. *In* Neckache and Backache. Springfield, Charles C Thomas, 1970, pp. 108-117.

32. Wickstrom J, LaRocca H: Management of patients with cervical spine and head injuries from acceleration forces. Current Practices in Orthopaedic Surgery, *6*:83-98, St. Louis, CV Mosby, 1975.

34

Spinal Cord Injuries

DANIEL RUGE

MODERN man, by virtue of both his occupational exposure and his leisure activities, is predisposed to spinal cord injuries. It can be said, then, that such injuries occur in those who are most active and physically fit. Public information has not properly stressed the consequences of injury to the central nervous system. Instead, it is presented to delight the reader and viewer with miracles which so far exclude neural regeneration. The consequences of spinal cord injury extend far beyond the domain of the orthopedist and neurologic surgeon, involving practically every discipline of medicine as well as many lay endeavors.

HISTORICAL BACKGROUND

The Edwin Smith surgical papyrus contains descriptions of five cases of injuries to the cervical vertebrae and differentiates between those having paralysis due to vertebral injury and those who have only cervical strain or vertebral injury without paralysis. There is even a statement in the papyrus that certain of these ailments are not to be treated, implying the hopelessness of the effort.

Early in the twentieth century, Allen experimentally determined that an impact of 340 gram-centimeters would produce paraplegia, which he assumed to be due to either destruction of axon cylinders or edema and hemorrhage.[3] His proposal to treat human victims by prompt deep vertical myelotomy at the site of injury, in order to drain the hemorrhage, was certainly heroic for the times.

This generation's interest has been stimulated by the heroic efforts of the military during World War II. The current interest is worldwide; old treatments that had failed are being used again, and methods of therapy that have some success in cerebral injury have been adapted to the spinal cord. The rate of success, regardless of treatment, is small, and so it is only natural that the search for better treatment continues. Although every patient with a spinal cord injury probably should be considered for a surgical procedure, it is not in the best interest of all patients that an operation be carried out.

INJURY TO THE SPINAL COLUMN

Most patients who have sustained injury to the spinal cord have had a fracture or dislocation of the spinal column; however, not all individuals who have had a fracture or dislocation of the spinal column have sustained injury to the spinal cord. Nonetheless, the latter group deserves careful observation to prevent further injury, because all who have injury to the spinal column are predisposed to spinal cord injury if there is either dislocation or instability.

There are occasional fractures of the spinal column that do not affect stability, do not encroach upon the vertebral canal, and are not potentially hazardous to the spinal cord or cauda equina. One such fracture is the "clay shovelers" fracture, in which avulsion of the seventh cervical or first thoracic spinous processes has occurred. Another such fracture is that of the transverse processes, which may result either from direct trauma or from torsion of the trunk, as may occur if an individual carries a heavy weight on one shoulder, and the opposite quadratus lumborum muscle, in its effort to keep the spine erect, contracts sufficiently to avulse transverse processes from the lumbar spine. Other fractures are more likely to result from trauma to the head or spine.

Cervical Spine

The patient who has sustained a craniocerebral injury may also have an injury to the cervical spine, particularly if there has been a blow to the back of the head causing extreme flexion of the neck. Severe hyperextension injuries may also injure the spinal cord, even though radiologic studies show neither fracture nor dislocation. Likewise trauma to the top of the head may cause injury to the spine, particularly at the junction of the occiput and atlas.

OCCIPITO-ATLANTAL DISLOCATION. The proximity of the convex occipital condyles to the superior surface of the atlas, plus the reinforcement of the ligaments that join the rim of the foramen magnum to the upper two cervical vertebrae create a very stable occipito-atlantal junction. Even so, dislocation may occur, particularly if the head is forced backward.

FRACTURE OF THE ATLAS. Jefferson drew attention to this type of fracture and believed that it occurred from a force transmitted to the top of the head, particularly if the head were held erect.[16] Diving or other accidents that cause a direct force to the vertex are usually responsible. The force is transmitted from the occipital condyles through the two lateral masses of the atlas, forcing them apart, so that the anterior arch, or posterior arch, or both, are fractured. The spinal cord is usually spared because the fragments are forced away from the cord, increasing the lumen of the vertebral canal at this point.

X-ray studies of the cervical spine may show little evidence of the atlas if the destruction is extensive; the axis will appear to have taken the position of the atlas (Fig. 34-1 A).

The atlas may dislocate without being fractured. The absence of stability between atlas and axis accounts for the frequency of atlanto-axial dislocation. The relationship of the atlas to the axis depends considerably on the transverse ligament of the atlas and the dens of the axis. If the ligament is torn, the atlas may dislocate forward, and if the dens is fractured, the atlas may dislocate either forward or backward. Should forward dislocation occur without simultaneous fracture of the dens, the cord would be impaled between the posterior arch of the atlas and the dens, resulting in death. There are, however, instances in which there is forward displacement of only one lateral mass of the atlas over the corresponding articular facet of the axis, and in such a situation, the spinal cord would be spared even though the dens remained attached to the axis.

FORWARD DISPLACEMENT OF THE DENS. Mobility of the upper cervical spine is possible because the lateral joints of the first two cervical vertebrae lie roughly in a horizontal plane. A flexion injury may cause the head to move or slide forward. Because the atlas is firmly attached to the occipital condyles, the subluxation is more likely to occur between atlas and axis, and as the strong transverse ligament carries the dens forward, it becomes dislocated anteriorly (Fig. 34-1 B). Fortunately, the lumen of the vertebral canal at this level is quite adequate and the cord is frequently spared.

BACKWARD DISPLACEMENT OF THE DENS. In extreme extension injuries, the anterior arch of the atlas may transmit enough force on the dens to fracture it and carry it posteriorly (Fig. 34-1 C). In such instances, the condition of the spinal cord is dependent on the integrity of the transverse ligament of the atlas and the space between this ligament and the posterior arches of both atlas and axis.

OTHER FRACTURES OF THE AXIS. Fracture of the main portion of the body of the axis occurs rarely. Occasionally a hyperextension injury spares the dens, and a fracture occurs through either the laminae or pedicles, producing a fracture that resembles the "hangman's fracture." The resemblance of the "hangman's fracture" is only radiologic; the spinal cord usually escapes injury because the lumen of the vertebral canal has actually increased (Fig. 34-2 A).

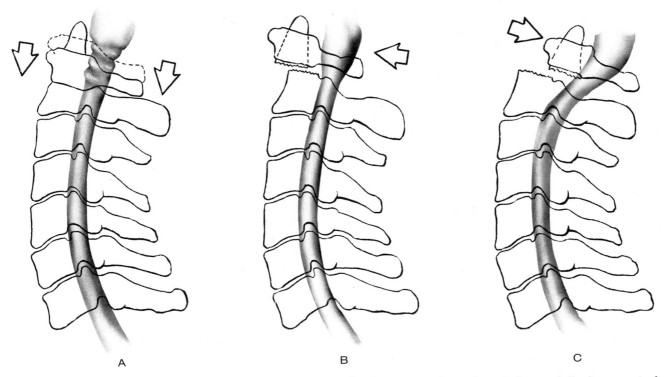

FIG. 34-1. *A*, Fracture of the atlas due to direct force transmitted to vertex of cranium; *B*, forward displacement of dens with atlas; *C*, backward displacement of dens with atlas.

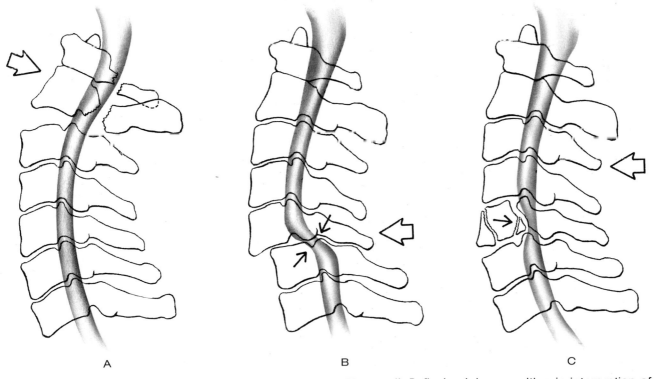

FIG. 34-2. *A*, Hyperextension injury resembling hangman's "fracture"; *B*, flexion injury resulting in interruption of ligaments, dislocation, and locking of facet joints; *C*, flexion injury resulting in bursting fracture and retropulsion of posterior fragment of vertebral body.

FRACTURE OF THE CERVICAL SPINE BETWEEN C3 AND C7. The classification of Whitley and Forsyth is very inclusive and is based on the mechanism of injury.[40]

Flexion Injuries. Even though the occiput and deep posterior cervical muscles provide good protection for the cervical spine, a blow to the occiput is the most common cause of flexion injury. If the force is adequate, it will produce interruption of ligaments, which allows dislocation with locking of the facet joints. The lumen of the vertebral canal becomes reduced as the arch of the superior vertebra approaches the body of the vertebra below (Fig. 34-2 *B*). Occasionally, flexion injuries without vertebral fracture or dislocation may cause retropulsion of fragments of the intervertebral disc. If the force is great enough to produce a bursting fracture, a posterior fragment of the body may also be forced into the vertebral canal (Fig. 34-2 *C*). The most severe injuries to the spinal cord occur with this type of injury, and the neurologic deficit is usually sudden and reduction of the fracture very difficult.

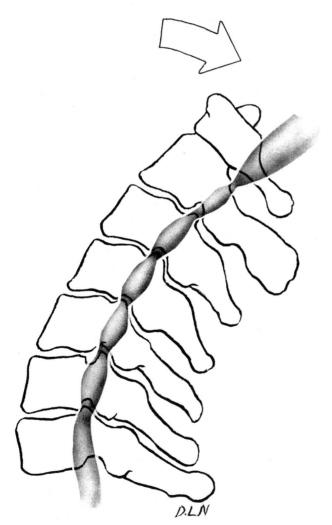

FIG. 34-3. Hyperextension injury.

Extension Injuries. Since the anterior cervical muscles are considerably weaker than are the posterior cervical muscles, a force transmitted to the face will permit marked extension. Older people who have an increase in the cervical lordosis are particularly prone to injuries of this type. If the anterior longitudinal ligament ruptures and the force is sufficient to carry the superior vertebra backward, it will separate from the vertebra. The radiologic evidence may be minimal, but because of the previously compromised vertebral canal, only slight bony displacement may produce disasterous results (Fig. 34-3). It is believed that most patients showing signs of central cervical cord syndrome have had such an injury.

Combined Injuries. If either a flexion or an extension injury has lessened ligamentous support and produced an unstable fracture, the spine is vulnerable to additional forces in the same accident. The effects of a to-and-fro injury are enhanced where instability exists.

Lateral Flexion Injuries. Forces directed to the lateral aspect of the skull or cervical spine may cause wedging of the lateral aspect of the vertebral body and disruption of the posterior elements on the side opposite the blow. Such injuries occur more commonly in children and may be associated with injuries to the brachial plexus, making diagnosis difficult.

Thoracic and Lumbar Spine

Most injuries below the cervical spine occur at T12 and L1. Any single or combination injury involving these vertebrae is possible. Thoracolumbar fractures are classified under four main types: anterior-wedge fracture, lateral-wedge fracture, fracture-dislocation, and isolated fracture of the neural arch.

ANTERIOR-WEDGE FRACTURE. Minor wedge fractures may occur without disruption of the posterior elements, but if the vertebral body loses one-third of its height anteriorly, the posterior ligaments have probably been ruptured, resulting in an unstable fracture.

LATERAL-WEDGE FRACTURES. These fractures result from a flexion-rotation injury. Occasionally, they are accompanied by fracture of the transverse process on the side opposite the wedging and injury to the posterior elements on the side of the wedging.

FRACTURE-DISLOCATION. The mechanism is extreme flexion and rotation, resulting in rupture of the posterior interspinous ligaments. There may be several degrees of displacement, such as simple forward subluxation of the facets, forward dislocation with fracture of the facets or neural arch, and forward dislocation with locking of the facets. Severe destruction of the posterior elements is associated with greater destruction of the vertebral body, resulting in severe impingement on the spinal cord both anteriorly and posteriorly.

NEURAL ARCH FRACTURE. The association of neural arch fractures with fractures of the transverse processes suggests that a rotation injury is responsible. The fractures are usually through the inter-articular portion of the lamina, and if this is accompanied by displacement, the superior facet slides forward while the inferior facet retains its normal position.

Injuries to the Spinal Column Secondary to Missile Wounds

Experience with missile wounds has shown the neurologic deficit to be greater than one would anticipate from the radiologic examination. Ricochet may cause neural injury without entering the vertebral canal. Penetrating missiles may pass through the vertebral canal or may become lodged within it.

Stable and Unstable Fractures

The posterior supporting complex, consisting of the interspinous and supraspinous ligaments, the ligamentum flavum, and the capsules of the facet joints can usually retain integrity with a pure flexion injury. Rotation or flexion-rotation is required to rupture the posterior elements and produce an unstable spine. If the posterior complex survives, the spine may be considered stable.

INJURIES OF THE SPINAL CORD

TRANSITORY NEUROLOGIC DEFICIT. Temporary interruption of physiologic function of the spinal cord may be seen in patients with or without radiologic evidence of injury. One generally assumes that there is neither mechanical pressure on such a cord nor gross anatomic change within it, but Scheinker has given experimental and pathologic evidence to show that cytologic change may be present even though the functional loss is transitory.[29] Recent observations have suggested that the gray matter is most involved because of its predominantly vascular and neuronal composition in contrast to the tough myelinated white matter. We have seen such patients, particularly after thoracic trauma has produced areflexia in the lower extremities, paraplegia, and sensory loss corresponding with the level of their injuries.

PERMANENT DISTURBANCE OF FUNCTION. Most patients who have a spinal cord injury reveal maximal signs of damage instantly. Holdsworth has reported on a series of 100 patients (out of a total group of 1,000) who had examinations carried out immediately, and only three of this group progressed from partial to total lesions.[13] He concluded that the cord damage is caused by sudden distortion of the vertebral canal rather than by slowly increasing pressure on the cord, as might be caused by edema or hemorrhage. The possibility that spinal shock conceals a progressive anatomic lesion must be considered. The unresolved question is the pathologic state of the spinal cord immediately after the trauma. Is the clinical state indicative of the anatomic or pathologic state? For each individual, does the initial paralysis result from a condition akin to the transitory disturbance of the cord, and does the ultimate permanent paralysis occur as a result of mechanical, anoxic, ischemic, or chemical effects which progressively destroy neural tissue?

According to Ducker et al., the greatest neurologic deficit occurs immediately and may be followed by clinical improvement, even though the pathologic anatomy worsens during the ensuing week.[12] They make no easy explanations, but show that in mild trauma, the initial damage is to the central gray matter and gradually involves the surrounding white matter, while in severe trauma the changes spread to include both gray and white matter promptly.

It is difficult to state the exact nature of most spinal cord injuries in pathologic terms, even after surgical exploration, because the pia mater and surrounding spinal fluid, plus other membranes, offer rather good protection to the visible external surface of the cord. A spinal cord may be neither contused nor lacerated on gross inspection, but the gray matter, which is rich in blood supply, is prone to early hemorrhage, and as the clot increases, destruction of white matter ensues. The pia mater is no protection against progressive injury occurring from within.

ISCHEMIA OF THE SPINAL CORD. Collateral circulation of the spinal cord is considered to be very limited, and certain areas, particularly the mid-thoracic region, are noted for their minimal vascularity. The anterior spinal artery is particularly prone to compression in flexion injuries, and opportunities for ischemia are particularly great when a fracture-dislocation has produced compromise of this vessel.

SYMPTOMS AND SIGNS. The great unknown about each patient at the time of injury and initial examination is the state of his spinal cord. One cannot know the current histologic state or ultimate histologic state based on the presence or absence of paralysis. The unparalyzed may become paralyzed and the paralyzed may improve even though experience of many supports that there is little hope for recovery in "complete" lesions one day old.

Symptoms and signs of spinal cord and cauda equina injury are seldom subtle. The presence of sensory or motor deficit in a conscious patient who has sustained injury will certainly suggest neural injury, but most serious injuries to the spinal cord follow direct trauma to the head resulting in a combination of overlapping craniocerebral and spinal cord symptomatology.

Injuries to the spinal column without neural sequelae pose a diagnostic and therapeutic dilemma. The possibility that cervical cord injury may occur deserves consideration in instance of head injury, and cervical spine films should be obtained if the patient has had a head injury. Damage to the thoracic and lumbar portions of the cord and cauda equina may be associated with extreme flexion and extension of the trunk.

If the injury to the spine is severe enough to cause neurologic deficit, accurate evaluation of the injury should include appraisal of motor and sensory modalities as well as evaluation of bladder, bowel, and autonomic functions.

The mechanism of injury may be determined by the history and by inspection for points of impact. Even though there is paralysis, careful sensory examination may show that a lesion is incomplete. One of the most important parts of this examination is to examine the saddle area to determine whether there is any sacral sparing. Any voluntary movements are helpful in determining the motor state. The presence of deep tendon reflexes probably indicates an incomplete injury, whereas the absence of reflexes is to be anticipated in the period of spinal shock.

Gentle palpation over the spinous processes may reveal a gibbus or increased separation of adjacent spinous processes. Location of pain over the spinous processes and surrounding area will also aid a great deal in determining the level. Motor power may be studied by observing the nature of breathing and the position assumed by the extremities. The presence of both intercostal and diaphragmatic breathing speaks for no injury above the mid-thoracic spine, but the absence of intercostal breathing will suggest a cervical or high thoracic injury. The patient, while lying on his back, may be asked to move his toes; and if this can be done, the lesion is either very low or incomplete. Other movements of the ankles, the knees, or hips may be requested and finer movements of the upper extremities may also be determined. Reference to the charts in Chapter 4 will aid in localization of the level.

Radiologic evaluation is not to be delayed until exhaustive history and examination are complete. A lateral radiograph of the spine is very important and should be made at the time of the initial examination. If at all possible, these films should be made with portable equipment, so that movement and handling of the patient may be kept to an absolute minimum. Films cannot be expected to demonstrate every fracture present, but it is important to localize dislocations and gross fractures early.

Occasionally, spinal fluid studies are indicated in the patient with a spinal cord injury. If there is marked dislocation, there is no point in subjecting the patient to a lumbar puncture because the result can probably be anticipated. In the past, great reliance was placed on the Queckenstedt test. There is still help to be gained from this study; if the test is positive, one can assume that there is pressure on the spinal cord, but one cannot assume absence of pressure on the cord if the test is negative. There is particular value in performing the Queckenstedt test on the patient who has motor and sensory deficits and normal radiographs. Should the presence of a block be shown, it would be desirable to introduce 1 cc. Pantopaque into the subarachnoid space, withdraw the needle, and then obtain radiologic localization. If the Queckenstedt test is negative, one may require more than 1 cc. of Pantopaque for an adequate study.

ACUTE CERVICAL CORD SYNDROME

Some patients with injury to the cervical cord have shown symptoms and signs that implicate the brain and autonomic nervous system. Rosenbluth and Meirowsky described the acute cervical cord syndrome, which is characterized by coma or disorientation, hypotension, bradycardia, and hypothermia.[27] One's first reaction might be that the coma is due to head trauma and that the vascular and temperature changes are secondary to muscarinic responses of cerebral tissue injury, but the condition has been observed in patients who had no head injury.

The bradycardia and hypotension have been attributed to interruption of sympathetic influences, permitting the parasympathetic system to go unchecked. Hypothermia is believed to occur in the absence of shivering, but this is an unpredictable effect being influenced by environmental factors as well. This state requires prompt treatment, for continued hypotension increases ischemia at the site of the injury.

ASSOCIATED INJURIES

Seldom is injury of the spinal cord or cauda equina produced without other serious complications. Cervical fractures are frequently associated with head injury, thoracic fractures with pulmonary and cardiovascular injury, and lumbar fractures with abdominal and long bone injuries.

Beginning immediately, it is imperative that respiration receive attention. Not only is an open airway essential, but steps to increase respiratory exchange are also important. Hypotension may result from the acute cervical syndrome or from blood loss related to associated injuries, and even several minutes of hypotension may increase the progression of cord destruction.

In spite of these complicating factors, which may frequently require attention, re-establishment of proper alignment should be given early consideration in order to preserve neural function.

SURGICAL TREATMENT

Indications for operative treatment and the type of operation being proposed are constantly changing. At the present time, many surgeons and physicians who have been responsible for large numbers of patients and have seen the progress of those treated surgically and nonsurgically, favor attention to early rehabilitation without primary surgical attention to the spinal cord or cauda equina. At the same time we are witnessing a renewed interest in the spinal cord and the hope that intervention in the first hours after injury will preserve neurologic function or actually reverse what appears to be permanent paralysis. Current therapeutic efforts which are expected to yield favorable results include the application of cold as described by Negrin,[23] and by Albin et al.[1]; vertebral realignment using tongs, traction, and manipulation via an anterior or lateral approach; and medication such as mannitol and steroids. Osterholm and Mathews have experimentally employed alpha methyl tyrosine to block norepinephrine synthesis in the injured spinal cords of cats.[24] Although this substance has proved to be a toxic agent, not recommended for human usage, they believe that monoamine antimetabolites may someday be effective in retarding the self destructive nature of the catecholamines that are released in the injured spinal cord. This type of investigation certainly deserves to be encouraged.

The goals of any spinal operation should include one or more of the following: (1) return of neural function; (2) retention of surviving neural function; (3) maintenance or restitution of a stable spinal column; (4) comfort; and (5) early physical and vocational rehabilitation.

Compression, produced by mechanical deformation, and ischemia (or anoxia) resulting from compression are the frequently cited causes of paralysis in the anatomically intact spinal cord. Tarlov stated that mechanical deformation was the critical factor and favored laminectomy, even for patients with a central cervical cord syndrome, if the neurologic deficit was great and accompanied by a spinal fluid block.[39] Mechanical deformation also affects circulation to the cord, and its correction will aid in combating ischemia.

It is to be remembered that laminectomy does not always ensure decompression. All too frequently the operation provides only the elimination of normal laminae, without actually removing the cause of the pressure, and may preclude the opportunity of later carrying out a stabilization procedure which may be very essential for proper rehabilitation. It is unnecessary and probably disastrous to employ suboccipital craniectomy and laminectomy of atlas and axis for injuries to the upper cervical spine.

Fortunately, the surgeon has available to him other means of correcting the mechanical deformation. This correction seems to be essential, regardless of conditions within the vertebral canal, and is the first step toward the goals enumerated above.

Reduction of Cervical Dislocation by Skeletal Traction

Barring extensive injury to the scalp and calvarium, there is a prominent place for skeletal traction. Prompt reduction not only corrects mechanical deformation, but may enhance vascular supply. Crutchfield has devised convenient tongs to apply to the skull. They may be applied in the emergency room or the patient's room, thus minimizing unnecessary transfer from hospital bed or stretcher to operating table and back.

TECHNIQUE. Stab incisions, requiring no sutures, are made in the parietal scalp, and special drill points are used to penetrate the outer table of the skull (Fig. 34-4 A). The site of placement is usually in the line of the mastoids, but can either be fore or aft, depending on the desired direction of pull. Crutchfield advocates slow reduction, believing that it protects the spinal cord and surrounding supporting tissues (Fig. 34-4 B). Fifteen pounds of traction is recommended for a dislocation of the upper third of the cervical spine and 25 pounds for dislocation of the middle and lower thirds of the cervical spine.

Roentgenograms may be obtained the day after traction is begun and may be repeated daily until one is certain that satisfactory realignment has occurred. If reduction takes place very promptly, one should anticipate an unstable spine requiring prolonged immobilization and possibly fusion.

With the current emphasis on more vigorous early management, there may be justification for using more pull to bring about more rapid reduction, but this should be reserved for patients who have serious neurologic deficit.

Gardner has recently devised tongs that do not require incision of the scalp or perforation of the calvarium. It is possible that they may be placed prior to transfer to the hospital (Fig. 34-4 C). The current general interest in spinal cord injury undoubtedly will focus more attention on immediate on-the-spot treatment.

Reduction of Cervical Dislocations Resistant to Skeletal Traction

If there is persistent locking of the facets, with the inferior facet of the vertebra above riding over the superior facet of the vertebra below, open reduction can bring about proper alignment.

TECHNIQUE. Through a posterior vertical incision, one can expose the spinous processes and laminae. Rongeurs may be used to remove a portion of the superior facet of the inferior vertebra, and gentle manipulation will bring about a proper reduction. The re-approximated spinous processes may then be wired toward each other and bone grafts may be placed to ensure fusion.

Indications for Other Decompressive Procedures

Until recently, laminectomy was considered the only feasible decompressive procedure. It has the disadvantage of not always accomplishing decompression and, with the popularization of anterior and lateral approaches, is utilized less frequently today. The advantages of laminectomy are that it doesn't require

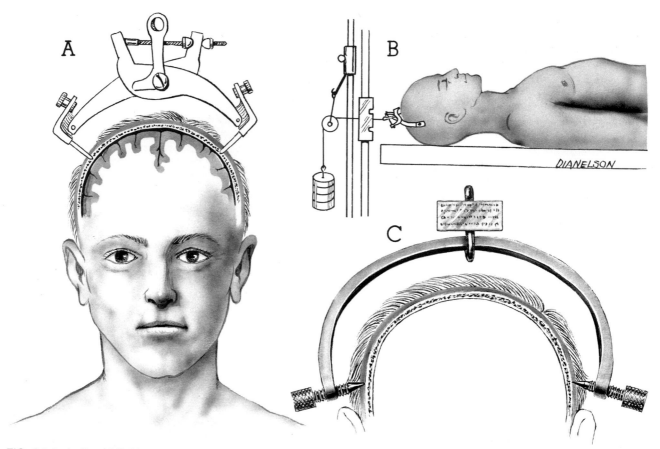

FIG. 34-4. *A*, Crutchfield tongs; *B*, traction with Crutchfield tongs; and *C*, Gardner-Wells tongs.

retraction of important vessels and viscera, and the potential exists for superior and inferior extension of the exposure. Regardless of the elected approach, the following are generally recognized as proper surgical indications: (1) progression of neurologic deficit; (2) partial or complete cerebrospinal fluid block (most surgeons would be guided by the expected effect of cervical traction); (3) penetrating wounds; (4) bone, disc, or foreign fragment within the vertebral canal; (5) posterior dislocation of gross nature; and (6) anterior cervical cord syndrome.

Recent laboratory studies seem to show that if serious neurologic deficit is not to result, surgical intervention must occur in less than four or five hours. Although the logistics of patient transfer make this an ideal difficult to achieve, this is an enormous problem worthy of every reasonable effort. Perhaps more reliable tools will aid in distinguishing physiologic from anatomic cord separation. Croft et al. have obtained such information in the laboratory via cortical evoked responses from scalp electrodes resulting from stimulation of a peripheral nerve.[6] Larson is gathering similar information from patients.

It is quite uncommon to find that a patient has lost sensation but retained motion. Degrees of paralysis are easily recognized and patients seem to sense any

decrease in motor power. The same is not true of sensation. If sensation is preserved, it is most likely going to be found in the sacral dermatomes (saddle area). Pinprick sensation usually remains longer than other sensations and motor power, and its presence early after injury is a rather good prognostic sign. If it is absent after one or two days and if there are no other signs of improvement, the prognosis for useful recovery is poor. It is not likely that a surgical procedure will alter the outcome in the patient who has been devoid of all sensation below the level of injury for several days.

In spite of the pessimism with which such a situation is viewed, attempts at relocation of vertebrae are probably justified because of ultimate stability and comfort, as well as the resulting increase in the lumen of the canal. Manometric or Pantopaque block, coexisting with normal radiographs, is worthy of decompression and exploration.

An increase in neurologic signs is justification for open surgery, including laminectomy, because one may be able to relieve pressure from fragments of disc or bone or remove a subdural or extradural hematoma. One need not be surprised if exploration does not reveal a pre-existing hematoma, and it is wise to anticipate that surgical exploration may cause a large amount of fresh bleeding if it is done within several days of the injury. Lausberg observed that the prognosis is better in the patient who develops signs slowly, but that laminectomy should not be delayed if there are any signs of progression.[21]

Wounds that penetrate the dura are deserving of early attention. Bony or foreign fragments within the vertebral canal are not necessarily cause for immediate operation. Jacobs and Berg reported poor restoration of neurologic function, even with prompt surgical attention judiciously applied in a war zone.[15] Yashon et al. were also surprised with the poor results obtained following removal of bullets in a civilian practice, but advocate laminectomy and cooling if the operation can be done within five or six hours of injury.[42]

Pain resulting from irritation of spinal roots by bone fragments or herniated discs may be justification for a decompressive procedure but is not an immediate consideration.

Attempts should be made to perserve stability of the spinal column, and if either the injury or the operation about the cord or cauda equina have caused instability,

spinal fusion will permit participation in rehabilitation procedures and possibly prevent further neurologic disability.

Surgery for Upper Cervical Fractures and Dislocations

There is no place for laminectomy in the patient who has had a fracture-dislocation at C1–C2. Immobilization with traction and some type of brace may be effective, but there is always the risk of latent subluxation.

The base of the odontoid process is the most common site of fracture and this may result in either forward or backward dislocation of the atlas. Should it be deemed necessary to surgically facilitate proper alignment and fusion, the surgeon has several options. Again, it is important to fit the operation to the patient. Ideally, one would prefer to secure the laminae of C1 to C2 (perhaps also C3), and this requires passing wires under the laminae (Fig. 35-5 A, B, C, D). Should this not be feasible one may fuse occiput to C2. Burr holes are

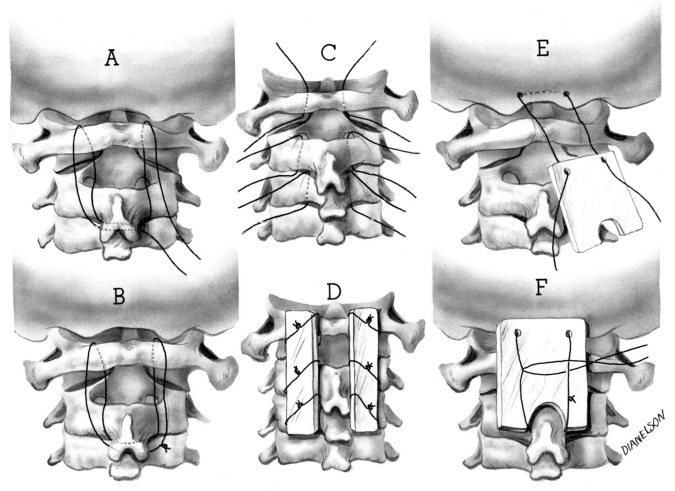

FIG. 34-5. A, B, Wiring used to immobilize C1 and C2; C, D, Fusion with autogenous bone graft and wiring of C1–C3; and E, F, Occipital-axial fusion with autogenous iliac bone graft and appropriate wiring.

placed in the occiput on either side of the midline several centimeters from the posterior rim of the foramen magnum. A wire is passed into one burr hole, passed extradurally to and out the other burr hole (Fig. 35-5 *E, F*). The iliac bone graft will have been perforated, and the two ends of the wire passed through the perforations, so that the superior portion of the graft is in contact with the occiput. After one end of the wire has been brought under the prominent spinous process of the axis, the two ends of the wire are tightened, causing the graft to make firm contact with occiput and axis. Slivers of bone may be placed under the graft to obliterate any space between graft and the posterior arch of the atlas.

Surgery for Middle and Lower Cervical Fractures

When skeletal traction does not bring about reduction, one may resort to open reduction as described on page 363. Should it be deemed proper to perform a laminectomy or foraminotomy, it may be done, but fusion will then require a longer strut of bone graft. The anterior approach as described by McFadden (see Chapter 36) is also worthy of consideration in dealing with this problem.

Management of Penetrating Wounds of the Spinal Canal

If the patient is seen within a few hours of injury, and if his condition permits, debridement and laminectomy may be done immediately. If seen later, it may be wise to simply debride the wound in order to perform a laminectomy safely at a later time. Unless the wound of entry is exactly in the midline, it is probably wiser to treat it separately from the laminectomy incision. Great effort may be required to remove all foreign material, and one should attempt to remove foreign objects and spicules of bone from the vertebral canal but not necessarily from the vertebral body.

Whether or not one opens the dura mater is dependent on many factors. It is opened if one suspects a foreign body, bone fragment herniated disc, or hematoma underneath it. If the dura is opened, reasonable effort at suture is advised, and if that is not feasible, a very snug muscle and fascia closure is essential to prevent appearance of a cerebrospinal fistula.

ANTIBIOTICS

Antibiotics should be administered if either the injury or the operation has penetrated the dura mater.

References

1. Albin MS, White RJ, Acosta-Rua G: Study of functional recovery produced by delayed localizing cooling after spinal cord injury in primates. J Neurosurg *29*:113–120, 1968.
2. Alexander E, Davis CH: Reduction and fusion of fracture of the odontoid process. J Neurosurg *31*:580–582, 1969.
3. Allen AR: Surgery of experimental lesion of spinal cord equivalent to crush injury or fracture dislocation of spinal column. JAMA *57*:878–880, 1911.
4. Bovill EG Jr, Eberle CF, Day L, Aufranc OE: Dislocation of the cervical spine without spinal cord injury. JAMA *218*:1288–1290, 1971.
5. Breasted JH: The Edwin Smith Surgical Papyrus. Chicago, U of Chicago, 1930.
6. Croft TJ, Brodkey JS, Nulsen FE: Reversible spinal cord trauma: a model for electrical monitoring of spinal cord function. J Neurosurg *36*:402–406, 1972.
7. Crutchfield WG: Skeletal traction for dislocation of the cervical spine. Report of a case. South Surg *2*:156–159, 1933.
8. Crutchfield WG: Treatment of injuries of the cervical spine. J Bone Jt Surg *20*:696–704, 1938.
9. Dohrmann GJ, Wagner FC, Bucy PC: Myelinated fibers in transitory paraplegia. J Neurosurg *36*:407–415, 1972.
10. Ducker TB, Assenmacher DR: Microvascular response to experimental cord trauma. Surg Forum *20*:428–432, 1969.
11. Ducker TB, Hamit HF: Experimental treatment of acute spinal cord injury. J Neurosurg *30*:693–679, 1969.
12. Ducker TB, Kindt GW, Kempe LG: Pathological findings in acute experimental spinal cord trauma. J Neurosurg *35*:700–707, 1971.
13. Holdsworth FW: Acute injuries of the cervical spine with cord damage. In Proceedings of the Third International Congress of Neurological Surgery. Excerpta Medica Foundations, 1966.
14. Holdsworth FW, Hardy A: Early treatment of paraplegia from fractures of the thoracolumbar spine. J Bone Jt Surg *35-B*:540–550, 1953.
15. Jacobs GB, Berg RA: The treatment of acute spinal cord injuries in a war zone. J Neurosurg *34*:164–167, 1971.
16. Jefferson G: Fracture of the atlas vertebra. Brit J Surg *7*:407–422, 1920.
17. Jefferson G: Remarks on fractures of first cervical vertebra. Brit Med J *2*:153–157, 1927.
18. Jefferson G: Treatment of spinal injuries. Practitioner *130*:332–341, 1933.
19. Kelly DL, Lassiter KRL, Calogero JA, et al.: Effects of local hypothermia and tissue oxygen studies in experimental paraplegia. J Neurosurg *33*:554–563, 1970.
20. Larson SJ: Personal Communication, 1973.
21. Lausberg G: Laminectomy in traumatic paraplegia. In Proceedings of the Third International Congress of Neurological Surgery. Excerpta Medica Foundation, 1966.
22. Matson DD: The management of acute compound battle-incurred injuries of the spinal cord. In Surgery in World War II, Vol. 2. Washington, Office of the Surgeon General, Department of the Army, 1959.
23. Negrin J Jr: Local hypothermia in spinal cord traumatic lesions. In Proceedings of the Third International Congress of Neurological Surgery. Excerpta Medica Foundation, 1966.
24. Osterholm JL, Mathews GJ: Altered norepinephrine metabolisms following experimental spinal cord injury. J Neurosurg *36*:386–394, 1972.
25. Rogers WA: Treatment of fracture dislocation of the cervical spine. J Bone Jt Surg *24*:245–258, 1942.
26. Rogers WA: Fractures and dislocations of the cervical spine. An end-result study. J Bone Jt Surg *39-A*:341–376, 1957.

27. Rosenbluth PB, Meirowsky AM: Sympathetic blockade, an acute cervical cord syndrome. J Neurosurg *10:*107-112, 1953.

28. Ruge DA (ed): Spinal Cord Injuries. Springfield, Ill. Charles C Thomas, 1969.

29. Scheinker IM: Neurosurgical Pathology. Springfield, Ill. Charles C Thomas, 1948.

30. Schlesinger EB, Taveras JM: Lesions of the odontoid and their management. Amer J Surg *95:*641-650, 1958.

31. Schneider RC: The syndrome of acute anterior spinal cord injury. J Neurosurg *12:*95-122, 1955.

32. Schneider RC: Surgical indications and contraindications in spinal cord trauma. Clin Neurosurg *8:*157-184, 1962.

33. Schneider RC: Cervical spine and spinal cord injuries. Mich Med *63:*773-786, 1964.

34. Schneider RC, Cherry G, Pantek H: The syndrome of acute central cervical spinal cord injury with special reference to the mechanisms involved in hyperextension injuries of the cervical cord. J Neurosurg *11:*546-577, 1954.

35. Schneider RC, Crosby EC: Vascular insufficiency of brain stem and spinal cord in spinal trauma. Neurology *9:*643-656, 1959.

36. Schneider RC, Kahn EA: Chronic neurological sequellae of acute trauma to the spine and spinal cord. J Bone Jt Surg *38-A:*985-997, 1956.

37. Schneider RC, Schemm GW: Vertebral artery insufficiency in acute and chronic spinal trauma. J Neurosurg *18:*348-359, 1961.

38. Schneider RC, Thompson JM, Bevin J: The syndrome of acute central cervical cord injury. J Neurol Neurosurg Psychiat *21:*216-227, 1958.

39. Tarlov IM: Acute spinal cord compression paralysis. J Neurosurg *36:*10-20, 1972.

40. Whitley JE, Forsyth HF: A classification of cervical spine injuries. Amer J Roentgen *83:*633-644, 1960.

41. Wilson CB, Bertan V, Norrell HA, et al.: Experimental cervical myelopathy. II. Acute ischemic myelopathy. Arch Neurol *21:*571-589, 1969.

42. Yashon D, Jane JA, White RJ: Prognosis and management of spinal cord and cauda equina bullet injuries in sixty-five civilians. J Neurosurg *32:*163-170, 1970.

35

The Halo

VERNON L. NICKEL

METALLIC fixation applied to the cranium as a means of stabilizing and controlling the position of the cervical spine should be credited to Crutchfield, who introduced calipers for spinal traction in 1933.[1,2] Crutchfield tongs are the most widely used fixation device throughout the world. Subsequent modifications by Vinke[3] and Barton[4] improved management of some of the inherent difficulties including complexity of application, the attainment of precise oblique positioning, and maintenance of tautness so that tongs do not slip. In 1936, Hoen attempted to accomplish skeletal cranial control by means of paired wire loops passed through burr holes in the skull.[5] All of these devices, however, are most effective in only one direction (traction) and are limited in their ability to position in several planes.[6]

In the early 1950s, Rancho Los Amigos Hospital and other respiratory centers had large numbers of patients with poliomyelitis, many of whom had suffered severe respiratory paralysis. With the use of improved respiratory equipment and increased knowledge of the physiology underlying its use, larger numbers of patients were surviving and the problem was now fixation. Many of these patients had severe paralysis of the cervical musculature and were unable to hold their head upright. The position of the cervical spine also affected deglutition, phonation, airway patency, and their ability to better use their accessory muscles for respiration. In some cases there was direct compression of a deformed cervical spine upon the respiratory mechanism.

At that time, patients were kept supine, with pads and pillows carefully positioned to maintain the head and cervical spine in optimum alignment. Dr. Jacquelin Perry, in 1955, was assigned the complex and difficult task of attempting to improve the care of these patients. She had had some experience with Hoen wires and her first attempts utilized this type of fixation to get patients upright. However, plaster of Paris, with its attendant difficulties, had to be used as a supplement for precise positioning. Some of the patients had paralysis that was confined to the bulbocervical area with relatively normal lower trunk and lower extremity function. It soon became obvious that an easy to apply, three-plane adjustment type of fixation would be optimum.

After speaking on this particular problem at the Houston Orthopedic Club in 1956, I was approached by Dr. FA Bloom, who suggested that he might have an idea that would be of help to us. Several orthopedists, including Paul Harrington and me, accompanied him to his home where he showed us a device he had been working on for some years. The idea had been originally conceived in the South Pacific during World War II when he was working with maxillofacial surgeons who needed a device that attached to the cranium to solidly fix crushed faces that had also been burned. He had learned that threads could be changed and several holes were needed for each screw (Fig. 35-1).[7] The shape of the screws was important; they had been designed with a sharp pin tip that readily penetrated into, but not through, the outer table of the skull. In addition, a broad bevel made further penetration difficult unless excessive force was applied. The screw has changed very little throughout the years except at Rancho Los Amigos Hospital, where the width of the bevel was increased.[8]

Those of us from Rancho Los Amigos Hospital immediately saw that the idea had great practical application, and we began utilizing the device. It soon became apparent that a complete ring provided more strength and rigidity than the reinforced partial ring employed

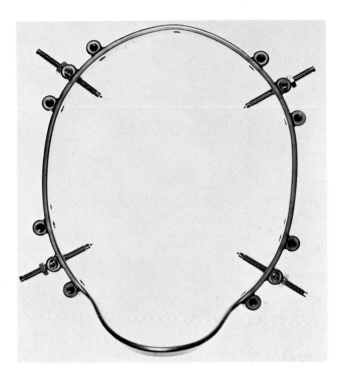

FIG. 35-2. The halo, showing four screws.

by Dr. Bloom. A fourth screw was also added to the original design (Fig. 35-2).

The halo, as it was quickly dubbed, was tremendously useful in our practice, and has gradually won recognition throughout the world. I believe it is superior and will probably replace other types of cranial fixation.

An interesting sidelight occurred in my private office some years after the development of the halo. I saw a device that had been developed in 1935 by my associate, Dr. Alonzo Neufeld, while working with Dr. Hubb Childs, a maxillofacial surgeon, for use in a depressed maxillary injury. The device was an incomplete ring in a coronal rather than a horizontal plane that used ordinary bone screws. Various versions of the halo have undoubtedly been used in other circumstances unknown to us, and I remember vaguely an early reference I have been unable to relocate in which it was used under similar circumstances.

The first publication on the use of the halo in its more modern sense was written by Perry and me and appeared in 1959.[9] A later, more detailed primary review in 1968 reported on 204 cases in which the halo was applied at Rancho Los Amigos Hospital.[10]

APPLICATIONS

Applications for the halo appear to be expanding,[11-13] but in general, use may be divided into four main categories.

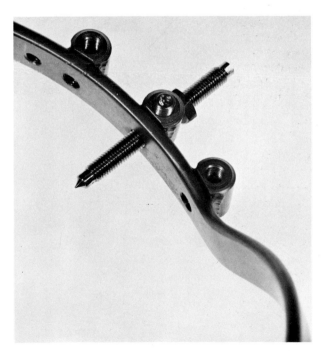

FIG. 35-1. The halo pin.

TRAUMA. In injuries to the cervical spine, such as fracture or fracture dislocation, the halo can be applied in bed as the traction device. Exact positioning can be achieved without excessive pressure on the skull. The halo is easy to apply. The sometimes serious complication of pressure ulcers of the occiput, which can occur when a patient is in one position for a long time (as when Crutchfield tongs are utilized), can be prevented because the halo suspends the cranium and eliminates direct pressure on the skin. Rollers may be applied to the halo with a board under the portion of the cervical spine just above the shoulders that may be used to more precisely control the degree of traction. Angulation can be exactly controlled by lengthening or shortening several ropes attached to the halo.

Exact positioning for flexion, extension, rotation, and right and left side bending can be performed most easily with the halo. With attachment of the halo to a body cast (Fig. 35-3) and more laterally to a Milwaukee brace or plaster jacket, a patient can become ambulatory at an early date reducing both time and cost of rehabilitation.[14] An additional benefit that greatly stimulated our use of the halo was the fact that the long periods of recumbency, which were formerly used, resulted in marked muscle atrophy as well as psychologic changes. These effects are much less severe as the patient is permitted to be out of bed at an earlier date.

The usefulness of the halo decreases rapidly as the injury site approaches the thoracic spine, and is of little use in patients with injuries below T5 or T6.

SPINE DEFORMITIES (Scoliosis). The use of the halo in scoliosis has been well described in a number of papers,[15,16] and has been of great benefit in all types of scoliosis involving the upper cervical to lower thoracic spine. It must be repeatedly emphasized that the halo is a powerful tool and must be carefully controlled to guard against the use of excessive traction. With appropriate distal fixation, as for instance through the femoral shafts, a method of correction of the deformed pelvis is now available.

The halo has been used with a variety of devices. Initially it was attached to a body cast well fitted over the iliac crest. Dr. Blount and his associates in Milwaukee broadened this application by attaching the halo to a Milwaukee brace and using it as a traction

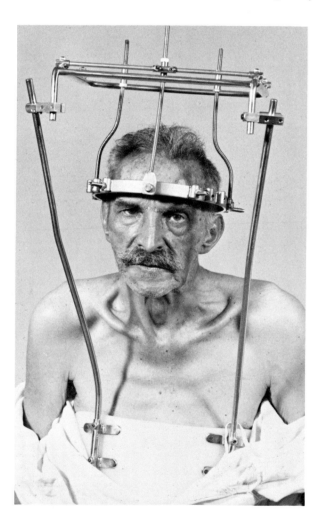

FIG. 35-3. Halo attached to body cast.

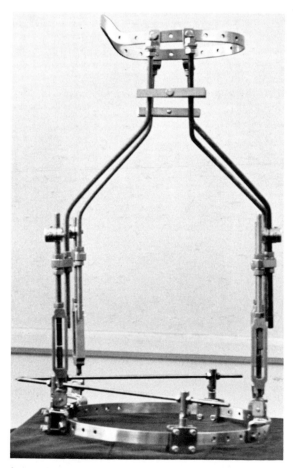

FIG. 35-4. The pelvic halo.

device. Halo femoral traction was developed by Dr. Moe and his associates in Minneapolis.

Halo pelvic fixation that eliminated the cast would appear to be an obvious development (Fig. 35-4). Many years ago at Rancho we attempted several methods of pelvic fixation utilizing pins similar to those employed for cranial fixation. The pins were inserted bilaterally into the posterior and iliac spines, but they had a tendency to creep and cause excessive skin irritation. In another method, Dr. Alice Garrett employed fixation of wire over buttons attached to the iliac crest, and in one case these proved quite successful. At the time, however, the use of bicycle loops attached to plaster appeared to be more feasible than the pelvic halo.[17] The bicycle loops were used in a number of patients on the Scoliosis Service at Rancho Los Amigos Hospital.

A number of groups around the world have successfully re-instituted the use of the pelvic loop including Dr. DeWald in Chicago[16] and Dr. O'Brien and his associates in Hong Kong.[18]

PARALYSIS OF THE NECK. The paralyzed neck requires precise positioning to obtain stabilization.[19] The halo is unquestionably the best device yet developed to manage this type of problem.

MAXILLOFACIAL INJURIES. The halo has continued to be used for the purpose for which it was designed by Dr. Bloom in the treatment of maxillofacial depressed fractures or burns about the face. No other device fulfills the requirements as well.

METHOD OF APPLICATION

The application of the halo is relatively simple, although precision of alignment is required for prolonged stability. The halo may be applied under local or a light general anesthetic depending on the tolerance of the patient. Usually a general anesthetic is used in children to allay their apprehension.[20] Visits to other patients wearing a halo aids in reducing anxieties about the device and helps the patient to understand the purpose and general comfort of the device.

The head need not be shaved, as was originally done. We now advise only a betadine scrub applied to the scalp in the immediate area.

It is important that the tips of the screws of the halo are just below the maximal circumference of the cranium, so that upward traction tightens rather than loosens the device. This placement directs the force into a thick mass of bone. Posteriorly, the halo is placed about one-eighth inch above the ear, but should not touch the pinnae which are very sensitive. Slightly more space is left posteriorly than anteriorly to compensate for possible low-grade edema which can develop in supine patients.

Some physicians place pin insertions in the most lateral channels to avoid visible scarring; however, this placement penetrates the temporalis muscle and its overlying fascia and can make chewing painful. Also, the bone is thinner in this area and fixation is less secure.

No skin incision is required as the screw itself will make an appropriate hole. A front pin and a diagonally posterior pin are tightened simultaneously. The tautness of the pin is most important and a torque screwdriver will give the degree of torque accurately so the pin will not penetrate the cranium. The final tension required in preadolescent children or those with an obviously thin cranium is 4 Kg-cm for each of the four screws, whereas in adults it should be 5.76 Kg-cm.[19] When the desired tension is obtained, the lock nuts are fastened tightly to avoid pins working loose.

After application of the halo, the support frame may be attached immediately or at some later date. The area about the pins should be cleansed daily with a mild antiseptic. Some minor discomfort may be felt by the patient for a day or two, but is usually controlled with mild analgesics. All nonambulatory patients must be turned periodically to protect the skin and alternate maximum pin pressure areas.

The halo and frame should be checked periodically for signs of looseness. Inflammation, discomfort, or a "clicking" sound are signs of a loose pin. Only then should the pins be tightened, not as a routine, because this will hasten erosions and penetration. If on tightening the pin appears to be penetrating too deeply, or if there is excessive inflammation about the pin, this pin should be replaced in an adjacent hole. The new pin should be inserted before the old pin is removed.

The removal of the halo is the reverse of the initial application and does not cause patient discomfort. The pin sites generally heal promtly, even where there has been considerable irritation and infection. The initial red welt shrinks and only a small white dimple remains.

COMPLICATIONS

Complications from the use of the halo are minimal.[21] There have been no long-lasting, serious complications in over 400 cases at Rancho Los Amigos Hospital. Infection of the pin site is the most frequent problem, as in any case in which a wire crosses the skin barrier. The development of persistent drainage or inflammation indicates the necessity of changing the pin position. Again it should be emphasized that the second pin is inserted before the first is removed. Serious deep-seated infection has occurred in four of our cases, necessitating the removal of small sequestra. Once this was done, the wounds all healed uneventfully.

Slippage of the halo occurs most frequently in cases in which the surgeon does not have extensive experience in its use and the halo is applied where the diameter of the cranium is decreasing rather than increasing.

In one of our cases it was thought that the pin had

probably penetrated the cranium, but new pins were attached through adjacent poles and the first pins removed without sequelae. We have heard of at least two cases in which brain abcess developed following the use of pins, but these cases were resolved without serious sequelae once they were treated.

Certain patients have oily scalps that require more frequent cleansing. Other patients have more pointed heads and the halo has to be applied more proximally. We facetiously refer to these types of problem cases as "fat heads" and "pin heads."

It is important to recognize that the halo is a powerful tool and that excessive traction can cause serious damage. In patients with scoliosis, this damage is usually to the cranial nerves. Among patients with congenital deformities, the greatest danger is in patients with diastematomyelia, in which results of excessive traction can be serious.

In summary, the halo is comfortable, effective, and easily applied. Complications of its use, especially considering its great potential, are minimal.

References

1. Crutchfield WG: Skeletal traction for dislocation of the cervical spine. South Surg 11:156, 1933.
2. Crutchfield WG: Skeletal traction in treatment of injuries to the cervical spine. JAMA 155:29, 1954.
3. Vinke TH: A skull traction apparatus. J Bone Joint Surg 30A:522, 1948.
4. Barton LG: The reduction of fracture dislocation of the cervical spine by skeletal traction. Surg Gynec Obstet 67:94, 1938.
5. Hoen TL: A method of skeletal traction for treatment of fracture dislocation of cervical vertebrae. Arch Neurol Psychiat 36:168, 1936.
6. Wells T: Personal communication.
7. Bloom FA: Personal communication.
8. Perry, J: Personal communication.
9. Perry J and Nickel VL: Total cervical spine fusion for neck paralysis. J Bone Joint Surg 41A:37, 1959.
10. Nickel VL, Perry J, Garrett A and Heppenstall M: The halo. A spinal skeletal traction fixation device. J Bone Joint Surg 50A:1400, 1968.
11. Welply WR: Fractures and dislocations of the cervical spine: early treatment. Manit Med Rev 46:175, 1966.
12. Pieron AP and Welply WR: Halo traction. J Bone Joint Surg 52B:119, 1970.
13. Prolo DJ, Runnels JB and Jameson RM: The injured cervical spine. Immediate and long-term immobilization with the halo. JAMA 224:591, 1973.
14. Tunback S: The use of the halo cast for treatment of cervical injuries. In Orthopedic Seminars. Downey, California, Rancho Los Amigos Hospital, 1972.
15. Winter RB, Moe JH and Ellers VE: Congenital scoliosis: a study of 234 patients treated and untreated. Part II. J Bone Joint Surg 50A:15, 1968.
16. DeWald RL and Ray RD: Skeletal traction for the treatment of severe scoliosis. J Bone Joint Surg 52A:233, 1970.
17. Garrett AL, Perry J and Nickel VL: Stabilization of the collapsing spine. J Bone Joint Surg 43A:474, 1961.
18. O'Brien JP, Yau ACMC, Smith TK and Hudgson DR: Halo-pelvic traction. A preliminary report on a method of external skeletal fixation for correcting deformities and maintaining fixation of the spine. J Bone Joint Surg 53B:217, 1971.
19. Nickel VL, Perry J, Garrett AL and Snelson R: Application of the halo. Orthopedic and Prosthetic Appliance Journal March 1960, p. 32.
20. Kopits SE and Steingass MH: Experience with the "halo cast" in small children. Surg Clin North Am 50:935, 1970.
21. Perry J: The halo in spinal abnormalities. Orthop Clin North Am 3:69, 1972.

36

Anterior
Open Reduction
of the Fractured
Cervical Spine

J. T. McFADDEN

OPEN reduction of flexion fractures of the cervical spine by the anterior approach fulfills all of the major requirements for adequate treatment: protection of the threatened cord, decompression of the vertebral canal, realignment of the displaced bony segments, and stabilization of the injured joints. Unfortunately, not all cervical spine fractures can be treated easily from this direction: dens fractures, obviously, do not lend themselves readily to repair by the anterior interbody fusion method, and C2-C3 fractures lie in a less accessible anatomic position than the lower cervical spine joints. Injuries that compromise the vertebral canal posteriorly with penetrating or impinging bone fragments require laminectomy for decompression.

PROTECTION OF CORD FUNCTION

The futility of applying conventional bone-setting methods to realign the fractured and dislocated cervical spine has been recognized since antiquity. Yet, no satisfactory alternative to hand traction and manipulation was devised until 1932 A.D., when Crutchfield reported his initial experience with skull calipers. In the ensuing 41 years, skull traction has had wide acceptance, principally on the premise that it is less dangerous than hand traction to the intact or partially destroyed cord. Recently, the advent of anterior interbody fusion methods has stimulated a revival of hand traction techniques for several reasons. Primarily, hand traction is less dangerous with open reduction than it was when used to attempt closed reduction of the spine. Also, traction with tongs requires a preliminary operation, followed by a relatively long period of incremental traction and adjustments to reduce

373

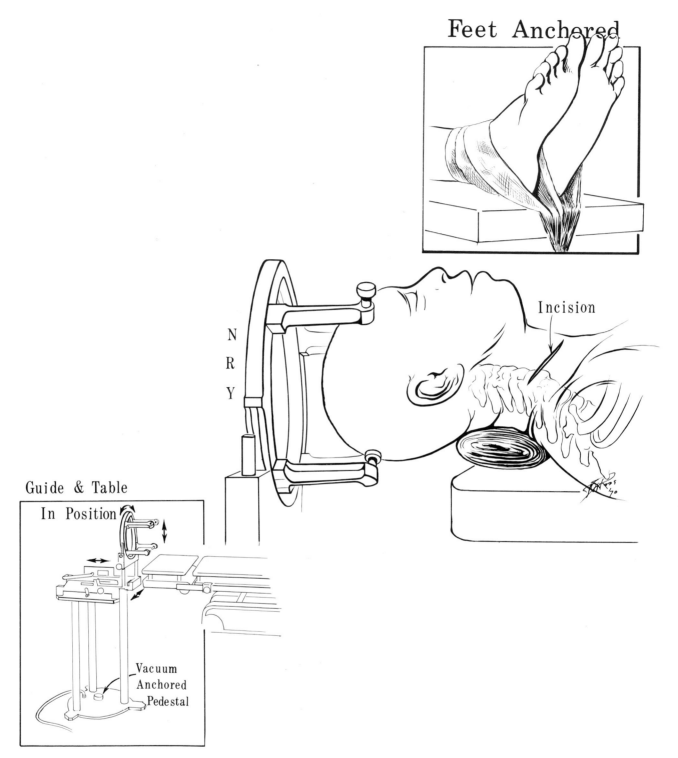

FIG. 36-1. Stereotaxic reduction of cervical spine dislocation: *A*, patient in position for operation; *B*, feet anchored; *C*, guide and table in position. Demonstrates eight motions inherent in guide system for manipulating fractured and dislocated cervical spine with body anchored to operating table. (From McFadden JT: Stereotaxic realignment of the dislocated cervical spine. Surg Gynec Obstet *133:*262–264, 1971)

the dislocation, whether or not in preparation for spinal fusion. It has been a matter of much concern to those who use caliper traction preliminary to fusion, that what has been accomplished with the calipers can be lost in anesthetizing and positioning the patient for operation. Both the hand and the caliper techniques offer uncertain directional control as well as poor incremental stretching and holding. For these reasons, from January 1970 to October 1975, a stereotaxic guide system was used for controlled traction and realignment in a series of 35 patients undergoing interbody fusion for fracture dislocations. The technical descriptions to follow will be based largely on this experience.

Rigid immobilization with a tight-fitting cervical collar adequately splints the neck for the trip to the operating suite, for the anesthetic induction, and for the endotracheal intubation. Aqueous Zephiran (benzalkonium chloride) copiously applied to the scalp eliminates the necessity to remove hair in that it probably prevents infection of the scalp puncture wounds made by the head holder pins of the stereotaxic device. After intubation of the patient and proper alignment of the operating table, in relation to the vacuum-anchored pedestal supporting the stereotaxic guide, the patient is then lifted and carefully moved by at least four assistants while the surgeon supports the splinted neck and guides the head into the head holder and secures it without changing the cervical malalignment (Fig. 36-1).

An inflatable bag under the neck serves as a fulcrum for realignment of fracture displacements. The fulcrum must be placed caudal to the lesion.

DECOMPRESSION AND REALIGNMENT

An oblique incision along a skin fold allows adequate exposure and causes less scarring on the neck (Fig. 36-1). For additional axial exposure, skin flaps can be developed over the surface of the platysma muscle. After incising the platysma muscle crosswise to the skin incision, the surgeon resects the omohyoid muscle, if it lies across the surgical field, and then develops the connective tissue plane between the carotid artery and thyroid gland sheaths down to the prevertebral fascia. A spinal needle inserted into the disc correctly identifies the space on Polaroid x-ray films or with image intensification. The deformity, however, usually is obvious. Indigo carmine, injected into the disc, trickles through and deeply stains disc fragments and tissue crevices created by the trauma, and apparently causes no damage to the spinal cord or peripheral nerves. (Caution: Methylene blue, on the other hand, permanently destroys spinal cord and nerve function.)

The longus colli muscles retract easily with blunt dissection. Hemorrhage responds adequately to bipolar coagulation. Unipolar coagulation and the cutting cautery are too dangerous to be used safely in this location. Retraction of the carotid artery laterally and the esophageal-tracheal complex medially seldom causes significant complications when performed skillfully and intermittently by hand. Sustained self-retaining retraction in this area is contraindicated because it endangers blood supply to the brain on the one side of the wound and esophageal and tracheal patency on the other side of the wound.

Decompression and realignment can now be accomplished simultaneously and progressively. That is to say, progressive debridement of the fractured joint facilitates progressive realignment of the broken bony segments. As the surgeon removes fragments of cartilage, nucleus pulposus, bone, and ligament, the anesthesiologist, when requested, exerts horizontal traction on the head with the rack and pinion mechanism on the floor of the stereotaxic guide (Fig. 36-1). Removal of the broken tissue further loosens the joint, allowing it to be stretched open, thus improving visualization of the wound floor (Fig. 36-2). At this point, the surgical microscope serves to identify remaining blood clot, fragments of bone, and disc material along the ramifications of indigo carmine seeping into the ravines of the anatomic disruptions (Fig. 36-3). Only with magnification is it possible to identify the various tissues accurately. Extruded disc material separating the longitudinal ligament from the posterior vertebral margins is extracted by dissecting around these corners (Fig. 36-3). Rents in the ligaments are enlarged to facilitate the retrieval of material extruded into the canal space. Hypertrophic spurs along the posterior vertebral margins are removed with fine drills and angled punches.

Thus decompressed, the joint and the vertebral canal are ready for realignment of the fractured and dislocated bony segments. The stereotaxic guide controls head movements in three dimensions and eight directions—up and down, side to side, head to foot, and clockwise and counterclockwise (see Fig. 36-1). These motions are reflected principally in that segment of the spine above the fracture after debridement. Manipulations of the operating table, on the other hand, with the head fixed rigidly on a separate pedestal, move the spine principally below the fracture. The combined motions, extension (lowering) of the head segment and elevation of the body segment, usually accomplish realignment easily, (see Fig. 36-2). Most flexion deformities, as a matter of fact, respond to stretching and extension (lowering) of the head segment with the stereotaxic guide alone. Any manipulations, whether with the vertical rack and pinion mechanism of the stereotaxic guide, or with operating table, are performed only when the floor of the joint and the longitudinal ligament or the vertebral canal are in full view of the surgeon. Thus, he can avoid additional encroachment on the canal and the cord by dislocated segments of bone.

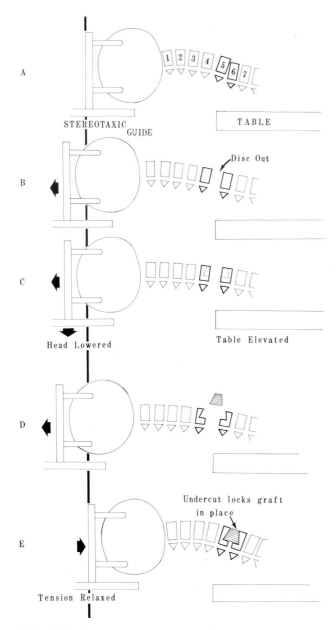

FIG. 36-2. Stereotaxic reduction of cervical spine dislocation: *A*, patient positioned without changing the alignment; *B*, disc removed with joint stretched slightly open; *C*, spine realigned by lowering the head and raising the body and by using any of the eight motions inherent in the head holder device as needed; *D*, joint stretched open to receive the graft; *E*, tension on the spine released to lock the trapezoid graft. This is a schematic drawing with the degree of stretching and joint opening exaggerated for emphasis. (From McFadden JT: Stereotaxic realignment of the dislocated cervical spine. Surg Gynec Obstet *133:*262–264, 1971)

The Locked Facet

A facet locks when the forces causing a flexion fracture are sufficiently violent to carry the inferior articular process of a vertebra so far in the cephalo-anterior direction that it escapes the confining resistance of the superior articular interface of the vertebra below, and slides forward and downward to rest against the anterior surface of the same superior articular process (Fig. 36-3). Obviously this displacement cannot be reduced by extension forces alone, which serve, in this case, only to tighten the bone lock. First, traction must be exerted along the long axis of the dislocated craniospinal segment until the posterior surface of the dislocated inferior articular process bypasses the superior surface of the locking superior articular process of the vertebral body below (Fig. 36-3); then extension of the cranial segment of the spine will bring the displaced inferior articular process back into its proper anatomic plane so that it can be released to resume its normal position (Fig. 36-3). Usually, only one articular facet is locked, the displacement having occurred by rotatory flexion to one side or the other. It may be necessary then to loosen the set screws of the head holder ring (see Fig. 36-1) and to turn the ring by hand to unlock the facets by a rotatory motion opposite to that which caused the injury. The facet will then slip back into place (Fig. 36-3). Image intensification can be used to monitor these realignment maneuvers.

STEREOTAXIS

Even though the stereotaxic apparatus is used to perform open reduction of a fracture dislocation of the cervical spine, the use of the word *stereotaxic* to describe this operation might be questioned on the grounds that the probe guide is not employed to direct an instrument to a target invisible to the naked eye.

Stereotaxis is a biological term synonymous with thigmotaxis, which describes the trophism of an organism to the stimulus of a solid surface. How it acquired its new (1908) meaning related to surgery is not clear.[1] As to the derivation, the prefix stereo- comes from the Greek word *stereos*, meaning both solid and having three dimensions. The suffix -taxic comes from the Greek word *tasso*, meaning to arrange.[2,3] Clarke, who invented and patented the first stereotaxic instrument, failed to give it a name in his original publication.[4] In the second publication, the adjective *stereotaxic* appeared without interpretation although Horsley and Clarke outlined the geometrical and mathematical concepts of this surgical approach in laboratory animals to some extent.[1] In Clarke's provisional patent specifications (18,297-British) of 1912, he refers to the device as a stereotaxic apparatus and describes his functional concept which pertained to an arrangement of three mutually perpendicular assumed planes intersecting within an enclosed space interpreted as a solid. In his complete specifications (22,455-British) he makes it abundantly clear that the solid means the cranium, and that the instrument was intended to supply mechanical ordinates for anatomical targets not only in the labora-

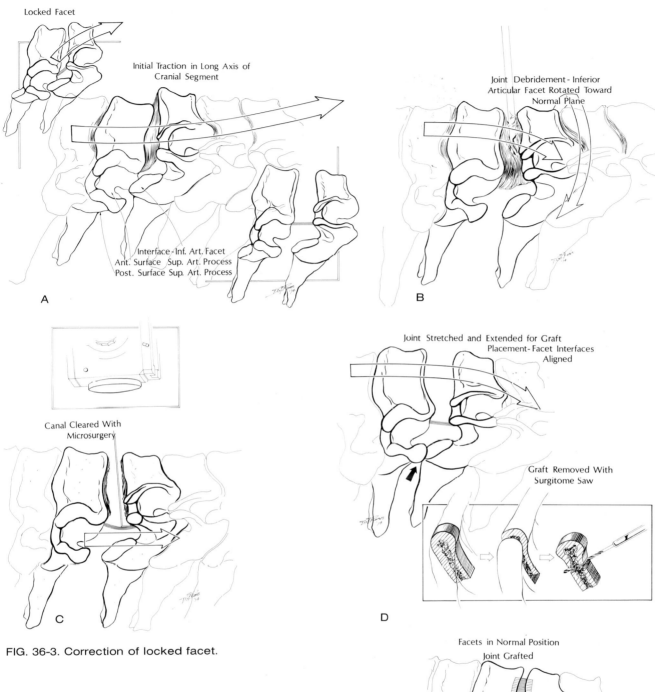

Locked Facet

Initial Traction in Long Axis of
Cranial Segment

Interface-Inf. Art. Facet
Ant. Surface Sup. Art. Process
Post. Surface Sup. Art. Process

A

Joint Debridement-Inferior
Articular Facet Rotated Toward
Normal Plane

B

Canal Cleared With
Microsurgery

C

FIG. 36-3. Correction of locked facet.

Joint Stretched and Extended for Graft
Placement-Facet Interfaces
Aligned

Graft Removed With
Surgitome Saw

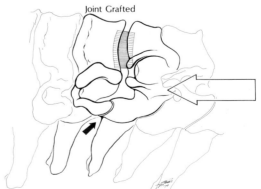

D

Facets in Normal Position
Joint Grafted

E

tory animal but also in the human brain. It appears from Clarke's description in his patent specifications that he used the name stereotaxis quite literally in the sense of a geometrical arrangement within a solid. Clarke and Horsley used only the adjectival form, but the noun *stereotaxis* has come to be used to name the science of stereotaxic surgery.[5] The term stereotrophism likewise has been used in reporting stereotaxic procedures.[6] Neither of these terms is given any surgical meaning whatsoever in contemporary standard dictionaries. Although stereotaxis was given its surgical meaning no later than 1908,[1] it did not appear in Dorland's Medical Dictionary until the 24th Edition (1965), where it is given a meaning related to a precise positioning in space. Both adjective and noun forms appear only in the latest complete supplement to the Oxford English Dictionary (1961) where it is described as related to thigmotaxis, but the apparatus of Clarke is also mentioned, as a mathematical instrument of physiology.[1] The word taxis alone is an old surgical word, having on philological evidence, the following meaning, very apropos to this new use: "a manipulative operation employed for replacing parts which have quitted their natural situation. . . .".[7] In view of its old meanings and in view of the newer concepts of stereotaxic devices, it seems most likely that the surgical meaning inherent in the word *stereotaxis* connotes three-dimensional control of an anatomical goal. Thus, the use of the term in this concept—to control realignment of the spine in three-dimensions—not only is justified, but actually broadens the spectrum of sterotaxic surgery.

Furthermore, Clarke described two distinctly separate functional components of his instrument: (1) the stereotaxic indicator for determining the ordinates and (2) the stereotaxic operative instrument for passing the probe or other instruments to the target. Well's adjustable stereotaxic head holder serves a comparable function to Clarke's stereotaxic indicator, albeit in an entirely different and far simpler manner. It therefore deserves the title stereotaxic no less than does the device of Clarke, its control of neck motions in three-demensions being incidental and, in the case of a broken neck, indeed fortuitous.

1. Horsley V and Clarke R: The structure and functions of the cerebellum examined by a new method. Brain *31:*45-124, 1908.

2. Lidell GH and Scott R: A Greek-English Lexicon. Oxford at The Clarendon Press. Vol. II, pp. 1640-1756.

3. Oliver L: Parkinson's Disease. Springfield, Ill. Charles C Thomas, 1967.

4. Clarke RH and Horsley V: On a method of investigating the deep ganglia and tracts of the central nervous system (cerebellum). British Med. J. *2:*1799-1800, 1906.

5. Cooper IS: Involuntary movement disorders. New York, Harper & Row, Hoeber Medical Division, 1969.

6. Adams JE: The future of stereotaxic surgery. JAMA, *198:*180-184, 1966.

7. The Oxford English Dictionary. Oxford at the Clarendon Press. Reprinted 1961, Vol. XI, page 122.

Commentary

The three commonly used methods for realignment, hand traction, halter traction, and caliper traction, can be used to accomplish open reduction. In our experience, however, these methods offer considerably more diffi-

culty than the stereotaxic method, principally because the surgeon has far less control over what is being done to the joint by a second person exerting uncontrolled traction on the cranial segment of the fractured spine.

STABILIZATION OF THE INJURED JOINT

Stabilization requires bone grafting in or across the joint by one of three general techniques: (1) a flat wafer-type graft countersunk into the disc space between intact cortical interfaces (Fig. 36-3); (2) the hole and dowel techniques; and (3) a free form graft tailored to fit a particular bony defect created by the injury and the necessary debridement (see Fig. 36-1).

The flat graft has been used when the cortical interfaces of the displaced joint have not been fractured. After debridement and removal of the cartilaginous interfaces by curettage, the joint is allowed to return to its neutral position in the horizontal plane by carefully releasing the horizontal traction. Caliper measurements of the joint space are then made, and a graft slightly larger than the disc space, cut from the iliac crest with a burr saw or a sagittal saw. Horizontal traction again is exerted to open the joint. The graft is gently tapped into the interspace and countersunk beyond the lips of the anterior vertebral borders. Traction is then released. Within the somewhat oval disc cavity, the snugly fitted graft cannot migrate past the lips of either the anterior or the posterior vertebral borders (Figs. 36-3 and 36-4).

The hole and dowel techniques have been abandoned in our series of anterior interspace fusions for cervical spine fractures because of a high incidence of angulation at the fused joint postoperatively.

Free form grafting has been used when bone has been fragmented by the injury. A trapezoid-shaped bed

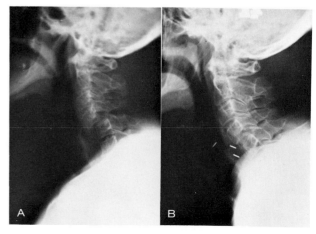

FIG. 36-4. *A,* Fracture dislocation. *B,* Fracture dislocation realigned, and joint fused by bone wafer (Smith-Robinson).

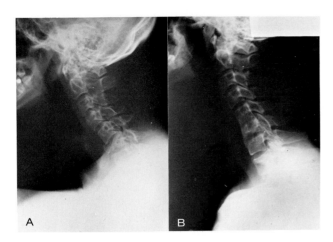

FIG. 36-5. *A*, Crush fracture of vertebral body. *B*, Trapezoid graft across 2 discs and damaged vertebral space.

with the long side down is cut into the two contiguous vertebral bodies across a disc space, or across two disc spaces and bridging an entire vertebral body, when the anterior border of a vertebral body has been crushed by the injury (Fig. 36-5). The interspace, after debridement, is measured with calipers, and the graft is sawed from the crest of the ilium, fitted into place and countersunk with the injured area stretched and extended open. When released the joint locks the trapezoid graft into place, where it acts much as a keystone in an arch (see Fig. 36-2).

Wound Closure and Postoperative Care

Methodical hemostasis prevents most of the complications of the anterior interbody fusion operations. A hematoma in the floor of the neck wound will compress the soft wall of the laryngotracheal complex which resists pressure less effectively than the overlying muscle and skin layers. The respiratory difficulty that ensues may progress to obstruction and strangulation unless the patient is rescued with endotracheal intubation and evacuation of the hematoma. Ill-advised tracheostomy in this situation carries grave danger of wound infection and serious secondary complications

such as osteomyelitis at the fracture site. A small siphon drain in the floor of the neck wound will prevent hematoma in the rare case with a hemostasis problem. Wound closure is accomplished in anatomic layers with suture materials of the surgeon's choice.

The donor site usually produces more postoperative discomfort than the neck wound. Two factors, in our opinion, contribute to the pain. Removal of bone graft with an osteotome or chisel produces a fine hair-line fracture proceeding across the ilium ahead of the instrument blade. Hematoma or seroma in the donor site distends the wound. These two contributing factors to pain can be diminished if the graft is taken with a high speed burr saw or sagittal saw and the tissues carefully approximated across the bone defect created at the donor site.

Careful and continuous neck support with a plastic collar or with a four-poster brace is mandatory until the joint fuses. Poor support contributes to graft slippage, joint angulation, progressive malalignment, aseptic graft necrosis, and exuberant spur formation.

Serial radiographs, lateral views, at intervals indicate the progress of joint healing and stabilization.

References

1. Crutchfield WG: Skeletal traction for dislocation of the cervical spine. Surgeon *2*:156–159, 1933.
2. Grant JCB: Grant's Atlas of Anatomy. Baltimore, The Williams & Wilkins Co, 1962, ed 5.
3. Howorth MD, Petrie JG: Injuries of the Spine. Baltimore, The Williams & Wilkins Co, 1964.
4. Loeser JD: History of skeletal traction in the treatment of cervical spine injuries. J Neurosurg *33*:54–59, 1970.
5. McFadden JT: Stereotaxic realignment of the dislocated cervical spine. Surg Gynec Obstet *133*:262–264, 1971.
6. Raynor RB: Severe injuries of the cervical spine treated by early anterior interbody fusion and ambulation. J Neurosurg *28*:311–316, 1968.
7. Ruge D: Spinal Cord Injuries. Springfield, Charles C Thomas, 1969.
8. Verbiest H: Anterior operative approach in cases of spinal cord compression by old irreducible displacement or fresh fracture of cervical spine. J Neurosurg *19*:389–400, 1962.
9. Wilkinson M: Cervical Spondylosis, It's Early Diagnosis and Treatment. Philadelphia, WB Saunders, 1971, ed 2.

37

Treatment of Fractures of the Thoracolumbar Spine

E. SHANNON STAUFFER

APPLIED ANATOMY OF THE THORACOLUMBAR SPINE

THE FOUR VERTEBRAE that comprise the thoracolumbar junction—T11, T12, L1, and L2—constitute a vulnerable site for fracture dislocations secondary to rotary forces. The thoracic vertebrae above this level are quite stable owing to the attachments of the ribs, intercostal muscles, and circular structure of the chest cavity. The configuration of the facets in the coronal plane absorbs rotatory forces in the thoracic area. The lumbar vertebrae below this level—L3, L4, and L5—become increasingly more stable and resistant to trauma owing to the larger vertebral body and dorsal element bony structure, the large psoas muscle, the heavy interspinous and supraspinous ligaments, and the lumbosacral fascia. The configuration of the lumbar facet joints is in the sagittal plane and prevents rotation. As the rotary forces descend through the thoracic vertebrae, they are obstructed at the T12-L1 facet joint. The vertebral body and dorsal elements are smaller than the lumbar vertebrae. Without the support of the rib cage or the psoas muscle and lumbosacral fascia, the rotary forces are dissipated at the T12-L1 junction by fracture (Fig. 37-1).

The stability of the spine depends on the anatomic configuration of the vertebral bodies, intervertebral discs, posterior facet joints, and intervertebral ligaments consisting of the anterior longitudinal ligament, posterior longitudinal ligament, interspinous ligament, and supraspinous ligament, and facet joint capsules. The posterior ligaments are of sufficient tensile strength to resist rupture with flexion, but they rupture when flexion is combined with rotation (Fig. 37-2).

The nervous system enclosed in the dural tube in the vertebral canal at this level consists of two types of neural tissue: (1) The sacral segments of the spinal cord are in the conus medullaris, which terminates at the lower border

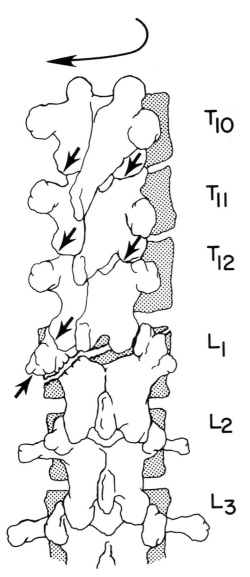

FIG. 37-1. Diagram of facet configuration of thoracic and lumbar vertebrae. Coronal facets in thoracic vertebrae allow rotation; sagittal facets of lumbar vertebrae prevent rotation. Rotary forces produce fracture at T12 due to abrupt change of facet configuration.

of the L1 vertebral body (Fig. 37-3). (2) All the lumbar roots (L1 to L5) traverse the T12-L1 junction intradurally. The conus medullaris responds to injury as central nervous system tissue. The anterior and posterior lumbar roots contained in the dural sheath are more resistant to injury and their response is similar to that of peripheral nerves.

The anterior and posterior roots join to form the lumbar nerve at the neural foramen, which is the site of the sensory dorsal ganglion cells. Injury to nerve roots proximal to these ganglion cells has a poorer prognosis for recovery of sensation than for recovery of motor function.

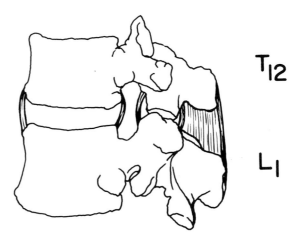

FIG. 37-2. Diagram of intervertebral ligaments at thoracolumbar junction.

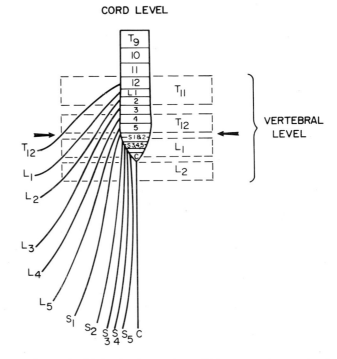

FIG. 37-3. Neural elements within neural canal at T12–L1 junction. Spinal cord segments of S1, S2, and S3, as well as cauda equina lumbar roots, L1, L2, L3, L4, and L5, may be injured by fracture.

MECHANISM OF INJURY OF FRACTURE-DISLOCATIONS

FLEXION. Flexion forces produce a compression fracture of the vertebral body without dislocation or fracture of dorsal elements. The spongy cancellous bone in the vertebral body will compress, dissipating the forces. This type of fracture is usually stable and without ligamentous injury, and there is no danger of late instability.

FLEXION OF THE BODY WITH DISTRACTION FORCES APPLIED TO THE SPINE. When a person is subjected to rapid deceleration while wearing a seat belt, the trunk forcibly flexes with the axis of rotation anterior to the vertebral canal, causing a distraction force on the posterior elements of the vertebra. The strong supraspinous and interspinous ligaments resist the distraction force, but since there is no compression force on the vertebral body, the force is dissipated by a fracture through the dorsal element extending from the spinous process down through the laminae and pedicles and a fracture through the body to the anterior longitudinal ligament. All the ligamentous structures remain intact. With recoil to the anatomic position, the fracture appears to be almost completely reduced. This fracture is unstable in the upright position, but stable in the recumbent position. These patients seldom have neurologic injury.

AXIAL-LOADING BURST FRACTURE. When an axial load is placed on the vertebra with minimal flexion or extension, the vertebral body becomes trapped between the hydraulic noncompressible forces of the discs above and below. The vertebral end plate fractures and the disc is forced into the interior of the vertebral body, pushing the fragments posteriorly, anteriorly, and laterally. The smaller upper lumbar vertebrae, without the stability of the rib cage, absorb these forces and either L1 or L2 may be fractured. Many of these fractures have significant neurologic injury owing to the rapid posterior protrusion of the posterior part of the vertebral body into the neural canal. These fractures are stable if the dorsal elements are not removed and usually heal without resultant late instability.

FLEXION ROTATION. This is the most common mechanism of fracture dislocation of the thoracolumbar spine. Flexion forces, coupled with rotation of the thorax in one direction and the pelvis fixed or rotating in the opposite direction, cause a fracture of the T12-L1 facet joint. The fracture travels down through the pedicles and produces a slice fracture of the top of the vertebral body. The opposite trailing facet dislocates with avulsion of the facet joint capsule. The posterior ligamentous complex is not efficient in resisting rotational forces when coupled with flexion. This fracture dislocation is unstable, and usually the patient has severe neurologic injury. If displaced, this fracture dislocation is difficult to reduce by closed methods and frequently heals with gross displacement and malunion.

PHYSICAL EXAMINATION OF THE PATIENT

The examination of a person with a suspected thoracolumbar fracture begins with a rapid assessment for possible injury to other systems. Vital signs must be recorded, along with results of examination for possible airway obstruction, rib fractures, upper extremity fractures, and soft tissue injuries. The lower extremities must be palpated for possible dislocation or fracture. Local tenderness is noted at the fracture site, as is a gap between the affected spinous processes in the midline. The patient resists any motion of the back when he is recumbent in the supine or prone position. There may be bruises over the shoulder or buttock which will indicate possible mechanisms of injury. The abdomen should be elevated for possible intra-abdominal injury and bleeding as well as paralytic ileus. It is of particular importance to examine the feet if the patient has fallen from a high place. Fractures and dislocations of the os calcis and talus are often associated with fractures of the lumbar spine.

Neurologic Examination

Serial examination is necessary to assess function of lumbar nerve root distribution and function of the sacral segments of the spinal cord, which are at the anatomic level of the fracture. Examination of the lumbar innervated areas documents cauda equina root function. The lumbar segments and roots provide sensation over the anterior aspect of the thigh, anterior and medial aspect of the calf, and the medial aspect of the foot. Motor function is supplied by the lumbar roots to the active hip flexors, iliopsoas, quadriceps, medial hamstrings, anterior and posterior tibialis, and extension of the great toe. The function of the spinal cord adjacent to the fracture is determined by examination of the sacral segments. Sensation in the saddle area around the genitalia and perineal skin signifies the presence of sacral sparing, an indication that the conus is under voluntary control from the brain. The motor power of the sacral area is reflected in voluntary control of rectal and vesicle sphincters and short toe flexor muscles.

It is important to evaluate perineal reflexes, the presence of which indicates an intact reflex arc through the sacral segments of the conus medullaris. These reflexes will be absent if there is a conus medullaris or root injury involving the sacral cord segments or roots, but may be present if the sacral roots and conus medullaris are intact in spite of a complete cord transection superior to the sacral segments. Injured lumbar roots traversing the fracture dislocation area have a good prognosis for future recovery. Progressive recovery may occur for as long as six months. Muscle strength that is detectable six months after injury tends to improve for 18 to 24 months, but muscles that are still completely paralyzed at the end of that six-month period cannot be expected to return to function.

The absence of sacral sparing (perianal sensation or voluntary sphincter control) signifies a complete spinal cord injury at the conus medullaris, and the prognosis

TABLE 37-1. Basic Patterns of Possible Neurologic Loss

Physical Examination	Lesion and Prognosis	
	Spinal Cord	*Roots*
1. No voluntary motor power distal to T12; no sensation distal to T12; no reflexes in lumbar or sacrally innervated areas.	Complete conus lesion (possible supraconus lesion with the conus in spinal shock); prognosis: poor.	Complete root lesion; prognosis: recovery of lumbar root function may occur.
2. No voluntary motor power; no sensation in lumbar or sacral areas, bulbocavernosus reflex present.	Complete cord supraconus lesion. Conus out of spinal shock and transmitting reflexes. Prognosis: nil for recovery of conus function.	Complete lumbar root lesion; prognosis: fair for recovery of lumbar root function.
3. Lumbar sensation or voluntary muscle activity present; no sacral sensation or sphincter control and no bulbocavernosus reflex.	Complete conus injury; prognosis: nil.	Lumbar roots have escaped complete injury; prognosis: good for progressive recovery of motor power and poor for recovery of sensation, since injury is proximal to the dorsal root ganglion.
4. Lumbar motor and sensory innervation present, no sacral sensation or sphincter control, and the bulbocavernosus reflex is present.	Complete supraconal lesion out of spinal shock; prognosis: nil for recovery of sacral innervation (bladder and bowel control); good for development of automatic bowel and bladder reflex emptying.	Lumbar root escape; prognosis: good for recovery of motor power in lumbar roots and improvement of sensation, due to escape of both anterior and posterior roots.
5. Lumbar sensation or motor function intact; sacral sensation or motor intact (sharp-dull discrimination in perianal skin area or voluntary control of rectal sphincter).	Incomplete conus lesion; prognosis: good for recovery of bowel and bladder control.	Root escape; prognosis: good for recovery of lumbar sensory and motor control.

for recovery is poor. There are five basic patterns of possible neurologic loss, each with definite physical findings and with definite prognoses (Table 37-1).

Prognosis for Developing Reflex Emptying of the Bladder

It is of utmost importance to ascertain whether emptying of the paralyzed bladder is based on upper motor neuron or lower motor neuron paralysis. If the patient has a complete paralysis of voluntary control of his sphincters and a positive bulbocavernosus reflex, the sacral reflex arc is intact, divorced from voluntary control. This is an upper motor neuron paralysis of the bladder and sphincter, and one may anticipate development of automatic filling and emptying on a reflex basis.

If the patient has a flaccid, paralyzed anal sphincter and no perineal bulbocavernosus reflex, he has a lower motor neuron areflexic paralysis of the bladder and automatic filling and reflex emptying cannot be expected. The lower motor neuron paralyzed bladder must be emptied by abdominal pressure (Crede) and Valsalva straining of the abdominal muscles.

X-RAY EVALUATION

If a fracture of the lumbar spine is suspected, the person should be taken to the Radiology Department on the original Emergency Room stretcher. A lateral roentgenogram, including the lower thoracic and the entire lumbar spine, can be taken without moving the patient from the stretcher (Fig. 37-4). Following examination of this roentgenogram, a large x-ray plate is carefully placed under the patient and an anterior-posterior film is obtained. This limited study will reveal any bony injury of serious magnitude. If fractures or dislocations are seen, treatment can be recommended on the basis of these films. Obliques are rarely of value and rotation of the patient to obtain oblique films may cause further injury. If no fracture or dislocation is seen on the lateral and AP views, a full series of oblique films may be obtained. Evaluation of the roentgenograms includes counting of the vertebrae to be sure all vertebrae in the suspected area are included in the exposure. This usually is T9 to L5. The anterior-posterior films should be examined for any malalignment of the spinous processes. Each lamina and facet should be carefully examined for evidence of dorsal element fracture. The width of the interspinous process space should be

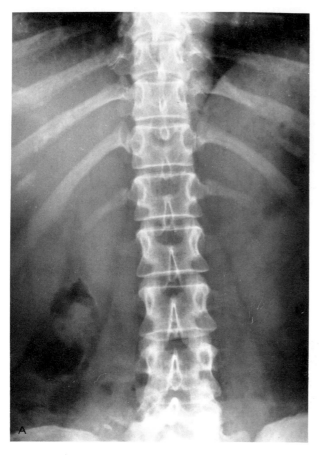 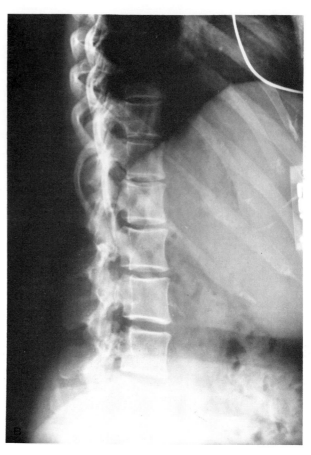

FIG. 37-4. Normal roentgenogram of thoracolumbar junction. *A*, Anteroposterior; *B*, lateral.

measured to ascertain possibility of ligamentous rupture and dislocation. The pedicles should be examined for possible widening at one level, indicating fracture of the vertebral body. The end plates of the vertebrae should be carefully evaluated for parallelism; any angulation would indicate suspicion of a fracture of the body. The height of the vertebral body should be measured to ascertain any compressed vertebral bodies. The transverse processes and ribs should be examined for possible fractures and displacement. On the lateral film the structure and form of the vertebral bodies should be carefully noted and any possible interruption of the cortical outline of the vertebral end plates or anterior portion of the body carefully noted. Any malalignment of the posterior portion of the vertebral bodies should be noted as well as any decrease in the height of the vertebral body.

On the lateral projection the dorsal elements, especially spinous processes, should be examined for possible fracture or widening of the interspinous process space.

TREATMENT

Treatment is based on the presence or absence of neurologic function and the radiographic evaluation of displacement and instability of the vertebrae.

COMPRESSION FRACTURES (Fig. 37-5). Compression fractures of the vertebral bodies without displacement, posterior protrusion of fragments, dorsal element fracture, or ligamentous rupture rarely have neurologic complications and are stable injuries. This injury is quite painful, however, and the patient should be admitted to the hospital for neurologic observation and observation for possible paralytic ileus. After several days he may begin extension exercises of the spine and isometric exercises of the abdominal muscles. After approximately one week of bed rest, the patient may be fitted with a thoracolumbar orthosis or body jacket and discharged, ambulatory, to be followed as an outpatient. The reduction of the fracture is unimportant, and reconstitution of vertebral height is possible to accomplish but virtually impossible to maintain. The body jacket or brace should be worn for four to six weeks and then only occasionally or not at all, as symptoms allow. If the magnitude of compression is severe, the increased kyphosis at the fracture site produces a compensatory hyperlordosis in the lower lumbar spine and may give rise to early lumbosacral disc degeneration in the future. This should be suspected if the patient develops low back complaints.

TRANSVERSE PROCESS FRACTURES (Fig. 37-6). Fractures of the transverse process in the absence of

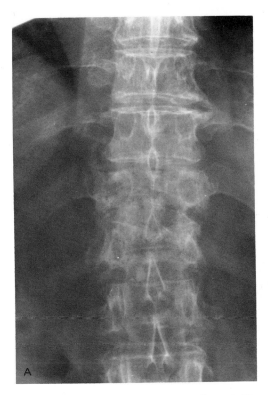

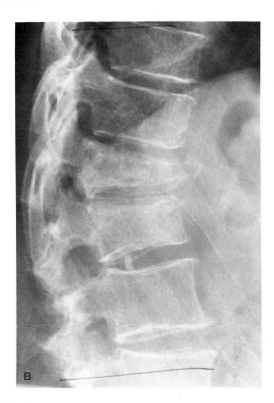

FIG. 37-5. Roentgenogram demonstrating stable compression fracture.

other vertebral disruption are caused by avulsion by the psoas muscle. These fractures cause considerable pain, which is best treated with bed rest and analgesics. Ileus must be considered, but is rare. The patient may be mobilized from bed as soon as symptoms permit. A light canvas corset will facilitate early ambulation.

DISTRACTION FRACTURE (Chance seat-belt injury). This fracture frequently reduces with the patient in the prone or supine recumbent position. Some separation of the spinous process fracture and transverse process fracture may remain, but is usually inconsequential. In the majority of cases healing proceeds without surgical intervention, since this is a pure cancellous bone fracture without ligamentous disruption dislocation. Six to eight weeks of bed rest, followed by six to eight weeks in a suitable orthosis, usually results in firm union at three to six months following the injury. If there is gross displacement and this cannot be reduced, or if there is injury to the lumbar roots, open reduction and internal fixation with spinous process wiring or Harrington compression rods may be indicated. Kaufer has suggested spinous process wiring; however, Harrington compression rods with hooks beneath the laminae afford much firmer fixation and allow early mobilization to an ambulatory status.

AXIAL LOAD BURST FRACTURE (Fig. 37-7). The patient with no neurologic loss rarely has sufficient displacement of the fracture to warrant open reduction. He may be treated with bed rest until the fracture becomes stable. The vertebral body fracture usually

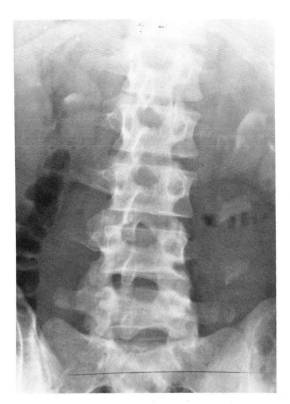

FIG. 37-6. Roentgenogram demonstrating fractures of transverse processes.

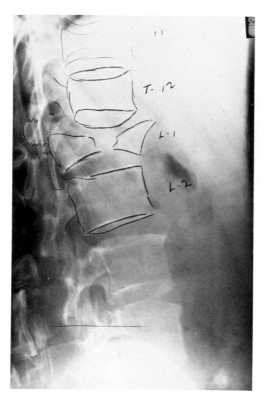

FIG. 37-7. Roentgenogram demonstrating burst fracture.

stabilizes with soft tissue healing at six to eight weeks. He may then be mobilized with a proper orthosis until solid bony union occurs at three to six months. Fractures through the dorsal elements, especially the laminae and facet joints, may persist with slow union or nonunion. This is usually of little significance so long as the vertebral body fracture heals and stability on flexion and extension occurs. If the patient has gross neurologic loss with displacement of the fragments, efforts should be made to reduce the fractures as soon as possible. This is rarely accomplished by closed methods of postural reduction. It may be done with halo-femoral traction, but only with difficulty in the paralyzed, anesthetic patient. Pressure sores and joint contractures are overriding complications to be avoided. Open reduction with Harrington distraction rods encompassing two vertebral bodies above and two vertebral levels below the burst body fracture is a method of reducing and providing internal fixation (Fig. 37-8). The anterior longitudinal ligament and the anulus fibrosis are rarely disrupted, and with distraction forces placed upon the laminae above and below the fractured vertebra, these ligamentous structures usually realign the vertebral body into near-normal alignment.

SLICE FLEXION ROTATION FRACTURE (Fig. 37-9). The neurologically intact patient rarely has significant displacement of the fracture (more than one-third body width or 30 degrees angulation) and can be treated by

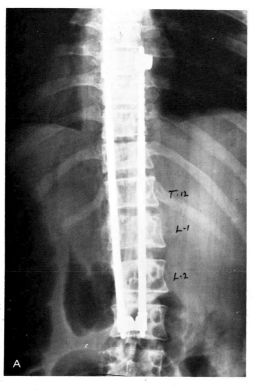

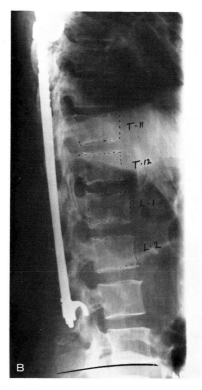

FIG. 37-8. Open reduction and internal fixation by Harrington distraction instruments accomplishes reduction of burst fracture.

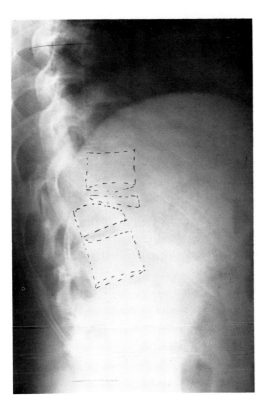

FIG. 37-9. Roentgenogram demonstrating slice fracture dislocation caused by flexion rotation injury.

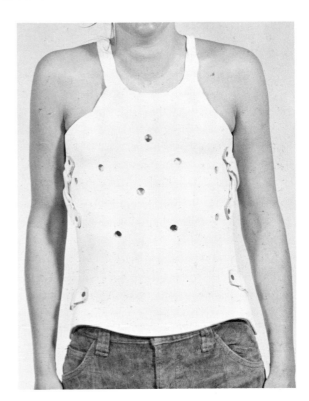

FIG. 37-10. Kydex body jacket used for ambulation for eight weeks following initial eight weeks of bed rest.

nonoperative means of bed rest with careful log-rolling side-to-side until the fracture becomes stable. Soft tissue healing and early bony union occur at about eight weeks, at which time the patient may become ambulatory in a body jacket for eight weeks (Fig. 37-10). Solid bony union occurs at three to six months. If the patient has gross neurologic loss with displacement of the spine, early correction of the dislocation is indicated. Incomplete conus and cauda equina lesions often recover and complete cauda equina lesions may improve if appropriate steps are taken to decompress the cauda. A complete conus injury with complete perianal anesthesia and no perineal reflexes, and complete paralysis of sphincters and toe flexors, has a poor prognosis and will not be affected by treatment. Pure conus injury without injury to the cauda equina is rare; therefore, reduction should be attempted in all patients with gross neurologic loss due to mixed injury of the conus and cauda equina.

REDUCTION

Reduction may be done by either closed methods of postural reduction with hyperextension at the fracture site or by nursing the patient on bolsters. Closed methods are difficult, however, owing to the tenderness and pain at the fracture site and the necessity to move the patient every two hours to provide adequate skin care (Fig. 37-11). It is recommended that the patient be nursed in a regular bed if he is going to be treated by nonoperative methods. A regular bed allows a patient's turning from side to side as well as his lying prone and supine, whereas frames allow only prone and supine positions. Because of the conical shape of the rib cage, there is gross motion of the fractured area at the thoracolumbar junction each time the patient is turned from the prone to the supine position. Circle-electric beds should never be used in the treatment of unstable thoracolumbar fractures because they load the body weight down through the fracture with each turning. Reduction is easily lost and displacement may increase as the patient is turned through the upright position (Fig. 37-12).

If the patient has gross displacement and it cannot be reduced by nonoperative methods, surgical reduction with internal fixation should be used. In the past, Mehrig-Williams plates have been used, with bolts through the spinous processes. However, the spinous processes are weak structures, and the plates may loosen causing poor fixation and reduction. With Harrington instrumentation, firmer internal fixation may be obtained, permitting early ambulation. The fracture dislocation without comminution, lateral displacement, or angulation can be reduced manually by open reduction, and the reduction can be maintained with Har-

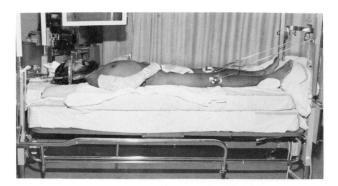

FIG. 37-11. Photograph of patient in bed with postural reduction.

rington compression rods (Fig. 37-13). The anterior longitudinal ligament is intact and, with the facets used as a fulcrum, accurate reduction can be obtained. It is important not to remove the facets in any debridement of the fractured posterior elements. If the body of the vertebra is comminuted or laterally displaced, compression rods will increase the scoliosis and distraction rods are required for reduction with lateral displacement or traumatic scoliosis. The firm fixation afforded by compression rods cannot be duplicated by distraction rods when there is a combination of the comminuted vertebral body and/or loss of facet joints. After reduction, it is evident that there is not persistent dural compression caused by the dorsal elements. Laminectomy offers little in the treatment of fracture dislocation of the thoracolumbar spine. Reduction to near anatomic position removes compression of the dural tube by a lamina.

Myelography on patients with fracture dislocations of the thoracolumbar spine is seldom beneficial. One may anticipate a block in most instances. Patients with incomplete lesions who demonstrate a block recover in the face of a persistent block. If a patient has a complete conus injury, removal of the block may not affect the prognosis. Examination of lateral myelographic films will reveal that the block results from projection of the vertebral body posteriorly into the vertebral canal. This protruding portion of the vertebral body is removed by reduction of the fracture. If it persists, the appropriate method of removing the block would not be laminectomy, which would in fact allow more angulation and increase the protrusion of the vertebral body into the canal. An anterior transthoraco-abdominal removal of the offending vertebral fragment from the anterior part of the vertebral canal would be more effective. This is only indicated in burst fractures that have a portion of the body protruding into the canal which is not reduced by distraction rodding of the posterior elements. The most common fracture dislocation, the slice fracture of the anterior superior aspect of the vertebral body, can be more easily reduced and rigidly fixed by the posterior open reduction method.

Treatment of the Comminuted Burst Fracture

This fracture is more frequent in the midlumbar spine (L2–L3). If the posterior part of the body has been forced into the vertebral canal, it is important to reduce this fracture to remove compressive elements causing compression on the nerve roots and the radicular arteries supplying the lumbar part of the spinal cord. Closed methods are not effective in reducing the displacement of the comminuted vertebral body. Compression forces with Harrington compression rods will worsen the fracture displacement. The preferred method of treatment of these fractures with neurologic loss due to impingement of the cauda equina is open reduction with Harrington distraction fixation.

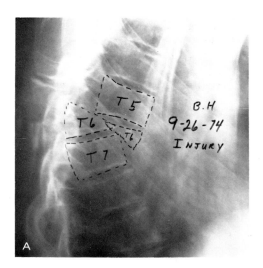

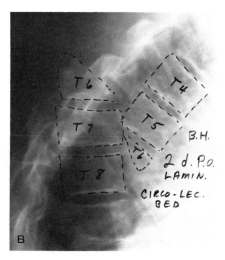

FIG. 37-12. Roentgenograms demonstrating re-displacement of fracture treated with circle-electric bed.

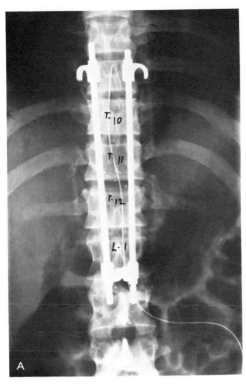 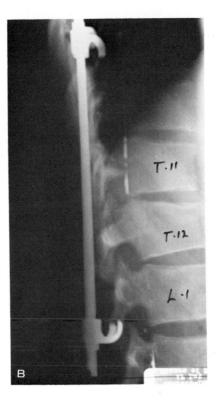

FIG. 37-13. Roentgenogram demonstrating open reduction and internal fixation with Harrington compression instruments.

The use of laminectomy is limited to the patient who demonstrates deterioration of his neurologic condition, as might occur with an epidural hematoma. Even though this is rarely a cause of the deterioration, a laminectomy should be performed, as evacuation of the hematoma may reverse the neurologic deterioration. The usual cause of such deterioration, however, is infarction of the lumbar and sacral segments of the cord due to progressively diminishing blood supply by the radicular arteries, which cannot be influenced by laminectomy.

REHABILITATION OF THE PARAPLEGIC

LOW THORACIC PARAPLEGIA. Rehabilitation of the paraplegic patient is based on his neurologic level. If he has a complete injury at the T12 level and demonstrates pelvic control through the abdominal muscles and the spinal extensor muscles, while muscles in the lower extremities are not innervated by the lumbar or sacral nerves, he will be trained to be independent in his wheelchair. He will be able to transfer in and out of the wheelchair, in and out of an automobile, drive an automobile, dress himself, and function independently in the wheelchair. Crutch and brace ambulation is feasible only for exercise. He may be fitted with crutches and long leg braces and encouraged to stand daily and to walk with the aid of parallel bars or walker, but in the absence of sensation, proprioception, or motor power in the lower extremities, purposeful ambulation cannot be anticipated.

UPPER LUMBAR PARAPLEGIA. If the patient has the use of muscles across the hips, such as flexors (iliopsoas), adductors, and sartorius of the L1-L2 nerve root distribution, he will have enough proprioception and control of the hips to be a functional ambulator in long leg braces. However, he will use the wheelchair for most activities, especially long-distance travel. This level is classified as Household Ambulation.

LOWER LUMBAR PARAPLEGIA, L3–4. Adequate root escape to allow the patient voluntary control of the quadriceps and hamstrings on one leg will allow the patient to ambulate with a short leg brace on that leg even though he has a long leg brace on the opposite leg. Thus he will become a Functional Ambulator. If he can ambulate with one free knee, he will have enough motor power, sensation, and proprioception to use crutches and braces to the exclusion of the wheelchair, and he is considered a Community Ambulator. Vocationally, however, he should be encouraged to pursue an occupation that will be performed mainly in the sitting position. Even though he is able to walk with crutches and braces, ambulation requires not only the use of his legs but also his arms and hands, and it is difficult to carry objects or walk for long distances with parcels.

BOWEL AND BLADDER REHABILITATION. With the higher level of lumbar paraplegia, T12–L1 functional level, the patient may have an upper motor neuron bladder, which means that he has an intact reflex arc through the S2–3 segments from the bladder to the spinal cord and back to the sphincters. If this reflex is intact, as demonstrated by the intact bulbocavernosus reflex, the patient will develop automatic reflex voiding even though he has no voluntary control. Most lumbar paraplegics, however, have a lower motor neuron bladder due to the interruption of the sacral nerve roots in the cauda equina or destruction of the S2–3 segments of the cord in the spinal canal posterior to the L1 vertebral body. Patients with lower motor neuron bladders will not develop reflex automatic voiding and will be required to void by abdominal strain and Crede suprapubic manual pressure. It is important, therefore, to obtain a cystometrogram early in the evaluation of paraplegia at the lumbar levels to ascertain the reflex activity possible by the bladder. The bowel program is best managed by suppositories every other night or every third night. Suppositories are effective in both upper motor and lower motor neuron paralysis by virtue of the local action on the bowel mucosa, which stimulates local peristalsis without a cord reflex being necessary.

LONG-TERM PROBLEMS OF PARAPLEGIA

The long-term problems of the patient with thoracolumbar or lumbar fracture with resultant paraplegia consist of:

1. Gradual production of pressure ulceration over the ischial tuberosities from prolonged wheelchair sitting. The person in a wheelchair must inspect his skin daily and use a proper seat cushion and wheelchair to prevent pressure ulcers from occurring.

2. Urinary tract deterioration. It is important that an annual urologic examination include an intravenous pyelogram and a search for vescico-ureteral reflex, hydroureter, progressive hydronephrosis, or the formation of urinary calculi.

3. The problem of late instability occurs if the patient has had an early destructive laminectomy in the face of a grossly displaced spine. Lateral flexion and extension films of the spine should be taken periodically at three-month intervals during the first year to ensure that a patient does not have a gradually collapsing instability of his fracture dislocation. If this is present, and the patient has a large laminectomy defect posteriorly which includes the facets, the operation of choice to prevent the instability from causing progressive angulation is an anterior interbody fusion.

Patients with lumbar fractures associated with neurologic loss must be accurately evaluated and carefully managed to prevent progression of the neurologic loss and provide the environment for maximum recovery. Reduction of marked displacement is important.

Realistic rehabilitation goals are necessary, and annual follow-up evaluations may prevent life-threatening complications.

References

1. Chance GQ: Note on A type of flexion fracture of the spine. Brit J Radiol 21:452–53, 1948.
2. Holdsworth F and Chir M: Fractures, dislocations, and fracture-dislocations of the spine. J Bone Joint Surg 52-A:1534–1551, 1970.
3. Smith WS and Kaufer H: Patterns and mechanisms of lumbar injuries associated with lap seat belts. J Bone Joint Surg 51-A:239, 1969.

Section X

Pain

38

Psychologic Aspects of Pain

D. KAY CLAWSON

WHAT is pain? Pain equals a noxious stimulus plus a disquieting emotion. In treating patients with complaints of low back pain, the practitioner must look as closely at the disquieting emotions as he does at the noxious stimuli. Failure to do so can only lead to numerous treatment failures, unnecessary operative procedures, and iatrogenic back cripples.[1]

Let us look at two patients with an identical problem. Patients A and B are both carpenters, age 40; each is married with three children. Both men have mild degenerative disc disease of the lumbar spine and on a given day experience a sudden onset of severe back pain with radiation into the foot. Bed rest, traction, and other conservative measures fail, a diagnosis of a herniated intervertebral disc is made, and a sequestrated fragment removed at operation. One man returns to work at six weeks; the other man, despite all medical efforts, is unable to return to work and seeks continuing medical care. The natural inclination of the scientifically trained, pragmatic physician is to seek the explanation in an anatomic abnormality of the back. Multiple studies are carried out to identify further degenerative changes of the spine, nerve root compression or scarring, or postural or mechanical instability that can be corrected through physical therapy, bracing, or surgery. The surgeon will find ample cause for the patient's complaints of pain, but until he starts to search for the *cause of disability*, rather than the cause of pain, he is doomed to failure.

Let us look at some of the psychosocial factors at work in these patients. Patient A has worked for the past 15 years for a small contractor. He has a warm personal relationship with his boss and knows the other men on the job well. The job provides a social outlet, as well as a satisfying work experience. He is as concerned about the welfare of his fellow employees and his boss as he is his own well-being; he knows this is reciprocated. In the home there is a genuine concern for the welfare of each member and love for one another. While being supportive, the family limits their visits while the patient is experiencing considerable pain, so as to "allow him time to rest." As he begins to recover, the visits are prolonged, and with each step of improvement and rehabilitation, he is encouraged and praised.

Patient B works out of the union hiring hall. He works for multiple contractors and frequently will go on the job not knowing another carpenter. A certain level of performance is demanded of him, and subconsciously he is beginning to recognize that certain tasks are more difficult for him to perform than they were ten years earlier. He blames other employees, usually younger men on the job, for work failures and accidents. At home there is considerable bickering over minor things; his wife complains of inadequate finances to meet the rising expenses, and the children are largely independent of parental guidance, seeking their own ways through life. At the time of great pain and medical crisis, the family hovers constantly around the patient, but as he begins to improve, their visits are shorter and less frequent. Which patient recovered and returned to work?

From the earliest times, the emotional component of pain has been recognized. Aristotle considered pain a passion of the soul, a state of feeling the antithesis of pleasure and the epitome of unpleasantness. The Bible equates pain as synonymous with suffering. The Old Testament teaches that wickedness and sin are the causes of pain and suffering, but through suffering we can atone for our sins and obtain forgiveness. Such thought has deep roots in the Judeo-Christian philosophy. This type of thinking, often in the subconscious, is a part of our heritage. Psychodynamically, pain is associated with man's primitive organization as a moral being. In early life, pain becomes associated with discipline, and later the individual takes moral pride in suffering. Moral values are incorporated as conscience, which is associated with guilt feelings and frequently demands punishment as a means of maintaining psychic equilibrium.

Recent studies would suggest that the classic pain pathways are modified to the point that we can no longer think of a peripheral sensory end-organ with transmission of impulses through the spinothalamic tract to the thalamus and hence to the cortex, but must recognize modulating factors. In addition, in the brain stem, the oligosynaptic sensory pathways send collaterals to the reticular formation, which is composed of multiple synaptic relays. Hence, noxious impulses passing via the spinothalamic tract are projected into two major brain systems: (1) the spinothalamic fibers through the thalamus to the sensory cortex, and (2) into the reticular formation and then through the medial intralaminar thalamus and the limbic system. Melzack and Wall have proposed a concept of pain that is appealing because it explains certain pain phenomena as well as how emotions and other cerebral processes influence pain.[9,10] They theorize that pain is not due only to neural activity, which resides exclusively in the pain pathways, but, rather, is the result of activity of several interacting neural systems. In this system, the substantia gelatinosa functions as a gate control system that modulates the afferent patterns before they influence the central transmission (T) cells in the dorsal horn. The T cells activate neural mechanisms, which comprise the action system responsible for perception of a response to pain. The signal, which triggers the action system responsible for pain experience and response, occurs when the output of the T cells reaches or exceeds a critical level. This critical level of firing is determined by the afferent barrage that actually impinges on the T cells and has already undergone modulation by the substantia gelatinosa activity. This barrage, in turn, is determined by the relative balance of activity between large and small peripheral fibers. Multiple inputs from this system, both from the physical and psychologic standpoint, modulate the transmission and hence the pain perception. Hence, psychodynamic mechanisms brought about by fear, anxiety, apprehension, psychic disorders, cultural influence, strong beliefs, motivations, and other feeling states greatly influence pain.[3] Cultural patterns dictate how the individual should bear pain; in some societies toleration of pain without expression of suffering is required; in others, overt expression of suffering is encouraged. Conscious and unconscious motivations may either inhibit or aggravate pain, as can strong emotions and beliefs. Powerful descending inhibitory influences exerted on the dorsal horns of the spinal cord can affect the gate control system, so that the input may be modulated before it is transmitted to both the discriminative and motivational systems. The excitement of games or that of war appears to block pain. Thus, it becomes readily apparent that there is an established but less well understood anatomic basis for pain apart from that observed in the soma, and this aspect of pain may in fact be paramount as we investigate the causes of disability.

Up to this point, we have dealt largely with the psychosocial modulators of pain perception. Of equal importance are the psychophysiologic (psychosomatic) aspects of disease. Emotional reactions associated with pain can and frequently do cause alterations of body functions that can either aggravate existing pain or cause new pain through psychophysiologic mechanisms. One of the most common causes of low back pain is skeletal muscle spasm provoked by emotional problems. Its presence may then add to the individual's anxiety, thus increasing muscle tension and further intensifying the pain. Psychophysiologic mechanisms can also alter the function of the heart, gastrointestinal tract, and urinary and reproductive systems. Noxious impulses, regardless of the source, produce typical patterns of response. These include local tissue reactions, muscle spasm of both skeletal and smooth muscle, and glandular hyperactivity. Constant muscle spasm with its associated vasospasm produces hypoxemia and metabolite build-up that serves to stimulate sensory nerve endings and thus produces further stimulation through the classic pain pathways.[2] This in turn produces more anxiety, tension, and stress, and serves to set up a vicious cycle. Chronic stimulation serves to constantly bombard the nervous system to the point that normal functioning of the internuncial pool may be permanently damaged through loss of its integrating mechanism. Pain, per se, can thus be extended and perpetuated long after the original noxious stimulus has ceased or the lesion has healed.

Pain must also be understood as a behavioral response. For the most part, pain and pain-related events have been viewed from a disease model, which assumes that the symptoms of pain are responses from underlying organic stimuli. Although this assumption is undoubtedly true in a majority of instances, the response of the patient to these stimuli can in fact be part of a behavioral response. To understand this suggestion, it is necessary to look at pain from a learning model rather than a disease model. The disease model states there is a noxious stimulus. Therefore, to understand pain, it is necessary to identify the underlying pathologic condition, and hence to treat the cause rather than the symptoms and the pain. The alternate possibility is that of the learning model as it relates to pain behavior. This conceptual model is based on the principle of operant conditioning,[4,5] which notes that actions or responses by patients may be influenced by reinforcing consequences in the immediate environment. Thus, if some type of behavior in the individual is followed by what for him is a positive reinforcing experience, that behavior will be increased and may be maintained indefinitely. Conversely, when the behavior is followed by a negative reinforcement, this will tend to diminish or alter the response, and this will occur independently of what happens to the underlying disease. Hence, the pain behavior comes under the control of environmental consequences rather than underlying disease. This conceptual model is essential in the management of patients with chronic disease, but an understanding of it is most helpful in the prevention of prolonged disability, particularly when an organic complaint may be only a symptom of a greater social and psychologic disturbance. The physician must therefore make an assessment of the patient's problem based on both the organic or structural disability and the psychologic or social disability.

Psychologic and psychosomatic potentiation of a back disability is an important cause of disabling back pain. The psychologic aspects are active in *all* individuals, and any suggestion that one individual has solely organic problems while another has only psychologic problems is a grave mistake. The physician must sort out to which degree each is active in a given patient, recognizing that the role of the organic and psychologic or psychosomatic aspects may vary from time to time, but always as time passes the psychologic aspects will become increasingly prominent. The diagnosis of psychosomatic back pain or psychosocial perpetuation of back symptomatology should not be made as a rule-out diagnosis, but is a positive diagnosis that can and should be made with each patient at the initiation of treatment. Regardless of whether one views pain from the psychoanalytic approach (where pain is associated with danger, sympathy, punishment, guilt, or sexual feelings) or from the psychosomatic approach (where pain is associated with stress, tension, and muscle contracture with its associated build-up of metabolites producing a vicious cycle) or as a learned behavioral response, the diagnosis can generally be established quite clearly through history, physical examination, and simple psychologic testing.

DIAGNOSIS OF PSYCHOPHYSIOLOGIC ASPECTS OF PAIN

1. The patient will describe the pain in dramatic terms. Such descriptions as "as though a spear were jammed into my back" or "a bolt of lightning struck me and rendered me paralyzed" are early clues to the personality of the individual. The patient's pain will usually be continuous and not totally relieved by analgesics.

2. The chronicity of the complaint is helpful. A well-studied pain problem of greater than two years' duration is not likely to be explained by further physical investigations, assuming that the patient has undergone adequate study by several different competent specialists.

3. The past history reveals a surprising amount of violence, pain, or chronic disease in the family. In addition, it will be noted that the onset of symptoms coincides with a period of high life stress.[6-8] There is a positive correlation between life stress and injury or disease.

4. A systems review will uncover a multiplicity of complaints, in addition to the low back problem, indicating that many other systems are involved. Frequently, one complaint may be cured only to have a new one arise. Despite the multiple complaints, a denial mechanism is frequently operational, that is, the patient denies that problems other than a specific injury or illness could be contributing to the etiology of the disorder or failure to respond to treatment. This is seen in its characteristic form in a sickly wife who is

emphatic in stating that she has a perfect marriage and a wonderful, doting husband; or in the husband who, having always relied on physical prowess to assert his virility and as a means of making a living, reaches the stage where he recognizes consciously or subconsciously that he can no longer compete with his younger peers and utilizes the excuse of a major or, at times, minor injury for his failure to perform as effectively as he once could, rather than accepting the aging process.

5. Secondary gain factors are always operable. While financial gain is the easiest to quantitate, it is not the most frequent. Usually the patient's ability to manipulate the environment provides the maximum secondary gain. It often takes the form of a housewife who, unable to control her husband or dominate the children in health, finds that through disability she is able to obtain the companionship, love, and attention that she sought unsuccessfully as a healthy wife and mother. To the male, it frequently represents a way of obtaining love and attention through the family, while allowing alterations in employment status to avoid doing work that he has found distasteful.

6. Virtually all of the patients with chronic back disability on the basis of some functional overlay have a long history of avoidance patterns. Such individuals have attempted to avoid conflict and difficult situations in life through running away, and the back pain and disability problem usually come to the fore at a time when the individual finds he or she can no longer avoid the conflict or difficult situation.

7. Physical findings are usually inconsistent with the complaints, at least in degree. This is most commonly seen in the over-reaction to light touch or a stop-go (jerking reaction) to requests to flex or extend the spine or while conducting straight leg-raising examinations. The patient may also tolerate tests when distracted that cannot be tolerated when the patient is concentrating on what the examiner is doing.

8. Response to treatment such as nerve blocks or medications must be carefully assessed. Twenty to 30 per cent of patients with organic pain obtain the same degree of pain relief with a placebo as with a narcotic. It is, therefore, hazardous to make a diagnosis solely on the basis of a placebo response. While an evaluation of the patient under a low dose of short-acting barbiturate may be helpful in differentiating the true malingerer, it is not particularly useful in evaluating the average patient with organic pathology and a superimposed functional overlay.

9. Of the numerous psychologic tests available, the most helpful in evaluating back pain patients has been the Minnesota Multiphasic Personality Inventory (MMPI). This provides an inexpensive method of evaluating patients. To obtain maximal use, it should be utilized on all patients seen with nonresponsive back pain complaints. The MMPI in the hands of a skilled interpreter or when used in the form of a computer-based memory bank can help to identify the likelihood that the patient will over-respond to somatic sensations. Test scores can also indicate the likelihood of there being enough muscle tension to produce pain. Of equal importance is the ability of the MMPI to tell how depressed, anxious, worried, or disorganized the patient may be in the presence of the pain and associated disability.

TREATMENT

In planning a treatment program, it is essential to carefully assess what role is played by each component; i.e., the noxious stimuli, the underlying psychologic disability based on past experience and teaching, the psychosomatic aspects as shown by the high life stress index, and the degree to which the responses are behavioral or learned patterns. If the cause of disability is largely from the noxious stimuli and this can be removed, this is undoubtedly the treatment of choice. Too often, this in fact is not the case. When the physician has then turned to the psychiatrist, he has all too often been disappointed. While the psychiatrist is best able to handle deep-seated psychologic disease, the uncovering of this aspect of the patient's problem is oftentimes so threatening as to cause the patient to reject such treatment or actually be made worse by it. When successful, it is time-consuming and expensive.

The life stress index is easy to assess, and the treatment is to reduce these stresses to a tolerable range. While diagnosis is relatively easy, it is most difficult in many situations to alter the stress-producing factors, but every effort should be made to do so. The patient must understand how tension and anxiety created by his current life situation serve to aggravate his pain and increase his disability. To do so, the significance of the learned pain model should be recognized. In the simpler situations, a program can be provided subtly through the way the physician manages the patient and in the counseling he affords the patient and the patient's family. In the more difficult situations, treatment requires a complete understanding of the total problem of the disability, by the patient, his family, and at times loyal friends and the employer. It must be realized by all of the patient's contacts that if his expressions or demonstrations of discomfort are followed by attention even to the point of administering medication, it serves only to reinforce the response. A behavior plus a positive reinforcement (love and attention) produces an increase in that behavior. On the other hand, a behavioral response followed by negative or adverse reinforcers (deprivation of love and attention, insistence on completion of the task) will serve to decrease that behavior. All reinforcers are more effective when delivered immediately. The key to success of the program is selective attention by physicians, other medical personnel, and the family. This requires training, for it is easy to tune out complaints but difficult to provide attention as the positive reward.

The program is established around the following areas.

1. *Medication.* To manage medication in an operant conditioning program, it is essential to recognize that analgesics for the most part do not actually stop pain but alter the patient's response to it; hence, it does little good in the overall treatment program and can be habituating or addicting. The patient must continue his pain complaints in order to obtain medication and the associated attention that it brings. In an operant program it is essential to first identify by trial and error how much and what kind of medication is required to reasonably well control the patient's demand for medication over a typical 24-hour period. These medications are then produced in a liquid form in a taste-masking vehicle (such as cherry cough syrup). They are delivered to the patient on a fixed-time basis, rather than when the patient complains of pain or requests medication. The interval between dosage should be less than the period the patient typically waited for pain medication before asking. As the program progresses, the analgesic aspect of the medication is gradually reduced while the same dosage of the masking vehicle is continued until the patient is receiving only the vehicle. As the treatment program progresses, the patient usually asks first to omit the nighttime dosages, for which he is wakened, and then gradually withdraws from the vehicle altogether.

2. *Social reinforcement.* Having recognized that the patient's pain response is a signal to an unhappy environment, every effort is made to achieve as happy an environment as possible. After the basic urges to satisfy hunger and provide some shelter have been satisfied, the individual's greatest need is for love and attention. Every attempt possible is made to modify the environment so as to remove the causes of unhappiness and provide for the basic drives of the individual. All too often, the individual only receives attention when he is ill or complaining. It is necessary for the physician and all people who come in contact with the patient to be socially unresponsive to complaints of pain or discomfort, while lavishing attention when the patient is doing socially acceptable activities. This means providing rest, love, and attention when the individual is working or doing socially constructive activities, and withdrawing, rather than providing these for the individual, when he complains of pain.

3. *Increased activity schedule.* As part of the social reinforcement program as well as to meet the needs of every individual for physical activity, an active physical and social life is essential to increase the sense of well-being and decrease the necessity for pain behavior. When prescribing an exercise program, it is advantageous to avoid having the patient work to tolerance. Allow the patient to work just below this limit and award him for doing so with a rest period before complaints of pain. It is helpful to have the patient keep a chart or graph to show the increase (decrease) in daily activity. This is used to convince the patient he is improving but also provides a means for the family or medical staff to provide social reinforcement through praise of increased accomplishment. If exercise (work) produces pain behavior, which is followed by rest, medication, and attention, it only serves to reinforce that behavior. However, if work is limited, then followed by rest and attention, this will tend to reinforce the work activity.

4. *Physical treatments.* While dealing with the emotional aspects of pain, it is equally essential to treat the physical problems. This can be done in such a way as to reinforce the efforts being made in the social and psychologic spheres. Efforts should be made to reduce muscle spasm and improve the muscle blood flow. Heat, massage, local analgesic infiltration, or nerve blocks can all be used effectively to this end. It is essential, however, that these treatments should be prescribed on a time-schedule basis, not in response to the patient's complaints. When the patient is complaining, the treatments must be administered by a totally nonresponsive individual. When the patient is acting in a socially acceptable manner, the treatment period can be utilized for social reinforcement. These treatments should not be administered as the cure but merely to provide relief of symptoms, thus allowing the patient to increase his activities.

5. *Alteration of the environment.* Through the entire treatment program, it is essential to assist the patient in altering the environment, where it is possible to do so, and assist the patient through counseling and education as to what he can do to better cope with an unhappy situation. One of the greatest treatment hurdles to be overcome is found when the secondary-gain factors from the illness cannot be altered and are the overriding concern. This is particularly related to workmen's compensation or insurance programs, cases in which the individual is in fact not able to function effectively in his old wage-earning capacity and must rely on compensation for his own and family support. Until society recognizes that it is cheaper and better to provide such individuals with the necessities of life strictly because the individual is not able to perform as he once could, rather than making it contingent on his continued complaints and demonstrations of disability, this problem will remain the major hurdle to be overcome in rehabilitation of many back cripples.

References

1. Clawson D, Bonica J, Fordyce W: Management of chronic orthopedic pain problems. In The American Academy of Orthopedic Surgeons Instructional Course Lectures, Vol 21. St. Louis, CV Mosby, 1972, pp. 8–22.

2. Dorpat T, Holmes T: Mechanisms of skeletal muscle pain and fatigue. Arch Neurol Psychiat *74:*628, 1955.

3. Engel G: "Psychogenic" pain and the pain-prone patient. Amer J Med *26:*899, 1959.

4. Fordyce W: Operant conditioning as a treatment method in management of selected chronic pain problems. Northwest Med *69:*580, 1970.

5. Fordyce W, Fowler R, Lehmann J, DeLateur B: Some implications of learning in problems of chronic pain. J Chronic Dis *21:*179, 1968.

6. Holmes T: The Hazards of Change. (News Release) Time, p. 54, March 1, 1971.

7. Holmes T, Rahe R: The social readjustment rating scale. J Psychosomatic Res *11:*213-218, 1967.

8. Holmes T, Wolff H: Life situations, emotions, and back-aches. Psychomatic Med 14, No 1, Jan-Feb 1952.

9. Melzack R, Wall P: Pain mechanisms: a new theory. Science *150:*971, 1965.

10. Melzack R, Wall P: Psychophysiology of pain. Int Anesthesiol Clin *8:*3, 1970.

39

Cordotomy and Rhizotomy for Pain

N. ARUMUGASAMY

PAIN is subjective, and whereas there are considerable racial differences to pain tolerance, there is no doubt that its relief is sought by the most stoic. In these days of greater life expectancy and injury, aside from the implications of a more disconcerting era of pain and carcinomas, the eradication of pain has tested the ingenuity of many and continues to be the subject of ongoing interest in most neurosurgical centers. With a trend to establish pain clinics, a multidisciplinary attack has been brought to bear on this problem by oncologists, anaesthesiologists, neurologists, neurosurgeons, psychiatrists, and others. The myriad of analgesic drugs available today attests to the fruitless search for a possible therapy without addiction to our chronic pain sufferers. As such, the surgical relief of pain appears to be a rational approach to this problem for the present.

To this end, various neurosurgical procedures have been introduced since the first dorsal rhizotomy done by Abbe[1,2] in 1888 and the first thoracic cordotomy by Martin on the suggestion of Spiller[16] in 1911. Dorsal column electroanalgesia, mesencephalic tractotomy by stereotaxy, and the more recent, much-in-vogue, percutaneous cordotomy have contributed significantly to our understanding of pain, its pathways, and especially its neurophysiology. Be that as it may, the operations of rhizotomy and open cordotomy, which may be performed under direct vision with great precision, are not only simple enough to perform, but have stood the test of time.

The radiologic coordinates for the proper placement of the lesion and its precise sizing are difficult to follow in the relatively blind method of percutaneous cordotomy. Further, electrophysiologic correlates, with sufficient attention to impedance measurements, and knowledge of radio frequency equipment, with application of monofocal stimulation, require the presence of a competent team. The variability of anatomic substrates, notwithstanding individual and racial differences, have offset the advantages of advances in instrumentation in stereotaxic and percutaneous methods. Following an examination of 24 of 200 patients who underwent percutaneous cordotomy, in 85% of the patients the lesions were placed in the ventral quadrants of the spinal cord in an effort to interrupt the lateral spinothalamic pathway. There were also instances in which the lesions extended to the dorsal quadrant of the spinal cord.[10] The placement of lesions by current induces more reaction and edema than does a surgical incision. Consequently, a drop in the level of analgesia a few months postoperatively, resulting from recovery of the contused and edematous cord, is more common with lesions produced by current.

While not discounting the possibility of establishment of a new pathway for pain (e.g., the incorporation of the multisynaptic series of short internuncial neurons), even in open cordotomies, we believe that section of the cord must be carried deeply enough for satisfactory results, and agree with Jefferson that most failures result from superficial cuts.[5]

For the purposes of this chapter, therefore, we are going to confine ourselves to surgical procedures in which lesions are placed under direct vision and adequate control. We specifically will confine ourselves to operations on the spinal cord and its issuing nerves that have continued to show proven value in the management of our patients: rhizotomy, thoracic cordotomy, and high cervical cordotomy.

RHIZOTOMY

One of the primary functions of the posterior spinal root is the conduction of painful sensation to the central nervous system, hence posterior root section was the first surgical procedure proposed for the relief of intractable pain. At the suggestion of Dana, rhizotomy was performed by Abbe in 1888 for pain in an upper extremity. Almost simultaneously, a similar procedure was performed by WH Bennett on the advice of Sir Victor Horsley for the relief of pain in a lower extremity.

It is immediately apparent that posterior rhizotomy alters the perception of sensations other than pain, and this limits its application. Also to be considered is that the original pain may persist despite the presence of complete anesthesia in the principle distribution of the divided roots, suggesting that the irritation is central to the point of rhizotomy or that the mechanism of the pain is not understood.

One could reason that if the pain originated on a given nerve, division of the appropriate posterior root would afford relief. However, if the disease involves an area served by more than one root, division of 3 or 4 roots might be required; for pain involving an entire limb or more, the procedure is not feasible.

Retrogasserian trigeminal neurotomy and intracranial section of the glossopharyngeal nerve for pain are well-accepted procedures. We believe that the selective denervation of pain fibers by posterior spinal rhizotomy, especially at thoracic levels, is relatively simple to perform and carries with it little in the way of morbidity or mortality. It is to be preferred in selected cases, and should not be withheld as a simple and effective method of relieving upper abdominal and chest wall pain. Diagnostic blocks at thoracic levels, although of some use, are not a must and we do not employ them routinely.

In cases of pain in the lumbosacral areas, selective denervation can be difficult, and we generally do not employ posterior spinal rhizotomy for pain in these areas. The conus and its issuing nerves are far removed from their exit foramina, and rather extensive operations are required for proper identification of the roots. Short of electrical stimulation, which at best can only be poorly localizing from an observer's point of view at the time of operation, we believe a thoracic cordotomy would be more suited for the relief of such pain.

White, following an experience with 50 patients, reported good long-term results in 69% of his patients.[20] He attributed his failures to incomplete or inadequate sectioning of contiguous nerve roots above and below the level to be denervated. He showed that at least two roots had to be cut both above and below the level desired for adequate results. Ray, in 1943, recommended sectioning of at least three contiguous sensory nerves, especially when the pain was somewhat removed from the spine.[13] Interruption of radicular arterial supply to the cord and the possibility of regeneration were overcome when White and Sweet further advocated an intradural sectioning of these nerves.[17,20] Under these circumstances, the relief of pain, if good, was permanent.

More recent reviews on the subject of rhizotomy have, however, been less encouraging. The experiences of Loeser,[8] Echols,[4] and Onofrio[12] have documented a 40 to 50% failure rate on long-term follow-up of patients. Loeser, for instance, showed that of some 286 patients operated on for chest wall and abdominal pain between 1958 and 1969, only 33 to 50% experienced long-term relief. He agreed, however, that such rhizotomy should be the first line of treatment. Echols, after a 20-year experience, had a 40% failure rate. That he was dealing with patients who had undergone operations for chronic disc disease may have a bearing on his percentage of failures.

PROCEDURE. The procedure is done preferably with the patient in the prone position, although the lateral decubitus may also be used. After adequate separation of the muscles from the spine and laminae, roentgenograms are taken with one of the exposed spinous processes marked. The level having been confirmed, appropriate laminectomy is undertaken. The dura is then opened, and once this is done, it is quite simple to

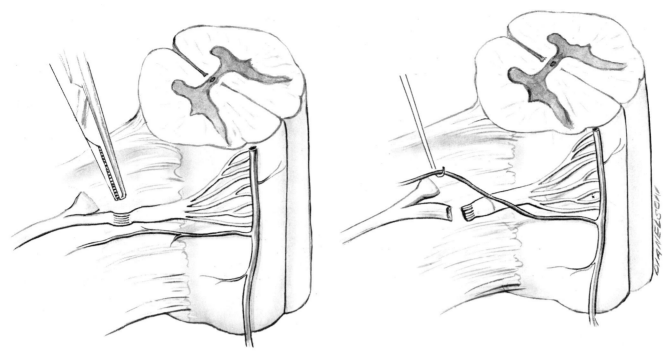

FIG. 39-1. Posterior rhizotomy. Posterior root is divided, and care is taken to spare segmental vessels.

follow the roots out to their exit foramina. Large radicular vessels, when present, are separated, and section of the nerve roots is undertaken between silver clips. This intradural section prevents any regeneration in the months to follow, and occurrence of infarction of the spinal cord is almost unknown with his procedure.

Adequate roots above and below the level being sectioned should be interrupted and the area carefully inspected for any remaining root filaments that may have escaped a cursory examination. We find that running a blunt hook alongside the cord at the level of sectioning serves as an adequate check on this possibility. The number of roots sacrificed is no doubt dependent on the type of pain being treated, and the proven overlap in innervation is a consideration. Following closure of the dura, the remainder of the incision is closed in layers.

THORACIC CORDOTOMY

Spiller is credited with having proposed section of the pain-mediating fibers in the anterolateral quadrant of the spinal cord. The incision into the cord may be made at several levels, the most common being in the upper thoracic segments. The pain-mediating fibers that enter the posterior roots cross to the opposite antero-lateral cord to form the lateral spinothalamic tract. The fibers of any given level reach the tract three to four segments higher than their point of entry. The tract is arranged in a laminated fashion, with the fibers of

caudal origin placed most superficially, and each subsequent layer of fibers representing higher levels placed more deeply.

Although it is generally realized that rhizotomy is preferred in individuals suffering from pain when a normal life can be expected, cordotomy has a real place in the treatment of patients with pain from carcinoma and other intractable varieties of pain. The possibility of paresthesias developing following cordotomies should in itself not be a deterrent to this procedure. When correctly performed, with a lesion of adequate size in the right place, it can be a gratifying procedure. Since individual variations in ascending fibers and variability in levels of crossing to the contralateral side occur, the lesions should be placed well above the level of analgesia preferred.

Although establishment of new pathways for pain, especially via the internuncial multisynaptic central core area and the ipsilateral tracts, is well known, misplacement of the lesion has also been responsible for a recurrence of the pain. The variability in the insertion of the dentate ligaments is sometimes responsible for the latter. By and large, failure in obtaining adequate effect is due to a small lesion when the incision into the cord is not carried sufficiently medially.[5] The dropping in the level of analgesia obtained with some recovery of a contused or edematous cord could also be a factor. Thus, when thoracic cordotomies are indicated, they should be done at high levels, preferably at T2 or T3.

The side to be sectioned will be opposite to that for pain relief. In operations at thoracic levels, bilateral

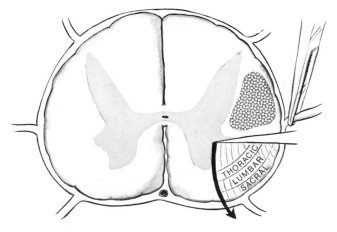

FIG. 39-2. Thoracic cordotomy. Note lamination of lateral spinothalamic tract. Lateral corticospinal tract, which must be avoided, is indicated by small circles.

cordotomies may be done at one sitting if desired, but we prefer to make one incision into the cord at least one segment lower than the first.

PROCEDURE. We perform the operation under general anesthesia with the patient in the prone position. When unilateral cordotomy is to be undertaken, the initial procedure is comparable to the one described for rhizotomy. Preliminary x-ray examination is not necessary, however. The dura is opened and care is taken to preserve the arachnoid and its contents of cerebrospinal fluid. Blunt separation of the nerve roots from the dentate ligaments is then undertaken. The dentate ligament is then divided close to its dural attachment. With traction on this ligament medially and toward the operator, it is possible to rotate the cord to get an excellent view of the anterolateral quadrant. An avascular zone of the cord is selected, and a section of the cord undertaken with a curved sharp blade. The blade is gently but deliberately plunged into the depths of the cord to almost the midline, and swept downward and outward to the level of the anterior root. Bleeding has not been a problem in our patients. Should this occur, it is generally in the form of a slight ooze that stops when a small cotton pledget is placed over the site. The operation is then terminated, and the incision closed in layers after adequate dural repair.

HIGH CERVICAL CORDOTOMY

Cervical cordotomy, when properly carried out, affords greater relief from painful conditions below the level of sectioning. It is superior to the procedures described heretofore for the relief of pain, but mortality and morbidity rates are higher than with thoracic cordotomy, especially when bilateral lesions are required.[11] The more medial and posterior placement of incoming pain fibers at cervical levels and the dorsal shift of the spinothalamic tract in the cervical cord are important considerations.[9] We agree with Kahn et al. that the section should be carried out just medial to the anterior root,[6,7] but have been compelled to place the lesion somewhat more dorsally than they did.

The results of open high cervical cordotomy are certainly equal to, and perhaps better than, those obtained by high cervical percutaneous cordotomy. Rosomoff noted complications of paresis, ataxia, sexual dysfunction, and respiratory difficulties when he performed bilateral high cervical cordotomies by the latter method.[14] Only 7 of 27 of his patients had complete relief of pain at the end of two years. In contrast, Schwartz records a 70% relief of pain in his series of 120 patients operated on by the open method.[15] His main reason for failures was an inadequate lesion. Thirty-four of his 45 survivors following bilateral open cordotomies had good relief of pain.

Because of the efficacy of high cervical cordotomy and the knowledge of a more dorsal disposition of sacral and lumbar segment pain fibers, this operation has been performed even in cases in which ordinarily a thoracic cordotomy would suffice. Further, pain in the gullet, arm, neck, and heart areas could not be expected to be relieved by thoracic cordotomies.

PROCEDURE. We perform this operation under general anesthesia, with the patient in the sitting position. An occasional patient complains of postoperative headaches from loss of cerebrospinal fluid at surgery, but this discomfort in itself is temporary and does not detract from the advantages of approach to the cervical area to be obtained with this position.

"Keyhole" surgery is not condoned. Cervical laminectomy is carried out from C1 to the upper border of C4. Every attempt is made to keep the arachnoid intact during incision of the dura. The dura is then anchored to the paraspinal muscles firmly. An avascular zone of cord between the C2 and C3 roots is selected. After division of the dentate ligament, medial and superior traction is applied on it toward the surgeon. This brings the anterolateral quadrant into view. Sectioning of the cord is identical to that performed at thoracic levels. However, the knife is usually directed some 20 degrees dorsal to the equator of the cord, toward the midline, and near the midline is swept to a point just medial to the anterior root. It is necessary to carry the incision significantly medialward, especially if pain is present at arm and cervical levels.

Should bilateral cordotomies be indicated, the operations are staged a week or so apart and done at least a segment or two lower than at the preceding operation. Bleeding from cord vessels has seldom posed a problem. It is usually quite self-limiting. Following hemostasis, and irrigation with saline, the dura is freed from the paraspinal muscles and closed. Apposition of the muscles is then concluded and the wound closed in layers.

References

1. Abbe R: Intradural section of the spinal nerves for neuralgia. Boston Med Surg J *135*:329-335, 1896.
2. Abbe R: Resection of the posterior roots of spinal nerves to relieve pain, pain reflex, athetosis and spastic paralysis —Dana's operation. Med Rec *79*:377-381, 1911.
3. Belmusto L, Brown E, Owens G: Clinical observations on respiratory and vasomotor disturbances as related to cervical cordotomies. J Neurosurg *20*:225-232, 1963.
4. Echols DH: Sensory rhizotomy following operation for ruptured intervertebral disc: A review of 62 cases. J Neurosurg *31*:335-338, 1969.
5. Jefferson G: The relief of pain. Lancet *2*:129-130, 1952.
6. Kahn EA, Peet MM: The technique of anterolateral cordotomy. J Neurosurg *5*:276-283, 1948.
7. Kahn EA, Rand RN: On the anatomy of anterolateral cordotomy. J Neurosurg *9*:611-619, 1952.
8. Loeser JD: Dorsal rhizotomy for the relief of chronic pain. J Neurosurg *36*:745-750, 1972.
9. Morin F, Schwartz HG, O'Leary JL: Experimental study of the spinothalamic and related tracts. Acta Psychiat Neurol Scandinav *26*:371-396, 1951.
10. Moossy J: The pathologist looks at cordotomy, (International Congress Series, No 193). Excerpta Medica, 1969, p. 28.
11. Ogle WS, French LA, Peyton WT: Experiences with high cervical cordotomy. J Neurosurg *13*:81-87, 1956.
12. Onofrio BM, Campa HK: Evaluation of rhizotomy: Review of 12 years experience. J Neurosurg *36*:751-755, 1972.
13. Ray BS: The management of intractable pain by posterior rhizotomy. Proc Ass Res Nerv Ment Dis *23*:391-407, 1943.
14. Rosomoff HL: Bilateral percutaneous cervical radiofrequency cordotomy. J Neurosurg *31*:41-46, 1969.
15. Schwartz HG: High cervical cordotomy, Clinical Neurosurgery. Vol 8. Baltimore, Williams and Wilkins and Company, 1962, pp. 282-290.
16. Spiller WS, Martin E: The treatment of persistent pain of organic origin in the lower part of the body by division of the anterolateral column of the spinal cord. JAMA *58*:1489-1490, 1912.
17. Sweet WH, White JC, Silverstone B, Nilges R: Sensory responses from anterior roots and from surface of interior of spinal cord in man. Trans Am Neurol Ass *75*:165-169, 1950.
18. Taren JA, Davis R, Crosby EC: Target physiologic corroboration in stereotaxic cervical cordotomy. J Neurosurg *30*:569-584, 1969.
19. Walker AE: The spinothalamic tract in man. Arch Neurol Psychiat *43*:284-298, 1940.
20. White JC, Sweet WH: Pain: Its Mechanisms and Neurosurgical Control. Springfield, Illinois, Charles C Thomas, 1955.

40

Percutaneous Cervical Cordotomy for Intractable Pain

RICHARD A. DAVIS

THE CLASSIC technique of spinothalamic cordotomy was pioneered in this country by Frazier and Spiller, while Foerster did the early operations in Europe. Although the risk of laminectomy is low in the patient with cancer, such a measure for pain relief often is not considered feasible for patients who have pulmonary or hepatic metastases and attendant nutritional problems. Therefore, there was real need for a "nonoperative" procedure to interrupt pain pathways. In 1963, Mullan reported the results of introducing a needle into the lateral spinal thalamic tract in the interlaminar space at C1-C2.[1] The first lesions were made with radioactive ytterium, but several years later, Rosomoff suggested the radiofrequency technique that is now used commonly.[4]

INDICATIONS

In the past it was customary to treat pain above the nipple line by posterior cervical rhizotomy, but percutaneous cervical cordotomy has changed this, because of the high dermatome levels that can be achieved. We now use the percutaneous technique for patients who have advanced malignant disease with bowel or bladder problems, and who probably would not return to work. It is our opinion that the motor and bowel-bladder difficulties after percutaneous cordotomy are too high to risk these untoward effects in patients who do not have preterminal disease. All other patients with intractable pain are treated by the classic open Spiller-Frazier cordotomy method, the complications of which are exceedingly rare. Frequently, we have done the open spinal cord procedure for unilateral pain, and three to six

404

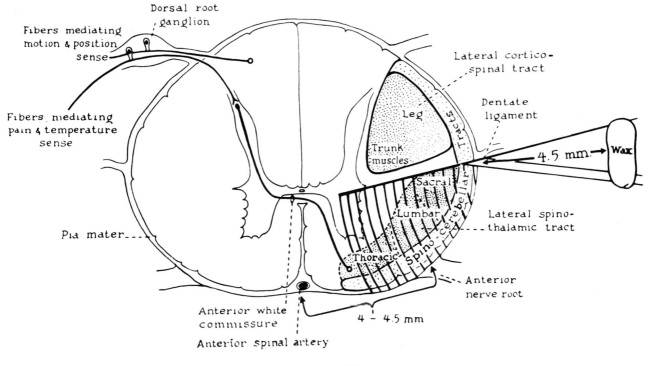

Thoracic II.

FIG. 40-1. Cross section of spinal cord with major sensory and motor pathways. (From Davis L Davis RA: Principles of Neurological Surgery. Philadelphia, WB Saunders Company, 1963.)

months later, when pain developed on the opposite side, a percutaneous lesion was made; this combination has been highly effective (Fig. 40-1).

TECHNIQUE

It is wise to have a profile of bleeding and clotting function in the cancer patient with pain who is to have a percutaneous cordotomy because of the possibilities of post-lesion edema and microscopic bleeding in and about the spinal cord. Many patients are unable to cooperate during the procedure because of extreme pain; therefore, heavy premedication is indicated which can be supplemented by short-acting narcotics given intravenously. We have felt that the anesthesia department should be present during the procedure to monitor the vital signs, to ensure an intravenous route, and to give narcotics or analgesics if needed. The patient is positioned supine with the head properly immobilized (Fig. 40-2). After the skin has been prepared below the mastoid process, it is infiltrated and a spinal needle is introduced under fluoroscopic control at the C1-C2 interlaminar space. After cerebrospinal fluid is obtained, the needle is immobilized in a carrier which can be advanced in the superior-inferior or anterior-posterior direction. A small

amount of Pantopaque is introduced to outline the dentate ligament, and the end of the needle must be superior to this point (Fig. 40-3). Once the dentate ligament is demonstrated, the active electrode is introduced through the spinal needle. The electrode is insulated except at the two ends, and the tip to be introduced into the spinal cord is approximately 2 mm. long. The position of the needle with its electrode is confirmed in the anterior-posterior direction under fluoroscopy and should not pass beyond the midpoint of the dens. Next, small bursts of radiofrequency current, 100 milliamps, are given at two- to three-second intervals and the sensory level to pain and temperature is determined. Impedance is of value to determine whether the electrode is in the cord substance; according to Ohm's Law, the effective milliamperage decreases rapidly with an increase in resistance, which is not evident when the electrode is bathed by cerebrospinal fluid. During the procedure, the hand and leg ipsilateral to the cordotomy are tested in terms of motor function, and if they become weak, the procedure should be discontinued. Generally, the sensory level can be carried to the desired dermatome, but often levels in the cervical region are obtained with radio-frequency current of short duration and less strength. After the sensory level is obtained, the needle is withdrawn and the patient is

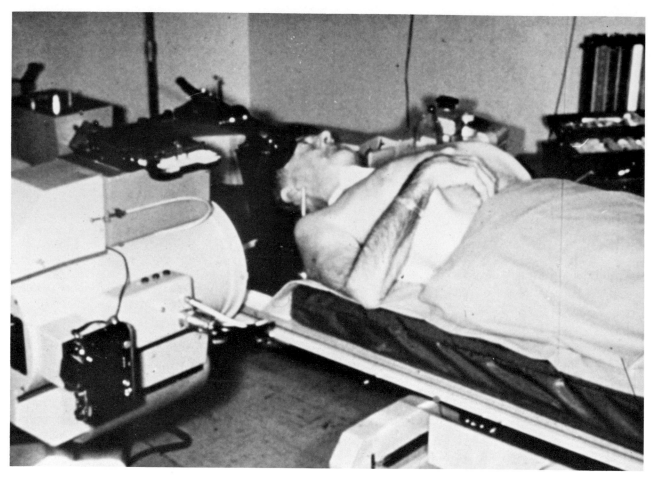

FIG. 40-2. Position of patient showing image-intensifier on left. Head and cervical spine are immobilized, but patient is otherwise free to cooperate.

observed in the recovery ward for a matter of two or three hours, particularly for any respiratory or further motor deficit.

COMPLICATIONS

The overall complication rate in over 100 percutaneous cervical cordotomies done at the Hospital of the University of Pennsylvania since 1966 has averaged approximately 25%. The most disturbing event has been the onset of motor weakness during the procedure, because the tip of the needle has impinged on the corticospinal tract, and this occurred in 10 patients. If recognized early and the procedure is terminated, they are usually reversible. There have been two deaths; one a so-called "sleep paralysis" in which the desired sensory level was obtained and the patient had no motor complications, but was found dead in bed, having been, apparently, perfectly fit only one-half hour before. Autopsy showed no cardiovascular or pulmonary com-

plications, and examination of the spinal cord revealed no extensive demyelinization or injury, but death twenty-four hours after the lesion was made probably would not show any histologic alteration in the cord. The second patient was not sent to the recovery ward and had a marked fall in blood pressure and was given vasopressors as an emergency measure, following which he had a coronary occlusion. Three cases complicated by meningitis have been treated successfully with antibiotics, and all patients had excellent recoveries. In approximately 20% of patients, the procedure had to be repeated because the sensory level could not be obtained with the first attempt. About 10% of patients have some bowel or bladder deficit after unilateral percutaneous cordotomy and require a catheter. This is usually a short-term problem, and with physical activity and the use of urecholine, the urinary retention is overcome before the patient leaves the hospital. We have performed seven bilateral percutaneous cervical cordotomies at staged intervals of six weeks to nine months. Fortunately, there have been no respiratory

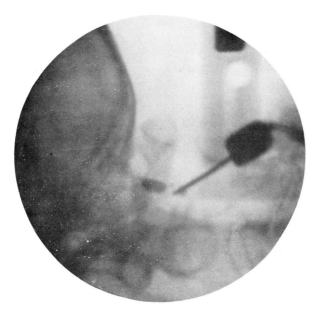

FIG. 40-3. Pantopaque is layered along dentate ligament, which is critical landmark in the performing of percutaneous cordotomy.

complications in these patients, and if both levels are kept below T1, there is no danger of diaphragmatic paralysis. The obvious hazards of doing a bilateral procedure at the same sitting, or before an adequate time period has elapsed, is evident and is comparable to making staged lesions in stereotaxic surgery of the basal ganglia.

RESULTS

Eighty per cent of patients experienced immediate relief of pain following percutaneous cervical cordotomy and could state this fact in the Radiology Department almost immediately after the lesion had been made. Reasons for unsatisfactory relief of pain were technical failure to make a cervical cord lesion, a level which was below the dermatome level of pain, and addiction to drugs. It can be said, therefore, that if the sensory loss to pain and temperature is adequate, the patient will have good pain relief in the great majority of cases. The problem of a falling sensory level was not a feature after percutaneous cervical cordotomy, and approximately 30% had levels which actually ascended several dermatomes. White has pointed out in a series of 50 upper thoracic cordotomies for pain of benign origin that half of the patients at the end of the year had inadequate pain relief, and that the cause of this was inadequate sensory levels.[5] Only six of our patients

have had percutaneous cordotomies performed for nonmalignant disease and have been followed for a period of more than three years. Two of these patients, unfortunately, have paresthesias which are extraordinarily annoying in the cervical dermatomes homolateral to the lesion, but all six have maintained a high sensory level which had not fallen over this period of time.

Approximately 10% of the patients in our series with percutaneous cervical cordotomies have had transient difficulty with bowel and bladder function. They have required a catheter for short periods of time, and then bladder function has recovered with the use of parasympathomimetic agents before hospital discharge. Bowel training has been more easily regulated. It was interesting that in the seven patients with bilateral percutaneous cordotomies, which were performed at staged intervals, none had bowel or bladder dysfunction. Approximately 10% of patients developed one or more paretic limbs, homolateral to the lesion, and half of these promptly recovered with physical therapy and training.

It is probable that the radiofrequency lesion more completely destroys the laminated fibers in the lateral spinothalamic tract, whereas with the usual surgical cordotomy, often the more medial fibers of the thoracic dermatomes are contused and only partially demyelinated by the knife or hook which is used. This undoubtedly accounts for the falling level which has been observed after the classic surgical cordotomy.

One of the most challenging present problems of percutaneous cordotomy is the respiratory paralysis that may result; fortunately, this is not a frequent complication, and as stated, we have not seen this in any of our bilateral percutaneous lesions, but only once following a unilateral cordotomy. Nathan has pointed out that the fibers of the descending respiratory tract in man probably lie in the most anterior part of the lateral column of the upper cervical cord, and that these fibers may form a part of the reticulospinal tract or that they may run with the olivospinal tract.[3] It is most probable that the respiratory paralysis seen after high percutaneous cervical cordotomy results from extension of the lesion into the anterior and medial part of the lateral columns. Most of the reported respiratory deaths have occurred during sleep when the patient "forgets to breathe," and most certainly some of the information carried by the reticulopetal system in this region is not reaching the upper midbrain and thalamus. Mullan et al., in a series of over 400 high cervical percutaneous cordotomies, stated that in addition to the danger of bilateral lesions that encroach upon the anterior quadrants of the upper cervical cord, patients with unilateral lesions and pre-existing pulmonary function are also likely to have respiratory paralysis.[2] It should be emphasized that these respiratory hazards of high cervical cordotomy are infrequent, and only nine patients in Mullan's series had this complication.

The development of the technique of percutaneous cervical cordotomy has added flexibility and ease to the relief of intractable pain in patients with advanced cancer. In the debilitated and preterminal state, the criteria for cordotomy have been vastly broadened, so that pain relief should be available to any patient in the modern clinic. Approximately 80% of all patients with intractable pain should be relieved by percutaneous cervical cordotomy; the chief hazard is respiratory paralysis which has an incidence of less than 1%. Approximately 25% of patients have some weakness of an extremity or difficulty with bowel or bladder function, both of which complications are reversible.

References

1. Mullan S et al: Percutaneous interruption of spinal pain tracts by means of a Strontium needle. J Neurosurg *20:*931-939, 1063.
2. Mullan S, Hosobuchi Y: Respiratory hazards of high cervical percutaneous cordotomy. J Neurosurg *28:*291-297, 1968.
3. Nathan PW, Smith MC: Long descending tracts in man. 1. Review of present knowledge. Brain *78:*248, 1955.
4. Rosomoff HL et al: Modern pain relief: percutaneous cordotomy. JAMA *196:*482-486, 1966.
5. White JC, Sweet WH: Pain and the Neurosurgeon: A Forty-Year Experience. Springfield, Charles C Thomas, 1969.

41

Spinal Implants for Relief of Pain

SANFORD J. LARSON

THE APPLICATION of electrical currents to the spinal cord through electrodes chronically implanted over the dorsal columns has been followed by relief of pain in a substantial number of patients.[2,3] The dorsal columns were initially selected as the site for the electrodes on the basis of the gate theory proposed by Melzak and Wall.[1] Activation of dorsal column axons may or may not be the explanation for relief of pain following application of current; nevertheless the method works. Certainly it is much simpler to implant electrodes over the dorsal columns than, for example, anterior to the spinal cord. However, when pain is located in the perineum and lower limbs, our patients have reported greater relief of pain when currents are applied through electrodes placed anterior to the spinal cord. Implantable units are manufactured by several companies. Although these units differ with respect to electrode configuration, they have certain features in common. Each is of unitary construction with a small subcutaneous receiver connected by cable to the electrode set. The currents are transmitted through the skin, picked up by a passive receiver implanted subcutaneously, and delivered to the cord. As the level of applied current is increased, the patient notices paresthesias below the level at which the electrodes were placed. Some patients have developed a sensory level with ankle clonus, increased deep reflexes, and pathologic reflexes. These findings have always disappeared after the currents were shut off. When currents are applied through the anterior electrodes paresthesias are not experienced, although perception of pain is diminished.

The surgical technique for implantation is not complicated. Since the electrode sets are relatively small, an extensive laminectomy is not required. For example, if it is desired to place the implant at the T7–T8 level, it is only necessary to remove the inferior portion of the spinous process and lamina of

T7 and superior portion of T8. The laminectomy need only be wide enough to admit the electrodes. A midline dural incision is made, and if possible, the arachnoid is not penetrated. Next a small incision is made either in the flank or over the anterolateral aspect of the chest wall, and a subcutaneous pocket created for the receiver. A gently curved, blunted Steinmann pin with a transverse drill hole near the tip is passed from the laminectomy incision to the incision in the flank or chest. The electrode set is placed in a small plastic or metal capsule in which a small hole has also been drilled transversely near the tip. The capsule and pin are connected with heavy wire suture material, and the capsule is then drawn into the laminectomy incision.

After removal from the capsule, the electrode set is implanted in the subdural space. The method of fixation to the dura depends on the type of unit to be implanted. For implants on the dorsal columns we use a set of 5 in-line platinum iridium disc electrodes embedded in a thin sheet of silastic, 20 mm. long by 6 mm. wide. A silastic keel is attached to the sheet on the side opposite the electrodes. The leads from each electrode are gathered together in a central cable that leaves the implant at a 45-degree angle. The keel serves to support the central electrode and also to facilitate fixation of the unit to the dura. Horizontal mattress sutures placed through the keel near its base above and below the cable provide snug approximation of the dura to the electrode set. For the anterior implant we use the 5 in-line electrode array but without a keel. The cable is incorporated in the silastic sheet in which the electrodes are embedded, and is oriented at right angles to the electrode array. The implant is autoclaved around a test tube 1 cm. in diameter to provide approximate conformity to the contour of the spinal cord. A wide laminectomy is necessary, with exposure of the nerve root sheaths bilaterally above and below the level of implant. A parasagittal dural incision is made on the left side of the spinal canal without opening the arachnoid. The dentate ligament is divided at its point of attachment to the dura, and the arachnoid is separated from the dura anterior to the spinal cord. On the left side two roots are divided, one above and the other below the level of implant. This can be done between extradural ligatures if the radicular arteries are small, or intradurally. Two roots are also divided on the right between extradural ligatures. If desired, an examination of the radicular vessels may be made through a dural incision over the preganglionic portion of the root prior to ligation and division.

The two-level rhizotomy is necessary because the amount of current that can be applied through the electrodes may otherwise be limited by the development of muscle contractions induced by electrical stim-

ulation of these roots. The dentate ligament is grasped, the cord slightly rotated, and the electrode set slipped anterior to the cord sufficiently far to place the electrode sets in the midsagittal plane. The distance to which the electrode sets are introduced is determined by a preliminary measurement of the spinal cord. The location of the electrode set is then checked by an anteroposterior x-ray film. If the electrode position is satisfactory, the set is fixed to the dura by horizontal mattress sutures above and below the central cable. After the muscle and fascia have been closed over the laminectomy, a relaxing loop of cable is placed subcutaneously and the skin closed. A similar procedure is followed for closure of the other wound. It is possible to begin transcutaneous transmission of current to the receiver within a few days following operation. Occasionally, if the arachnoid has been penetrated, cerebrospinal fluid will collect along the cable and about the receiver. This situation can be corrected by making short incisions under local anesthesia over the cable and parallel to it. Circumferential sutures are placed in the soft tissue around the cable and tied down to occlude the passageway for cerebrospinal fluid.

More recently we have used an implant in which electrode sets are placed anterior and posterior to the spinal cord, as previously described, but with the posterior electrodes connected to the positive pole of the receiving unit and the anterior electrodes to the negative pole. This type of unit has been used for control of pain in the upper limbs secondary to carcinoma of the lung. The posterior unit is placed at C2 and the anterior unit at about C3. In the cervical area, only one root and the corresponding dentate ligament need be divided for placement of the anterior electrode set. With application of current these patients have developed a dissociated sensory loss, usually extending from C2 to approximately T8 or 10. The relief of pain and the dissociated sensory loss have persisted for as long as several hours after cessation of current.

The procedure for spinal implant is not lengthy, entails minimal blood loss and tissue trauma, and if necessary, could be performed under local anesthesia. The method appears to hold considerable promise for relief of pain in those patients who would otherwise require a cordotomy.

References

1. Melzack R, Wall PD: Pain mechanisms: a new theory. Science *150*:971-979, 1965.
2. Nashold BS Jr, Friedman H: Dorsal column stimulation for control of pain. J Neurosurg *36*:590-597, 1972.
3. Shealy CN, Mortimer JT, Hagfors NR: Dorsal column electroanalgesia. J Neurosurg *32*:560-564, 1970.

Section XI

Special Categories

42

Neurosurgical Management of Spastic Conditions

EDIR B. SIQUEIRA

SPASTICITY

SPASTICITY resulting from lesions of the spinal cord is a complex syndrome which presents a characteristic picture regardless of its cause. Typically, violent contractures of the abdominal and psoas muscles are suddenly followed by simultaneous flexion of the hips and knees and adduction of the thighs. Finally, dorsiflexion of the feet occurs, accompanied by extension of the great toes and fanning of the other toes. After the initial contraction phase, the muscles relax partially, and after several weaker contractions, the extremities return to incomplete extension. Autonomic discharges with emptying of the bladder and bowel, pilo-erection, and sweating frequently accompany the muscular contractions (the pilo-erection and sweating being limited to areas of anesthesia).

Spinal lesions implicated in the etiology of spasticity include trauma, neoplasms, vascular abnormalities, and degenerative diseases, trauma being the most common. If recognized and treated early, some neoplasms of the spinal cord need not lead to spasticity. Primary vascular abnormalities such as arteriovenous malformations and arteriosclerotic occlusive disease are quite rare. By contrast, degenerative diseases such as multiple sclerosis are common and spasticity becomes a prominent feature in the course of the illness.

Isolation of the distal segment of the spinal cord from the controlling mechanism located in higher centers of the central nervous system results in spasticity.[8] Though the spasticity itself is not harmful, in the neglected patient pressure sores and urinary tract infections are sources for continuous irritation, causing reflex spastic contractures of the extremities. In turn, the spasticity may aggravate the pressure sores and urinary tract infections and interfere with medical management. On the other hand, under certain

413

circumstances spasticity can be used positively in the emptying of the urinary bladder and in the rehabilitation of paraplegics.

Cleanliness, dietary regulation, and careful attention to all details of the patient's life are of the utmost necessity, since neglect of these precautionary measures may predispose to breakdown of skin, formation of kidney and bladder calculi, fistulas in the urethra and distal alimentary tract, and urinary tract infections, all of which contribute to the appearance of flexion spasms. Nonetheless, severe spasms may occur despite scrupulous care of the patient, and should pressure sores develop, spasticity may interfere with their treatment.

The treatment of a patient with spasticity should begin with pharmacotherapeutics, such as diazepam (Valium). This has been extensively investigated by Nathan and co-workers.[1,3,15] Unfortunately, drugs are ineffective in the treatment of severe spasm and may sedate a patient too heavily if given in dosage sufficient to decrease or abolish the spasms.

Local blocks may be employed if the most disabling spasticity is confined to a small group of muscles. For instance, obturator neurectomy is indicated in some patients with adductor spasms, and its simplicity allows it to be employed even in a severely debilitated patient. Properly chosen tenotomies are another useful alternative. Destruction of nerves supplying a specific muscle group by peripheral phenol block requires specialized equipment, techniques, and training, but it may be helpful in the treatment of a limited spastic condition.[9]

With failure of pharmacotherapeutics and local blockade techniques, more destructive procedures are required. Naturally, both patient and surgeon are reluctant to utilize procedures that preclude neurologic recovery. Unfortunately, the assessment of potential for neurologic recovery is difficult, since neurologic recovery has been noted in some patients with severe flexor spasms. We know of no patient, however, who has made useful functional recovery after developing marked spasticity. The final decision to eliminate spasticity must be made with participation from the patient, and special care should be taken to explain to him that while spasmotic pain and subjective sensations not directly related to spasticity will not be alleviated, elimination of spasticity will prepare him for opportunities for rehabilitation.

Subarachnoid injection of 95% aqueous solution of alcohol[4,18] or of phenol[10,16] may be used to achieve a chemical rhizotomy. Shortly after the injection the patient is relieved of spasticity, and this relief persists for at least several months and is frequently permanent.

ALCOHOL-MEDIATED RHIZOTOMY. Since the 95% aqueous alcohol solution is less dense than cerebrospinal fluid, the foot of the bed must be elevated after lumbar puncture has been performed in order to prevent the cephalad migration of alcohol to a dangerous level.

Seven to 12 ml. of alcoholic solution is slowly injected (not more than 1 ml. per minute) until testing reveals that either spasticity has subsided or the sensory level has risen above its previous position. The foot of the bed should be kept elevated for 24 hours.

PHENOL-MEDIATED RHIZOTOMY. Lowrie and Vanasupa demonstrated that a solution of 1.5 phenol:Pantopaque provided permanent or prolonged relief, while lesser concentrations of phenol were inadequate.[10] As suggested by Ruge, 1.25 g. phenol mixed with 5 ml. Pantopaque (larger quantities of phenol may elicit a febrile reaction) should be introduced into the subarachnoid space under fluoroscopic control while the patient is in a lateral position.[16] The phenol Pantopaque solution is directed to a level as high as T10 bathing all the spinal roots from that level caudalward (Fig. 42-1), and since it is of higher density than cerebrospinal fluid, it will accumulate on the dependent side and effect a unilateral rhizotomy. After the phenol Pantopaque material has been injected, the patient should be kept in lateral decubitus position for six hours, after which time, if desirable, the Pantopaque can be removed.

Adhesions from any cause may render alcohol or phenol injection impossible. In these instances, as well as when chemical rhizotomy fails to provide prolonged relief from spasticity, an open surgical approach is indicated. Föerster advocated posterior rhizotomy to alleviate spasticity.[5] Tarlow has reviewed the failures of posterior rhizotomies and has reported on two patients whose spasticity remained after appropriate posterior rhizotomy.[19] He concluded that an apparently complete deafferentation may actually be incomplete because afferent impulses from intact neighboring posterior roots may spread along axonal branches to motoneurons in segments deprived of sensory innervation. Alternatively, he suggests that hypertonus may result from spontaneous discharge of motoneurons.

In lieu of posterior rhizotomy, anterior rhizotomy from T10 to S1 has been advocated for relief from severe flexor spasms.[6,7,12,14] Munro states that the anatomic key to localization of nerve roots is the relationship of the first lumbar roots to the last dentate ligament. After removing the laminae of T11 and T12 and opening the dura mater, one should see the conus and the origin of the cauda equina. If these are below the exposure, one removes L1; if above, T10. With this exposure and proper identification of the L1 nerve roots, Munro believes one can identify the anterior nerve roots from T10 to S1.

A more radical procedure devised by MacCarty is selective cordectomy.[11] In high thoracic injuries, he recommends leaving an isolated segment of spinal cord to maintain the reflex tone of the abdomen to aid bladder and bowel evacuation. In low thoracic injuries, he removes the lumbar and sacral portions of the cord. In both instances removal includes the conus.

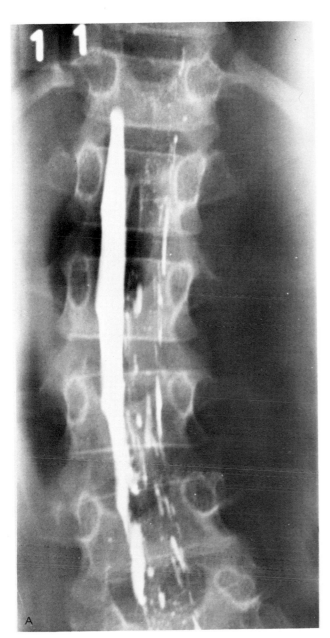 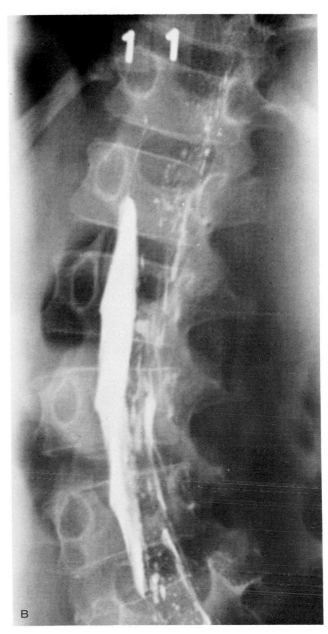

FIG. 42-1. The Pantopaque and phenol mixture is visualized radiographically as it bathes nerve roots in the vertebral canal at the level of T10 during a chemical rhizotomy. Right and left lateral decubitus positions are shown.

Longitudinal myelotomy (Yamada, Perot and Ducker 1972) has also been advocated for the control of mass spasms.

A level of T10 should be achieved in order to eliminate spasms and contractures of the psoas muscles. This is best achieved by an anterior or total rhizotomy distal to T10 or a cordectomy that detaches the cauda equina from the conus medullaris and produces a permanent lower motor neuron lesion. The exact consequence on bladder function is unknown, but it is generally believed that lower motor neuron lesions create fewer bladder complications than do upper motor neuron lesions.

SPASMOTIC TORTICOLLIS

A brief discussion of this condition is undertaken here, not only because of its similarity to spasticity, but also because its treatment may include laminectomy.

In spasmodic torticollis there are recurrent contractions of the cervical muscles, causing an abnormal posture of the neck, which may lead to contracture of the involved muscles, causing continuous torsion of the neck.

The differential diagnosis includes emotional disturbances, fracture-dislocations of the cervical spine, herniation of a cervical intervertebral disc, osteomyelitis of the cervical spine, tumors of the spine or of the spinal cord, and disease of the muscles themselves.

Etiologically, torticollis is probably a "local form" of dystonia. In some instances, it represents the initial stage of dystonia, which eventually will involve the upper extremities and the trunk. Spasmodic torticollis may also be a sequela of epidemic encephalitis.

Spasmodic torticollis is most commonly seen in young and middle-aged women. Usually the sternocleidomastoid muscle is initially involved and continues to be the muscle most severely affected in the late states of the disease. As the sternocleidomastoid muscle contracts, it pulls the head over to one side and rotates the chin in a spasmodic intermittent manner. The other muscles involved include the posterior and lateral neck muscles, as well as the upper portion of the trapezius.

The severity of spasmodic torticollis varies from patient to patient. In the same patient it worsens with emotion, observation, and fatigue, but disappears during sleep.

The treatment of spasmodic torticollis depends on its severity. In mild cases no treatment is indicated. Probably the use of a "tranquilizing" drug, such as diazepam, might be helpful in such patients.

In the severe and disabling cases of spasmodic torticollis, surgical intervention is indicated. Unfortunately, stereotaxic surgery (such as destruction of the ventrolateral nucleus of the thalmus) ordinarily gives only temporary relief.

In severe cases probably the most effective surgical therapeutic approach consists of the technique described by McKenzie.[13] He advocated section of the intraspinal portion of the spinal accessory nerves and of the upper three or four anterior roots of the cervical spinal cord. The operation has to be done bilaterally and is carried out through an upper cervical laminectomy. It is important that the first cervical anterior root be sectioned. This root is often hidden by the first dentate ligament, and success of the operation requires that it be identified and sectioned.

References

1. Cook JB, Nathan PW: On the site of action of diazepam in spasticity in man. J Neurol Sci 5:33-37, 1967.
2. Dimitrijevic MR, Nathan PW: Studies of spasticity in men. I. Some features of spasticity. Brain 90:1-30, 1967.
3. Dimitrijevic MR, Nathan PW: Studies of spasticity in men. II. Analysis of stretch reflexes in spasticity. Brain 90:333-358, 1967.
4. Dogliotti AM: Traitement des syndromes douloureaux de la peripheric par l'alcoholisation subarachnoidienne des racines posterieures a leur emergence. Presse Med 39:1249-1252, 1931.
5. Föerster O: Uber eine neue operative methode der behandlung spasticher lähmungen mittels resektion hinterer rüchenmarkswurzen. Z Orthopadische Chirurgie 22:203-223, 1908.
6. Freeman LW, Heimburger RF: The surgical relief of spasticity in paraplegia patients. I. Anterior rhizotomy. J Neurosurg 4:435-443, 1947.
7. Freeman LW, Heimburger RF: The surgical relief of spasticity in paraplegic patients. II. Peripheral nerve section, posterior rhizotomy and other procedures. J Neurosurg 5:556-561, 1948.
8. Heimburger RF: Spasticity resulting from trauma. In Neurological Surgery of Trauma. Edited by JB Coates and AM Meirowsky. Washington, Office of the Surgeon General, Department of the Army, U.S. Army Medical Service, 1965.
9. Khalili AA, Betts HB: Management of spasticity with phenol nerve block. Dept. of Health, Education and Welfare publication, 1970.
10. Lowrie H, Vanasupa P: Comments on the use of intraspinal phenol-Pantopaque for relief of pain spasticity. J Neurosurg 20:60-63, 1963.
11. MacCarty CS: The treatment of spastic paraplegia by selective spinal cordectomy. J Neurosurg 11:539-545, 1954.
12. MacDonald IB, McKenzie KG, Botterell EH: Anterior rhizotomy. The accurate identification of motor roots the lower end of the spinal cord. J Neurosurg 3:421-425, 1946.
13. McKenzie KJ: Intrameningeal division of the spinal accessory and roots of the upper cervical nerves for the treatment of spasmodic torticollis. Surg Gynec Obstet 39:5-10, 1924.
14. Munro D: Rehabilitation of patients totally paralyzed below the waist, with special reference to making them ambulatory and capable of earning their living. I. Anterior rhizotomy for spastic paraplegia. New Eng J Med 233:453-461, 1945.
15. Nathan PW: Spasticity and its amelioration. In Modern Trends in Neurology. Edited by D Williams. Vol 5, New York, Hoeber, 1970.
16. Ruge D: Spasticity in spinal cord injuries. In Spinal Cord Injuries. Edited by D Ruge. Springfield, Charles C Thomas, 1969.
17. Poppen JL, Martinez-Niochet A: Spasmodic torticollis. Surg Clin N Amer 31:883-890, 1951.
18. Sheldon CH, Bors E: Subarachnoid alcohol block in paraplegia. Its beneficial effect on mass reflexes and bladder dysfunction. J Neurosurg 5:385-391, 1948.
19. Tarlow IM: Deafferentation to relieve spasticity or rigidity: reasons for failure in some cases of paraplegia. J Neurosurg 25:270-274, 1966.
20. Yamada S, Perot PL, Ducker TB: Longitudinal myelotomy for control of mass spasms. Personal communication, 1972.

43

Biomechanics of the Spine and Orthoses

ROBERT D. KEAGY

MOST DISEASE or injury of the spine can be treated while the patient is ambulatory and performing many of his usual daily living activities. Treatment is most successful if the biomechanical import of daily living activities is considered. These physical requirements involve both what a patient does and how he does it. An orthosis is a force system which can effect how a patient performs, but it is only part of the guidance that a patient needs.

CERVICAL SPINE

Control of motion, position, and internal forces is most critical in the neck.

Biomechanics of the Cervical Spine

The cervical muscles position the head in relation to the cervical spine, while the cervicodorsal muscles position the head in relation to the thorax. Cervicodorsal, lumbosacral, and hip muscles determine the relationship of the head-chest axis to the vertical. When the head is balanced vertically over the thorax, the muscles of the neck are relatively silent, but tilting the head up or down requires muscle activity and increases loadings on the spine. On the other hand, if the head is forward of the thorax, as may occur with (1) neck flexion, (2) sitting without a backrest, or (3) leaning forward at the hips, muscles throughout the spine must act, because gravitational balance does not exist.

Head forward postures are frequent and occur, for instance, as we drink soup, bend over the work bench, or strain to read a book lying on a flat desk.

Intense interest, concern, depression, or pain are all portrayed in "body language" by combinations of forward body tilt or slump with the head forward of the thorax. If emotional tensions are added, the scapulae rise on the thorax. If these postures persist for several hours, pain will be felt over the dorsal paraspinal muscles, in the neck, or at the muscular insertions at the skull, and suboccipital headache with referral down the arm may ensure.

Commonly right-handed patients lean slightly to the right, using their left hand to position an object on which they may be working, and this combination of postural imbalance plus isometric muscle contraction in the left shoulder girdle probably accounts for the pain experienced along the medial border of the left scapula.

CERVICAL COLLARS. Cervical collars reduce neck motion and control the distance of the chin or occiput from the chest (without regard for any specific part of the chest). Sizable displacements of the head on the thorax are possible with ordinary collars, although the patient ordinarily settles on a restricted range of head position. However, if the patient leans forward or slumps, the major muscle forces are not reduced and the neck muscles are working under even greater isometric conditions, resulting in aggravation of the self-propagating postural pain syndrome. If the chin is held up too high for the patient to look downward, he is forced to tilt at the hips to see his work.

CERVICAL BRACES. Gross instability of the cervical spine is best managed with the patient horizontal and in traction, or in the "halo" type of device. If the spine is not intrinsically stable or if stringent control of head-thorax position is desired, then a brace of the type shown in Figure 43-1 is indicated. Special care is required to make the occipital piece comfortable if the patient is to sleep in this brace.

Ambulatory Management

Since the major forces on the neck occur during the transitional functions of getting up, lying down, or bending over, but do not occur when the head is vertically balanced or when the patient is supine, head balance is the key to ambulatory treatment for most patients. "Military" posture is not needed, but rather the patient must stand, walk, and work in a vertically balanced manner, so that the head is over the thorax, the thorax over the pelvis, and the pelvis over the feet. Work must also be positioned at a height allowing comfortable hand placement and easy vision, so that the head does not hang forward continuously. One can and should bend, reach, or turn, but none of these postures should be persistent. When sitting the patient must have a comfortable backrest against which to relax, for without a backrest he will soon slump, resulting in forward head displacement. Thus "neck" patients should never eat meals while sitting on the edge of their beds, and paper work and books should be tilted up (e.g., tilted drawing tables or propped up spiral transcription pads). In addition, a table or desk should

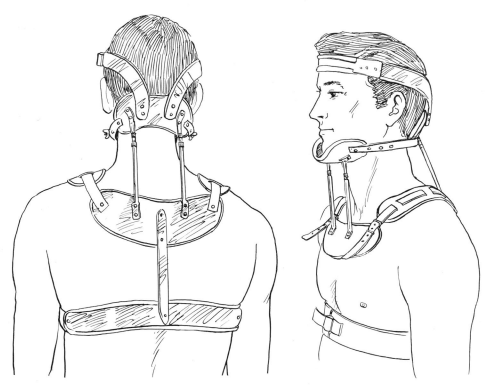

FIG. 43-1. Cervical brace.

permit one to get his feet and knees under it, so that he is not required to lean forward. The aching neck should be kept warm and protected from drafts, since the response to chilling is to tighten the muscles, elevate the shoulders, and thrust the head forward.

THORACIC AND LUMBAR SPINE

Biomechanics of the Thoracic and Lumbar Spine

The spine is a semi-flexible rod subjected to bending, twisting, shearing, and axial compressive loading forces, which are least when the spine is horizontal and fully supported along its length. Consequently a comfortable firm bed or reclining backrest may be the optimal orthosis, especially in patients with disc space infections or unstable spinal fractures, which will heal only when spared mechanical stress.

In balanced vertical posture, the normal spine can support the superimposed weight of the head, arms, and trunk with very little activity required of the trunk or spinal muscles, and the electromyogram is relatively silent (Fig. 43-2). The observed activity is related to prompt corrections which maintain the balanced position. As soon as the distribution of the suspended weight changes to an unbalanced position, gravity makes the spine bend, as may occur when an arm reaches forward or when the hip flexors tilt the pelvis and spine forward. Muscular activity controlling spinal flexion appears as soon as the load on the spine is off vertical balance (Fig. 43-3), and increases the axial loadings on the vertebrae and discs to levels greatly exceeding those that exist during quiet standing in a balanced "EMG silent" position. These high-pressure, nonbalanced positions are the transitional positions required to change from the lying to sitting or standing positions.

Between vertical balance and the fully bent position, there are an infinite number of unbalanced transitional positions that require muscular control. Persistence in an unbalanced posture requires continuous isometric contractions of muscle, which may interfere with circulation within the muscle owing to the unremitting increase in internal pressure. This persistent deficiency of the blood supply may result in muscular inflammation and pain. Since variations in muscle contraction during normal motion permit adequate blood flow, this muscle pain may be prevented by frequent change in position, avoidance of prolonged postural imbalance, or partial support of one's weight with the arms.

When the spine is flexed to the limit, motion is controlled by the ligaments, and the muscles can be relaxed. For the thoracic and lumbar spine, this occurs in the fully bent-over "rice planter" or "rag doll" position and in the relaxed or "slumped" sitting position. High loadings occur in these end-point or slumped

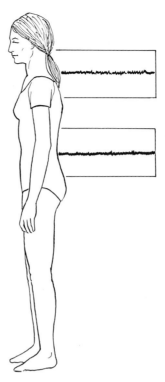

FIG. 43-2. In balanced vertical posture electromyogram is relatively silent.

positions despite EMG silence of the muscles due to the ligamentous constraints.

Although forward flexion of the spine is controlled by the paraspinal muscles, hip muscles control the position of the pelvis over the femur. As the pelvis tilts forward the entire spine tends to tilt and the paraspinal muscles contract strongly (to counteract the force of gravity), resulting in lordosis. The paraspinal and abdominal muscles control the position of the thorax over the pelvis. Either the hip muscles or the abdominal muscles can initiate spinal flexion. Spinal flexion is not the same thing as "bending over" (forward bending). Bending over is something the whole patient does whether the spine flexes or not. Forward bending requires hip flexion controlled by the hip extensors, but the amount of associated spinal flexion is independent of hip flexion and determined by the paraspinal muscles. Hence a ballerina can tie her shoe laces without flexing her spine by controlling trunk position with her hip extensors and preventing spinal flexion with her paraspinal muscles (Fig. 43-4). This paraspinal muscle action adds a compressive load to the spinal elements whether or not spinal flexion occurs.

In normal relaxed sitting, without a backrest, the pelvis tilts backward and the thoracolumbar spine assumes the C-shaped curve of the fully flexed spine (Fig. 43-5). The top of the C is stationed over the hip joints; the mid part of the C, the lower thoracic area, is well posterior to the hips; and the head and neck, on the

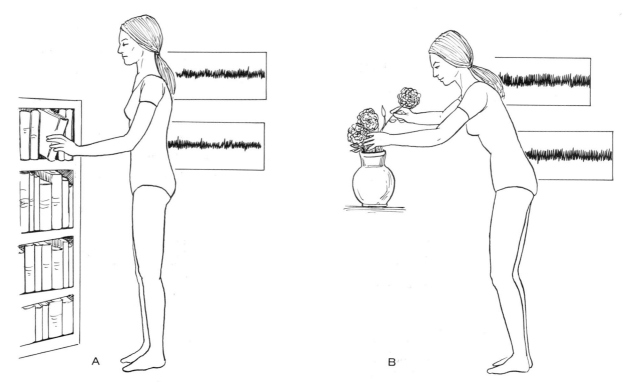

FIG. 43-3. Muscular activity controlling spinal flexion appears as soon as load on spine is off vertical balance, as when arm reaches forward (*A*) or hip flexors tilt the pelvis and spine forward (*B*).

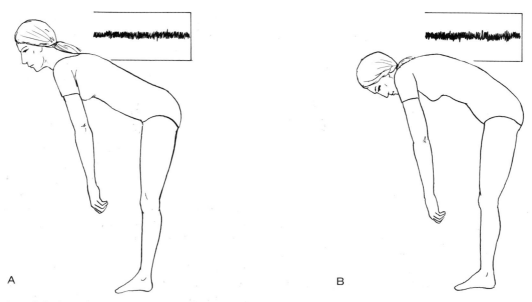

FIG. 43-4. *A and B,* Increase in muscular activity during forward bending.

upper end of the arc, are thrust forward as a counterbalance. In this position, the lumbar muscles can relax and the weight of the torso hangs on the spinal ligaments (as in the "rice planter's" position). The compressive loads and bending moments are relatively high, and the abdominal contents are compressed, making diaphragmatic respiration difficult.

In a chair, the "sitting base" is maximized when the ischia are fully back. If the backrest is vertical, it holds the middle of the spine over the hips (Fig. 43-6), and the "C" configuration of the relaxed spine is then forced to tilt forward, causing the weight of the upper torso to be forward of the hip joints. This is an unbalanced position, and hip extensor activity is required to prevent

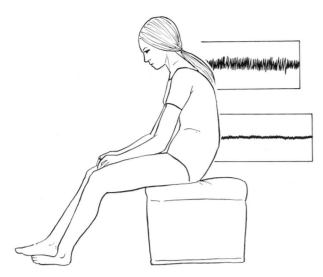

FIG. 43-5. C-shaped curve of fully flexed spine.

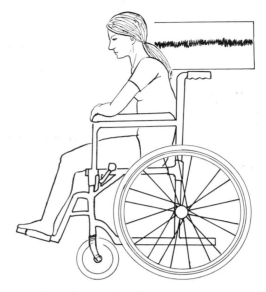

FIG. 43-7. Use of shoulder depressors to control posture with vertical backrest.

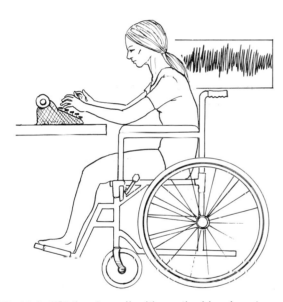

FIG. 43-6. "Sitting base" with vertical backrest.

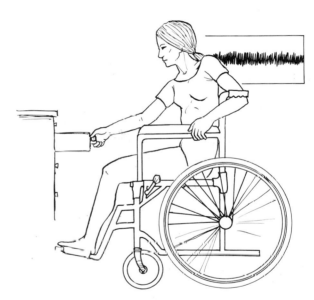

FIG. 43-8. In absence of shoulder depressors, patient loops one arm around handle of chair to prevent his falling forward.

the patient from falling forward. Forward hand placement adds to the imbalance and breathing is difficult. Thus the vertical backrest is extremely uncomfortable because it prevents the patient's leaning back. Many wheelchairs have this fault, a vertical backrest, and since the ischia are placed back in the chair to increase the sitting base for fear of ischial pressure sores, the patient who lacks spinal muscle activity is condemned to rest his elbows on the armrest and use his shoulder depressors to control his posture (Fig. 43-7). Lacking shoulder depressors, as many quadriplegic or dystrophic patients do, the patient will loop one arm around the handle of the chair to prevent his falling forward (Fig. 43-8), making bimanual hand use impossible. Sometimes a chest restraint is used on the chair to support

the upper torso to free the hands for other uses. A more restful position of support can be achieved, even in a straight backed chair, if the buttocks can move forward, away from the backrest, so that one can lean back on the backrest.

If the backrest is tilted backward approximately 15 degrees, the spine can rest back against it (Fig. 43-9). The thoracic spine straightens because the chest is now behind the pelvis and forward imbalance is not present. The backrest controls the posteriorly imbalanced position, and neither ligaments nor muscles are needed. In this position compressive loads and bending moments

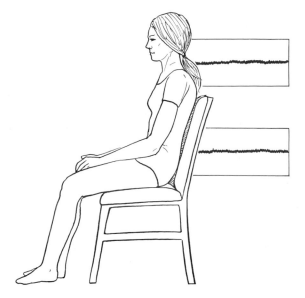

FIG. 43-9. Backrest tilted backward approximately 15 degrees.

are low, bilateral hand function is possible, and the straighter dorsal spine increases respiratory capacity and facilitates diaphragmatic respiration. Patients who have diseases of the spine compatible with vertical management should always sit where there is a backrest and should rest against it (Fig. 43-10).

PRINCIPLES OF THE USE OF ORTHOSES. Orthoses are force systems that exert a mechanical effect by applying pressure at prescribed points. Because of the anatomic packaging, the spine is directly available to

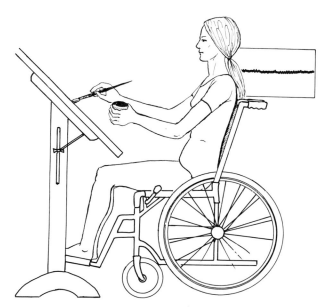

FIG. 43-10. When disease of spine is compatible with vertical management, patient should always rest against backrest.

external forces only in the midline posteriorly and thus orthoses frequently exert their forces indirectly by pressing on the skin of the torso or head, at some distance from the spine itself. Pressures exist only to the extent that the body presses back on the brace.

When an external force presses on the skin, nerves are stimulated. While light pressures, such as a wrist watch band, elastic waist band, ring, or brassiere strap, can be tolerated for prolonged periods and are easily relegated to subliminal consciousness, greater degrees of pressure elicit painful neurologic stimuli. If the contact force exceeds capillary pressure, blanching and ischemia occur. Such pressure concentrations become first annoying, then intolerably painful. Thus, strong forces must be distributed over wide areas to remain below the threshold pressure for discomfort or ischemia.

Since patients respond to pressures by withdrawal to a different position to decrease the pressure, orthoses, when fitted, must permit the patient to withdraw to a "low pressure" position. Devices designed for "immobilization" must have a full set of orthotic pressures, which can constrain any deviation from the desired position so that the patient, having found the low pressure position, will experience the discomfort of mechanical restraint if motion toward any other position occurs. The orthotic system can be planned so that some motions are permitted while other motions result in increased pressures or discomforts.

Effects of an orthosis are not necessarily entirely mechanical. If someone feels a few stitches let go in a tight garment when bending over, he probably will spend the rest of the time in that garment avoiding that bending activity. In that situation, the garment does not "hold the person up" mechanically, but rather it constrains the person through psychologic effects. An orthotic device can similarly encourage a patient to maintain a given position without exerting mechanical force beyond those minimal pressures inherent in simply suspending the device on the patient. These psychophysiologic constraints are dependent on an intact sensory and motor system and are not available when the patient lacks the ability to detect position or is deficient in motor coordination.

Spinal orthoses can modify spinal motions and establish the relations of the chest to the pelvis, but an orthosis cannot limit the stresses on the spine that occur during forward bending as a result of hip flexion. Therefore, it is imperative that patients be instructed not to bend. The thorough physician will instruct the patient on how to accomplish daily living activities without bending. For example, to pick up something, the patient should squat rather than bend. If the patient has arthritis or weak knees, a long handled "grabber" will reduce the need to bend. The forward bend associated with getting out of a chair can be prevented if the patient can use his arms and has full length arm rests (not short "desk arms") on his chair. Shoes and socks can be put on without bending over if the patient can lean back in a chair and bring his feet up. Eating and writing should be done from the backrest of a chair rather than by leaning forward. The patient should avoid the rear seat of a car because entering requires forward bending. To get into the front seat, he faces away from the doorway while he sits down. Once seated, he can turn to face the front.

Immobilization of a flail spine in the vertical position is a major problem. The ligamentous spine, devoid of muscles and ribs, can stand vertically without any support except the spinal ligaments, but it buckles when approximately five pounds of weight is applied vertically. When the spine is completely devoid of supporting musculature (e.g., trunk muscles, rib cage and associated musculature) as in advanced muscular dystrophy, or paralytic poliomyelitis, even rigid cylindrical body jackets will not completely prevent the spine from collapsing if the patient sits or stands. Skeletal fixation devices such as Harrington rods internally, or the halo device externally, are of only very limited and transient value in attempts to immobilize the upright flaccid spine.

Many patients with spinal disease also have respiratory problems. Motions essential for respiratory ventilation are: (1) chest expansion, (2) diaphragmatic motion with abdominal expansion, and (3) flexion and extension of the thoracic spine. To breathe, the patient must be able to perform at least one of these motions. If the patient has limitation of one or more of these motions, the orthosis must not interfere with the residual ventilatory capacity. Skeletal fixation or extensive spine fusion for scoliosis eliminates dorsal spine motion, and ankylosing spondylitis prevents both spine motion and rib motion. Patients with such conditions are particularly dependent on diaphragmatic respiration. Completely encircling the torso with rigid pressure points limits the expansion of the chest or abdomen. Corsets, casts, or braces must permit the epigastrium to expand as the diaphragm descends during inhalation. Some diseases cause paralysis of the abdominal muscles. Then, when the body is upright, the abdominal viscera are unsupported and their weight, sagging downward, pulls the diaphragm down so that diaphragmatic respiration cannot occur. Abdominal venous pooling also may occur. A low abdominal corset with an open epigastric area can support the visceral weight while permitting epigastric expansion. It also controls venous pooling, but if an abdominal corset is too tight, swelling occurs in the ankles.

During ordinary bending or lifting activities, there is an increase in intra-abdominal pressure due to abdominal muscle action. As lifted loads increase, there is progressively more abdominal muscle action, causing increased intra-abdominal pressure. This increase in pressure in the abdominal "balloon" provides a distracting lengthening or straightening effect on the flexed lumbar spine and reduces the requirement for paraspinal muscle action. The loading on the lumbosacral disc may be reduced by as much as 35%. A corset around the abdomen can produce a substitute source of intra-abdominal pressure and can reduce the activity of the abdominal muscles. To the extent that a corset substitutes for the abdominal muscles, these muscles become less active. Prolonged corseting causes marked abdominal muscle weakness. Also, there is an increase in axial rotation of the fifth lumbar vertebra on the sacrum while a person is walking in a corset. Since the vertical axis of rotation passes behind the body of L5, this increased rotation implies increased shear force through the L5 disc.

THREE-POINT PRESSURE SYSTEMS. Flexion of the spine can be limited by "three-point" pressure systems. A single set of three points limits bending of the spine in one direction. An example of a three-point system is the Jewett brace (Fig. 43-11). This type of device can theoretically be used in the management of anteriorly wedged flexion fractures of the dorsal or lumbar spine. Actual use of such orthoses is limited by several factors. First, the lower anterior pad rests on the abdomen above the pubic brim, which will not tolerate much pressure. Second, the distance from the pubis to the sternal notch while a person is standing or supine is about four inches greater than the distance between these points when he is seated. If adjusted to limit a person's forward bending while he is standing, the three-point "anterior motion control" orthoses (Jewett, Pipkin, Florida, etc.) are extremely uncomfortable while

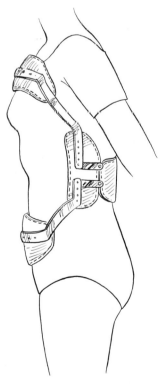

FIG. 43-11. Jewett brace.

he is sitting, especially when he is leaning forward to eat. Therefore, they are usually adjusted for sitting comfort and have little direct effect on the patient while he is standing or walking. For ordinary compression fractures of the lower dorsal and lumbar spine, a corset with flexible stays is a more realistic orthosis. The patient is also admonished to avoid forward bending and to seek assistance with daily living activities. The inadequately instructed patient will not be protected by the "three-point" AP motion control brace, whereas the adequately instructed, cooperative, and competent patient does well in a corset and does not need a rigid three-point brace.

END-POINT CONTROL. The bending characteristics of the spine, or any semi-flexible rod, can also be modified by control of the end-point conditions of the rod. Semi-flexible rods buckle when some specific amount of weight is applied axially. This critical load, for the human ligamentous spine, is about five pounds. Figure 43-12 shows that by changing the end-point conditions of a rod, the critical load can be increased by various factors—a factor of sixteen when the base is rigidly fixed and the top can neither sway nor tilt. This probably accounts for the greater success of the Milwaukee brace (Fig. 43-13), as compared against two thousand years of other techniques which applied forces to the scoliotic spine but ignored the end-point conditions. Although observers frequently assume that the Milwaukee brace is a distracting device like a "jack," the effect of the brace seems most likely to be due to the establishment and maintenance of end-point conditions. This is why a chin pad is not needed and can be replaced with the neck ring. This underscores the

necessity for insisting that the patient keep the pelvic girdle fitting snugly, so that the neck ring and occipital pad can have maximum benefit, yet there can always be room for a finger between the occiput and the pad. The Milwaukee brace is also remarkably effective in the correction (i.e., actual permanent change in alignment) of the spine in active Scheuermann's disease. The basic brace is the same as for the scoliotic patient, but for juvenile kyphosis the spinal pad is placed transversely just below the apex of the kyphosis. This combines a three-point pressure system with end-point control.

Correction of spinal deformity refers to a permanently retained change in structural alignment. The history of "correction" by bracing reiterates that orthoses fail to produce permanent change by forces applied for their magnitude alone. Although the uninjured spine can be casted or braced in many positions, it will not retain the imposed positions when the device is removed. "Correction" of alignment in scoliosis or kyphosis can only occur if spinal growth centers are still active or tissue healing is present (e.g., after operation or reduction of fractures). The correction of scoliotic or kyphotic alignment effected by bracing is retained when the brace has exerted its forces during growth or healing, and the orthosis modifies the conditions in which growth is occurring. The changes that can be produced during the "growth" period are out of all proportion to the magnitude of the applied pressures.

MANAGEMENT OF SCIATIC SCOLIOSIS, ABNORMAL LUMBAR LORDOSIS, AND THORACIC KYPHOSIS. "Sciatic scoliosis" is an acquired, nonstructural lateral curvature, or list, of the adult spine. There is a sudden gross disturbance of the righting reflex system with displace-

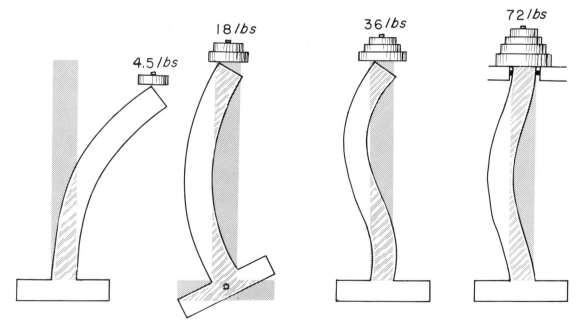

FIG. 43-12. Buckling loads with different end-point conditions.

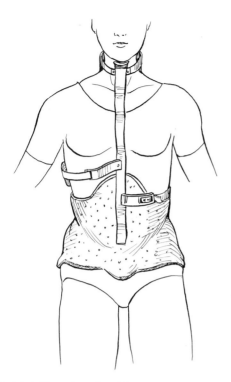

FIG. 43-13. Milwaukee brace.

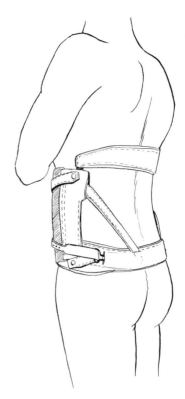

FIG. 43-14. Williams brace.

ment of the head and upper torso off the midline to a lateral or anterolateral position. The pathologic basis is not known and neither pain nor disc disease is dependably present. Spinal orthoses do not correct the disturbed alignment, but a heel lift frequently induces correction if it is used correctly. The temptation may be to put the lift on the side toward which the patient leans, as if to prop the spine upright by tilting the pelvis. This ignores the righting reflex disturbance, and the deformity usually remains unchanged despite the new pelvic elevation. Instead heel lifts should be placed on the opposite side since placement of the heel lift so that it tilts the spine further seems to stimulate the righting reflexes and frequently produces correction after the patient walks a short while. Thus, an applied force can induce an effect at a distance through the action of reflexes.

The righting reflexes are also used to manage lumbar lordosis and thoracic kyphosis. Lordosis of the upright lumbar spine exists only if the pelvis is tilted forward at the hips and the lumbar muscles are actively restoring the chest to a balanced position over the pelvis. If the hip extensors can be induced to change this tilt, the patient then is tilted backward unless the abdominal muscles act to reduce the lordosis and keep the torso upright. The lumbar muscles are then less active, the abdominal muscles more active, the spine straighter, and loadings at the lumbosacral level reduced.

WILLIAMS BRACE. Unfortunately, there is no lower extremity orthosis that controls hip flexion. However, if the lumbar spine is flexed by a three-point system, such

as a flexion body cast or a Williams brace (Fig. 43-14), the righting reflex system does not permit the patient to walk continuously bent. The flexion attitude created in the lumbar area induces an extensor activity both at the hips and in the dorsal spine to relieve the postural imbalance. This is desirable in the treatment of low back disease associated with lordosis. The straightening response induced in the thoracic spine by lumbar flexion orthoses has been used in the management of active juvenile kyphosis. Besides wearing the orthosis, the kyphotic patient should not lean forward continuously to eat or read. Rather the youth should sit back on a dependable backrest. Textbooks should be tilted up, vision tested, and illumination adjusted to preclude the need to place the head forward or "peer" while studying.

STRAPS. Figure-of-eight straps do not help juvenile round back. Scapulothoracic joint position has no effect on the spine because the scapulae are highly mobile on the thorax. Straps around the shoulders from behind, tightened enough to pull the shoulders back, seriously limit hand placement. Such straps have no effect on spine position.

The straps on dorsolumbar corsets (Fig. 43-15) also fail to control dorsal kyphosis at any age, especially the kyphosis of osteoporosis. Moreover, since shoulder straps run up and down from the shoulders to the corset, making the straps fit more snugly causes the entire garment to "ride up" unless perineal straps

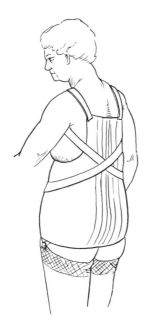

FIG. 43-15. Dorsolumbar corset.

are used. Perineal straps are badly tolerated if they are tightened. Comfortably adjusted, these corsets are only psychologic supports, and a lumbosacral corset and appropriate admonitions concerning bending are more effective and far less a nuisance to the patient and to the physician.

TAYLOR BRACE AND OUTRIGGERS. Other ineffective attempts to control the thoracic spine include the Taylor brace (Fig. 43-16) and the use of a "cow-horn" outrigger

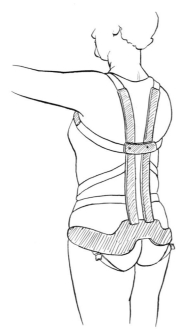

FIG. 43-16. Taylor brace.

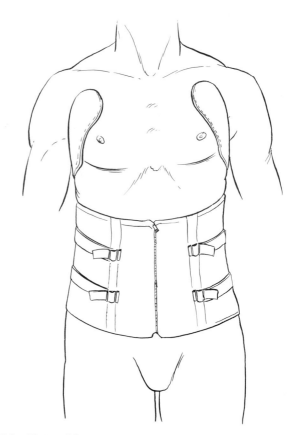

FIG. 43-17. "Cow-horn" outrigger on lumbar device.

(Fig. 43-17) on lumbar devices. The pectoral "cow-horn" is usually placed in the infraclavicular fossa at the deltopectoral groove superficial to the coracoid. Any effect is related to painful pressure on the coracoid or clavicle. Scapulothoracic motion and hand placement are limited more than spine position.

The standard Taylor brace uses shoulder straps and differs from the lumbosacral corset in being more rigid, longer, and more expensive. Being rigid, the long brace will be more uncomfortable if the patient flexes his spine while bending, and therefore the patient may not flex his upper lumbar spine as much during bending. However, the loads of holding the spine straight while bending at the hips will still be present. Further, since the brace grasps the upper torso only by the mobile shoulder girdle, the dorsal spine will not be immobilized. Lumbosacral motion may actually increase.

MANAGEMENT OF LOW BACK PAIN. Many physicians believe that the management of low back pain occasionally calls for the use of an orthosis. There are no proven criteria by physical findings or diagnoses to help in the selection of brace type or timing. A survey of orthopaedic surgeons revealed that the lumbosacral corset, chairback (Knight) brace (Fig. 43-18), Williams brace, flexion body cast, and Norton-Brown braces were all in use in patterns that seem more regional than rational.

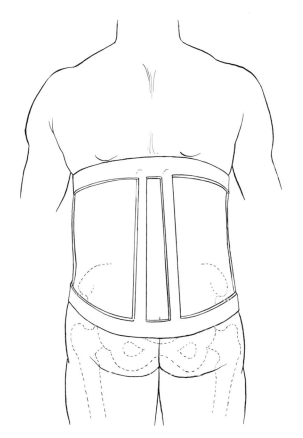

FIG. 43-18. Chairback (Knight) brace.

Spinal fusion procedures are most commonly performed at the lumbosacral and lower lumbar levels, and postoperative "immobilization" has been the goal of many devices. The studies of Norton and Brown show that none of the lumbar orthoses fully immobilize the lumbosacral junction. The longer spinal orthoses actually increased lumbosacral motion. None have been proven to produce a higher rate of bony union, and many experienced surgeons do not depend on an orthosis for "immobilization" after lumbosacral fusion. The patient is instructed to avoid bending and given positive suggestions on daily living activities.

Long orthoses have an additional disadvantage because, in normally efficient walking there are transverse rotations of the pelvis and counter-rotations of the shoulder girdle. The lower spine rotates with the pelvis, the upper spine with the shoulders. The nodal point at which this axial rotation changes is T8. Devices or operations that interfere with this counter-rotation by rigidly attaching the chest to the pelvis produce a "tin soldier" stiffness of the torso, which increases the energy cost of walking. While long spinal fusions may be needed for scoliosis, the long orthoses for the trunk are probably never indicated. Note that the Milwaukee brace grasps the pelvis firmly, but has only isolated pressure areas on the chest.

Degenerative disease of the lower lumbar discs is a common problem. The use of rigid orthoses gives equivocal results and long term abdominal muscle weakness. There is certainly no regular benefit from an orthosis for the patient after routine disc surgery and no proven benefit from these devices in the conservative or preoperative period.

Some patients with recurrent low back symptoms get some relief from the temporary use of a lumbosacral corset. These patients should be warned to wean themselves as soon as the acute episode is over. The best prophylaxis is an appropriate exercise and activity program. Patients need much instruction on techniques to accomplish activities of daily living without exceeding their capacities. At the same time the exercise program attempts to expand their capacity beyond the exigencies of daily living.

Faulty Bending Techniques

Whether the body is standing, bending, or lifting, its center of gravity must be over the feet. The center of gravity of the body represents the sum of all of the partial centers of mass of the parts of the body. In the cadaveric position—horizontal or vertical—this center is one-half inch in front of the second sacral vertebra. This "spot" is just behind the line joining the centers of rotation of the hips. The "weight-bearing line" from this center of mass to the ground passes between the feet and in the midline, and midway between the points at which the heels and the balls of the feet contact the ground. When the body is bending, the centers of mass for the head, arms, and chest move forward. The center of gravity of the body shifts owing to this redistribution of mass. If the weight-bearing line were to pass anterior to the metatarsal heads, the body would fall. When the body is bending normally, the pelvis shifts posteriorly (Fig. 43-19) to counterbalance the head, arms, and chest, so that the net center of gravity passes within the standing base.

There is an old parlor trick wherein a bet is made that an individual who stands with his heels against a wall cannot pick up a dollar bill on the floor without moving his feet or bending his knees. Since the wall prevents the necessary posterior weight displacement for forward bending over the available base, his efforts to bend forward are humorously futile and associated with heel elevation. He does not fall but he comes close to falling.

Some patients with back problems aver that they cannot bend. When requested to try, they bend forward at the hips but the buttocks do not shift back. Their heels leave the ground as they attempt to shift their standing base forward and they are unable to bend more than about 20 to 30% of normal. The complaint is that attempts to bend even this far cause a "pulling pain" in the low back. These people have lost the ordinary skill which shifts the buttocks posteriorly. The Burns test (page 307) positions the buttocks back on a

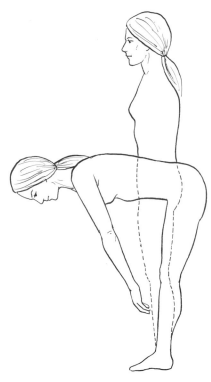

FIG. 43-19. When body bends normally, pelvis shifts posteriorly.

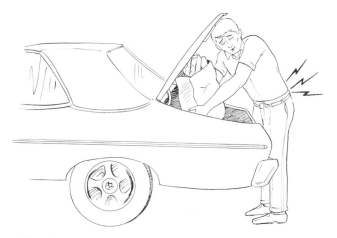

FIG. 43-20. Faulty bending technique: both feet and knees are anchored.

large base and facilitates bending. Bending, if it is to be done at all, must have an appropriate weight shift posteriorly. Lifted objects must be near the feet. Neither orthosis, muscle relaxants, nor surgery will permit bending if the bending technique is faulty.

Another faulty bending technique occurs when both the feet and the knees are anchored—as in putting groceries in the trunk of an automobile (Fig. 43-20). Here the pressure of the bumper prevents forward falling, thus permitting an unusual degree of bending of the trunk and hips. This results in tremendous strains on the hips, paraspinal muscles, and vertebral column, as the spine functions as the boom of a crane. No pill, orthosis, or operation can make this a safe or sensible maneuver. Placing one foot in the trunk of the car will make lifting things in or out much safer.

Exercises

Instructions and coaching in technique are essential to successful management of back pain. The orthosis cannot absolve the patient or the physician of responsibility for governing the techniques of use. Good coaching and intelligent cooperation can relegate orthoses to the role of reminders. Braces do not strengthen a "weak back," for the weak back is only strengthened by progressively graded exercise and physical activities. The most commonly successful exercises are abdominal muscle exercises of the Williams type. Since these exercises are intended to strengthen the abdomen, not the iliopsoas, they should be done with the hips and knees flexed. It is not necessary or useful to wear an orthosis while doing these exercises. Upright activity, such as walking and jogging, can be planned to add additional muscle strength and skills. Early in the program an orthosis may guide, or reinforce, weak muscles and so permit the patient to achieve a level of activity that can increase his capacity and ultimately relieve him of the need for external support. If the abdomen is weak, any straight leg raising exercise will produce painful lordosis.

Index

Page numbers in *italics* indicate illustrations; those followed by t indicate tables.

Abdominal pain, rhizotomy for, 400
Abscess, paravertebral, 99
    in spinal tuberculosis, 105, 106, 110
        radiographic features of, *337*
Abscess wall, in spinal tuberculosis, 109
Acceleration-deceleration forces, head and neck injuries
        from, 347-354
    delayed degenerative changes in, *348, 349, 351, 352, 353*
Achondroplasia, 244
Activity schedule, in operant conditioning program,
        psychologic aspects of pain and, 397
Adamkiewicz, artery of, 48
Adolescent thoracic scoliosis, 180
Age, anterior fusion in spinal tuberculosis and, 113t
Age/sex correlation, in spinal tuberculosis, 105t
Agenesis, sacral, 239, *239*
Albers-Schoenberg disease, fracture of pars interarticularis
        and, 199, *200*
Alcohol-mediated rhizotomy, 414
Alloplasty, scoliosis and, 187
Ambulation, household, 389
Ambulator, community, 389
    functional, 389
Ambulatory management, in cervical spine conditions, 418
Amphiarthrosis, 14, 27
Amyelus, 12
Amyotrophic lateral sclerosis, 61
Anatomy, radiographic, of cervical spine, 64-68, *64, 66, 67*
        of lumbar spine, 69, *69, 70, 70, 72*
    of sacrum, 70, *71*
    of thoracic spine, 68, *68, 69*
    of vertebral canal, 71, *72*
    spinal, 13-39
        blood supply and, 16, 36
        ligaments and, 24-27, *26, 27*
        muscles and, 28-36, *28, 30, 31, 33, 34*
        nerves and, *35, 36,* 37, *37, 38*
        review of features of, 62
        skin and, 13, *14*
        vertebrae and intervertebral discs and, 14-23, *15, 16, 17,
            18, 19, 20, 21, 22, 23, 24, 25*
Anesthesia, intubation, in spinal osteotomy for fixed flexion
        deformity, 169
Aneurysmal bone cyst, 275, 283, *283*
Aneurysmal syndrome, 108
Angle, lumbosacral, 23
    of inclination, in scoliosis, 182
Anomalies, bony, compressive lesions at foramen magnum
        and, 262-264
Anterior approach in spinal fusion, scoliosis and, 190
Anterior median fissure, of spinal cord, 10
Anterior spinal fusion, in spinal tuberculosis, 111, 112t. *See
        also* Lumbar spine, fusion of.
Anterior-wedge thoracolumbar fractures, 360
Anterolateral approaches to cervical spine, 125-131
Antibacterial agents, spinal infections and, 100
Anulus fibrosus, 15
Apophyses, 15
Arachnoid cysts, 290, 293
Arachnoid membrane, 40
Arch, vertebral, 4, 14, 62. *See also* Neural arch.

Arm. *See* Extremity, upper.
Arnold-Chiari malformation, *232*
  atlanto-occipital fusion and, 240
Arterial system of spinal cord, 47-49
  venous system and, *48*
Arteries, in embryo, 4
  nutrient, to vertebral body, 37. *See also* specific arteries.
Arteriography, compressive lesions at foramen magnum and, 252
Arteriovenous malformation of spinal cord, *297*
  operating microscope in surgery for, 297
Arthritis, radiographic features of, 341-344, *341, 343, 344, 345*
Arthrodesis, by Freebody technique, *149. See also* Spinal fusion.
Astroblastoma, 291
Astrocytomas, 291
  operating microscope in surgery for, 297
Athetoid patients, isthmic spondylolisthesis and, 197
Atlanto-axial dislocation, 358
Atlanto-axial fusion, 240
Atlanto-axial ligament, 27, *27*
Atlanto-occipital fusion, 240, *240*
  with Klippel-Feil deformity, *241*
Atlanto-occipital membrane, 27, *27*
Atlas, 16
  articulation between dens and, *26*
  assimilation of, 262, *263*
  axis and, *18, 19, 122*
  dens and, *123*
    and body of axis and, exposure of anterior arch of, 128
  fracture of, 358, *359*
  in embryo, 5
  occiput and, congenital fusion of, *240*
  ossification and, 6
  transverse ligament of, 26
Atrophy, sciatica and, 307
  Sudek's, 93
Attitude, in spinal tuberculosis, 106
Avoidance patterns, psychophysiologic aspects of pain and, 396
Axial-loading burst fracture of thoracolumbar spine, 382, 385, *386*
Axis, 18
  atlas, dens and body of, exposure of anterior arch of, 128
  atlas and, *18, 19, 122*
  dens of. *See* Dens.
  fractures of, 358, *359*
  in embryo, 5
  ossification and, 6

Bacilli, gram-negative, osteomyelitis and, 100
Back motion, test for, in painful low back, 306
Back pain. *See* Pain and Painful low back.
Backrest, backward tilting, 421, *422*
  vertical, 420, *421*
Bacteroides infections, paravertebral abscess and, 99
Basilar invagination, 262, *264*
  posterior decompression for, 264
Basivertebral veins, 25
Batson's venous plexus, spinal tuberculosis and, 103
Bending, faulty techniques in, 427, 428
  forward, in sitting position, evaluating painful low back and, 308
    muscular activity and, *420*
  normal, *428*
Bending films, solidity of lumbar spinal fusion and, 152
Biomechanics, of thoracic and lumbar spine, 419-422
  of spine, orthoses and, 417-428

Bladder function, bowel and, percutaneous cervical cordotomy and, 407
  rehabilitation in lumbar paraplegia and, 390
  reflex emptying of in fracture of thoracolumbar spine, 383
Blastemal stage, in spinal development, 3
Block vertebrae, 242, *242*
Blood supply, spinal, 16, 36
Body, vertebral. *See* Vertebral body(ies).
Body jacket, fracture of thoracolumbar spine and, *387*
Bone, anatomic patterns of loss of, *88*
  development of, 6
  healing of, biologic failure in, 95
    in osteomalacias, 92
    test for, in spinal tuberculosis, 107
  pseudofracture of, 90
  remodeling of, 90
  turnover of, 90
  undecalcified sections of, *91*
Bone age, establishment of, in scoliosis, 183
Bone cyst, aneurysmal, vertebrae and, 275, 283, *283*
Bone graft
  cervical vertebral body fractures and, 130, *131*
  dowel, in interbody fusion of lumbar spine, 151, *151*
  extent of, in paraspinal approach to lumbar spine, *156*
  fibula for, in interbody fusion of lumbar spine, 150, *150*
  horseshoe iliac, 149, *150*, 151
  iliac, in anterior lumbar interbody fusion, 163, *163*
    in anterior lumbar spine fusion by Freebody technique, 147
    in paraspinal approach to lumbar spine, *155*
    shaping of, to fit disc space, *127*
  in cervical disc space, 126-128, *128*
  in crush fracture of vertebral body, *379*
  in stabilization of fracture of cervical spine, 378
  rib for, in interbody fusion of lumbar spine, 151, *151*
  tapping into place of, *128*
  upper cervical, 123, *123*
Bone lesions of vertebrae, tumor-like, 275, 283
Bone sequestra, Pott's paraplegia and, 113
Bone tumors. *See* Tumors, bone.
Bony anomalies, compressive lesions at foramen magnum and, 262-264
Bony union, test for, in spinal tuberculosis, 107
Bony wall, tumors arising from, *268, 269*
  compressive lesions at foramen magnum and, 264-267
Bowel and bladder function, percutaneous cervical cordotomy and, 407
  rehabilitation in lumbar paraplegia and, 390
Brace(s), cervical, 418, *418*
  chairback, *427*
  hyperextension back, spinal osteotomy for fixed flexion deformity and, 171
  Jewett, *423*
  Knight, *427*
  Milwaukee, *425*
    scoliosis and, 185, *185*
  Taylor, 426, *426*
  Williams, 425, *425*
Brachial plexus, 38
  lumbosacral and, development of, 8
Brain injury, subclinical, 348
Breathing, abdominal, positioning for spinal osteotomy for fixed flexion deformity and, *170*
Bronchopleural fistula, 139
Brown-Sequard syndrome, 60
  spinal cord tumors and, 288
Brucella infections, spinal, 100
Burns test, in evaluating painful low back, 307

C1, C2 and, *66, 122. See also* Atlas.
Canal, vertebral, 71
    narrow lumbar, 320
Capital erectors, posterior, 32
Capital muscles, oblique, 32
Carcinoma
    metastases of, to spinal cord, 289
        to vertebrae, 281, 282, *282*
            radiographic features of, 340, *340*
    percutaneous cervical cordotomy in, 404
    primary osteogenic, radiographic features of, 340, *340*
    thoracic cordotomy in, 401
Cast, body, evaluation prior to lumbar fusion and, 332, *332*
    halo and, *370*
    scoliosis and, 186
    spinal osteotomy for fixed flexion deformity and, 171, *172, 173*
Cauda equina, 9
    decompression of, 158, *158*
    hemisected lumbar spine and, *37*
    lesions of, 60
    tumor of, *292*
Cell specialization, in neural tube, 8, *8*
Central arteries, 49
Central canal, hernial protrusions of, 290
Central cord lesions, 60
Central nervous system, examination of, scoliosis and, 182
Central veins, 49
Centrifugal arteries of spinal cord, 49
Centripetal arteries of spinal cord, 49
Cerebellospinal tract, 47
Cervical braces, 418, *418*
Cervical collars, 418
Cervical cord lesions, diagnosis of, 60
Cervical cord syndrome, 60, 360, 362
Cervical cordotomy. *See* Cordotomy, cervical.
Cervical curve, delayed degenerative changes in, acceleration-deceleration force injuries and, *348, 349, 351, 352, 353*
Cervical disc, herniated, surgical treatment of, *318*
Cervical operations, transoral and transinfrahyoid, 121-124
Cervical plexus, 38
Cervical segments, exposure of fifth and sixth, *126*
Cervical spine, abnormalities of, 72-75, *73, 74, 75*
    anterolateral approaches to, 125-131
    articulated, *17*
    as osteotomy site, 169
    biomechanics of, 417
    dislocation of, resistant to skeletal traction, reduction of, 363
        skeletal traction in, 363
        stereotaxic reduction in, *374, 376*
    exposure of entire anterior, *129*
    exposure of transverse process of, *130*
    extension injuries to, 360, *360*
    flexion injuries to, between C3 and C7, *259*, 360
    fracture of. *See* Fracture(s), cervical spine.
    fracture-dislocation of, *378*
    hemisected, cord and, *35*
    hyperextension injury to, *350, 359, 360*
    injury to, 358-360
        from acceleration-deceleration forces, *348, 349, 350, 351, 352, 353*
        halo and, 370
    lateral approach to, 132-136, *134, 135*
    lateral flexion injuries to, 360
    middle and lower, surgery for fractures of, 366
    radiographic anatomy of, 64-68, *64, 66, 67*
    spondylolisthesis in, 206

upper, craniovertebral junction and, anomalies of, 239-241
    surgery for fractures and dislocations of, 365, *365*
    transoral and transinfrahyoid approaches to, 121-124.
    See also Atlas and Axis
Cervical spondylosis, 316-318
    surgical treatment of, 317
Cervical-thoracic neural arch defect, kyphoscoliosis and, *225*
Cervical vertebrae, 16-19
    fourth, 17, 18
Chairback brace, *427*
Chemical rhizotomy, spasticity and, 414
Chemonucleolysis, 212
Chest wall pain, rhizotomy for, 400
Chiari type 1 malformation, 267-269, *269*
    clinical features of, 268t
Children, disc space infections in, 97, *98*
    latent period of spinal tuberculosis in, 104
    sacroiliac joint fusion in, 159, *160*
    scoliosis in, 181
    spondylolisthesis in. *See* Spondylolisthesis, in children.
    transoral and transinfrahyoid operative approaches and, 124
Chisel, midline approach in lumbar spinal fusion and, 143
Chondrification, centers of, in embryo, *5*
Chondrogenous stage in spinal development, 4
Chondro-osteodystrophy, 243
Chordoma(s), spinal cord, 7, 289
    vertebral column, 279
Chronicity, psychophysiologic aspects of pain and, 395
Chymopapain, 143
Circle-electric bed, thoracolumbar spine fracture and, *388*
"Clay shovelers" fracture, 358
Cleft spine, 7
Cleft vertebrae, coronal, 242, *242*
    sagittal, 243, *243*
Cloward interbody fusion of lumbar spine, 151
Cluneal nerves, iliac crest and, *145*
Cobb technique, measurement of curvature in scoliosis by, 183, *183*
Coccygeal vestige, 9
Coccyx, 23
    sacrum and, *23, 24, 25*
Collapse, concertina, Pott's paraplegia and, 113
    spinal tuberculosis and, 108, *109*
Collars, cervical, 418
Comminuted burst fracture of thoracolumbar spine, 388
Community ambulator, 389
Compensation claims, failure of lumbar spine operations and, 329
Compensatory lordosis, in spinal tuberculosis, 105, 109
Compression by redundant nerve roots, 321
    of nerve roots, disc protrusion and, *319, 320*
Compression fractures. *See* Fracture(s), compression.
Compressive lesions at foramen magnum. *See* Foramen magnum, compressive lesions at.
Concertina collapse. *See* Collapse, concertina.
Congenital anomalies of spine, 223-245. *See also* specific anomalies.
Congenital scoliosis, 180
Congenital spondylolisthesis, *201*
Contrast studies, compressive lesions at foramen magnum and, 252
Conus medullaris, 40
    lesions of, 60
    tumor of, *292*
Cord, spinal. *See* Spinal cord.
Cord syndrome, cervical, 60, 360, 362
Cordectomy, spasticity and, 414

Cordotomy, cervical, high, 402
    percutaneous, dentate ligament and, *407*
        for intractable pain, 404-408
        patient position and, *406*
    rhizotomy for pain and, 399-403
    thoracic, 401, *402*
Cornua, vertebral, in embryo, 5
Coronal cleft vertebrae, 242, *242*
Corsets, painful low back and, 304, 427
Corticospinal tract, lateral, 45, 46
    destruction of, 60
    determining extent of involvement of, 55
    ventral, 46
Corticosteroid injection, 302
Costotransverse joint, 324
Costotransverse ligaments, scoliosis and, 178
Costotransversectomy, in spinal tuberculosis, 111
Costovertebral joint, 324
Costovertebral syndrome, 325, 327
Craniospinal tumors, diagnosis of compressive lesions at
        foramen magnum and, 250
    surgical treatment of, 255
Craniovertebral junction and upper cervical spine, anomalies
        of, 239-241
Cruciate paralysis, 61
Crutchfield tongs, *364*, 368
    cervical dislocation and, 363
Cuneocerebellar tract, 45
Curette, midline approach in lumbar spinal fusion and, *143*
Curvature, measurement of, in scoliosis, 183, *183*
Cushing's osteoporosis, 93
Cutaneous dimple, spina bifida occulta and, 226
Cyst(s), aneurysmal bone, 275, 283, *283*
    arachnoid, 290, 293
    dermoid, 234, 290
    enterogenous, 238
    ependymal, 261, *261*
    epidermoid, 234, 290
    hydatid, 290
    intramedullary and juxtamedullary, surgical treatment of,
        293
    neurenteric, 238
    pilonidal, 234
    teratomatous, 290

Decompression
    and realignment, in anterior open reduction of fractured
        cervical spine, 375
    Chiari type 1 malformation and, *269*
    degenerative spondylolisthesis and, 215, *216*
    excision of loose lamina and, in spondylolisthesis, 218-222,
        220
    narrow lumbar vertebral canal and, 320
    of cauda equina and nerve roots, paraspinal approach to
        lumbar spine and, 158, *158*
    posterior, for basilar invagination, 264
    spinal cord injuries and, 363-365
    spinal stenosis and, 215
    syringomyelia and, 270t, 270-273, *273*
Deep muscles, anatomy of spine and, 29-34
Deformity(ies), 175-245. *See also* specific deformities.
    fixed flexion, correction of, *172, 173, 174*
    osteotomy of spine for, 168-174
Degeneration, spondylotic, *316*
    subacute combined, 61
Degenerative changes, delayed, injuries from acceleration-
        deceleration forces and, *348, 349, 351, 352, 353*
Degenerative diseases, of thoracic spine, 323-327
Degenerative spondylolisthesis. *See* Spondylolisthesis,
    degenerative.

Denervation, fibrillations of, 78
Dens
    and body of axis, atlas and, exposure of anterior arch of,
        128
    anomalies of, 241
    articulation between atlas and, *26*
    displacement of, 358, *359*
    in embryo, 5
    ossification and, 6
    relationship of, to atlas, *123*
Dentate ligament(s), 41
    percutanous cervical cordotomy and, *407*
Dermal sinus, congenital, 234-236, *235*
Dermatomes, sensory, *54, 55*
Diagnosis, 51-84. *See also* specific procedures and conditions.
Diarthroses, 14
Diastematomyelia, 236-238, *237*
Dimple, cutaneous, spina bifida occulta and, 226
Disability, low back problems and, 329
Disc, intervertebral, 14
    blood supply to, 16
    degeneration of, in spondylolisthesis and, 207·
    excision of, 330
        anterior intervertebral interbody fusion and, in
            acceleration-deceleration injury, 352
        cervical, 126
        lumbar fusion and, 329
    flexion and, *163*
    great vessels and, in anterior lumbar fusion, *164*
    hemisected mid-lumbar, *16*
    herniated, 15, *316*
        cervical, surgical treatment of, *318*
        lumbar, surgical treatment of, *320*
    in embryo, 4
    lumbar, spinal fusion in disease of, 142
        surgical treatment of herniated, *320*
    lumbosacral, 15
    narrowing of, following solid posterior lateral fusion,
        146, *146*
    nerve roots and, *38*
    orthoses in degenerative disease of, 427
    protrusion of, nerve root compression and, *319, 320*
    protrusion or herniation of, in spondylolisthesis, 218
    sequestrated, in spinal tuberculosis, 108
        Pott's paraplegia and, 113
    thoracic, derangement of, 323, 325-327
    vertebrae and, 14-23
Disc disease, lumbar, spinal fusion and, 142
Disc space infections. *See* Infections, disc space.
Disc spaces from C3 through C7, vertebral bodies and,
    exposure of, 125-128
Discharges, electromyographic, 79, *79*, 80
Discitis, radiographic features of, 336, *337*
Discogenic disease, anterior interbody fusion of lumbar
    spine in, 147
Discography, acceleration-deceleration injury and, 352
Diseases, metabolic and infectious, 85-114
    neuromuscular, electrodiagnosis of, 76-84
    osteoporosis as, 88. *See also* specific diseases.
Disintegrated motor unit potentials, 77
Dislocation(s), atlanto-axial, 358
    cervical, resistant to skeletal traction, reduction, 363
        skeletal traction in reduction of, 363
        stereotaxic reduction of, *374, 376*
    occipito-atlantal, 358
    spinal, Pott's paraplegia and, 113
    upper cervical fractures and, surgery for, 365, *365*
Displacement, of dens, 358, *359*
Dissectomy, thoracic, 326
Distraction, in spondylolisthesis, 210, *211*

Distraction fracture, of thoracolumbar spine, 385
Distraction rod, Harrington, scoliosis and, *188*
Disuse osteoporosis, 94
Dorsal column gray matter, 42
Dorsal white column, 45
Dowel grafts, 151, *151*
Dura mater, 40
   exposure of, in laminectomy, *119*
   opening of, 120
   penetration of, Pott's paraplegia and, 113
Dwyer correction and stabilization, 187, *189*
Dysgenesis, sacral, *239*
Dysplastic spondylolisthesis, 201, *201*, 213

Efferent pathways, motor, *46*
Ehlers-Danlos disease, scoliosis and, 181
Electrical silence, 80
Electrodes, spinal implantation of, for pain relief, 409
Electrodiagnosis of neuromuscular disease, 76-84
Electroencephalogram, subclinical brain injury and, 348
Electromyogram, 80
Electromyographic concepts, 77-80
Electromyography, 76-81
Ely test, in evaluating painful low back, 309
Empyema, scoliosis and, 181
End-plate noise, 80
End-point conditions, buckling loads with, *424*
End-point control, of spinal flexion, 424
Enterogenous cysts, 238
Entrapment syndrome, posterior primary ramus, 325, 327
Environment, alteration of, psychologic aspects of pain and, 397
Enzymatic studies, vertebral column tumor diagnosis and, 276
Eosinophilic granuloma, 275, 284, *284*
Ependymal cyst, at foramen magnum, 261, *261*
Ependymal layer, of neural tube, 8
   of spinal cord, 10
Ependymoma, at foramen magnum, 255, *256*
   of spinal cord, 290, *297*
      surgery for, 297
Epidermoid cyst, 234, 290
Epiphysial centers, secondary vertebral, 6
Epistropheus, 18
Equilibrium, maintaining, 47
Erector spinae, 29-31
Escherichia coli, vertebral osteomyelitis and, 97
Evoked sensory responses, 82
Ewing's tumor, 280
Examination, radiologic, 62-75
Exercises, back pain and, 428
   painful low back and, 303, *304, 305*
   scoliosis and, 185
Extension injuries, to cervical spine, 360, *360*
External spinal veins, 49
Extradural neoplasm, *292*
Extradural tumors. *See* Tumors, extradural.
Extramedullary tumors. *See* Tumors, extramedullary.
Extraperitoneal approaches, lateral extrapleural and, to thoracic and lumbar spine, 137-141
Extrapleural and extraperitoneal, approaches, lateral, to thoracic and lumbar spine, 137-141
Extrapyramidal systems, destruction of, 60
Extravertebral congenital scoliosis, 180
Extremity, upper, cordotomy for pain in, 402
   descending motor and motor facilitory tracts and, 47
   diagnosis of spinal cord lesions and, 60
   sweating of, 47
   voluntary movement of, 46
Extrinsic muscles of spine, *28*

Facet, locked, in cervical spine fracture, 376, *377*
   thoracic and lumbar vertebral, configuration of, *381*
Facial expression, in spinal tuberculosis, 105
Failure, of lumbar spine operations, approach to, 328-333, *331*
Familial tendencies, congenital anomalies of spine and, 224
   isthmic spondylolisthesis and, 194, 195, *197*, 198, *198*
Fasciculations, 79
Fasciculi proprii, 47
Fasciculus, medial longitudinal, 47
Fasciculus cuneatus, 45
Fasciculus gracilis, 45
Fatigue fracture of pars interarticularis, 198, 199, *200*
Ferguson technique, 183
Fibrillation potentials, 78, *78*
Fibrocartilaginous mass, spondylolisthesis and, 207, 218, *221*
Fibula, as bone graft site, 150, *153*, 163, *163*
Films, bending, solidity of lumbar spinal fusion and, 152
Filum terminale, 9, 40
Fissure of spinal cord, anterior median, 10
Fistula, bronchopleural, 139
Flexed thigh test, in evaluating painful low back, 308
Flexibility, spinal, in scoliosis, 182, 183
Flexion, injuries from, fracture dislocations of thoracolumbar spine and 381
   with distraction forces to spine, 382
   to cervical spine between C3 and C7, *359*, 360
   plantar, of foot, in evaluating painful low back, 308
   spinal, disc and intervertebral foramen and, *163*
      end-point control of, 424
      muscular activity and, *420*
      three-point pressure systems limiting, 423
Flexion deformity, fixed. *See* Deformity(ies), fixed flexion.
Flexion rotation, fracture-dislocations of thoracolumbar spine and, 382
Flip test, in evaluating painful low back, 307, *308*
Fluoroscopy, 68
Foot drop, anterior tibial test for, in evaluating painful low back, 309
Foramen, intervertebral, effects of flexion on, *163*
   unroofing of, in spinal osteotomy for fixed flexion deformity, *171*
   neural, transverse processes, pedicles and, exposure of, *130*
Foramen magnum, *250*
   compressive lesions at, 249-273
      diagnosis of, 250-253
      surgical treatment of, 253-262
Fracture(s)
   axial-loading burst of thoracolumbar spine, 382, 385, *386*
   cervical spine, anterior open reduction of, 373-379
      between C3 and C7, 360
      surgery for, 365, *365*
      vertical compression, 130, *131*
   "clay shovelers," 358
   comminuted burst, of thoracolumbar spine, 388
   compression
      of cervical spine, 130, *131*
      of thoracolumbar spine, 384, *385*
      of vertebral body, 276
      vertebral giant cell tumor and, 279
   crush, of vertebral body, *379*
   distraction, of thoracolumbar spine, 385
   fatigue, of pars interarticularis, 198, 199, *200*
   gross vertebral, 276
   middle and lower cervical, 366
   neural arch, in thoracic and lumbar spine, 360
   of atlas, 358, *359*
   of pars interarticularis, acute, *196*, 199, 213
      fatigue, 198, 199, *200*
   slice flexion rotation, of thoracolumbar spine, 386
   stable and unstable, of spinal column, 361

Fracture(s) (*continued*)
  stable compression, of thoracolumbar spine, *385*
  thoracolumbar, circle-electric bed and, *388*
    classification of, 360
    patterns of neurologic loss in, 383t
      reduction of, 387–389, *388*
    treatment of, 380–390
  transverse process, 358, 384, *385*
  vertebral body, caused by tumors, 276
    cervical, 130, *131*
    crush, *379*
  vertical compression, of cervical spine, bone graft for, 130, *131*
Fracture-dislocation, of cervical spine, *378*
  of thoracic and lumbar spine, 360
  of thoracolumbar spine, mechanism of injury of, 381
  slice, of thoracolumbar spine, *387*
Fractures and dislocations, upper cervical, surgery for, 365, *365*
Frazier's cycles, 287
Freebody grafting, *148*
Freebody technique, of anterior lumbar spine fusion, 147, *149*
  spondylolisthesis and, 212
Friedreich's disease, 61
Froin's syndrome, 289
Function, permanent disturbance of, spinal cord injuries and, 361
Functional ambulator, 389
Fusion, atlanto-axial, 240
  atlanto-occipital, 240, *240*
    with Klippel-Feil deformity, *241*
  congenital, 240, *241*, *242*
  rib, thoracic hemivertebra with, *244*
  sacroiliac joint, in children, 159, *160*
    surgical technique in, 313, *314*
  spinal. *See* Spinal fusion.
Fusion time, anterior fusion in spinal tuberculosis and, 112t

Gain factors, psychophysiologic aspects of pain and, 396
Gait, in diastematomyelia, 236
  in spinal tuberculosis, 105
Ganglioneuroma, 291
Garner-Wells tongs, 363, *364*
Gelpi retractors, 155, *156*
Giant cell tumor, vertebral, 279
Giant motor unit potentials, 78
Glioblastoma multiforme, 291
Glioma(s), of medulla oblongata and spinal cord, surgical treatment of, 253–255, *254*
  of spinal cord, 291
Goldthwaite irons, 171, *172*
Graft, bone. *See* Bone graft.
Gram-negative rods, vertebral osteomyelitis and, 97
Granulation tissue, Pott's paraplegia and, 113
  tuberculous, permeation of vertebral body by, *108*
Granuloma, eosinophilic, 275, 284, *284*
  in spinal tuberculosis, 107
Gray matter, 42, 43, *43*
Gray substance, of spinal cord, 10
Great vessels and disc, handling of, in anterior lumbar fusion, *164*
Growth plates, vertebral, scoliosis and, 178
Gullet, high cervical cordotomy for pain in, 402

Halo, 368–372, *369*
  attached to body cast, *370*
  pelvic, *370*
  scoliosis and, 187, 370

Hamstrings, tight, spinal fusion in children and, 159
Harrington compression and distraction fixation, fractures of thoracolumbar spine and, 386, *386*, 387, 388, *389*
  scoliosis and, 187, *188*, 189
Head, descending motor and motor facilitory tracts and, 47
  neck and, injuries from acceleration-deceleration forces and, 347–354
    delayed degenerative changes in, *348, 349, 351, 352, 353*
Healing, bone. *See* Bone, healing of.
Heart, high cervical cordotomy for pain in, 402
Heel lift, in sciatic scoliosis, 425
Height, measurement of, in scoliosis, 182
Hemangioma, vertebral, 276, *277*
Hemangiopericytomas of spinal cord, *296*
  operating microscope in surgery for, 296
Hematomas, extradural, 289
Hemi-arch, vertebral, ossification in, 6
Hemiplegia cruciata, 61
Hemivertebra, 243, *244*
Heredity, scoliosis and, 178. *See also* Familial tendencies.
Herniated disc syndrome, 15. *See also* Disc, intervertebral, herniated.
Hibbs spinal fusion, *157*
High-frequency discharges, 79, *79*
  bizarre, 80
High turnover osteoporoses, 94
Hips, flexion deformity of, spinal osteotomy and, 168
History, psychophysiologic aspects of pain and, 395
  scoliosis in children and, 181
Horner's syndrome, 60
Horseshoe iliac grafts, 149, *150*, 151
Household ambulation, 389
Hurler's syndrome, 244
Hydatid cysts, 290
Hydrocephalus, postoperative, 233
  spina bifida and, 229
Hydromyelia, atlanto-occipital fusion and, 240
Hyperelastosis, scoliosis and, 181
Hyperextension back brace, spinal osteotomy for fixed flexion deformity and, 171
Hyperextension body cast, Goldthwaite irons and, spinal osteotomy for fixed flexion deformity and, *172*
Hyperextension injury, to cervical spine, *350, 359, 360*
Hypocalcemia, osteomalacias and, 92
Hypophosphatemic osteomalacias, 95
Hysteria and malingering, painful low back and, 306–309. *See also* Pain, psychologic aspects of.

Iatrogenic spondylolisthesis, 198, *200*, 213
Idiopathic scoliosis, 180
Iliac crest, cluneal nerves and, *145*
  for bone graft, in anterior lumbar interbody fusion, 163, *163*
  in paraspinal approach to lumbar spine, *155*. *See also* Bone graft; iliac.
Iliacus, 34
Iliocostalis, 29
Iliopsoas, 34
Ilium, obtaining bone from, through midline incision, *145*
Immunologic methods, vertebral column tumor diagnosis and, 276
Implants, spinal, for pain relief, 409
Incision, in anterior lumbar interbody fusion, 163
  in anterior open reduction of fractured cervical spine, 375
  in exposure of anterior arch of atlas, dens, and body of axis, 128
  in exposure of anterior vertebral bodies and disc spaces from C3 through C7, 126, *127*
  in exposure of transverse process and pedicles of C3 through C7, 129

Incision (*continued*)
 in Freebody technique of lumbar spinal fusion, 147
 in laminectomy, 118, *118*
 in lateral approach to cervical spine, 133, *134*
 in lateral extraperitoneal approach to lumbar spine, 139, *139*
 in lateral extrapleural approach to thoracic spine, 137, *138*
 in midline approach in lumbar spinal fusion, 143, *143, 145*
 in paraspinal approach to lumbar spine, 154, *155*
 in spinal osteotomy for fixed flexion deformity, 170
 in surgery for compressive lesions at foramen magnum, *254, 255, 257, 259, 267*
 in transinfrahyoid cervical operations, 123
 in transoral cervical operations, 122, *122*
 left flank, in lumbar spinal fusion, 149
Inclination, angle of, in scoliosis, 182
Industrial patient, painful low back in, 301
Infantile thoracic scoliosis, 180
Infection(s), disc space, 96
 in children, 97, *98*
 postoperative, in adults, 99, *99*
 pelvic, vertebral osteomyelitis and, 97
 spinal, 96–101
  antibacterial agents and, 100
  Bacteroides, paravertebral abscess and, 99
  pyogenic, 98
  radiographic features of, 336, *337–339*
  treatment of, 100. *See also* Tuberculosis of spine.
 transoral operative approach and, 121
 urinary tract, vertebral osteomyelitis and, 97
Infectious diseases, metabolic and, 85–114. *See also* specific diseases.
Inflammatory disorders, radiographic features of, *343*, 344
Infrahyoid muscles, 33
Injury(ies), associated, spinal cord injuries and, 362
 cervical spine. *See* Cervical spine.
 chance seat-belt, 385
 head and neck, from acceleration-deceleration forces, 347–354
  delayed degenerative changes in, *348, 349, 351, 352, 353*
 maxillofacial, halo and, 371
 mechanism of, in fracture-dislocations of thoracolumbar spine, 381
 penetrating, of spinal canal, 366
 spinal column, 358–361
  secondary to missile wounds, 361
 spinal cord, 357–367
  surgical treatment in, 362–366
 thoracic and lumbar spine, 360
Insertional activity, 79
Instrumentation, spinal, scoliosis and, 187
Interbody fusion. *See* Spinal fusion.
Intercostal nerves, 38
Interference, electromyographic, 77
 patterns of, *80, 81*
Intermediate column gray matter, 42
Intermedullary neoplasms at foramen magnum, 250
Intersegmental pathways, 47
Interspinal ligaments, 25
Interspinales, 32
Interspinous ligaments and spinous processes, excision of, degenerative diseases of thoracic spine and, 327
Intertransversarii, 32
Intertransverse ligaments, 26
Intervertebral disc. *See* Disc, intervertebral.
Intervertebral foramen, effects of flexion on, *163*
Intervertebral ligaments, at thoracolumbar junction, *381*
Intervertebral spaces, 62
Intradural extramedullary tumors. *See* Tumors, intradural, extramedullary.

Intradural intramedullary tumors. *See* Tumors, intradural, intramedullary.
Intramedullary cysts of spinal cord, juxtamedullary and, surgical treatment of, 293
Intramedullary glioma, *254*, 291
Intramedullary tumors. *See* Tumors, intramedullary.
Invagination, basilar, 262, *264*
 posterior decompression for, 264
Ischemia of spinal cord, 361
Isthmic spondylolisthesis. *See* Spondylolisthesis, isthmic.

Jacket, Kydex body, slice flexion rotation fracture of thoracolumbar spine and, *387*
 plaster, following posterior spinal fusion for scoliosis, 190
 plastic and, in scoliosis, 186
Jewett brace, *423*
Joint(s), anatomy of spine and, 27
 costotransverse, 324
 costovertebral, 324
 in embryo, 5
 sacroiliac. *See* Sacroiliac joint.
Juvenile thoracic scoliosis, 180
Juxtamedullary cysts of spinal cord, intramedullary and, surgical treatment of, 293

Kidney, as infection focus in spinal tuberculosis, 103, *104*
 lateral deviation and, 105
Klebsiella, vertebral osteomyelitis and, 97
Klippel-Feil syndrome, 241, *241*
Knight brace, *427*
Kuskokwim disease, 204
Kyphoscoliosis, 179
 cervical-thoracic neural arch defect and, *225*
 in diastematomyelia, 236
Kyphosis, compression fractures of thoracolumbar spine and, 384
 congenital, spinal fusion in, 146
 in spinal tuberculosis, 105, *106, 107*
  anterior fusion and, 112
  secondary changes with, 109
 thoracic, management of, 424

Lamina(e)
 loose, decompression and excision of, in spondylolisthesis, 218–222, *220*
  fusing part of, to sacrum, 158, *158*
 removal of, to expose dura mater, *119*
Laminectomy, 117–120
 cervical spondylosis and, 317
 low back pain following, *330*
 lumbar spondylosis and, 320
 spinal cord injuries and, 363
 spinal implants for pain relief and, 409
 spinal tuberculosis and, 112
 spondylolisthesis due to pars interarticularis elongation and, 213
Latent period, in spinal tuberculosis, 104
Lateral approach to cervical spine, 132–136, *134, 135*
Lateral deviation, in spinal tuberculosis, 105, *106*
Lateral extrapleural and extraperitoneal approaches to thoracic and lumbar spine, 137–141
Lateral flexion injuries, to cervical spine, 360
Lateral retroperitoneal approach to lumbar spine, *139–141*
Lateral retropleural approach to thoracic spine, *138*
Lateral-wedge thoracolumbar fractures, 360
Latissimus dorsi, 28
Left flank approach, in lumbar spinal fusion, 149
Leg, measurement of, in scoliosis, 182

Lesions, compressive, at foramen magnum. *See* Foramen magnum, compressive lesions at.
  of cauda equina, 60
  segmental distribution of, in Pott's disease, 112t
  spinal cord, 60, 61
    assessment of, 53
  tumor-like bone, of vertebrae, 275, 283
    bone tumors and, 274-286
Levator scapulae, 29
Lidocain hydrochloride injection, 302
Life stress index, psychologic aspects of pain and, 396
Ligament(s), anatomy of spine and, 24-27
  costotransverse, scoliosis and, 178
  dentate, 41, percutaneous cervical cordotomy and, *407*
  interspinous, excision of spinous processes and,
    degenerative diseases of thoracic spine and, 327
  intervertebral, at thoracolumbar junction, *381*
  pain in spondylolisthesis and, 208
  spinal, in embryo, 5
Ligamentum(a) flavum(a), *26*
  removal of, in laminectomy, 119
Ligamentum nuchae, 25
Lipman-Cobb technique, curvature in scoliosis and, 183, *183*
Lipomas, 291
Lipomeningocele, 291
List, in evaluating painful low back, 308
Living pathology, in spinal tuberculosis, 107
"Localizer," Risser, 186
Locked facet, in cervical spine fracture, 376, *377*
Longissimus, 29
Longitudinal ligaments, 24
  posterior, *26*, 27
Longus capitus, 34
Longus colli, 34
Lordoscoliosis, 179
Lordosis, abnormal lumbar, 424
  compensatory, in spinal tuberculosis, 105, 109
Low back, pain in. *See* Pain, low back and Painful low back.
  problems with, disability and, 329
  sensory areas in, *144*
Low turnover osteoporoses, 94
Lumbago, acute attack of, 302
Lumbar cord, lesions of, 60
Lumbar disc, herniated, surgical treatment of, *320*
Lumbar disc disease, spinal fusion and, 142
Lumbar interbody fusion. *See* Lumbar spine, fusion of.
Lumbar lordosis, abnormal, 424
Lumbar nerves, posterior primary divisions of, sensory areas in low back supplied by, *144*
  transverse processes and, *144*
Lumbar plexus, 38
Lumbar puncture, spinal tumor diagnosis and, 288
Lumbar spine, articulated, *22*
  as osteotomy site, 169
  fusion of, 142-153
    anterior, *148*
      Freebody technique for, 147-149
      left flank approach in, 149
    anterior interbody, 146, 162-167, *148, 149, 150, 151*
      following laminectomy, *166*
      primary, *166*
      technique of, 163-165
    indications for, 329
    midline approach in, 143-146, *145*
    other techniques for, 150-152
    postoperative care in, 152
    solidity of, 152
  hemisected, cauda equina and, *37*
  lateral retroperitoneal approach to, *139-141*
  operations on, approach to failure of, 328-333, *331*

paraspinal approach to, 154-161
  radiographic anatomy of, 69, *69*, 70, *70, 72*
  surgical treatment of, indications for, 328-330
  thoracic and. *See* Thoracic spine; Thoracolumbar spine.
  tuberculosis of, lateral deviation in, *106*
Lumbar spondylosis. *See* Spondylosis, lumbar.
Lumbar vertebra(e), 20-22
  ligaments and, *26*
  spondylolisthesis defect of pars and, *195*
  third, *22, 23*
  thoracic and, facet configuration of, *381*
Lumbar vertebral canal, narrow, 320
Lumbosacral angle, 23
Lumbosacral area, in spondylolisthesis, at operation, *219*
  postoperative infection in, *99*
Lumbosacral disc, 15
Lumbosacral nerve plexus, brachial and, development of, 8
Lumbosacral pain, thoracic cordotomy for, 400
Lung, as infection focus in spinal tuberculosis, 103
  penetration of, abscess in spinal tuberculosis and, 106
Lytic type of isthmic spondylolisthesis, 194-197
  treatment of, 208-212

Male sexual dysfunction, anterior lumbar interbody fusion and, 147, 165
Malignant bone tumor, primary, 280
  secondary, 281-283
Malignant disease. *See* name of specific diseases and structures.
Malingering, hysteria and, painful low back and, 306-309. *See also* Pain, psychologic aspects of.
Mantle layer, of neural tube, 8
  of spinal cord, 10
Marfan's syndrome, 181
Marginal layer, of neural tube, 8
  of spinal cord, 11
Mass, fibrocartilaginous, spondylolisthesis and, 207, 218, *221*
Maxillofacial injuries, halo and, 371
Median nerve, evoked sensory responses and, 82, *83*
  motor nerve conduction velocity and, 81, *82*
Medication, in operant conditioning program, psychologic aspects of pain and, 397
Medulla oblongata, spinal cord and, surgical treatment of glioma of, 253-255, *254*
Medullary arteries, 48
Medulloblastoma, 291
Mehrig-Williams plates, 387
Membrane, arachnoid, 40
  atlantooccipital, 27, *27*
  tectorial, 27
Meninges, development of, 11
  spinal cord, 40
Meningioma, at foramen magnum, surgical treatment of, 255, *257, 258*, 260
  of spinal cord, 290
    surgical treatment of, 293
      operating microscope in, 296
Meningocele, 12, *12*, 227, *227*
  anterior sacral, 234
  cervical, *227*
  intrathoracic, 233
  lumbar, *228*
Meningomyelitis, tuberculous, 113
Meningomyelocele, 12
Metabolic diseases, infectious and, 85-114. *See also* specific diseases.
  radiographic features of, 335-336, *336*
Metabolism, scoliosis and, 178

Metastases, carcinoma, to spinal cord, 289
  to vertebrae, 281, 282, *282*
Microbiologic considerations, in infections of spine, 97, 100
Microfractures, vertebral, 276
Microscope, operating, in spinal cord surgery, 295-298
  in transoral operative approach, 122, *122*, 123
Microscopy, vertebral column tumor diagnosis and, 275
Mid-dorsal spine, hemisected, cord and, 36
Midline approach, in lumbar spinal fusion, 143-146, *143*, *145*
Midline incision, in paraspinal approach to lumbar spine, *155*
Milwaukee brace, *425*
  scoliosis and, 185, *185*
Minnesota Multiphasic Personality Inventory,
    chemonucleolysis and, 329
  psychophysiologic aspects of pain and, 396
Monamine antimetabolites, spinal cord injuries and, 363
Morquio's disease, 243
Motion, cervical intersegmental, 15
  in thoracic spine, 19
  spinal, 27
Motor and motor facilitory tracts, descending, 45-47
Motor efferent pathways, *46*
Motor nerve conduction velocity, 81, *82*
Motor pathways, major sensory and, of spinal cord, *405*
Motor unit, 77
Motor unit potentials, 77, *77*
Motor weakness, percutaneous cervical cordotomy and, 406
Movement, voluntary, 47
Mucopolysaccharidosis 1, 244
Multifidus spinae, 32
Multiple myeloma, 280, *281*
Multiple sclerosis, 61
Muscle fiber disease, electromyogram in, 81
Muscle tone, control of, 47
  of flexor muscle groups, 46
  pathways for sensation of, 45
Muscles, anatomy of spine and, 28-36
  action of, 34-36
  contraction of, electromyography and, 80
  deep, 29-34
  examination of, spinal cord lesions and, 55
  extrinsic, acting on spine, 33
    of spine, *28*
  innervation of, spinal segments and, 56-59t
  intervertebral, in embryo, 4
  intrinsic, of spine, *30*, *31*
  spasm of, test for, in painful low back, 306
  suboccipital triangle and, *33*
  weakness of, test for, in painful low back, 307
Muscular activity
  forward bending and, *420*
  spinal flexion and, *420*
Myelin, in spinal cord, 11
Myelin sheath, of peripheral nerve fibers, development of, 8
Myelitis, tuberculous, 108
Myelography, acceleration-deceleration injury and, 352
  compressive lesions at foramen magnum and, 252
  fracture dislocations of thoracolumbar spine and, 388
  spinal cord tumors and, 289
Myeloma, multiple, 280, *281*
Myelomatosis, 280, *281*
Myelomeningocele, 12, 227
  Arnold-Chiari malformation and, *232*
  repair of, *231*
  sessile lumbar, *228*, *229*
Myelotomy, longitudinal, spasticity and, 415
Myokymia, 79
Myopathic motor unit potentials, 77
Myopathy(ies), 77
  fibrillations of, 78

Myotome, 3
Myotonic discharges, 79

Nascent motor unit potentials, 78
Neck, head and, injuries from acceleration-deceleration
    forces and, 347-354
  delayed degenerative changes in, *348*, *349*, *351*, *352*, *353*
  high cervical cordotomy for pain in, 402
  paralysis of, halo and, *370*
  trunk and, control of, 46
Neoplasm, extradural, *292*
  intermedullary, diagnosis of compressive lesions at
    foramen magnum and, 250
  intradural extramedullary, *292*
  intradural intramedullary, *292*. See also Tumor(s).
Nerve action potentials, 80
Nerve plexuses, brachial and lumbosacral, development of, 8
Nerve roots, 62
  compression of, disc protrusion and, *319*, *320*
  redundant, compression by, 321
  relations of, to disc, *38*
Nerve stimulation studies, 81-84
Nerve(s), anatomy of spine and, 37
  cluneal, iliac crest and, *145*
  evoked sensory responses of, 82
  lumbar, posterior primary divisions of, sensory areas in
      low back supplied by, *144*
    transverse processes and, *144*
  motor, conduction velocity of, 81, *82*
  segmental, in embryo, 4
  severence of, electromyography in, 80, 81
  spinal, cutaneous branches of, *14*
    development of, 8
    neuroblasts and, growth of, *9*
    origin of, 41
    posterior primary divisions of, midline and paraspinal
      approach to lumbar spine and, 159
    spinal cord and, organization of, *8*
    spinal cord segments and, relation to vertebral spinous
      processes of, *42*
Neural arch, 14, 62
  absent, congenital fusion and, *241*
  with posterior osseous tubercle, *240*
  defect of, cervical-thoracic, kyphoscoliosis and, *225*
    lumbar, *233*
    meningocele and, *228*
    thoracic hemivertebra and, *244*
  fracture of, in thoracic and lumbar spine, 360
Neural canal, at T12-L1 junction, neural elements within,
    381
Neural crests, neural tube and, origin of, *7*
Neural foramen, transverse processes, pedicles and, exposure
    of, *130*
Neural tube, 7
  cell specialization in, 8, *8*
  neural crests and, origin of, *7*
Neurenteric cysts, 238
Neurilemomas, 290, *296*
Neurinomas, 290
Neuroanatomy, 40-50
Neuroblast(s), development of, 8, *9*
  spinal nerve and, growth of, *9*
Neuroblastoma, scoliosis secondary to radiation and, 181
Neurofibroma, anterolateral at foramen magnum, surgical
    treatment of, 258-260, *259*
  intradural, myelogram of, *341*
  of spinal cord, 290
    surgical treatment of, 293
      operating microscope in, 296

Neurofibromatosis, scoliosis and, 181
Neurologic deficit, transitory, spinal cord injuries and, 361
Neurologic evaluation, 53-61
Neurologic loss, thoracolumbar spinal fractures and patterns of, 383t
Neuromuscular disease, electrodiagnosis of, 76-84
Neuromuscular scoliosis, 180
Neuron series, tumors of, 291
Neuropathy(ies), 77, 81
  fibrillations of, 78
Nodes, Schmorl's, *316*
Noise, end-plate, 80
Notocord, 4
Nucleus pulposus, herniation of, *316*

Oblique capital muscles, 32
Obliquus externus, 34
Obliquus internus, 34
Occipital bone, hyperplasia or hypertrophy of, surgical treatment of, 264, *265*
Occipital vertebra, 240
Occipito-atlantal dislocation, 358
Occipito-atloid articulation, hyperplasia or hypertrophy of, 264
Occiput, atlas and, congenital fusion of, *240*
Oligodendrogliomas, 291
Omohyoid muscle, 33
Open reduction, anterior, of fractured cervical spine, 373-379
Operating microscope, in spinal cord surgery, 295-298
  in transoral operative approach, 122, *122*, 123
Operative approaches, 115-174. *See also* specific operative approaches.
Orthoses, biomechanics of spine and, 417-428
  principles of use of, 422-428
Ossification, centers of, in thoracic vertebra and ribs, 5, *5*
Osteoarthritis, radiographic features of, 341-344, *341*
Osteoblastoma of bone, vertebral benign, 278, *278*
Osteochondrodystrophies, scoliosis and, 181
Osteodystrophy, posttraumatic, 93
Osteogenesis imperfecta, 244
  scoliosis and, 181
Osteogenous stage, in spinal development, 5
Osteoid, 89
  increased, conditions associated with, 92t
Osteoid border, 89
Osteoid seam, 89
Osteoid-osteoma, vertebral, 277, *278*
Osteolytic carcinoma metastases, 281, *282*
Osteomalacias, 89-92
  clinical features of, 93t
  features of surgical import in, 94t
  osteoporoses and, in spinal surgery, 87-95
  radiographic features of, 335, *336*
  specific conditions of, 95
Osteomyelitis, vertebral, 96, 98, *98*
Osteophytosis, radiographic features of, *342*, 344
Osteoplastic carcinoma metastases, 282, *282*
Osteoporosis(es), 87-89
  anatomic patterns of bone loss in, *88*
  clinical features of, 89t
  osteomalacias and, in spinal surgery, 87-95
  prognosis and therapy in, 90t
  radiographic features of, *88*, 335, *336*
  specific conditions of, 92-95
Osteotomy of spine for fixed flexion deformity, 168-174
  anatomy of, *169*
Outriggers, 426, *426*

Pachymeningitis externe, 108
Pain, 391-410
  abdominal, rhizotomy for, 400
  back, exercises for, 428
  chest wall, rhizotomy for, 400
  cordotomy and rhizotomy for, 399-403
  interbody fusion of lumbar spine and, 147
  intractable, percutaneous cervical cordotomy for, 404-408
    thoracic cordotomy for, 401, *402*
  low back, following laminectomy, *330*
    lumbar interbody fusion and, 152
    management of, orthroses in, 426
    of sacroiliac joint origin, 311-314. *See also* Painful low back.
  lumbar spinal fusion and, 142
  lumbosacral, thoracic cordotomy for, 400
  perceptions of, spinal cord lesions and, 53
  psychologic aspects of, 393-398
  psychosocial factors in, 393
  radicular, in spondylolisthesis, 218
  spinal implants for relief of, 409
  spinal tuberculosis and, 104
  spondylolisthesis and, 207, 218
  temperature and, pathways for, 43
  thoracic radicular, 323
  treatment program in, 396
  upper abdominal and chest wall, rhizotomy for, 400
  visceral, pathways for, 44
Painful low back, acute attack of, treatment of, 302
  hysteria and malingering and, 306-309
  lumbar interbody fusion and, 147
  nonoperative treatment of, 301-310
  routine instructions for care of, 303.
  tests for evaluating, 306-309. *See also* Pain, low back.
Paralysis, cruciate, 61
  muscular, scoliosis and, 178
  of neck, halo and, *370*
  respiratory, percutaneous cervical cordotomy and, 407
  spinal cord injuries and, 361, 363
Paraplegia, anterior fusion in spinal tuberculosis and, 112t
  long-term problems of, 390
  Pott's, spinal tuberculosis and, 105, 108, 113
  rehabilitation in, 389
Paraspinal approach to lumbar spine, 154-161
Paravertebral abscess, 99
Pars interarticularis, acute fracture of, *196*, 199, 213
  defects of, *196*
  elongation of, without separation, 197, *199*, 212
  fatigue fracture of, 198, 199, *200*
  high-grade spondylolisthesis and, *195*
  isthmic spondylolisthesis and, 194, *195*
  lesions of, in twins, *198*
  unilateral separation of, treatment of, 212
Pathways, ascending sensory, 43-45
  for sensation of muscle tone, 45
  intersegmental, 47
  major sensory and motor, *405*
  motor efferent, *46*
  pain and temperature, 43
  sensory afferent, *44*
  touch, pressure, and position sense, 45
  visceral pain, 44
Patient description, psychophysiologic aspects of pain and, 395
Pedicles, 62
  transverse process and, of C3 through C7, exposure of, 129, *130*
Peduncular spondylolisthesis, 204, *204*
  treatment of, 216

Pelvic halo, *370*
Pelvic infections, vertebral osteomyelitis and, 97
Pelvic obliquity, in scoliosis, 182
Pelvis, leveling of, painful low back and, 305
Peritoneal contents, handling of, in anterior lumbar
     interbody fusion, *164*
Peroneal nerve, motor nerve conduction velocity and, 81
Phase lag pool loss, 94
Phenol-mediated rhizotomy, in spastic conditions, 414
Phenomenon, revascular, 109, *110*
Photographic examination, in scoliosis, 182
Physical findings, psychophysiologic aspects of pain and,
     396
Physical treatments, in operant conditioning program,
     psychologic aspects of pain and, 397
Pia mater, 40, 41
Pilonidal sinus, 12, 234
Plantar flexion of foot test, in evaluating painful low back,
     308
Plaster jacket, following posterior spinal fusion for scoliosis,
     190
     plastic and, in scoliosis, 186
Plexus(es), brachial, 38
     lumbosacral and, development of, 8
     cervical, 38
     lumbar, 38
     sacral coccygeal, 38
Polyphasic motor unit potentials, 77, *77*
Position, in laminectomy, 117
     in osteotomy of spine for fixed flexion deformity, *170*
     sense of, pathways for touch, pressure and, 45
Positive potentials, 79
Positive sharp waves, 79
Positive waves, 79, *79*
Posterior approach in spinal fusion, scoliosis and, 187-190
Posterior interbody fusion, reduction of spondylolisthesis
     and, 210, *212*
Posterior median septum, 10
Posterior midline approach, in interbody fusion of lumbar
     spine, 151
Posterior primary divisions of lumbar nerves, sensory areas
     in low back supplied by, *144*
     transverse processes and, *144*
Post-laryngeal wall, midline incision of, *122*
Postmenopausal osteoporosis, 92
Postoperative care, anterior lumbar interbody fusion, and,
     164
     lumbar spinal fusion and, 152
     paraspinal approach to lumbar spine and, 161
     spinal osteotomy for fixed flexion deformity and, 171
Postoperative infection, 96, *99*, 99
Posttraumatic osteodystrophy, 93
Postural reduction, in fractures of thoracolumbar spine, *388*
Posture, balanced vertical, *419*
     control of, with vertical backrest, *421*
Potential(s), fibrillation, 78, *78*
     motor unit, 77, *77*
     nerve action, 80
     positive, 79
Pott's disease, segmental distribution of lesions in, 112t
Pott's paraplegia, spinal tuberculosis and, 105, 108, 113
Pressure, touch, position sense and, pathways for, 45
     yielding of spine upon, in spinal tuberculosis, 107
Primordium, vertebral, 4
Prostate, carcinoma metastases and, 281
Pseudoarthrosis, posterior, bone graft position and, *163*
     posterior spinal fusion for scoliosis and, 189
Pseudofracture, 90
Pseudomonas aeruginosa, vertebral osteomyelitis and, 97

Pseudo-myotonic discharges, 80
Pseudo-retrospondylolisthesis, *205*
Pseudospondylolisthesis, 202
Psoas major, 20, 34
Psoas minor, 34
Psychologic and social factors, failure of lumbar spine
     operations and, 329
Psychologic aspects of pain, 393-398
Psychologic tests, psychophysiologic aspects of pain and, 396
Psychophysiologic aspects of pain, 394
     diagnosis of, 395
Psychosocial factors, pain and, 393
Pulmonary evaluation, in scoliosis, 184
Pus, Pott's paraplegia and, 113
     spinal tuberculosis and, 108
Pyogenic infection, spinal, 98
Pyramidal tract, destruction of, 60

Quadratus lumborum, 20, 34
Queckenstedt test, 289

Rachischisis, 7, 228
Radial nerve, evoked sensory responses and, 82
Radiation, scoliosis and, 181
Radicular arteries, 48
Radicular pain, in spondylolisthesis, 218
     thoracic, 323
Radicular veins, 49
Radioactive scanning, vertebral column tumor diagnosis and,
     276
Radiologic examination, 62-75
     compressive lesions at foramen magnum and, 252
     fractures of thoracolumbar spine and, 383
     injuries from acceleration-deceleration forces and, 349
     lytic type of isthmic spondylolisthesis and, 194
     osteoporosis of spine and, *88*
     scoliosis and, 183
     spinal cord tumors and, 288
     transoral operative approach and, 122, 123
     vertebral column tumors and, 275
Rami, anterior and posterior primary, 324
Ramus entrapment syndrome, posterior primary, 325, 327
Raney technique for anterior lumbar spine fusion, 162-167
     retractors for, *149*
Realignment, decompression and, in anterior open reduction
     of fractured cervical spine, 375
Rectus abdominis, 34
Rectus capitis anterior, 34
Rectus capitis lateralis, 34
Reduction, anterior open, of fractured cervical spine, 373-379
     fractures of thoracolumbar spine and, 387-389, *388*
     spondylolisthesis and, 209-212
Reflex activity, 47
Reflexes, righting, 425
Rehabilitation of paraplegic, 389
Reinforcement, social, in operant conditioning program,
     psychologic aspects of pain and, 397
Remodeling, of bone, 90
Renal failure, chronic, osteomalacia of, 95
Respiratory impulses, 47
Respiratory paralysis, percutaneous cervical cordotomy and,
     407
Reticulospinal tract(s), 47
     destruction of, 60
Retractors, Gelpi, in paraspinal approach to lumbar spine,
     155, *156*

Retractors, Gelpi (*continued*)
  in anterior fusion of lumbar spine, *149, 152*
  midline approach in lumbar spinal fusion and, *144*
  obtaining bone from ilium and, *145*
Retroperitoneal approach, lateral, to lumbar spine, *139-141*
Retropleural approach, lateral, to thoracic spine, *138*
Retrospondylolisthesis, 204-206, *205, 206*
Revascular phenomenon, 109, *110*
Reverse spondylolisthesis, 204-206, *205, 206*
Rheumatoid arthritis, radiographic features of, *343,* 344, *344, 345*
Rhizotomy, alcohol-mediated, in spastic conditions, 414
  cordotomy and, for pain, 399-403
    phenol-mediated, in spastic conditions, 414
    posterior spinal, 400, *401*
    spasticity and, 414, *415*
Rhomboid muscles, 29
Rib(s), fusion of, thoracic hemivertebra with, *244*
  interbody fusion of lumbar spine and, 151, *151*
  removal of, in anterior approach in spinal fusion, 190
  spinal tuberculosis and, 109
  vertebra and, chondrification centers in, in embryo, *5*
Rib hump, in scoliosis, 182, *182*
Righting reflexes, 425
Rigidity, in spinal tuberculosis, 105
Risser "localizer," 186
Robinson approach, in exposure of anterior vertebral bodies
  and disc spaces from C3 through C7, 125-128
Roentgen survey, 335-346. *See also* Radiologic examination.
Root cycle, spinal cord tumors and, 288
Rotation, vertebral, in scoliosis, 184, *184*
Rotator spinae, 32
Rotatores, 32
Rubrospinal tract, 46

Sacral agenesis, 239, *239*
Sacral bar, in spondylolisthesis, *210*
Sacral coccygeal plexus, 38
Sacral dysgenesis, *239*
Sacral sparing, in thoracolumbar fracture, 382
Sacroiliac joint
  fusion of, in children, 159, *160*
    surgical technique in, 313, *314*
  injection of, 311, 312, *312, 313*
  low back pain and, 311-314
Sacrospinalis, 29-31
Sacrospinalis-splitting approach to lumbar spine, 154-161
Sacrum, 22
  coccyx and, *23, 24, 25*
  fusing part of loose lamina to, 158, *158*
  radiographic anatomy of, 70, *71*
  wide open, pars interarticularis defect and, 195
    pars interarticularis elongation and, 198
Salmonella, antibacterial agents and, 100
  vertebral osteomyelitis and, 97
Saw-tooth waves, 79
Scalenes, 34
Scapula, anatomy of spine and, 29
  trapezius muscle and, 28
Schmorl's nodes, *316*
Schwannomas, 290.
Sciatic scoliosis, management of, 424
  spondylolisthesis in children and, 207
Sciatica, tests for evaluating, 306-309
  traction and, 305
Sclerosis, amyotrophic lateral, 61
Sclerotome, 3, *4*
Scoliosis, 177-192
  clinical evaluation in, 181-185

halo and, 187, 370
  pathogenesis of, 178
  radiographic features of, 336, *339*
  sciatic, management of, 424
  spondylolisthesis in children and, 207
  terminology and classification of, 179-181
  treatment of, 185-191
Scoliosis Research Society, classification of structural spine
  deformity of, 179
Seat-belt injury, 385
Semispinalis muscle group, 32
Senile osteoporosis, 93
Sensory afferent pathways, *44*
Sensory and motor pathways, of spinal cord, *405*
Sensory areas, in low back, supplied by posterior primary
  divisions, *144*
Sensory dermatomes, *54, 55*
Sensory latencies, median, *83*
Sensory level, percutaneous cervical cordotomy and, 407
Sensory pathways, ascending, 43-45
  major motor and, of spinal cord, *405*
Sensory responses, evoked, 82
Sensory tests, spinal cord lesions and, 53
Septum, posterior median, 10
Sequestra, Pott's paraplegia and, 113
  spinal tuberculosis and, 108, *110*
Sequestrated discs, in spinal tuberculosis, 108
Serratus muscles, 29
Sexual dysfunction, male, in anterior lumbar interbody
  fusion, 147, 165
Shoe lifts, painful low back and, 305
Shoulder depressors, posture control with vertical backrest
  and, *421*
Sinovertebral nerves, 38
Sinus, congenital dermal, 234-236, *235*
  formation of, in spinal tuberculosis, 106
  pilonidal, 12, 234
Sitting base, vertical backrest and, *421*
Skeleton, osteomalacic state of, 90
  osteoporotic, 87
    radiographic features of, *88*
Skin, anatomy of spine and, 13
Slice flexion rotation fracture, of thoracolumbar spine, 386
Slice fracture dislocation, of thoracolumbar spine, *387*
Slip, Hibbs spinal fusion and, *157*
  spondylolisthesis and, 193, *197, 200, 203, 205, 206, 208, 215, 216*
  paraspinal approach in lumbar spinal fusion and, 157, 158, *159*
Social factors, psychologic and, failure of lumbar spine
  operations and, 329
Social reinforcement, in operant conditioning program,
  psychologic aspects of pain and, 397
Spasm, muscle, test for, in painful low back, 306
Spasmotic torticollis, 415
Spastic conditions, neurosurgical management of, 413-416
Spina bifida, 7
  dysplastic spondylolisthesis and, 201
  elongation of pars interarticularis and, 198
  hydrocephalus and, 229
  pars interarticularis defect and, 195
Spina bifida cystica, 227-233
  operation in, 230-233, *231*
Spina bifida occulta, 224-227, *225, 226*
  treatment of, 226
Spinal arteries, 47-49
Spinal canal, penetrating wounds of, 366
Spinal column
  injury to, 358-361
    secondary to missile wounds, 361

Spinal column (*continued*)
  stable and unstable fractures of, 361
Spinal cord, anatomy of, 40-50
  anomalies of, 11, *12*
  anterior median fissure of, 10
  arterial system of, 47-49
    venous system and, *48*
  cervical, diagnosis of lesions of, 60
  development of, 7-12, *8, 9, 10*
  extent of, *41*
  in three month embryo, *9*
  injuries of, 357-367
    surgical treatment in, 362-366
  ischemia of, 361
  lesions of, 60, 61
    assessment of, 53
    in vertical compression fracture of cervical spine, 130, *131*
  major sensory and motor pathways of, *405*
  medulla oblongata and, surgical treatment of glioma of, 253-255, *254*
  meninges of, 40
  operating microscope in surgery on, 295-298
  Pott's paraplegia and, 113
  protection of function of, in anterior open reduction of fractured cervical spine, 373-375
  segments of, spinal nerves and, relation to vertebral spinous processes of, *42*
  spinal nerve and, organization of, *8*
  spine and, development of, 3-12, *9*
  sulci, and gray and white matter of, *43*
  tumors of, 287-294
    pathologic classification of, 289-291
    radiographic features of, 340, *340*
    surgical treatment of, 291-293
      operating microscope in, 295-298
Spinal fusion, anterior, in spinal tuberculosis, 111, 112t
  congenital, *241, 242*
  congenital kyphosis and, 146
  Hibbs, *157*
  interbody, anterior intervertebral disc excision and, acceleration-deceleration injury and, 352
  lumbar. *See* Lumbar spine, fusion of.
  osteotomy for fixed flexion deformity and, 171
  posterior interbody, reduction of spondylolisthesis and, 210, *212*
  postoperative use of orthroses and, 427
  scoliosis and, 187-191
  spondylolisthesis and, 198, 209, 212
  tight hamstrings in children and, 159
Spinal implants, for pain relief, 409
Spinal instrumentation scoliosis and, 187. *See also* specific devices.
Spinal nerves. *See* Nerves.
Spinal osteomyelitis, 98
Spinal shock, spinal cord tumors and, 288
Spinal stenosis, decompression and, 215
Spinal tuberculosis. *See* Tuberculosis of spine.
Spinalis group, 29
Spine, anatomy of. *See* Anatomy.
  anomalies of, 7, *7*
  biomechanics of, orthoses and, 417-428
  congenital anomalies of, 223-245. *See also* specific anomalies.
  cervical. *See* Cervical spine.
  cleft, 7
  deformity(ies) of, 175-245. *See also* specific deformities.
    fixed flexion, correction of, *172, 173, 174*
      osteotomy of spine for, 168-174
    halo and, 370

  development of, 3-7
  distraction forces to, flexion of body and, in fracture-dislocations of thoracolumbar spine, 382
  fully flexed, *421*
  hemisected, cord and, *35, 36, 37*
  infections of. *See* Infection(s) and Tuberculosis of spine.
  ligaments and. *See* Ligament(s).
  lumbar. *See* Lumbar spine.
  muscles of. *See* Muscles.
  osteotomy of, for fixed flexion deformity, 168-174
  roentgenogram of, in osteoporosis, *88*
  segments of, muscle innervation and, 56-59t
  spinal cord and, development of, 3-12, *9*
  thoracic. *See* Thoracic spine.
  thoracolumbar. *See* Thoracolumbar spine.
  tuberculosis of. *See* Tuberculosis of spine.
  yielding upon pressure of, in spinal tuberculosis, 107
Spinocerebellar tracts, 45
Spinotectal tract, 44
Spinothalamic tracts, 43, 45
  destruction of, 60
Spinous processes, interspinous ligaments and, excision of, degenerative diseases of thoracic spine and, 327
  removal of, in laminectomy, 119, *119*
  spinal nerves and spinal cord segments and, *42*
Splenius muscles, 29
Splint, posterior spinal fusion for scoliosis and, 190
Spondylitis, ankylosing, radiographic features of, 343, 344
  tuberculous, radiographic features of, *338*
Spondylolisthesis, anterior interbody fusion of lumbar spine in, 147
  chemonucleolysis and, 212
  classification of, 194t
  degenerative, 202-204, *202, 203, 215*
    isthmic and, occurrence of, 203t
    treatment of, 213-216, *216*
  dysplastic, 201, *201*, 213
  etiology of, 194-208
  in children, 194, 206
    reduction of, 209-212, *211*
    surgical treatment of, 209
  isthmic, degenerative and, occurrence of, 203t
    treatment of, 208-213
    types of, 194-201
  lumbosacral area in, at operation, *219*
  pain in, 207, 218
  pars interarticularis and. *See* Pars interarticularis.
  peduncular, 204, *204*
    treatment of, 216
  radiographic features of, 336
  treatment of, 208-222
    conservative, fusion with and without reduction, 208-217
    excision of loose lamina and decompression in, 218-222, *220*
Spondylolisthesis acquisita, 198, *200*
  treatment of, 213
Spondylosis, 299-333
  cervical, 316-318
    surgical treatment of, 317
  lumbar, 318-320
    laminectomy in, 320
    wedge removal in, *321*
Spondylotic degeneration, *316*
Spongioblastoma, 291
Stabilization, Dwyer correction and, 187, *189*
  in cervical spine fracture, 378
Staphylococcus aureus, vertebral osteomyelitis and, 97
Stenosis, spinal, decompression and, 215
Stereoscopy, 63
Stereotaxic reduction, of cervical spine dislocation, *374, 376*

Sternocleidomastoid muscle, 33
Sternohyoid muscle, 33
Sternothyroid muscle, 33
Sterotaxis, 376
Straps, 425
Strength-duration curves, nerve stimulation studies and, 83, *83*
Stress index, psychologic aspects of pain and, 396
Subacute combined degeneration, 61
Subcostal nerve, 38
Subependymal gliomas, 291
Subluxations, Pott's paraplegia and, 113
Suboccipital muscles, 32
Suboccipital triangle and muscles, *33*
Subperiosteal dissection, in laminectomy, *118,* 119
Sudek's atrophy, 93
Sulci, spinal cord, gray and white matter and, *43*
Sulcocommissural arteries, 49
Sulcus limitans, in neural tube, 8
Superficial spinal muscles, 28
Supraspinal ligament, 25
Sural nerve, evoked sensory responses and, 82
Surcingle system, Von Lackum, 186
Sweat glands, facial, 47
Sweating, on trunk and extremities, 47
Swimmers view, 67
Syndrome, aneurysmal, 108
    Brown-Sequard, 60
        spinal cord tumors and, 288
    cervical cord, 60, 360, 362
    costovertebral, 325, 327
    Froin's, 289
    herniated disc, 15. *See also* Disc, intervertebral, herniated.
    Horner's, 60
    Hurler's, 244
    Klippel-Feil, 241, *241*
    Marfan's, 181
    posterior primary ramus entrapment, 325, 327
Syringomyelia, 60, 269-273, *271, 272,* 290
    atlanto-occipital fusion and, 240
    decompression surgery in, 270t, 270-273, *273*
Systems review, psychophysiologic aspects of pain and, 395

Tailbone. *See* Coccyx
Taillard's criteria, 219
Taylor brace, 426, *426*
Tectorial membrane, 27
Tectospinal systems, 46
Tectospinal tract, 46
Tectotegmentospinal tract, 47
Tegmentospinal systems, destruction of, 60
Temperature, pain and, pathways for, 43
Teratomatous cysts, 290
Tests, in evaluating painful low back, 306-309
Thoracic cord, lesions of, 60
Thoracic cordotomy, 401, *402*
Thoracic disc derangement, 323
    differential diagnosis in, 325
    treatment of, 325-327
Thoracic dissectomy, 326
Thoracic hemivertebra, with rib fusion, *244*
Thoracic kyphosis, management of, 424
Thoracic radicular pain, 323
Thoracic spine, articulated, *20*
    as osteotomy site, 169
    degenerative diseases of, 323-327
    lateral retropleural approach to, *138*
    lumbar and, biomechanics of, 419-422
        fracture-dislocation of, 360

injury to, 360
    lateral extrapleural and extraperitoneal approaches to, 137-141. *See also* Thoracolumbar spine.
    radiographic anatomy of, 68, *68,* 69, *69, 72*
Thoracic vertebra(e), 19
    lumbar and, facet configuration of, *381*
    ribs and, centers of ossification and, *5*
    seventh, *21*
Thoracoabdominal approach, anterior, spinal fusion in scoliosis and, 191
Thoracolumbar junction, intervertebral ligaments at, *381*
    normal roentgenogram of, *384*
Thoracolumbar spine, anatomy of, 380, *381*
    fractures of. *See* Fracture(s), thoracolumbar.
    mechanism of injury of fracture-dislocations of, 381
    slice fracture-dislocation of, *387. See also* Thoracic spine, lumbar and.
Thorax, rotation of, in scoliosis, *182*
Three-point pressure systems, limiting spinal flexion and, 423
Thyrohyoid muscle, 33
Tibial nerve, motor nerve conduction velocity and, 81
Tomography, 63, 71
Tongs, Crutchfield, *364,* 368
        cervical dislocation and, 363
    Garner-Wells, 363, *364*
Torticollis, spasmotic, 415
Touch, pressure, position sense and, pathways for, 45
Tracheostomy, exposure of anterior arch of atlas, dens, and body of axis and, 128
    transinfrahyoid operative approach and, 123
    transoral operative approach and, 122
    upper cervical spine surgery and, 121
Tract(s), cerebellospinal, 47
    corticospinal. *See* Corticospinal tract.
    cuneocerebellar, 45
    motor and motor facilitory, descending, 45-47
    reticulospinal, 47
        destruction of, 60
    rubrospinal, 46
    spinocerebellar, 45
    spinotectal, 44
    spinothalamic, 43, 45
        destruction of, 60
    tectospinal, 46
    tectotegmentospinal, 47
    vestibulospinal, 47
Traction, cervical dislocations and, 363
    exposure of anterior vertebral bodies and disc spaces from C3 through C7 and, 125
    injuries from acceleration-deceleration forces and, 350
    laminectomy and, 117
    preoperative, scoliosis and, 186
    sciatica and, 305
    thoracic disc derangement and, 325
Transinfrahyoid cervical operations, transoral and, 121-124
Transinfrahyoid operative approach, 123
Transitory neurologic deficit, spinal cord injuries and, 361
Transoral and transinfrahyoid cervical operations, 121-124
Transoral operative approach, 122
Transthoracic operative approach, to tuberculous spine, 111
Transverse abdominis, 34
Transverse ligament of atlas, 26
Transverse process(es), and pedicles of C3 through C7, exposure of, 129, *130*
    fracture of, 358, 384, *385*
    in embryo, 4
    posterior primary divisions of lumbar nerves and, *144*
Transversospinal muscles, 32
Trapezius muscle, 28

Trauma, 355-390. *See also* specific injuries.
  halo and, 370
  osteodystrophy due to, 93
  phase lag pool loss and, 94
  radiographic features of, 344, *345, 346*
  scoliosis and, 181
Treatment(s), physical, in operant conditioning program,
    psychologic aspects of pain and, 397
  response to, psychophysiologic aspects of pain and, 396
Trunk
  measurement of alignment of, in scoliosis, 181, *182*
  neck and, control of, 46
  sweating on, 47
Tubercle bacillus, types of, in spinal tuberculosis, 102
Tuberculosis of spine, 102-114
  age/sex correlation in, 105t
  differential diagnosis in, 110
  kyphosis in, 105, *106, 107*
  lateral deviation in, 105, *106*
  living pathology in, 107-110
  pathogenesis of, 102
  Pott's paraplegia and, 113
  radiographic features of, 336, *337-339*
  secondary changes with, 109
  site of, *105*
  statistics in, 103
  symptoms and signs in, 104-107
  treatment of, 111-113
    anterior fusion and, 111, 112t
Tuberculous meningomyelitis, 113
Tuberculous myelitis, 108
Tumors, 247-298
  arising from bony wall, *268, 269*
    compressive lesions at foramen magnum and, 264-267
  benign vertebral, 276-279
  bone, and tumor-like lesions of vertebrae, 274-286
    primary malignant, 279, 280
    secondary malignant, 281-283
  craniospinal, diagnosis of compressive lesions at foramen
    magnum and, 250
    surgical treatment of, 255
  differential diagnosis of extradural, intradural
    extramedullary, and intradural intramedullary, 288
  Ewing's, 280
  extradural, at foramen magnum, 251
    of spinal cord, 289, *292*
      differential diagnosis of intradural extramedullary,
        intradural intramedullary and, 288
      intradural and, 291
      intradural extramedullary, intradural intramedullary,
        and, differential diagnosis of, 288
      operating microscope in surgery for, 296
      surgical treatment of, 291
  extramedullary, at foramen magnum, diagnosis of, 251
    surgical treatment of, 255-261
    of spinal cord, intradural, 289
  intradural, of spinal cord, extradural and, 291
  intradural extramedullary, of spinal cord, 289, *292, 296*
    extradural, intradural intramedullary, and, differential
      diagnosis of, 288
    operating microscope in surgery for, 296
    surgical treatment of, 293
  intradural intramedullary, of spinal cord, 290
    extradural, intradural extramedullary, and, differential
      diagnosis of, 288
    surgical treatment of, 293
  intramedullary, at foramen magnum, surgical treatment
    of, 253-255
    of spinal cord, *297*
      operating microscope in surgery for, 297

of cauda equina, *292*
of conus medullaris, *292*
of neuron series, 291
spinal cord. *See* Spinal cord, tumors of.
vertebral giant cell, 279
Wilm's, 181
Tumor-like bone lesions of vertebrae, 275, 283
Turnbuckle cast, in scoliosis, 186
Turnover, of bone, 90
Twins, identical, scoliosis and, 178
  isthmic spondylolisthesis and, 195
  pars interarticularis lesions in, *198*

Ulnar nerve, evoked sensory responses and, 82
  motor nerve conduction velocity and, 81
Urinary incontinence, in diastematomelia, 236
Urinary tract, congenital anomalies of, vertebral anomalies
    and, 180
  infections of, vertebral osteomyelitis and, 97

Vein(s), basivertebral, 25
  of spinal cord, 49
Venous plexus, vertebral, spinal tuberculosis and, 103, *103*
Venous system of spinal cord, 49
  arterial system and, *48*
Ventriculography, compressive lesions at foramen magnum
    and, 252
Ventriculostomy, postoperative hydrocephalus and, 233
Vertebra(e), at typical levels, *63*
  block, 242, *242*
  cervical, 16-19
    fourth, *17, 18*
  coronal cleft, 242, *242*
  fractures of, pathologic, caused by tumors, 276
    cervical, 130, *131*
    crush, *379*
  in embryo, *4*
  intervertebral discs and, 14-23
  lumbar. *See* Lumbar vertebra(e).
  occipital, 240
  pars interarticularis of. *See* Pars interarticularis.
  ribs and, chondrification centers in, in embryo, *5*
  sagittal cleft, 243, *243*
  scoliosis and, 178
  thoracic. *See* Thoracic vertebra(e).
  transverse process and pedicles of C3 through C7, 129
  tumors of, benign, 276-279
    bone, and tumor-like lesions of, 274-286
Vertebral arch, 4, 14, 62. *See also* Neural arch.
Vertebral body(ies), 14, 62
  anterior, disc spaces and, from C3 through C7, exposure
    of, 125-128
  arteries to, 37
  fracture of. *See* Fracture, vertebral body.
  in spinal tuberculosis, 107, *108,* 109
Vertebral canal, 71
  narrow lumbar, 320
Vertebral column. *See* Spine.
Vertebral congenital scoliosis, 180
Vertebral growth plates, scoliosis and, 178
Vertebral hemangioma, 276, *277*
Vertebral interspaces, infection of. *See* Infection(s), disc
    space.
Vertebral muscles, 33, 34, *34*
Vertebral osteomyelitis, 96, 98, *98*
Vertebra prominens, 18
Vertebral rotation, in scoliosis, 184, *184*
Vestibulospinal tracts, 47

Vestige, coccygeal, 9
Virus studies, vertebral column tumor diagnosis and, 276
Visceral pain pathways, 44
Vitamin D, osteomalacias and, 92, 95
Von Lackum surcingle system, 186
V-waves, 79

Wedge, double posterior, in spinal osteotomy for fixed
    flexion deformity, *169*
    removal of, in lumbar spondylosis, *320*

Whiplash, 347
White column, dorsal, 45
White matter, 43–47
    sulci and gray matter of spinal cord and, *43*
Williams brace, 425, *425*
Wilm's tumor, 181
Wounds, missile, injuries to spinal column secondary to, 361
    penetrating, of spinal canal, 366

X-ray examination. *See* Radiologic examination.
Xylocaine, injection of, in sacroiliac joint, 311, 312, *312*, *313*